Health Care Issues

Selections from *CQ Researcher*

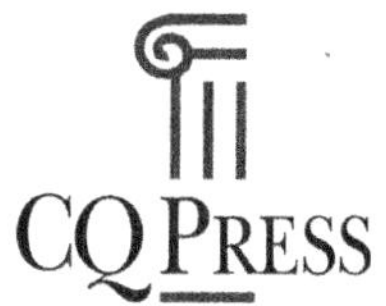

A Division of SAGE
Washington, D.C.

CQ Press
2300 N Street, NW, Suite 800
Washington, DC 20037
Phone: 202-729-1900; toll-free, 1-866-4CQ-PRESS (1-866-427-7737)
Web: www.cqpress.com

Contents

Annotated Contents

The 12 *CQ Researcher* reports reprinted in this book have been reproduced essentially as they appeared when first published. In the few cases in which important developments have since occurred, updates are provided in the overviews highlighting the principle issues examined.

HEALTH SYSTEM AND REFORM ISSUES

Health-Care Reform

The health-care reform legislation signed into law by President Barack Obama in March 2010 marked the biggest attempt to expand access to health care since Medicare and Medicaid were launched in the 1960s. The massive legislation will help 32 million Americans get health insurance coverage and bans insurers from denying coverage to those with preexisting illnesses. It also expands Medicaid to all poor people — except illegal immigrants — and gives subsidies to low- and low–middle-income people to buy insurance. But opponents, including every Republican member of Congress, say the coverage expansion is simply too expensive, at a price tag of about $1 trillion over 10 years. They also say new fees and taxes to help pay for the coverage place too big a burden on currently insured people. Meanwhile, a group of state attorneys general is challenging the constitutionality of the law's requirement that everyone buy health insurance.

Medication Abuse

Michael Jackson's shocking accidental death in June 2009 was only the latest in a string of high-profile fatalities from multiple prescription medications. Actor Heath Ledger and model and sex symbol Anna Nicole Smith died in comparable circumstances. But celebrities aren't the only abusers of painkillers, sedatives and stimulants. Prescription drug abuse has become a growing problem in the United States, even as illegal drug use has gradually declined. In 2005, for example, more people ages 45 to 54 died from drug overdoses — mostly prescription painkillers — than in car crashes. Many people believe prescription drugs are safer than illegal drugs, so changing public attitudes is a challenge. Also, many prescription narcotics are being diverted to dangerous, recreational use, but doctors, dentists and nurses are poorly informed about the potential for abuse. Meanwhile, government drug-education programs focus on illegal drugs while largely ignoring the risks of prescription abuse.

Caring for Veterans

Veterans often spend more time waiting for decisions from the Department of Veterans Affairs (VA) on their disability claims than they spent at war. At least 500,000 veterans have waited an average of six months for a decision on a disability claim and another 200,000 have waited an average of five years for a decision on an appeal. New VA Secretary Eric Shinseki — himself a disabled Vietnam vet — vows to unblock the huge claims backlog, but it may take until 2015. That's partly because the VA has expanded the number of compensation-worthy illnesses from the Vietnam War. Veterans' organizations laud Shinseki but disagree over how deeply VA changes should run. Meanwhile, lawmakers in Congress are close to passing legislation to compensate relatives and friends caring for veterans with catastrophic, lifelong disabilities such as traumatic brain injuries arising from improvised explosive devices — the homemade bombs that are the hallmark of the wars in Iraq and Afghanistan.

Legalizing Marijuana

From statehouses to the White House, attitudes toward marijuana laws are changing. California's top tax collector is endorsing proposed state legislation to legalize and tax pot, and Republican Gov. Arnold Schwarzenegger says he'd like the idea debated. More than a dozen other states have enacted or are considering laws to permit medical-marijuana use or remove criminal penalties for possession. In Congress, Democratic Sen. Jim Webb of Virginia — a hard-nosed Marine combat veteran — wants marijuana legalization considered in a top-to-bottom review of sentencing and drug laws. Full-scale, nationwide legalization still seems distant, but the Obama administration has declared a hands-off approach toward California's medical-marijuana outlets, unless the state-sanctioned sites are determined to be trafficking operations. Opponents of marijuana legalization object on moral and health grounds, but the opposition appears to be weakening, especially in a time when the economic crisis is cutting into police and prison budgets nationwide.

Prison Health Care

A high percentage of the more than 2 million inmates in U.S. jails and prisons suffer from mental illness, addiction or infectious and chronic diseases like HIV/AIDS and diabetes. About a quarter suffer from major depression and a fifth from psychosis. Many had little or no health care before being incarcerated. Providing treatment and preventive care for prisoners who eventually return to society can help stem the spread of infectious disease in communities and keep those with mental illness and addiction from landing back in jail, say public-health officials. While prisoners are, ironically, the only Americans who have a constitutionally guaranteed right to health care, most prison health-care systems are underfunded and understaffed, making the care they provide spotty at best. Meanwhile, strict sentencing guidelines and three-strikes-and-you're-out laws have created a burgeoning — and aging — prisoner population, which is driving skyrocketing health-care costs even higher.

Reproductive Ethics

Nadya Suleman, an unemployed, 33-year-old, single mother from Southern California, felt her six children weren't enough. In January 2008, after a fertility doctor implanted six embryos she had frozen earlier, Suleman gave birth to octuplets — and was quickly dubbed "Octomom." Many fertility experts were shocked that a doctor would depart so far from medical guidelines — which recommend implantation of only one, or at most two, embryos for a woman of Suleman's relatively young age. Multiple births often do result from in vitro fertilization (IVF) and other assisted-reproduction technologies; however, the number of multiples has dropped over the past few years. Analysts note that government statistics show a large percentage of clinics frequently ignore the guidelines on embryo implantation. In response, lawmakers in several states have introduced proposals to increase regulation of fertility clinics.

Abortion Debates

The abortion wars are heating up again. Anti-abortion groups strongly opposed President Obama's health-care overhaul, insisting that the plan's insurance coverage provisions opened the door to public subsidies for abortions. They remain opposed even after Obama issued an executive order that regulations be issued barring use of federal funds for abortion services except in limited circumstances. For their part, abortion-rights groups say the restrictions leave reproductive freedoms worse off than before. Anti-abortion groups are now pressing state legislatures to similarly bar coverage for abortion under the insurance exchanges to be established under the new health-care law. In addition, they are pushing new restrictions on abortion procedures, including a requirement that a woman be shown an ultrasound image of her fetus before the procedure. Abortion-rights advocates say the proposals amount to political interference with women's constitutionally protected right to make their own medical decisions.

PREVENTIVE AND PUBLIC HEALTH ISSUES

Breast Cancer

Breast cancer is the second most common cancer among women in the United States, after skin cancer, and the second-leading cause of cancer death, after lung cancer. Yet breast cancer mortality rates have been declining, most probably the result of early detection and better treatment. Advances in hormone therapy and discoveries of antibody treatments have markedly improved the outcome for breast cancer patients, along with the development of genetic tests on tumor tissue to determine which patients will best benefit from chemotherapy. While progress is being made, some debates never seem to fade. There continue to be disagreements about the age at which women should begin mammography screening, how to treat the increasing number of "zero stage" breast cancers that screening detects and the extent to which environmental pollutants cause breast cancer. In addition, disparities in treatment and racial outcomes continue to be documented.

Preventing Cancer

Deaths from cancer and new cancer cases have decreased slightly in the past few years. It's the first time the statistics have declined over an extended period and the best piece of news yet to come out of the nation's 38-year-old "war on cancer." Despite scientists' early optimism that the discovery of an actual cancer cure was imminent, most recent gains have come instead from earlier detection and cancer-prevention achievements, especially lower smoking rates. Those gains have prompted calls for a shift in federal cancer programs toward prevention and detection and away from research, which has been funded much more generously. Prevention proponents say focusing more on prevention and detection makes sense because cancer biology now demonstrates that individuals' cancers vary so widely and contain so many cell mutations that new, widely effective treatments will be even harder to come by than previously expected.

Battling HIV/AIDS

Two-thirds of the world's 40 million HIV/AIDS cases are in impoverished sub-Saharan Africa, which also has 12 million children orphaned by the disease. In the United States, the toll is heaviest on African-American women. Rich countries and private donors are now spending billions to fight AIDS in developing countries. But only 2 million people in those countries receive life-prolonging antiretroviral medications, while millions more are newly infected. With an HIV vaccine years away, public health experts say a renewed focus on prevention is the best way to stem the epidemic. Prevention turns on two stubborn issues: behavior change and shifts in generations-old patterns of poverty and gender inequality. Meanwhile, in 2008 President Bush reauthorized the President's Emergency Plan for AIDS Relief (PEPFAR) for up to $48 billion over the next five years. While the program has pumped billions into overseas AIDS programs, AIDS groups want PEPFAR broadened to cover additional health and development issues, and the reauthorized program does incorporate funding for tuberculosis and malaria programs.

Fighting Superbugs

Antibiotics — the wonder drugs of the 20th century — are gradually losing their clout. Bacteria naturally develop resistance to antimicrobial drugs. In recent years, overuse of antibiotics has caused a growing number of staphylococcus bacteria to evolve into disease-causing "superbugs" resistant to drugs like methicillin. Hospital patients with MRSA — a potent antibiotic-resistant staph infection — are four times as likely to die as other patients. Moreover, while most superbugs once thrived only in hospitals, new strains outside health facilities are killing healthy people. Adding to the concerns of public-health officials, drug companies are developing few new antimicrobials. Some activists urge strong curbs on all antimicrobial use, including those to promote fast growth in farm animals. Others oppose legal requirements for animal or human antibiotics, arguing that voluntary efforts are better able to keep pace with the fast-evolving world of microbes.

Regulating Toxic Chemicals

Chemicals are integral to many everyday products, from electronics and toys to building materials and household goods. But environmental, health and consumer advocates say the agencies responsible for protecting Americans from exposure to harmful chemicals are allowing too many dangerous substances into the market without testing them for toxicity. Some goods, such as medicines, are tested for safety before they can be sold, but many common products do not go through premarket safety screening. Many concerns focus on infants and young children, who are especially sensitive to toxic hazards. Chemical manufacturers say the existing regulatory system works effectively and can be tightened to address new concerns, but critics argue that a precautionary approach — which would require producers to show that materials are safe before they can be marketed — would protect consumers more fully.

Preface

Is the new health-care reform law a good idea? Does the Veteran's Administration adequately serve wounded vets? Should marijuana be treated like alcohol and taxed? These questions — and many more — are at the heart of health care policy. How can instructors best engage students regarding these crucial issues? We feel that students need objective, yet provocative examinations of such issues to understand how they affect citizens today and will for years to come. This annual collection aims to promote in-depth discussion, facilitate further research and help readers formulate their own positions on crucial issues. Get your students talking both inside and outside the classroom about *Health Care Issues*.

This first edition includes 12 up-to-date reports by *CQ Researcher*, an award-winning weekly policy brief that brings complicated issues down to earth. Each report chronicles and analyzes executive, legislative and judicial activities at all levels of government. This collection is divided into two policy areas — health system and reform issues and preventive and public health issues — to cover a range of issues found in most health policy courses.

CQ RESEARCHER

CQ Researcher was founded in 1923 as *Editorial Research Reports* and was sold primarily to newspapers as a research tool. The magazine was renamed and redesigned in 1991 as *CQ Researcher.* Today, students are its primary audience. While still used by hundreds of journalists and newspapers, many of which reprint portions of the reports, the *Researcher*'s main subscribers are now high school, college and public libraries. In 2002, *Researcher* won the American Bar Association's coveted Silver Gavel award for magazine excellence for a series of nine reports on civil liberties and other legal issues.

Researcher staff writers — all highly experienced journalists — sometimes compare the experience of writing a *Researcher* report to drafting a college term paper. Indeed, there are many similarities. Each report is as long as many term papers — about 11,000 words — and is written by one person without any significant outside help. One of the key differences is that writers interview leading experts, scholars and government officials for each issue.

Like students, staff writers begin the creative process by choosing a topic. Working with the *Researcher*'s editors, the writer identifies a controversial subject that has important public policy implications. After a topic is selected, the writer embarks on one to two weeks of intense research. Newspaper and magazine articles are clipped or downloaded, books are ordered and information is gathered from a wide variety of sources, including interest groups, universities and the government. Once the writers are well informed, they develop a detailed outline, and begin the interview process. Each report requires a minimum of 10 to 15 interviews with academics, officials, lobbyists and people working in the field. Only after all interviews are completed does the writing begin.

CHAPTER FORMAT

Each issue of *CQ Researcher*, and therefore each selection in this book, is structured in the same way. Each begins with an overview, which briefly summarizes the areas that will be explored in greater detail in the rest of the chapter. The next section chronicles important and current debates on the topic under discussion and is structured around a number of key questions, such as "Is prescription-drug abuse as serious as illegal drug abuse?" and "Is mammography being oversold and overused?" These questions are usually the subject of much debate among practitioners and scholars in the field. Hence, the answers presented are never conclusive but rather detail the range of opinion on the topic.

Next, the "Background" section provides a history of the issue being examined. This retrospective covers important legislative measures, executive actions and court decisions that illustrate how current policy has evolved. Then the "Current Situation" section examines contemporary policy issues, legislation under consideration and legal action being taken. Each selection concludes with an "Outlook" section, which addresses possible regulation, court rulings and initiatives from Capitol Hill and the White House over the next five to 10 years.

Each report contains features that augment the main text: two to three sidebars that examine issues related to the topic at hand, a pro versus con debate between two experts, a chronology of key dates and events and an annotated bibliography detailing major sources used by the writer.

CUSTOM OPTIONS

Interested in building your ideal CQ Press *Issues* book, customized to your personal teaching needs and interests? Browse by course or date, or search for specific topics or issues from our online catalog of *CQ Researcher* issues at http://custom.cqpress.com.

ACKNOWLEDGMENTS

We wish to thank many people for helping to make this collection a reality. Tom Colin, managing editor of *CQ Researcher*, gave us his enthusiastic support and cooperation as we developed this first edition. He and his talented staff of editors and writers have amassed a first-class library of *Researcher* reports, and we are fortunate to have access to that rich cache. We also thankfully acknowledge the advice and feedback from current readers and are gratified by their satisfaction each volume.

Some readers may be learning about *CQ Researcher* for the first time. We expect that many readers will want regular access to this excellent weekly research tool. For subscription information or a no-obligation free trial of *Researcher*, please contact CQ Press at www.cqpress.com or toll-free at 1-866-4CQ-PRESS (1-866-427-7737).

We hope that you will be pleased by the first edition of *Health Care Issues.* We welcome your feedback and suggestions for future editions. Please direct comments to Charisse Kiino, Editorial Director, College Publishing Group, CQ Press, 2300 N Street, NW, Suite 800, Washington, D.C. 20037, or ckiino@cqpress.com.

—*The Editors of CQ Press*

Contributors

Thomas J. Colin, managing editor of *CQ Researcher*, has been a magazine and newspaper journalist for more than 30 years. Before joining Congressional Quarterly in 1991, he was a reporter and editor at the *Miami Herald* and *National Geographic* and editor in chief of *Historic Preservation.* He holds a bachelor's degree in English from the College of William & Mary and in journalism from the University of Missouri.

Nellie Bristol is a veteran Capitol Hill reporter who has covered health policy in Washington for more than 20 years. She now writes for *The Lancet*, the *British Medical Journal* and the *Journal of Disaster Medicine and Public Health Preparedness*. She graduated in American studies from George Washington University, where she is now working toward a master's degree in public health.

Marcia Clemmitt is a *CQ Researcher* staff writer and a veteran social-policy reporter who previously served as editor in chief of *Medicine & Health* and staff writer for *The Scientist.* She has also been a high school math and physics teacher. She holds a liberal arts and sciences degree from St. John's College, Annapolis, and a master's degree in English from Georgetown University. Her recent reports include "Gridlock in Washington" and "Reproductive Ethics."

Kenneth Jost, associate editor of *CQ Researcher*, graduated from Harvard College and Georgetown University Law Center. He is the author of the *Supreme Court Yearbook* and editor of *The Supreme Court A to Z* (both from CQ Press). He was a member of the *CQ Researcher* team that won the American Bar Association's 2002 Silver Gavel Award. His previous reports include "Bilingual Education vs. English Immersion" and "Testing in Schools." He is also author of the blog Jost on Justice (http://jostonjustice.blogspot.com).

Peter Katel is a *CQ Researcher* staff writer who previously reported on Haiti and Latin America for *Time* and *Newsweek* and covered the Southwest for newspapers in New Mexico. He has received several journalism awards, including the Bartolomé Mitre Award from the Inter-American Press Association for coverage of drug trafficking. He holds an AB in university studies from the University of New Mexico. His recent reports include "New Strategy in Iraq," "Rise in Counterinsurgency" and "Wounded Veterans."

Barbara Mantel is a freelance writer in New York City whose work has appeared in *The New York Times*, the *Journal of Child and Adolescent Psychopharmacology* and *Mamm Magazine.* She is a former correspondent and senior producer for National Public Radio and has won several journalism awards, including the National Press Club's Best Consumer Journalism Award and the Front Page Award from the Newswomen's Club of New York for her April 18, 2008, *CQ Researcher* report "Public Defenders." She holds a bachelor's degree in history and economics from the University of Virginia and a master's degree in economics from Northwestern University.

Jennifer Weeks is a *CQ Researcher* contributing writer in Watertown, Mass., who specializes in energy and environmental issues. She has written for *The Washington Post, The Boston Globe Magazine* and other publications, and has 15 years' experience as a public-policy analyst, lobbyist and congressional staffer. She holds an AB from Williams College and MAs from the University of North Carolina and Harvard University.

CHAPTER

1

Health-Care Reform

By Marcia Clemmitt

Excerpted from the CQ Researcher. Marcia Clemmitt. (June 11, 2010). "Health-Care Reform." *CQ Researcher*, 505-528.

Health-Care Reform

By Marcia Clemmitt

The Issues

Enactment of the most far-reaching health-care law in at least four decades pumped emotions to a fever pitch among opponents and supporters alike.

"Today, after almost a century of trying; today, after over a year of debate; today, after all the votes have been tallied — health insurance reform becomes law in the United States of America. Today," President Barack Obama proclaimed at the March 23 White House signing ceremony. [1]

With equal passion, Republicans unanimously rejected the landmark Patient Protection and Affordable Health Care Act, refusing to award it even a single vote.

The law "is an historic betrayal of the clear will of the American people," scolded Republican National Committee Chairman Michael Steele. Referring to the new requirement that all Americans carry health-insurance coverage, he said the law represented "an historic loss of liberty." [2]

The landmark law will extend coverage to about 32 million of the nation's 45 million uninsured people by:

• Expanding Medicaid;

• Providing subsidies to help low- and middle-income families buy insurance;

• Creating regulated insurance markets where people without employer-sponsored insurance can buy subsidized coverage; and

• Using Medicare's economic clout to cut health care costs.

While supporters tout the law's multi-faceted approach to access and cost problems, conservatives argue the federal government has no right to require individuals to purchase insurance or states to participate in coverage-expansion programs. At least 20 state attorneys general and several private groups are suing to stop the law.

The law has two main facets — expanding health coverage and developing cost-control measures, says Judith Feder, a professor of public policy at Georgetown University and former staff director of the 1990 U.S. Bipartisan Commission on Comprehensive Health Care, which called for universal health coverage.

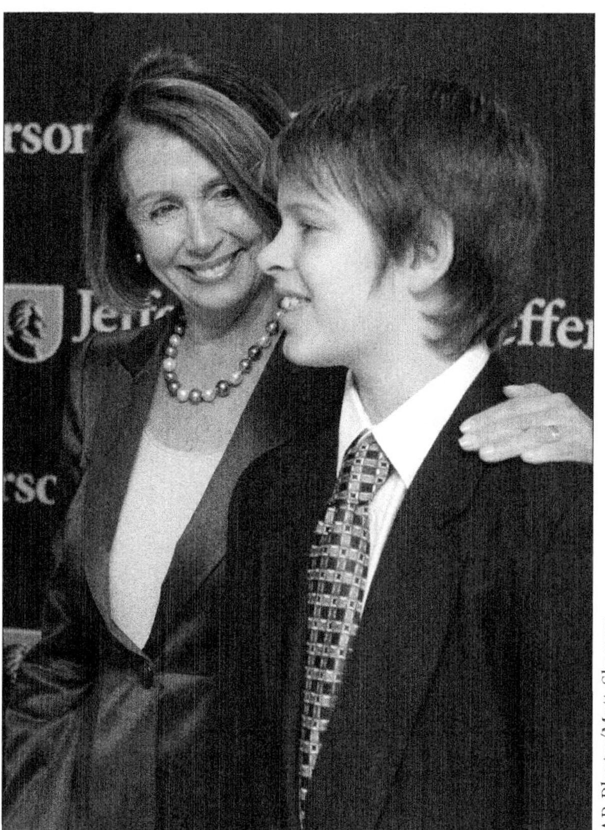

House Speaker Nancy Pelosi, D-Calif., greets 11-year-old Brian McCann during a news conference on health care in September 2009, months before she helped engineer passage of the landmark health reform law. The sweeping new law enables people with preexisting medical conditions, like Brian, to get affordable insurance.

For the first time in history, the law "establishes access to affordable health care as a national responsibility," with "the great bulk of the dollars coming from taxpayers" to fund the coverage expansion, says Feder. The cost-cutting sections contain provisions designed to essentially reengineer health care to favor efficient, effective treatments and preventive medicine over expensive but relatively ineffective services, she says. This is "urgent for a variety of reasons," including the fact that the high cost of health care is the main reason people are uninsured, says Feder.

The law launches a variety of "institutions and experiments" that policymakers hope can eventually slow the huge annual increases in health-care costs, says Michael E. Chernew, a professor of health policy at Harvard Medical School. Some are simple payment cuts to health-care players like private "Medicare Advantage" plans that most health-care economists agree have long been overpaid, he says.

But the law also will launch numerous demonstration projects aimed at developing ways to pay doctors, hospitals and other providers for delivering good health outcomes efficiently rather than continuing the current system, which mostly pays for services whether they are successful and necessary or not, Chernew explains.

"We can't be sure the [cost-cutting] things in the law will work, and critics can argue that they are not pursued aggressively enough or quickly enough," says Chernew. "Nevertheless, we have to do them, and from a pure cost-curve standpoint, [the law's framers] did whatever they could possibly do, what is politically possible."

Health Reforms Opposed in Majority of States

State lawmakers in at least 39 states have introduced legislation to limit, alter or oppose aspects of the health-reform plan. The measures largely seek to make or keep health insurance optional and allow people to purchase any type of coverage they choose. Such legislation passed and is in effect in three states — Idaho, Utah and Virginia — and legislation passed in Oklahoma and Georgia is ready for approval by the governors. The bills did not pass in 21 states.

State Legislation Opposing Certain Health Reforms, 2009-2010

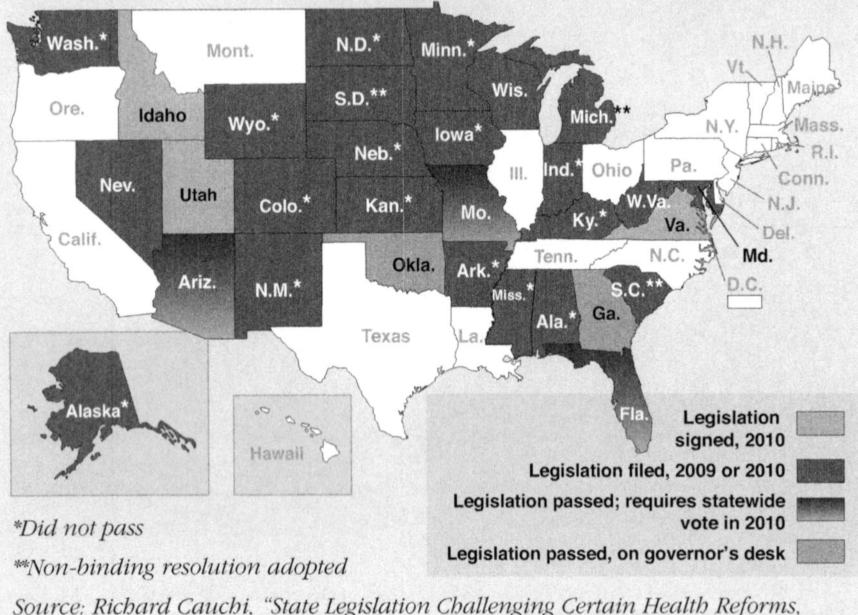

**Did not pass*

***Non-binding resolution adopted*

Source: Richard Cauchi, "State Legislation Challenging Certain Health Reforms, 2010," National Conference of State Legislatures, May 2010

The law also has some "pro-competitive" elements to encourage private insurers to emphasize cost and quality control as well, Chernew says. The "insurance exchanges" that will be set up in states to help people without employer coverage buy insurance "are very pro-competition" since they get insurers to compete against each other for individuals' business, Chernew says.

"It's very easy for those not in power to argue that those in power haven't done enough," Chernew says, but those in power "can only do what is politically possible" in a system where health-care providers and insurers hold enormous influence.

Ultimately, Chernew acknowledges, "the law could turn out to be a disaster" because, when the results are in from cost-cutting experiments, "the solution [to rising costs] may require tough choices" to impose cost-trimming measures that doctors and patients won't like.

If that happens "and we end up not having the political will" to impose the changes, the federal budget deficit will soar because, under the law, the nation has committed itself to "a new entitlement program" — subsidizing health coverage for most low- and middle-income Americans, Chernew says.

The law takes some good steps but also leaves a few important things undone, says Mark McClellan, a former chief of Medicare and Medicaid under President George W. Bush and now director of the Engelberg Center for Health Care Reform at the centrist Brookings Institution think tank. For example, McClellan says the law's tax on high-cost employer-provided health insurance with rich benefit packages is a good way to raise money for coverage, but the tax should kick in sooner.

"It got pushed back to 2018," after complaints about unfairness, he says. But he argues that it is fair to end the tax-favored status of the most benefit-rich coverage, in favor of spending those dollars to help lower-income people gain coverage. Currently, "we pay about $250 billion a year for those employer subsidies, and most of that goes to higher-income people," he says.

One set of conservative-backed cost-trimming provisions that didn't make it into the law are so-called "consumer-side" incentives for people to take steps on their own to reduce health spending, McClellan says. For example, private insurers are implementing "wellness plans" to give consumers financial incentives to take common-sense steps like stopping smoking or losing weight, which should save health-system dollars down the line, he says.

Limits on lawsuits against health-care providers also should have been included, says McClellan. Such reforms can trim 2-3 percent annually from medical spending, and while that amount may seem minimal, "it could add to the other reforms" and increase the law's cumulative cost-cutting effect, he says.

The new law also has its critics among proponents of guaranteed, universal access to health care.

"The law does not solve the problem," says Steffie Woolhandler, an associate professor of medicine at Harvard and longtime advocate of national, single-payer health care.

"If the bill works as planned, there will still be 23 million uninsured people in 2019, of whom about a quarter will be illegal immigrants," she says. Furthermore, many who get insurance under the bill will end up underinsured, she added, partly because about 16 million of the newly insured will be enrolled in Medicaid, which most doctors don't accept because of its lower payments. "They can go to the emergency room (ER), but they'll have trouble getting primary care for conditions like high blood pressure" and the like, where early treatment could keep ER-type health emergencies from happening, she says.

Many who buy insurance in the law's new exchanges also "will get woefully inadequate coverage," since the insurance available there "will cover only 60 percent" of medical costs, says Woolhandler.

"Because the law was sold largely on the basis of cost containment, the critics are able to fire at it by saying, 'It won't save as much money as you say,' " says Arthur L. Caplan, a professor of bioethics at the University of Pennsylvania. "If, instead, you had had the discussion of whether there is a right to health care, critics would have to explicitly make their arguments for why health care is not a right," bringing out into the open the real issue, which the country must face sooner or later, he says.

"Only critics looking for some way to derail reform give a hoot about details" like individual mandates or tax provisions, Caplan said. "No nation on Earth has ever reformed its health care system by asking the public to wallow around in the details of health reform." Instead, nations including Canada, Britain, Singapore, Taiwan, Germany and Australia "secured agreement that health care is a right and then, and only then, moved on to figure out how to guarantee that right to all citizens," he said. [3]

As health reform is implemented amid protests in Washington and the states, here are some of the questions being debated:

Is the new health-care reform law a good idea?

The new law's supporters say it puts in place most of the mechanisms for coverage expansion and cost control that are politically possible in the complex, private-sector-dominated American health system, but many conservative critics have called for the law's partial rollback or repeal. They argue that increased government involvement in health care can only damage the job market, interfere with individual freedom and worsen cost problems. Critics on the left, meanwhile, say there was little point in enacting provisions that will only temporarily lower the number of uninsured Americans without creating a permanent solution.

The bill's so-called "individual mandate," requiring everyone to purchase insurance, is unconstitutional, said Sen. Orrin Hatch, R-Utah.

The purpose of insurance is to spread costs across the population — with people paying in even in years when they don't use much health care. Those payments serve as a buffer against times when they are sick and use services — and if people wait until they become ill to sign up for insurance, insurers are unable to spread costs in this way.

For this reason, an individual mandate has been part of some Republican coverage-expansion proposals over the years, as well as the 1993 proposal by President Bill Clinton.

Hatch raised no objection to the individual mandates in the Clinton plan, "but . . . 17 years later . . . I looked at it and, constitutionally, I came to the conclusion . . . that this would be the first time in history that the federal government requires you to buy something you don't want," he said. "If we allow the federal government to tell us what we can or can't buy, then our liberties are gone." [4]

"Forcing employers to offer health insurance . . . will cost America jobs and revenue, and inhibit small businesses from growing," according to the small-business lobbying group National Federation of Independent Businesses. "It's a bad idea any time but is particularly destructive in the current economic environment." [5]

By requiring employers to pay a penalty if they don't offer workers substantial health-insurance coverage, the law "creates an incentive for employers to avoid hiring workers from low-income families, hurting those who need jobs the most," said Kathryn Nix, a research assistant at the conservative Heritage Foundation. (Low-income workers are the least likely to receive employer-based health insurance because its cost is more than most employers are willing to shoulder as an added cost of employing a worker.) [6]

Tax increases to pay for expanding coverage will damage the economy, Nix continued. For example, the law raises some taxes on investment income, a

Wealthy to Pay Higher Medicare Tax

Before passage of the health-care plan, middle-income families paid a higher Medicare tax than wealthy families. Under the plan, middle-income families will continue to pay a 2.9 percent tax but the tax on couples making $10 million annually would nearly triple.

Medicare Tax Under Health Reform

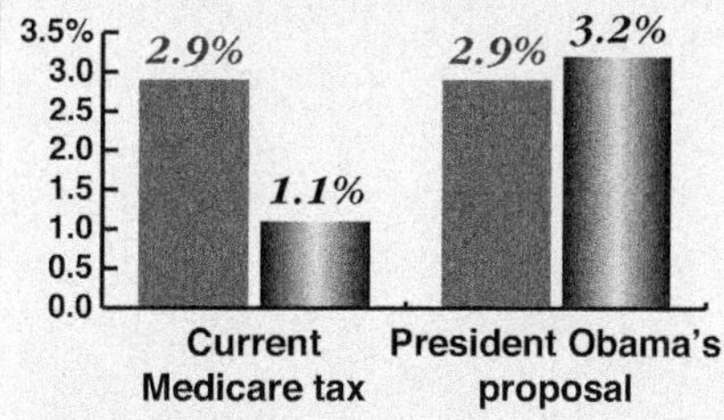

Middle-income family
Couple making $10 million annually

Source: Chuck Marr, "Changes in Medicare Tax on High-Income People Represent Sound Additions to Health Reform," Center on Budget and Policy Priorities, March 2010

Health Reforms That Begin This Year

A few programs expand coverage for the neediest.

Most Americans won't see many effects of the health-care reform law this year. However, the law does launch a few programs that start expanding coverage for some of the neediest people and some who are easier to cover. [1]

High-risk pool — Many people with preexisting medical conditions can't get affordable insurance under current laws. To help close that gap, this year a temporary "high-risk pool" will begin offering price-capped coverage to people with pre-existing illnesses. In 2014 the new law will require insurers to take all comers.

Young adult coverage —Young adults are one of the largest uninsured groups. Beginning this year, for the first time, young adults up to age 26 can get coverage under their parents' health insurance.

Benefit limits — In the past, patients with serious illnesses were likely to lose their insurance coverage when they ran into a lifetime limit on the dollar value of their coverage. Beginning this year, the law bans lifetime dollar limits on coverage and also bans insurers from canceling a patient's insurance policy for any reason except fraud by the patient. Also beginning this year, children may not be refused health insurance because of preexisting medical conditions.

Medicaid expansion — For the first time, states may offer Medicaid coverage to all poor people, not just to mothers and their young children or the disabled.

Business tax credit — Small businesses whose workers' annual wage is under $50,000 get tax credits if they provide health insurance.

Regulating insurance premiums — Insurers must report the proportion of premium dollars they spend on actual medical services, and the federal government will establish a process for judging whether annual premium increases are justified.

— Marcia Clemmitt

[1] See "Focus on Health Reform: Summary of New Health Reform Law," The Henry J. Kaiser Family Foundation, March 26, 2010, and "Timeline for Health Care Reform Implementation: System and Delivery Reform Provisions," The Commonwealth Fund, April 1, 2010.

move that "will discourage investment in the U.S. economy . . . reducing the potential for economic growth."

"Families with incomes greater than $250,000 will pay a higher Medicare payroll tax — up to 2.35 percent, plus a new 3.8 percent tax on interest and dividend income. With this stroke, Democrats have managed to punish both work and the savings of American families," wrote Sally C. Pipes, chief executive officer of the free-market-oriented Pacific Research Institute in San Francisco. [7]

Increasing government involvement in health care will likely drive some doctors out of Medicare and perhaps out of practice altogether, said Robert E. Moffit, director of health policy studies at Heritage. Having public and private insurers pay for health care rather than allowing individuals to pay directly out of their own pockets for it "already [compromises] the independence and integrity of the medical profession," and the new law "will reinforce the worst of these features," because "physicians will be subject to more government regulation and oversight," said Moffit. [8]

Some critics on the left also see more harm than good in the reforms.

The law "hurts many more people than it helps," wrote blogger Jane Hamsher of the liberal website Firedoglake. "A middle-class family of four making $66,370 will be forced to pay $5,243 per year for insurance," an amount that will leave many without enough discretionary income to cover other bills, she said. [9]

But reform supporters counter that expanding coverage is worth the law's cost and that its provisions are not unconstitutional.

"There is a long line of [Supreme Court] cases holding that Congress has broad power to enact laws that substantially affect prices, marketplaces and commercial transactions," including cases decided by the current conservative-dominated court, wrote Ian Millhiser, a policy analyst at the liberal Center for American Progress. "A law requiring all Americans to hold health insurance does all of these things," so its constitutionality is not in question, he said. The 2005 case *Gonzales v. Raich*, for example, "establishes that Congress can regulate even tiny insurance providers who serve only a handful of local residents because such local activity substantially affects a multistate market," said Millhiser. [10]

"The Supreme Court decades ago held that the business of insurance fell within Congress' regulatory authority under the Commerce Clause," wrote Simon Lazarus, public policy counsel to the National Senior Citizens Law Center. [11]

The court noted that "perhaps no modern commercial enterprise directly affects so many persons in all walks of life as does the insurance business," said Lazarus. Consequently, the 1944 finding "could hardly be more consonant with Congress' identical case for expanding federal regulation of health insurance in 2009," including the "individual mandate" to buy coverage, since "many independent experts, studies and analyses concur" that without such a require-

Health Reforms That Begin in 2011 and Beyond

Changes spread costs, reduce spending increases.

The health-reform law contains hundreds of provisions designed to expand insurance coverage, spread the tax burden of paying for the new coverage fairly and eventually tame steep annual increases in spending while improving care. Most of the provisions will be phased in over the next eight years. [1]

2011

Long-term care — People may enroll in an insurance plan to fund future long-term care needs, including services that can help them stay in their own homes.

Drug company fees — Annual fees paid by large pharmaceutical manufacturers will help pay for expanding health coverage.

Hospital-acquired illnesses — Medicare won't pay hospitals to care for infections caused by a patient's hospital stay.

OTC drugs —To raise money, the law bans paying for over-the-counter drugs from tax-favored accounts like flexible spending accounts unless a doctor has prescribed the drugs.

2012

Paying health-care providers — To hold down rising medical costs and improve care, Medicare will begin paying doctors and hospitals less when patients develop preventable illnesses and study other potential incentives to get medical providers to work together to deliver care more efficiently.

2013

Standardize insurance operations — To save money and set the stage for the new health-insurance exchanges that launch in 2014, health-insurance eligibility, enrollment and claims procedures will be standardized nationwide.

Higher Medicare taxes — To raise money to expand insurance coverage, individuals with adjusted gross incomes over $200,000 ($250,000 for couples who file jointly) will pay higher Medicare taxes.

2014

Individual mandate — U.S. citizens and legal residents must carry health coverage or pay a tax penalty.

Employer contributions — To help pay for coverage expansion, employers with more than 50 workers must either offer health coverage or pay a per-worker fee.

Insurance exchanges — State-based regulated markets will help individuals and small businesses buy health coverage that is tax-subsidized on a sliding scale for people earning up to 400 percent of the federal poverty level. The federal government will establish a minimum benefit package for health coverage.

Medicaid expansion — The federal government will pay to expand Medicaid to all non-elderly Americans earning up to 133 percent of the federal poverty level.

Insurance rules — Insurance companies will no longer be able to refuse new coverage or coverage renewal to anyone, regardless of preexisting conditions or other factors. To keep insurance affordable for all, older and sicker people can't be charged more than three times what the average person in the community pays for coverage. Annual dollar limits on benefits are banned.

Insurer fees — Insurance companies will pay fees based on their size.

2018

Benefit tax — To raise funds, tax breaks will end for health plans with annual premiums exceeding $10,000 for an individual (or $27,500 for a family). Such so-called Cadillac plans benefit only richer Americans and are believed to be inefficient.

— Marcia Clemmitt

[1] See "Focus on Health Reform: Summary of New Health Reform Law," The Henry J. Kaiser Family Foundation, March 26, 2010, and "Timeline for Health Care Reform Implementation: System and Delivery Reform Provisions," The Commonwealth Fund, April 1, 2010.

ment "overall health reform will be unsustainable," he said. [12]

The law is "an enormously positive step to expand access and put in tools" to begin driving down costs, says Jacob Hacker, a Yale University professor of political science who was the chief architect of a proposal — eventually dumped from the legislation — to include a public, government-run health insurance plan to compete against private insurers. "I was a very strong advocate of the bill even after the public-plan option was off the table," he says.

Supporters argue that by making it easier for people to get non-job-based health coverage and beginning to trim costs, the law will actual improve businesses' ability to create jobs. Inability to find affordable health coverage under current law "is one of the major reasons why small businesses close their doors and corporations ship jobs overseas," said Obama. [13]

By establishing a system in which fewer people experience breaks in insurance coverage, the law will improve health and trim some costs, according to Mathematica Policy Research, a consulting firm in Princeton, N.J. Studies show that "adults with continuous insurance coverage are healthier and at lower risk for premature death than those who are uninsured or whose coverage is intermittent," the firm reported in April. [14]

"Continuous coverage also can reduce administrative costs," Mathematica said. For example, "guaranteed eligibility for Medicaid and the Children's Health

Half of Unemployed Workers Are Uninsured

Out of nearly 6 million unemployed workers with incomes below 200 percent of the poverty level, more than 50 percent are uninsured. The new law will allow unemployed people and others without job-sponsored coverage to buy tax-subsidized insurance.

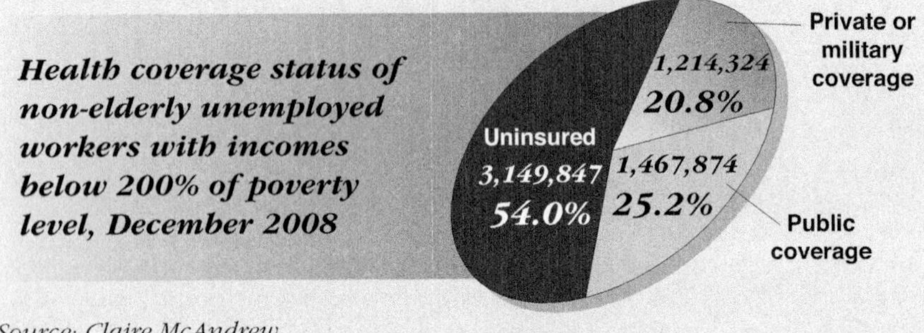

Source: Claire McAndrew, "Unemployed and Uninsured in America," Families USA, February 2009

Insurance Program for six or 12 months can lower states' administrative costs by reducing the frequent movement (called 'churning') of people in and out of the programs," drastically cutting paperwork and staff time. [15]

Will people with insurance lose out under the new law?

Critics say the new law will change things for the worse for people who have either public or private insurance today. Reform supporters argue, however, that while the law will change how many people get coverage and care, it will ultimately provide better options for everyone.

Many provisions that raise revenue to pay for coverage expansion will leave insured Americans worse off, said John Berlau, director of the Center for Investors and Entrepreneurs at the free-market think tank Competitive Enterprise Institute. For example, a provision to raise tax money to fund the law's coverage expansion will ban using pre-tax dollars from a flexible-spending account or health-savings account to buy over-the-counter drugs unless a doctor has prescribed them, creating "an effective tax increase of up to 40 percent on these items," said Berlau. [16]

About 7 million Medicare enrollees will lose the more generous benefits they now receive from "Medicare Advantage" private health insurers that serve the Medicare program, said Grace-Marie Turner, president of the Galen Institute, a free-market think tank in Alexandria, Va. Payments to those insurers will be cut under the law, based on recommendations by many economists that Medicare has long overpaid the plans. But the resulting pull-out of the plans from Medicare will be a significant hardship for the Medicare enrollees who've come to rely on the richer benefits Medicare Advantage plans provide, compared to traditional Medicare, Turner said. [17]

Before the law was enacted, the United States already faced a shortage of primary-care doctors and, with an estimated 32 million newly insured people by 2019 under the law, primary-care physicians will be stretched even thinner, according to *Kaiser Health News*. [18]

If Congress actually implements Medicare payment cuts named in the law, "15 percent of hospitals and other care facilities that rely on Medicare reimbursements would become unprofitable, meaning that they might drop Medicare patients," limiting "the availability of care for millions of seniors," the *Columbus* [Ohio] *Dispatch* editorialized. [19]

But health-reform supporters say that, contrary to critics' warnings, the law, on balance, will make it easier for virtually everyone to maintain continuous access to health insurance and care.

Rather than losing money, hospitals actually "come out winners" under the law, so access won't become a greater problem, said Maggie Mahar, a fellow at the liberal Century Foundation. [20]

Hospitals got in on early negotiations for the law and negotiated some payment rate cuts that they found acceptable, said Urban Institute senior fellow Robert Berenson. Now "hospitals are off-limits until 2020" from pay cuts proposed by the new board established by the law to make sure that Medicare hits its spending targets, Berenson said. [21]

Moreover, hospital payment cuts "will be offset by the fact that hospitals will be seeing an influx of paying patients" as more people gain insurance, Mahar said. [22]

And Medicare cuts will actually benefit enrollees, some analysts argue. Cutting payments for ineffective care such as hospital readmissions, for example, will not only make Medicare more economically sustainable over the long haul but help eliminate hospital stays that amount to unnecessary "hardship for the patient," said a report published by the liberal-leaning Commonwealth Fund in Manhattan. [23]

The law will help insured people avoid unwarranted insurance-premium rate increases by requiring annual review of premium increases in a public process that will, for the first time, require public input, not just explanations of their charges by the insurance company, according to the liberal consumer group Families USA. Before the law went into effect, many states had "no process for obtaining consumer input in the rate-review process," so state officials heard "only the insurers' side of the story" and often were unaware that the proposed rates were unaffordable. [24]

Changes brought about by the law "do not pose a risk to the public," says Georgetown University's Feder. "What insured people are currently at risk of is higher costs" that will force them out of their coverage, either because they lose a job, become self-employed or an employer stops offering it, she says. Under the new law, "if there's an employment change, now for the first time they'll have a real option," she says.

In another boon for patients, "beginning this year, if you become seriously ill, insurers won't be able to drop your coverage on the grounds that you forgot some detail of your medical history when you applied for insurance," as they could in the past, said Mahar. From now on, insurers "will be able to rescind your policy only if they can prove fraud, or that you intentionally set out to deceive them. This won't be easy." [25]

Will health care reform make care more affordable?

Supporters of the new law say its tax-funded subsidies will help low-income people afford health coverage and that health-provider payment initiatives will slow out-of-control health spending. But skeptics say that the law's affordability provisions are all unproven.

Using incentives and accountability, the new law tries to nudge doctors, hospitals and other health-care providers toward eliminating unnecessary illness and treatment, said David Kendall, a senior fellow at Third Way, a center-left advocacy group in Washington. For example, "the current system . . . lets doctors who cause infections through improper hand-washing send [insurers] more bills to treat" infections that patients may get as a result, Kendall explained. The new law institutes cost-saving provisions such as requiring hospitals to "effectively put a warranty on their care by limiting the payments they get from Medicare if a patient is readmitted" too soon or in circumstances that suggest his or her earlier care was ineffective or harmful. [26]

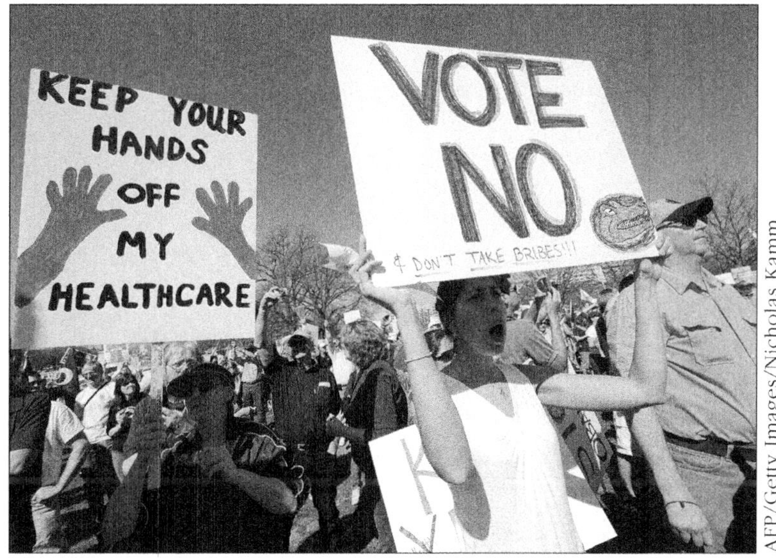

Supporters of the Tea Party movement demonstrate against the health care bill at the Capitol on March 20, 2010, just before a cliffhanger vote on the sweeping legislation the next day. Critics say the plan will cost too much and give the government too much control over Americans' health decisions.

If such an outcomes-based payment system — often referred to as a "bundled" payment system — can be developed "that providers can live with, we'll be in a much better place" than we are today when it comes to holding down costs, says Harvard Medical School's Chernew. Whether the law is making inroads should begin to become evident in about five years, he says.

Other proposed provider-payment measures "include just about everything we know" about cost control, making it a best effort at implementing cost savings on the provider side, says McClellan, the former Medicare and Medicaid chief under George W. Bush.

The "history of previous legislation is auspicious," because earlier laws that cut health-care provider payments have almost always had a bigger cost-cutting effect than analysts first predicted, said Peter Orszag, director of the White House Office of Management and Budget. [27]

In academic analyses of health-system reorganization plans that stamp out inefficient care — as the law aims to do — "the estimates of possible efficiency savings range up to 30 percent or more of medical spending," said Harvard University professor of economics David M. Cutler. Because previous analyses have underestimated the cost-saving effects of such measures, there's a good chance that "costs will fall more rapidly than expected," Cutler said. [28]

Nevertheless, even some analysts who see significant good in the law have doubts about its ability to make health care affordable.

"I suspect that the legislation is going to be more successful at coverage goals than at cost-containment goals," says Katherine Baicker, a professor of health economics at the Harvard School of Public Health. "You can throw money" at patients and providers and increase individuals' access to health care, "but we simply don't yet know how" to slow health-care cost growth, even though scholars do have ideas about what may work, she says.

Also unknown is "whether Congress will have the political will" to enforce cost-cutting measures that the law's demonstration projects find to be effective, says Baicker. Health-care providers always fight such changes because they affect income, and that means "all these things could easily be left to wither on the vine," she says. "While the demos may be promising, there is no built-in mechanism in the law to give them teeth."

For example, the law sets up a program for testing the "comparative effectiveness" of health treatments — with the goal of spending health-care dollars only for what works best, notes a report by Medicare's actuary. Requiring Medicare to base payments on comparative-effectiveness findings would reap "substantial savings," says the actuary's office. However, the law does not authorize establishment of a federal board "with authority over payment and coverage policies" to force Medicare and other programs to stop paying for less effective treatments, said the actuary. Instead, the legislation only requires dissemination of the research as a recommendation for payment changes. Because of lawmakers' reluctance to impose tough changes, therefore, a program that could save a lot of money will result only in "small savings," and even those will "take many years to develop," the report predicts. [29]

"If there were an FDA [Food and Drug Administration] of cost containment, none of these measures would be considered safe and effective," quipped Mark Pauly, a professor of health-care systems, business and public policy at the University of Pennsylvania's Wharton School. Nevertheless, a few provisions, such as reducing rates of hospital readmission by letting nurses counsel patients about staying healthy and requiring hospitals to take stringent steps to ward off hospital-acquired infections, likely will save money, Pauly conceded. [30]

But some conservative critics say the law's cost-cutting initiatives simply cannot work.

"You cannot control costs unless someone does the controlling. And there is nothing in the legislation that would free either patients or doctors to do that job," said John Goodman, president of the National Center for Policy Analysis, a free-market think tank in Dallas. Goodman is among conservatives who argue that the entire system of third-party insurance — not just public programs like Medicare — shields patients too much from the high cost of health care. Therefore, he argues that since the new law preserves an insurance system, it cannot succeed at cost control. Goodman argues that health costs will only be controlled when patients must fully confront the cost of the care they seek, so that they will bargain hard to force their medical providers "to use their intelligence, creativity and innovative ability to seek efficiencies the way people do in other markets." [31]

Furthermore, several provisions in the law "are sure to increase health-insurance premiums in the short term," says the Galen Institute's Turner. A ban on health insurers placing a lifetime or annual limit on the benefits an individual receives will raise premiums for all policyholders, she said. [32]

Meanwhile, liberal opponents say the law lacks the most powerful known means of holding down costs. For example, allowing Americans to buy prescription drugs from Canada "could have saved American consumers roughly $100 billion," but that didn't make it into the bill because drug manufacturers strenuously object to the practice, wrote liberal blogger Jon Walker. Creating a centralized federal government authority to negotiate payments with health-care providers would also lower payment rates, and requiring insurance-benefit packages to be standardized would reduce administrative costs and allow for better comparison shopping. But neither of those common-sense measures is in the new law either, Walker said. [33] ■

BACKGROUND

Exceptional America

Virtually all other industrialized countries have concluded that health care is a right that nations owe their people and have created taxpayer-funded public or combination public-private systems to provide it. By contrast, the U.S. Congress has never seriously debated establishing a universal right to care. [34]

"We had a little of this conversation after the Civil War," resulting in a basic guarantee of health care as a right for veterans, says University of Pennsylvania ethicist Caplan. Other nations have gone much farther, however. For example, after World War II, Britain explicitly discussed whether health care should be guaranteed as a right and decided that "it was part of what the nation owed to a people who had lived through the blitz" — Nazi Germany's sustained seven-month bombing of Britain during the early years of World War II, he says.

"Canada had the conversation and concluded that" a guaranteed right to health care "is part of what would bind [the geographically vast country] together as a nation," says Caplan.

"We're the only county that finds it quite this difficult to discuss" whether health care should be a right, in part because of historical struggles to harmonize a racially and ethnically diverse society, Caplan says. It's easier for a smaller, homogeneous nation to discuss using taxpayer dollars to offer health care to all, he says.

As a result, health insurance in America developed as a purely private enterprise in the first half of the 20th century. At first, there was limited concern about paying for coverage. Gradually, however, as care grew more expensive, employers began offering hospitalization insurance as a benefit for workers.

By the 1940s, large unionized companies dominated the American economy, and many used health-insurance benefits as a bargaining chip in labor negotiations. Employer-sponsored health plans successfully spread out health-care costs among large pools of workers and,

Continued on p. 516

Chronology

1880s-1930s

As the cost and effectiveness of health care increase, industrialized countries mull universal access, and Americans worry about affording health care.

1883
Germany creates first universal health-care system.

1929
School system in Dallas, Texas, launches first prepaid hospital insurance plan for employees.

1932
Committee on the Cost of Medical Care details Americans' growing difficulties in paying for care.

1935
Attempts fail to include health coverage in the Social Security Act.

1940s-1980s

Employer-sponsored insurance becomes the dominant form of U.S. health coverage. Congress enacts Medicare and Medicaid to fill coverage gaps for the elderly, the disabled and poor mothers with children.

1943
Wagner-Murray-Dingell bill for compulsory national health insurance is introduced in Congress. . . . National War Labor Board declares employer contributions to insurance are income-tax free, opening the way for companies to use health insurance packages to attract workers.

1946
United Kingdom launches fully nationalized universal coverage system — National Health Service.

1960
U.S. health spending totals $28 billion, or 5.2 percent of gross domestic product (GDP).

1965
President Lyndon B. Johnson signs Medicare and Medicaid into law.

1971
President Richard M. Nixon places wage and price controls on medical services.

1980
Health spending tops $255 billion, or 9.1 percent of GDP.

1990s-2009

Rising health costs force some Americans to drop coverage, prompting Congress to enact a public insurance program for children in working families.

1993
President Bill Clinton and first lady Hillary Clinton propose sweeping health-system reforms. Insurance industry launches opposition campaign.

1994
Senate abandons the Clinton health plan without debate.

1997
President Clinton signs State Children's Health Insurance Program (SCHIP) to provide coverage for children in working families.

2000
Health spending totals $1.4 trillion, or 13.8 percent of GDP.

2002
Congress enacts Health Care Tax Credit for those who lose their jobs to foreign competition.

2006
Massachusetts enacts mandatory, universal health-coverage program.

2009
Massachusetts officials consider implementing "payment bundling" — paying doctors and hospitals a flat fee upfront to cover patients — to control cost growth in their universal-coverage plan. . . . Congress votes to expand SCHIP program. . . . President Obama and congressional Democrats slowly push coverage-expansion plans through Congress in the face of heated opposition; bill passes Senate on Dec. 24.

2010s

Implementation begins of the most wide-ranging health-reform legislation in U.S. history.

2010
Health reform clears Congress on March 21; President Obama signs legislation intended to cover about 32 million uninsured people and re-engineer the health-care payment system to trim costs; the law's main provisions take effect in 2014. . . . The 2009 federal SCHIP expansion falters as state budgets suffer from recession. . . . Connecticut becomes first state to sign up for the 2010 reform law's option to immediately extend Medicaid coverage to poor adults outside the traditional Medicaid categories of disabled people and mothers and their young children. . . . At least 20 state attorneys general sue the federal government to stop the health-care law.

2014
Main provisions of the 2010 health law are slated to begin, including a requirement for all Americans to buy health insurance.

States Will Be Ground Zero for Many Changes

"A lot is resting on the shoulders of the states."

Public-policy experts agree that the states will play a crucial role in implementing the new health-care reforms, but they aren't all sure the states are up to the task.

"A lot is resting on the shoulders of the states" for the success of health-care reform, says Stan Dorn, a senior research associate at the Washington-based Urban Institute, a centrist think tank.

"This federalism aspect of the law is one of the biggest worries" in some respects "because reliance on states leads to enormous variation" in a program, which likely will leave some residents of the country with low benefits and little protection under the new law, says Georgetown University professor of public policy Judith Feder. Some analysts tout states as "laboratories of democracy," where innovative ideas are often pioneered and tested, but Feder argues that studies show that most states rarely innovate. "Federalism is overrated," she says.

Yale University professor of political science Jacob Hacker says ultimate success will heavily depend on the states and federal government working together. "To me, one of the biggest challenges of implementation is that the law creates dual authority in many areas," he says. "Hopefully, good partnerships will develop." Specifically, Hacker explains, the federal government will be funding subsidies for people without employer-based coverage to buy insurance in new markets, called exchanges, but the states are charged with setting up and running the exchanges.

Most of the money to fund actual new insurance coverage under Medicaid and in the new exchanges will come from the federal government, which should prove a boon to states in some respects, since it's state and local authorities who often see the consequences as uninsured people develop severe medical problems. States will end up bearing a large share of administrative expenses for the programs, however.

"The states that do the least now" to provide Medicaid coverage "will get the most money from the expansion" of Medicaid to a new group of eligible people — everyone with incomes under 133 percent of the federal poverty level, says Judith Solomon, a senior fellow at the left-leaning Center on Budget and Policy Priorities.

States generally will benefit from the Medicaid expansion because currently "very, very large numbers of the low-income people" who will become eligible for the mostly federally funded Medicaid expansion "are currently in some state-funded programs," such as mental-health programs, Solomon says.

State officials who are fretting about the cost of the new programs tend to "assume that 100 percent" of eligible people will participate, "but we've never seen any such number" in previous programs, so it's unlikely to happen this time either, says Solomon.

"That's not to say that there won't be some expenses" for states, Solomon says. Just as in the current Medicaid program, states will pick up half the administrative costs for the new, much larger Medicaid population — beginning in 2014 — while the federal government will pay for the other 50 percent of the administration.

"I'm worried about the administration side, where there's only a 50 percent federal match," says Dorn. "No state person will want to brag about hiring more state employees" since all state governments are constrained by legal requirements to balance their budgets annually, he says.

Nevertheless, when it comes to getting high numbers of eligible people enrolled, intensive outreach is crucial, plus having as many as possible automatically enrolled based on information government agencies already possess, rather than requiring them to fill out application forms, Dorn says. That makes administrative "resources the greatest implementation question."

Unless they opt out of the responsibility, states also are supposed to set up and manage the health-insurance exchanges that in 2014 are slated to begin selling coverage to people without employer-sponsored health insurance.

"But if I were a state legislator or governor, the last thing I would want to do would be to run an exchange," says Dorn. "The federal money [to administer the exchanges] runs from 2014 to Jan. 1, 2015," and after that "each exchange must raise its own money by charging fees" to insurers or health-care providers, Dorn explains. All of these players "will want services the exchanges provide but won't want to pay." That will give states a difficult balancing act: raising money while also tightly regulating the health-care market, Dorn says.

If many states are leery, "the feds might end up doing it all, which might not be a bad outcome," he says, although it's not what the law anticipates.

— Marcia Clemmitt

Continued from p. 514

by doing so, allowed each individual to pay relatively low and consistent premiums, even in years when they had accidents or illnesses. Furthermore, since the sickest people are unlikely to be employed, private insurance companies prospered in an insurance market almost entirely made up of employer-sponsored coverage.

Hybrid Solutions

Beginning as early as the 1940s, however, some lawmakers grew troubled by the realization that vulnerable populations — such as the elderly and the disabled — did not have workplace-based coverage. Many of these people couldn't afford individual policies, which in most states insurers could price according to the individual's own health risk.

Members of Congress made unsuccessful attempts to launch discussion of health coverage for all in 1943, 1945, 1947, 1949 and 1957, and Presidents Franklin D. Roosevelt, Harry S. Truman, Richard M. Nixon and Clinton all proposed guaranteed universal coverage.

Ultimately, however, Congress backed off even debating such proposals because of strong opposition from big employers, insurers and health-care providers — who feared that increased government involvement in health care would mean less autonomy in practice and lower pay. Even organized labor opposed the discussions, largely because it liked bargaining for good health-care benefits.

But the growing size of the population without coverage eventually forced Congress to act. To supplement the private health-insurance system, which left many people behind, Congress launched two large public insurance programs in 1965, effectively creating a right — or "entitlement" — to health care for two specific groups of Americans. The Medicare program covers the elderly, while Medicaid covers poor mothers with young children and some poor and seriously disabled people.

Congress expanded public coverage one more time to reach another population that was increasingly priced out of employer-sponsored coverage. The State Children's Health Insurance Program (SCHIP), launched in 1997, covers children in low- and middle-income working families.

History, then, leaves the United States with a hybrid system — about half public and half private. While the arrangement matches the policy preferences of many Americans, who tend to be political centrists, it poses a complex challenge for lawmakers faced with high rates of uninsurance and fast-rising costs.

When Nixon and Democratic Presidents Jimmy Carter, in the 1970s, and Clinton, in the 1990s, proposed health-care overhauls intended to help provide affordable care for all Americans, all three plans were complicated by their attempts to leave both public and private coverage intact. Further, because of their hybrid nature, all invited harsh criticism both from conservative Republicans, who oppose taxpayer-financed, government-regulated health care, and from liberal Democrats, who often argue that private health-insurance markets simply don't work and ought to be replaced by all-public coverage.

The Clinton Plan

In 1993 and 1994, when Bill and Hillary Clinton, now Secretary of State, proposed their health-care overhaul plan, Congress came as close as it ever has to debating a full-fledged health overhaul. The times seemed to favor action. When the Clintons' Health Security Act was proposed, up to two-thirds of Americans told pollsters they favored tax-financed national health insurance.

The Clinton proposal attempted to thread the needle of the hybrid U.S. system by maintaining large public-coverage programs while creating new, tightly regulated private-insurance markets where people could buy coverage that was tax subsidized for low-income people. In an attempt to hold onto the private business dollars that had long financed health care in the United States for workers, the plan would have required all employers to contribute to the cost.

But the proposal's complexity helped make the plan an easy target for political opponents and businesses and health-care insurers and providers who feared its complicated rules and high costs. Less than a year after the proposal was announced, Congress informed the White House that it had no plans to move the plan forward.

"The failure of the Clinton health plan . . . vividly demonstrates . . . that most Americans — even the underinsured and the soon-to-be-uninsured, the potentially uninsurable and the one-illness-from-bankruptcy — can be scared into fearing that changing America's inadequate public-private patchwork means higher costs and lower quality," Yale's Hacker wrote. "This is the legacy of an insurance structure that lulls many into believing they are secure when they are not, that hides vast costs in quiet deductions from workers' pay, [and] that leaves government paying the tab for the most vulnerable and the least well," he said. "It is the very failings of our insurance system that make dealing with those failings so devilishly hard." [35]

But many conservatives continue to argue that too-strict government regulation of health care along with insurance and public programs like Medicare are the culprits that have hopelessly damaged the health-care market and made effective overhaul difficult.

"The problems in American health care have not been caused by a failure in the health care market, but mainly by distortions imposed on the market," such as "federal tax subsidies and programs that have created a third-party payment system," said Rep. Paul Ryan, R-Wis. The key to a successful overhaul is to convert to an all-private system, by means such as creating "a standard Medicare [cash] payment to be used for the purchase of private health coverage," he said. [36]

Massachusetts Plan

Over the years, many states have attempted to enact systemwide reforms on their own, frustrated by the federal government's reluctance even to discuss universal health care. The pioneers of sweeping reform included Tennessee, Oregon, Washington, Vermont and Minnesota.

Those states generally attempted to expand public coverage for the poorest residents and provide some form of tax-funded subsidies to help other low- to middle-income and sick people

Reforms Face Many Hurdles

"The war to make health-care reform an enduring success has just begun."

As the health-reform law is implemented, the number of things that can go wrong is as big as the health-care system is complicated. Besides the fact that not only states but also doctors and hospitals may balk at the new provisions, future Congresses must ante up continued funding to administer the law, never a certain outcome.

The law's coverage-expansion portions "are so state-based that the states can stymie a lot," says Judith Solomon, a senior fellow at the left-leaning Center on Budget and Policy Priorities. "There can be a great deal of stalling" on getting some initiatives like a large Medicaid expansion up and running. The law also will largely rely on increased state regulation of health insurers, which could lead to large variations" around the country in how tightly insurers are held to consumer-friendly standards.

Furthermore, "Medicaid rolls in some states will expand by 50 percent or more" beginning in 2014, and "it is unclear whether these states will be able to find enough providers who are willing to accept the anticipated payment rates," wrote Henry J. Aaron, a senior fellow at the centrist Brookings Institution think tank, and Robert D. Reischauer, president of the centrist Urban Institute. Will states "raise provider payment rates, curtail Medicaid benefits (as states are legally authorized to do), or simply let patients fail to find doctors who are willing to provide them with care?" they ask. [1]

One of the balancing acts that face lawmakers seeking to expand coverage in the employer-based U.S. system is keeping enough employer money in the game to avoid overwhelming taxpayers with new costs. Accordingly, the law was developed in hopes of limiting incentives for employers to drop workers' coverage.

But already "there are some troubling signs that employers will back off coverage because of the existence of the exchanges," where workers can buy insurance — using tax-funded subsidies — if their employers don't offer it, says Yale University professor of political science Jacob Hacker. If that happens on a large scale, "for society as a whole it might be a better thing and more fair, because having employers as the basis for coverage distorts labor markets" because the fear of losing health insurance often traps people in jobs or careers they don't want, Hacker says. "Nevertheless, it's not a direction that most people want to go in."

Federal agencies must transform the law's rather general language into specific rules, and some observers say that might produce rules that are unworkable. Moreover, there's evidence that the agencies are already falling behind in the process.

"They're not going to meet their deadlines, so they should push the whole thing back," says Joseph Antos, a scholar at the free-market American Enterprise Institute think tank and a former assistant director of the Congressional Budget Office. "It's going to take more than the three years" the law has set aside to get the massive coverage-expansion program up and running.

purchase coverage in more tightly regulated private insurance markets. But while the programs have increased coverage, at least temporarily, all have eventually foundered as costs continued rising while taxpayer willingness to fund coverage for sick or lower-income people waned.

Massachusetts first began expanding coverage to all its citizens in 1988 and enacted its latest plan in 2006. The law shifted Medicaid funding to provide more subsidies to individuals to get insurance; placed requirements to buy or help pay for coverage on both employers and individuals; and set up a statewide regulated insurance market — known as an insurance "Connector" — which state officials hoped would force insurers to compete for enrollees based on quality and price of benefits. [37]

Reactions to Massachusetts' latest initiative are mixed.

Costs are the big challenge, and it's not yet clear how state attempts to change the medical culture to favor efficiency over excess services and high price tags are working, says Chernew, of Harvard Medical School. "Some say that the culture in the state is changing, but others say we're on the verge of collapse."

People using the Connector to buy insurance "have had lots of different choices of health plans, and there's been good consumer service and information," says the Urban Institute's Dorn.

Furthermore, "they've been good at negotiating for low premiums" with insurers, he says. For example, Massachusetts has several extremely expensive hospital systems, which have had enormous clout in winning high payment from insurers over the years because patients want access to them, Dorn explains. But the Connector set up price competition by establishing a low-cost coverage option that didn't include the big-name systems, and consumers concerned with price, such as young people earning lower wages, have signed up for it, he says.

The state also has rewarded health insurers who keep premiums low by enrolling the most "default" enrollees — people who don't seek out the health coverage on their own — with the insurer who quotes the lowest premium. Default enrollees are often the healthiest, cheapest-to-cover people, thus helping that insurer hold down costs by having an extra helping of healthy people in their pool, Dorn says.

Advocates of single-payer systems, however, say Massachusetts' attempt at health-care expansion is doomed, just

Already there's evidence that agencies like the Centers for Medicare and Medicaid Services (CMS) are overwhelmed, Antos says. Neither CMS nor the Department of Health and Human Services (HHS) "is an insurance company" or has much experience in insurance, a serious lack since a massive insurance expansion is a central portion of the law, and Congress has relied on the agencies to flesh out virtually all the details, Antos says. HHS Secretary Kathleen Sebelius is a former Kansas insurance commissioner, "but she admitted that she doesn't have any particular influence in health-care reform."

Drafters of the law made little use of the expertise of the insurance industry and insurance analysts and regulators, "so there will be mistakes" in implementation, charges Antos. "It was done without consultation with the many, many experts, and HHS looks as if it's not going to ask experts now."

But Hacker says it's "too soon to be that critical of the implementation." The critical judgments will be made in the next year or so, when it will be possible to begin judging whether implementation will be smooth, he says. And while rules for how much premium revenue must fund health care "are inevitably going to be contentious, I don't believe it'll preclude insurers from participating," says Hacker. "The fact is that insurers were supportive of these things because they want the revenue" that will accompany expanded, subsidized coverage.

Nevertheless, "there's such a long time before the law goes fully into effect that critics can paint it any way they want," making it very easy for opponents to turn the public against the law, says Hacker. "The best thing advocates could do for themselves is not to trumpet their achievements but to make clear that the law is a first step."

In another setback to implementation, Senate Republicans are blocking the nomination of physician Donald Berwick, a professor of health policy and management at the Harvard School of Public Health, to head CMS. Conservatives say that Berwick's work with Britain's National Health Service is a sign he would use government to destroy American physicians' independence. Supporters argue that, to advance the health-reform law's cost-cutting initiatives, CMS must have a leader dedicated to emphasizing effectiveness and efficiency in U.S. medical practice. [2]

"The war to make health-care reform an enduring success has just begun" and "will require administrative determination and imagination and as much political resolve as was needed to pass the legislation," Aaron and Reischauer warn. [3]

— Marcia Clemmitt

[1] Henry J. Aaron and Robert D. Reischauer, "The War Isn't Over," *The New England Journal of Medicine online*, March 24, 2010, www.nejm.org.

[2] For background, see Linda Bergthold, "Who Is Don Berwick and Why Do the Republicans Want to Kill His Nomination," *Huffington Post blog*, June 1, 2010, www.huffingtonpost.com/linda-bergthold/who-is-don-berwick-and-wh_b_596859.html.

[3] Aaron and Reischauer, *op. cit.*

like earlier attempts. "Unfortunately, competition in health insurance involves a race to the bottom," said Harvard Medical School's Woolhandler. "Insurers compete by not paying for care: by denying payment and shifting costs onto patients or other payers." [38] ■

CURRENT SITUATION

Democrats in Power

With Democrats holding not only the White House but also substantial majorities in both the House and the Senate for the first time in three decades, advocates of health-care reform hoped that the 111th Congress — whose term runs from 2009 through 2010 — would finally be the one to debate a health-care overhaul for the entire population.

In his first address to a joint session of Congress, on Feb. 24, 2009, newly inaugurated President Barack Obama declared that "we must . . . address the crushing cost of health care" and thus "can no longer afford to put health-care reform on hold." High-cost health care "now causes a bankruptcy in America every thirty seconds. . . . In the last eight years, [health-insurance] premiums have grown four times faster than wages. And in each of these years, 1 million more Americans have lost their health insurance." [39]

Furthermore, he said, "already, we have done more to advance the cause of health-care reform in the last 30 days than we have in the last decade." For example, "when it was days old, this Congress passed a law to provide and protect health insurance for 11 million American children whose parents work full time" by using a cigarette tax to expand funding for the public-sector SCHIP program that covers children in working families, he said. [40]

"I suffer no illusions that this will be an easy process," said Obama. "But I . . . know that nearly a century after Teddy Roosevelt first called for reform, the cost of our health care has weighed down our economy and the conscience of our nation long enough. . . . Health-care reform cannot wait, it must not wait, and it will not wait another year." [41]

In the House, the legislation waited nearly 10 months, passing on a 220-215

Does Health Reform Create Winners and Losers?

More affordable coverage for sicker people will boost costs for healthier people.

Critics charge that the health-care reform plan makes some Americans winners and others losers. Some liberal critics charge that, by relying on private insurance for much of the tax-subsidized coverage expansion, Congress will essentially just direct more taxpayer dollars into the already bloated coffers of the insurance industry.

Other analysts aren't so sure, however.

Many of the people who will enroll in tax-subsidized coverage will not have had consistent insurance coverage for several years, and as a result often have developed significant health needs that will drive their spending up, said Maggie Mahar, a fellow at the liberal, New York City-based Century Foundation. [1]

According to recent analyses, around 11 percent of uninsured people are in "fair" or "poor" health, compared to only 5 percent of privately insured people who report poor health. Unlike in the past, "under the new reform law, insurance companies will not be able to charge these new customers more than they charge others in their community," said Mahar. This means that insurers are unlikely to reap a big windfall from the tax-funded subsidies, she argued. [2]

The same legislative provision that Mahar cites as making coverage more affordable for sicker people will cause health premiums to rise for younger, healthier people, however — an example of the way the law creates some winners and losers in the attempt to get more people covered, noted Trudy Lieberman, a longtime health-care journalist who is a contributing editor to the *Columbia Journalism Review.* [3]

"This is not national health insurance we're talking about, where everyone, no matter how old or young, is treated equally," Lieberman wrote. "We are talking about a private insurance market where companies have to make money to stay in business" and where one key way of making money in the past has been for companies to simply avoid insuring the sickest people so that healthier people can pay lower premiums.

Under the new law, however, insurance companies will be "required to take sick people who will file large claims" and also will be banned from charging them the extremely high premiums that they are liable for in the individual insurance market today, she said. Instead, older or sicker people will be on the hook for premiums that are "no more than three times what [insurers] charge a younger person," and as a result premiums for younger, healthier people will rise by an estimated 15 to 17 percent. Insurers "have to make up the revenue shortfall somehow, and they'll do it by increasing the premiums for younger people. It's a balancing act Congress has permitted," she wrote. However, for young adults earning $43,000 per year or less, some of the premium increase will be offset by a federal tax credit.

In another financial balancing act, lawmakers had to determine whether to offer larger taxpayer-funded subsidies to a smaller population of people — with lower incomes — or spread out the subsidies to a larger population. More subsidies might make the law more politically popular but also would require making subsidies for the lowest-income people smaller than they might have been otherwise. Some analysts fear that lawmakers came down on the wrong side of that question.

"One big worry that I have is affordability," says Stan Dorn, a senior research associate at the Urban Institute think tank. In the 2006 coverage expansion launched in Massachusetts, the state provided "much bigger subsidies" and "much more extensive coverage" to people with incomes up to 300 percent of the federal poverty level — the group most in danger of being priced out of coverage, says Dorn. (In 2009, for example, a family of four earning about $66,000 had an income 300 percent of the poverty level.)

But the federal law took a different tack, offering smaller subsidies for every income group — including the lowest — in order to provide some level of subsidy for people with incomes up to 400 percent of the poverty level, he says. "It would have been better to concentrate more on the people up to 300 percent of the poverty level rather than spread the subsidies so far."

— *Marcia Clemmitt*

---

[1] Maggie Mahar, "Myths & Facts About HealthCare Reform: Who Wins & Who Loses?" *Healthbeat* blog, April 6, 2010, www.healthbeatblog.com.

[2] *Ibid.*

[3] Trudy Lieberman, "The White House vs. the Associated Press," *Columbia Journalism Review online*, April 7, 2010, www.cjr.org.

vote on Saturday evening, Nov. 7, 2009, with one Republican voting in favor and 39 Democrats opposed. [42]

In the Senate, however, where the minority party wields much more power, debate dragged on into spring 2010, with the measure all but given up for dead on several occasions. Republican senators repeatedly threatened to filibuster — hold the floor without allowing the health-care legislation to come to a vote — forcing Senate leaders to muster 60-vote majorities five times to move the bill forward.

On Dec. 24, 2009, by a 60-39 margin, Senate Democrats finally passed their version of the legislation with no Republican votes. The Senate and House bills varied considerably, however, and, in such a case, both houses of Congress must — one way or another — pass identical bills before they can become law.

Thus, the cliffhanger continued for an additional three months as Democrats struggled to piece together a reform

Continued on p. 522

At Issue:

Will the health-care reform law harm the federal budget?

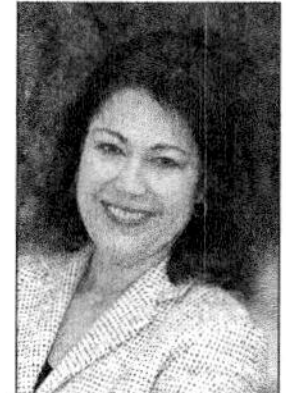

GRACE-MARIE TURNER
PRESIDENT, GALEN INSTITUTE

WRITTEN FOR *CQ RESEARCHER*, MAY 2010

President Obama's health overhaul law will have a devastating impact on the federal budget, both because of what it does and what it fails to do.

It does increase federal health spending, creates expensive open-ended entitlements and uses budget gimmicks to hide the true costs of the massive expansion of federal spending.

And it fails to lower health costs, bend the cost curve down or provide real solutions to the trillions of dollars in red ink facing existing entitlement programs, especially Medicare and Medicaid.

Nonetheless, to win passage of the health law, supporters insisted the law would be fiscally responsible and would reduce the deficit. Not a chance.

The Congressional Budget Office (CBO) recently said the law will cost $115 billion more than originally estimated, pushing the total cost above $1 trillion. But this underestimates the true costs by hundreds of billions — if not trillions of dollars — due to the law's deception and budget gimmicks.

Part of the true cost was concealed by delaying expensive subsidies until 2014 while starting many of the tax hikes and Medicare cuts much earlier. Further, the law is purportedly paid for with $569 billion in tax increases and $528 billion in cuts to Medicare. But these Medicare cuts are highly suspect given Congress' history of pushing them off to keep doctor payments level — and keep physicians in the Medicare program. Keeping payments just at current rates will cost $276 billion over 10 years, according to the CBO.

When these and other costs are included, the more accurate price tag for ObamaCare is $2.5 trillion over a decade.

Rather than helping contain escalating health spending, as promised, ObamaCare pushes it higher. Medicare's chief actuary, Rick Foster, says federal health spending will rise by $311 billion by 2019 thanks to the law.

And this estimate doesn't include tens of millions more people who could lose their health insurance at work. The law threatens employers with big fines and subjects them to unpredictable health insurance cost increases; many are considering dropping coverage. If they do, millions more workers would be dumped onto health exchanges where they'll be subsidized by taxpayers. If this happens, federal spending will explode.

Gimmicks, new entitlements and unrealistic assumptions are just some of the many ingredients in ObamaCare that will have a crippling impact on the federal budget. We simply can't afford this law.

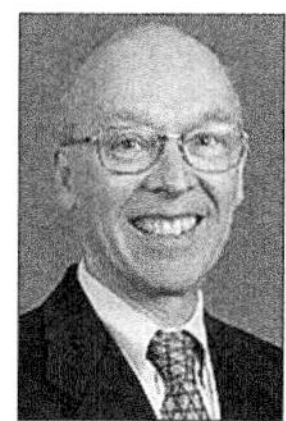

PAUL N. VAN DE WATER
SENIOR FELLOW, CENTER ON BUDGET AND POLICY PRIORITIES

WRITTEN FOR *CQ RESEARCHER*, MAY 2010

The Congressional Budget Office (CBO) estimates that the new health reform law will reduce deficits by $143 billion over the first decade (2010-2019) and by about one-half of 1 percent of gross domestic product, or about $1.3 trillion, over the second decade (2020-2029).

The law will extend coverage to over 30 million uninsured Americans and provide important consumer protections to tens of millions of insured Americans whose coverage may have critical gaps. It will more than pay for these improvements by making specific reductions in Medicare, Medicaid and other programs and by increasing tax revenues (such as by raising the Medicare tax on high-income people).

Despite CBO's finding that the law will reduce deficits, some people have argued that it will actually increase deficits, claiming that CBO's cost estimate includes savings that won't occur, omits costs that should be included, or both. Those claims don't withstand scrutiny (see "Health Reform Will Reduce the Deficit," www.cbpp.org/files/3-25-10health.pdf).

For example, some claim that the law's Medicare savings are unrealistic because Congress never lets Medicare reductions take effect. History shows this is untrue. Over the past 20 years Congress has enacted four pieces of legislation that include significant Medicare savings; virtually all of the savings in three of them (the 1990, 1993 and 2005 budget reconciliation bills) took effect, as did nearly four-fifths of the savings in the fourth piece of legislation (the Balanced Budget Act of 1997).

Some contend that the health-reform law should include the cost of permanently fixing Medicare's sustainable growth rate (SGR) formula for setting physician payments. The poorly designed formula turned out to require much larger cuts in physician payments than Congress intended when it enacted SGR, so Congress has regularly acted in recent years to prevent the full SGR cuts from taking effect. But the SGR cost is in no way a result of health reform — the government will incur this cost regardless of health reform, not because of it.

Because rising health-care costs represent the single largest cause of the federal government's long-term budget problems, fundamental health reform is key to their solution. Experts agree that slowing the growth of health-care costs will require an ongoing process of testing, experimentation and rapid implementation of what is found to work. The health-reform law begins that process. It starts to transform a system that delivers ever more services into one that provides effective, high-value health care.

Continued from p. 520

package that could win all the needed conservative Democratic votes in the Senate while retaining liberal support in the House. In addition, by 2010, Democrats' previous 60-vote, filibuster-stymieing Senate majority was reduced to 59 votes, as Sen. Scott Brown, R-Mass., was seated as the elected replacement of the late Sen. Edward M. Kennedy, D-Mass. — longtime ardent champion of health-care reform — who died of brain cancer on Aug. 26, 2009.

Ultimately, using several parliamentary maneuvers, Senate Majority Leader Harry Reid, D-Nev., and Speaker of the House Nancy Pelosi, D-Calif., engineered passage of a bill acceptable to Democrats in both houses. On March 21, the House passed the Senate's version of the bill. Then, under a process called "reconciliation," first the Senate and then the House passed a package of changes to the Senate legislation to make it acceptable to the generally more liberal House Democratic majority. Reconciliation bills — which are permitted to include only provisions that relate to the federal budget — may not be filibustered and thus require only a 51-vote majority in the Senate to pass. [43]

"Part of Obama's frustration" over health care "is that he thought that in the end some Republicans would approve" the legislation, "which is not as radical as the overhaul that Nixon proposed" in the early 1970s, says Bryan D. Jones, a professor of congressional studies at the University of Texas, in Austin.

The new law is "a much more conservative policy than was considered in the past," says the Urban Institute's Dorn. For example, in the Clinton plan, "we were going to leave behind our employer-based coverage, and there would have been a uniform benefit standard" for all health insurance. The Clinton proposal also included "explicit regulation of insurance premiums" to prevent them from rising too high and largely dictated what insurance benefit packages could contain, says Dorn. "This bill doesn't have any of that."

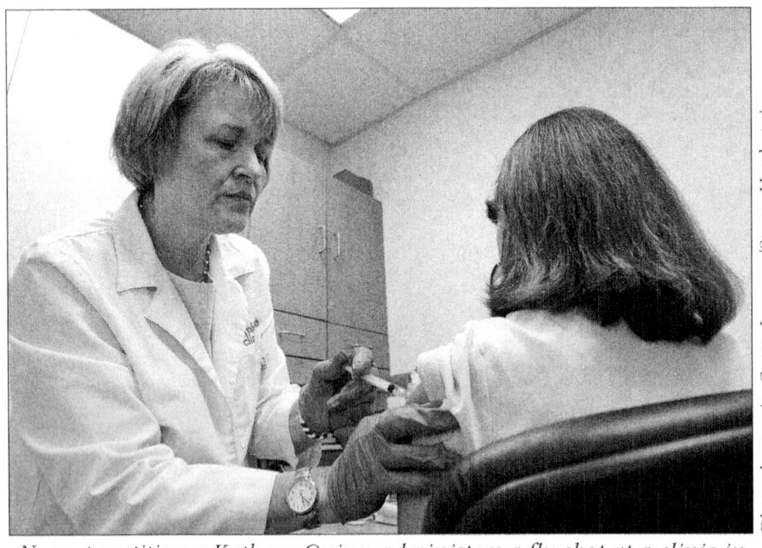

Bloomberg via Getty Images/Steve Hockstein

Nurse practitioner Kathryn Quinn administers a flu shot at a clinic in a CVS store in Wyckoff, N.J. Proponents of the health-reform law say using nurse practitioners for more tasks often performed by physicians will help keep health-care costs down.

In fact, many Democrats liken the bill to the 2006 Massachusetts plan, passed by a Democrat-dominated legislature and signed into law by then-Gov. Mitt Romney, a Republican.

"A lot of commentators have said . . . this is sort of similar to the bill that Mitt Romney . . . passed in Massachusetts," said Obama. [44]

Many conservatives, including Romney, heatedly deny that the Massachusetts plan has much in common with the 2010 federal law, however.

"We don't like . . . the intrusion of the federal government on the rights of states" in the federal law, which requires states to participate in health-coverage expansions, nor the taxes the law will raise to pay for coverage, said Romney. [45]

Implementing the Law

Perhaps the biggest difference the law will make for most people is that, beginning in 2014, it will provide a new, regulated insurance marketplace. People who cannot get employer-sponsored coverage can shop for health insurance at the so-called state exchanges. The law also will provide many people with subsidies to help pay for that coverage. [46]

Also in 2014, people with incomes up to 133 percent of the federal poverty level can get Medicaid coverage, paid for mostly by the federal government. Currently, only certain groups of people, mainly poor mothers and their young children and some severely disabled poor people, are eligible for Medicaid.

Health insurers will face a very different set of rules and expectations in the new system, says Georgetown University's Feder. Today U.S. health insurers compete for profits largely based on "risk selection" — trying to be the insurer whose benefit packages attract the healthiest people, because money that doesn't go to medical care can go to profits. While the law "doesn't stamp out risk selection, it sure as hell treads on it," she continues, mainly because, ultimately, it will require insurers to take all comers and will also require that a certain minimum percentage of premiums go towards medical care, she explains.

Many of the law's provisions aimed at cost containment involve "putting new [health-care-delivery and payment] arrangements in place and getting providers into them," says Feder. Under the new arrangements, providers like doctors and hospitals "would retain earnings if they're efficient and deliver high-quality care rather than delivering a high volume of care," as occurs under current systems, she says.

"It's going to take a lot of money and new resources for Medicare to implement and implement quickly" the law's many new programs, says former Medicare and Medicaid chief McClellan. "It normally takes seven to 10 years" for a good idea to actually become part of the Medicare program. "But we don't have that kind of time."

Furthermore, there's the fear that, as in the past when Medicare has proven that certain techniques for saving money worked, Congress may block nationwide rollout of the methods, because of providers who worry they'll lose money, McClellan says.

"The risk is not that the bill is repealed but that pieces of it" won't be supported by future Congresses, says Robert Blendon, a professor of health policy at the Harvard School of Public Health. For example, a Republican Congress that opposes taxes may cut funding for federal subsidies that are required to help people afford insurance, he says.

Meanwhile, congressional Democrats are mulling additional changes they say may be needed to improve the health-care system for patients, such as tightening government oversight of health-insurance premium price increases. [47]

Fighting the Law

Conservatives continue to argue that the law involves government too much in health care.

"The new law requires all Americans to purchase health insurance or pay a penalty . . . an unprecedented extension of congressional power," wrote the Heritage Foundation's Nix. Furthermore, she said, "the health-care overhaul . . . diminishes the federalist system upon which the U.S. was founded, which grants certain powers to the states in order to limit those of the federal government." The law requires that states expand their Medicaid programs, whether or not they want to, and also includes new federal regulations on health insurers, which have been largely state regulated, Nix said. [48]

One of the most prominent initiatives to halt the law is a lawsuit now backed by 20 states and the National Federation of Independent Business.

"After all the political deals were made, small businesses were left with a law that does little to address costs and instead is filled with new mandates, taxes and paperwork requirements that increase the cost of doing business," said Karen Harned, head of the federation's legal office. [49]

The Obama administration has already filed a brief in federal district court in Detroit in one of the earliest lawsuits against the law. The suit was filed by the Thomas More Law Center, a conservative legal group in Ann Arbor, which argues that the law's individual mandate to buy health insurance violates constitutionally protected freedoms.

The administration argues that decisions to opt out of health insurance are more than personal choices but have consequences for the entire country — thus making them suitable targets of federal lawmaking. The administration's brief argues that when uninsured people get sick, people who have been paying insurance, as well as taxpayers, pick up the bill for their care. Thus, "individual decisions to forgo insurance coverage, in the aggregate, substantially affect interstate commerce by shifting costs to health-care providers and the public," making them a fair target for federal legislation under the Commerce Clause. [50]

Ironically, former Gov. Romney — who signed Massachusetts' health-reform law — is among opponents who've called most loudly for stopping the new federal law. Rather than seeking judicial repeal, however, Romney this spring urged voters to support Republican candidates to win back a congressional majority in November. Then "we can clamp down on this bill . . . by not funding it," he said. [51] ■

OUTLOOK

Dealing with Rationing

Supporters argue that as people learn more about the new law, most will back it. However, expanding taxpayers' responsibility to help provide health coverage for most Americans will ultimately require wrestling with the toughest question: As costs rise, how should taxpayer-supported health benefits be limited — or rationed?

"As people come to understand the basic approach" of the new law, "they'll like most of it," says the Urban Institute's Dorn. Many already support "providing more help for people who can't afford insurance, requiring employers to help and setting up new rules that help people buy" insurance in a more transparent, regulated marketplace, he says.

"Once the law is implemented, people won't have to worry that, 'Oh, if I get laid off, I'll lose coverage for my asthmatic daughter' " because they will be able to buy subsidized coverage elsewhere, he says.

But single-payer advocate Woolhandler of Harvard says the new law will only temporarily slow momentum for much larger reform "because we didn't really solve anything. The cost curve was absolutely not fixed" by the legislation, "so a lot of middle-class people" will eventually find their coverage threatened again. "Very quickly people are going to see that nothing is solved."

With a program in place to ensure basic health coverage to most Americans, the next debate will be about "rationing" care, says Baicker of the Harvard School of Public Health. As the number of available health services — and their price tags — increases, "public programs, at least, almost certainly won't be able to pay for anything that has any benefit at all," but, eventually, "will need to have a higher threshold" — paying only for things that have a certain level of benefit — to avoid having health costs squeeze out all other government spending, she says.

Merely broaching the conversation — let alone reaching conclusions about what care to fund — will be extremely difficult, Baicker says.

Currently, our system rations care by pricing some people out of care altogether, except for emergencies treated in the emergency room, says University of Pennsylvania ethicist Caplan.

Because lawmakers "avoided any discussion of rationing" in the recent debate, the public is running around with the delusion that we don't ration now," Caplan says. "But the discussion we need to have should start now, because the public will need many years to accept" the notion of health spending limits, he says. ■

About the Author

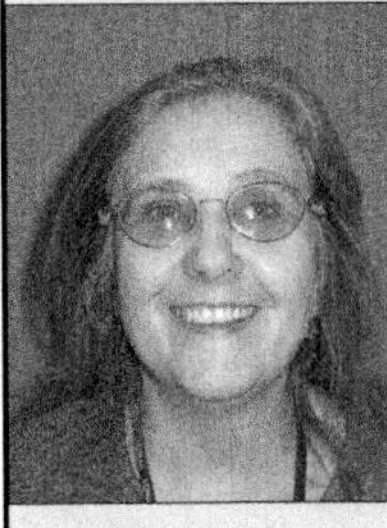

Staff writer **Marcia Clemmitt** is a veteran social-policy reporter who previously served as editor in chief of *Medicine & Health* and staff writer for *The Scientist.* She has also been a high school math and physics teacher. She holds a liberal arts and sciences degree from St. John's College, Annapolis, and a master's degree in English from Georgetown University. Her recent reports include "Preventing Cancer" and "Reproductive Ethics."

Notes

[1] Quoted in Scott Wilson, "With a Signature, Obama Seals His Health-care Victory," *The Washington Post*, March 24, 2010, p. A1.

[2] Steven Thomma and David Lightman, "Obama Signs Health-care Bill, but GOP Protests Continue," McClatchy Newspapers/*Miami Herald*, March 23, 2010, www.miamiherald.com/2010/03/23/1543254/obama-signs-health-care-legislation.html.

[3] Arthur L. Caplan, "Right to Reform," *The Journal of Clinical Investigation*, October 2009, p. 2862, www.jci.org.

[4] Quoted in Michael Sweeney, "Hatch Attacks Individual Mandate He Previously Supported," *TPM LiveWire, Talking Points Memo* blog, March 26, 2010, http://tpmlivewire.talkingpointsmemo.com.

[5] Quoted in "Health Care Reform: Not Ready to Be Discharged Yet," *Knowledge at Wharton* newsletter, March 31, 2010, http://knowledge.wharton.upenn.edu/article.cfm?articleid=2457.

[6] Kathryn Nix, "Top 10 Disasters of Obamacare," Web Memo, The Heritage Foundation, March 30, 2010, www.heritage.org.

[7] Sally C. Pipes, "Obamacare Wins: Now the Pain Begins," *New York Post*, March 22, 2010, www.nypost.com.

[8] Robert E. Moffit, *Obamacare: Impact on Doctors*, WebMemo No. 2895, The Heritage Foundation, May 11, 2010, www.heritage.org.

[9] Jane Hamsher, "Fact Sheet: The Truth About the Health Care Bill," *Firedoglake* blog, March 19, 2010, http://fdlaction.firedoglake.com.

[10] Ian Millhiser, "If at First You Don't Succeed, Hope for Activist Judges," Center for American Progress website, March 23, 2010, www.americanprogress.org; for background, see *Gonzales v. Raich*, 545 U.S. 1 (2005), www.law.cornell.edu/supct/html/03-1454.ZS.html.

[11] Simon Lazarus, "Mandatory Health Insurance: Is It Constitutional?" Issue Brief, American Constitution Society, December 2009, www.acslaw.org/node/15654; for background, see *United States v. Southeastern Underwriters Association*, 322 U.S. 533 (1944), http://supreme.justia.com/us/322/533/.

[12] *Ibid.*

[13] "President Barack Obama State of the Union Address, Feb. 24, 2009," About.com: US Politics website, http://uspolitics.about.com/od/speeches/l/bl_feb2009_obama_SOTU.htm.

[14] Jill Bernstein, Deborah Chollet and Stephanie Peterson, "How Does Insurance Coverage Improve Health Outcomes?" Issue Brief, Mathematica Policy Research, April 2010, www.mathematica-mpr.com.

[15] *Ibid.*

[16] John Berlau, "Health Care: Fix Middle-Class 'Medicine Cabinet Tax' in Reconciliation," Competitive Enterprise Institute, March 23, 2010, www.cei.org.

[17] Grace-Marie Turner, "Foster's Report Validates Fears," *National Journal Expert Blogs*, May 3, 2010, http://healthcare.nationaljournal.com.

[18] Quoted in "True or False? Top Seven Health Care Fears," msnbc.com/*Kaiser Health News*, April 2, 2010, www.msnbc.com.

[19] "Flaws of Health-care Overhaul Grow More Apparent Every Day," *Columbus* [Ohio] *Dispatch*, April 29, 2010.

[20] Maggie Mahar, "Myths & Facts About Health-Care Reform: The Impact on Hospitals, and Patients Who Need Hospital Care — Part 3," *Healthbeat* blog, April 21, 2010, www.healthbeatblog.com.

[21] Quoted in *ibid.*

[22] Mahar, *op. cit.*

[23] Stuart Guterman, Karen Davis, and Kristof Stremikis, "How Health Reform Legislation Will Affect Medicare Beneficiaries," The Commonwealth Fund, March 2010, www.cmwf.org.

[24] "Rate Review: Holding Health Plans Accountable for Your Premium Dollars," Families USA Issue Brief, April 2010, www.familiesusa.org.

[25] Maggie Mahar, "Myths & Facts About Health-Care Reform: Who Wins and Who Loses?" *Healthbeat* blog, April 6, 2010, www.healthbeatblog.com.

[26] David B. Kendall, "A Foundation for Cost Control," *National Journal* blogs, March 22, 2010, http://healthcare.nationaljournal.com.

[27] "In Search of a Fiscal Cure," *Newsweek*, May 10, 2010, p. 12.

[28] David M. Cutler, "Time to Prove the Skeptics Wrong on Health Reform," Center for

American Progress, April 23 ,2010, www.americanprogress.org.

[29] Richard S. Foster, "Estimated Financial Effects of the 'Patient Protection and Affordable Care Act' as Amended," Office of the Actuary, Centers for Medicare and Medicaid Services, April 22, 2010.

[30] Quoted in "Health Care Reform: Not Ready to Be Discharged Yet," *op. cit.*

[31] John Goodman, "The Most Important Feature of ObamaCare Is Something No One Is Talking About," John Goodman's blog, March 29, 2010, www.john-goodman-blog.com.

[32] Testimony before Senate Committee on Health, Education, Labor and Pensions, April 20, 2010.

[33] Jon Walker, "Former Obama Aide David Cutler Ignores Proven Cost Control ideas to Inflate Grade on President's Health Care Plan," *Firedoglake* blog, March 10, 2010, http://fdlaction.firedoglake.com.

[34] For background, see the following *CQ Researcher* reports by Marcia Clemmitt, "Rising Health Costs," April 7, 2006, pp. 289-312; "Universal Coverage," March 30, 2007, pp. 265-288; and "Health Care Reform," Aug. 28, 2009, pp. 693-716.

[35] Jacob S. Hacker, "Yes We Can? The New Push for American Health Security," *Politics & Society*, March 2009, p. 14.

[36] Paul Ryan, "A Roadmap for America's Future: Description of the Legislation," House Budget Committee Republican website, www.roadmap.republicans.budget.house.gov.

[37] For background, see John E. McDonough, Brian Rosman, Fawn Phelps and Melissa Shannon, "The Third Wave of Massachusetts Health Care Access Reform," *Health Affairs online*, Sept. 14, 2006, http://content.healthaffairs.org/cgi/content/full/25/6/w420.

[38] Testimony before House Energy and Commerce Subcommittee on Health, June 24, 2009, www.pnhp.org/news/2009/june/testimony_of_steffie.php.

[39] "President Barack Obama State of the Union Address, Feb. 24, 2009," About.com: US Politics website, http://uspolitics.about.com/od/speeches/l/bl_feb2009_obama_SOTU.htm.

[40] For background see Ceci Connolly, "Senate Passes Health Insurance Bill for Children," *The Washington Post*, Jan. 30, 2009, p. A1, www.washingtonpost.com/wp-dyn/content/article/2009/01/29/AR2009012900325.html.

[41] "President Barack Obama State of the Union Address, Feb. 24, 2009," *op. cit.*

[42] For background see "House Passes Health Care Reform Bill," CNN.com, Nov. 8, 2009, www.cnn.com/2009/POLITICS/11/07/health.care.

[43] For background see Timothy Noah, "Health Reform: An Online Guide," *Slate*, April 12, 2010, www.slate.com.

[44] Quoted in Eric Kleefeld, "Romney Spokesman: 'Romney Plan' Is Not Like Obama's Health Care Reform, Despite What Obama Says," *Talking Points Memo* blog, March 31, 2010, http://tpmdc.talkingpointsmemo.com.

[45] Quoted in Andrew Romano, "Mitt Romney on RomneyCare," *Newsweek online*, April 19, 2010, www.newsweek.com.

[46] For background see "Side-by-Side Comparisons of Major Health Care Reform Proposals," Focus on Health Reform website, Kaiser Family Foundation, April 8, 2010, www.kff.org/healthreform/sidebyside.cfm.

[47] For background see "Senate Democrats Seek Legislation to Regulate Insurer Rate Hikes," *Kaiser Health News* website, April 21, 2010, www.kaiserhealthnews.org/daily-reports/2010/april/21/insurers.aspx?referrer=search.

[48] Nix, *op. cit.*

[49] Quoted in Tom Brown, "States Joined in Suit Against Healthcare Reform," Reuters, May 14, 2010, www.reuters.com.

[50] Quoted in Ricardo Alonso-Zaldivar, "U.S. Files First Defense of Health Care Law in Court," The Associated Press, May 12, 2010, http://news.yahoo.com/s/ap/20100512/ap_on_bi_ge/us_health_care_challenge.

[51] Quoted in Jonathan Chait, "Could Republicans Repeal Health Care Reform?" *The New Republic online*, March 19, 2010, www.tnr.com.

FOR MORE INFORMATION

Alliance for Health Reform, 1444 I St., N.W., Suite 910, Washington, DC 20005-6573; (202) 789-2300; www.allhealth.org. Nonpartisan group providing information on all facets of health coverage and access, including transcripts and videos of Capitol Hill briefings from experts with a wide spectrum of views on reform.

The Commonwealth Fund, One East 75th St., NY, NY 10021; (212) 606-3800; www.commonwealthfund.org. Private foundation that supports research on and advocates for universal access to affordable, high-quality health care.

The Heritage Foundation, 214 Massachusetts Ave., N.E., Washington, DC 20002-4999; (202) 546-4400; www.heritage.org. Public-policy think tank provides analysis of health reform and health care from a conservative viewpoint.

John Goodman's Health Policy Blog, National Center for Policy Analysis, 12770 Coit Rd., Suite 800, Dallas, TX 75251-1339; (972) 386-6272; www.john-goodman-blog.com. Conservative analyst who advocates for free-market policies provides daily commentary on health care and health reform.

Kaiser Health News, www.kaiserhealthnews.org. Foundation-funded, editorially independent nonprofit news group provides information on current events affecting health care.

National Conferences of State Legislatures, 444 North Capitol St., N.W., Suite 515, Washington, DC 20001; (202) 624-5400; www.ncsl.org. Nongovernmental group that tracks proposed state legislation related to health-care reform.

National Journal Expert Blogs: Health Care, http://healthcare.nationaljournal.com. Reporters from the political magazine and a wide variety of health-care experts and analysts provide commentary.

The White House Blog: Health Care, www.whitehouse.gov/blog/issues/Health-Care. Obama administration officials comment on implementation of the new law.

Bibliography

Selected Sources

Books

Grater, David, *The Cure: How Capitalism Can Save American Health Care*, Encounter Books, 2008.

A psychiatrist who has practiced in the United States and Canada makes the conservative case for reforming the health care system by ending government regulation and third-party payment through insurance and instead having consumers pay directly for care.

Hacker, Jacob S., ed., *Health at Risk: America's Ailing System — and How to Heal It*, Columbia University Press, 2008.

A Yale University professor of political science who was chief architect of the proposal — eventually abandoned by Congress — to include a public, government-run insurance plan to compete with private insurers, assembles essays by health-policy scholars on topics including the state of health-care quality.

Reid, T. R., *The Healing of America: A Global Quest for Better, Cheaper, and Fairer Health Care*, Penguin Press, 2009.

A former foreign affairs correspondent for *The Washington Post* reports his impressions of a round-the-world tour to explore health care systems.

Articles

Cohn, Jonathan, "How They Did It," *The New Republic*, June 10, 2010, www.tnr.com, p. 14.

In the early days of his administration, President Obama switched from opposition to support of an individual mandate to buy insurance.

Meyer, Harris, "Group Health's Move to the Medical Home: For Doctors, It's Often a Hard Journey," *Health Affairs*, May 2010, p. 844.

At a private health plan that's trying to reengineer medical practice to favor primary and preventive care, as the new health-reform law seeks to do nationally, many physicians balk at the change.

Milligan, Susan, "GOP Targets Nominee to Run Health Agency," *The Boston Globe*, May 13, 2010, www.boston.com, p. 1.

In a move that could hamper implementation of the health-reform law, congressional Republicans have been blocking President Obama's nomination of Donald Berwick, a Massachusetts pediatrician, to head the Centers for Medicare and Medicaid Services, on the grounds that Berwick believes that cost controls and pay-for-performance are required.

Ostrom, Carol M., "Health-care Law Will Alter High-Risk Pool, but Just How Hasn't Been Worked Out," *Seattle Times*, April 18, 2010, p. A1.

Under the new health-care reform law, states and the federal government starting this summer will set up temporary programs to help people with serious illnesses obtain affordable coverage. In 2014, private insurers will be required to enroll people regardless of health status. Currently, 35 states already have such programs, and enrollees in those programs worry that Congress' legislative language may lock them out of the federal plan even though they might get more affordable coverage there.

Reichard, John, "After the Win, No Time to Lose," *CQ Weekly*, April 5, 2010, p. 814.

Federal health agencies face unprecedented challenges in developing rules for the huge, multifaceted health-reform law and making its multiple, complex programs work.

Reports and Studies

Butler, Stuart M., "Evolving Beyond Traditional Employer-Sponsored Health Insurance," The Hamilton Project, Brookings Institution, May 2007, www.brookings.edu/papers/2007/05healthcare_butler.aspx.

A health-policy scholar from the conservative Heritage Foundation, a Washington think tank, explains the legal, regulatory and business changes he believes would be required to create a stable health-insurance system based on conservative principles, as the current employer-based system crumbles.

Cauchy, Richard, "State Legislation Challenging Certain Health Reforms, 2010," National Conference of State Legislatures, May 2010, www.ncsl.org.

States and the federal government share a complex set of responsibilities for regulating health insurance and health care in the United States, which has often set some states at odds with the federal government. As federal health-reform legislation slowly moved through Congress over the past year, at least 39 state legislatures have proposed bills to limit, change or oppose certain federal actions on health care.

Lazarus, Simon, "Mandatory Health Insurance: Is It Constitutional?" American Constitution Society, December 2009, www.acslaw.org/node/15654.

A lawyer for the National Senior Citizens Law Center argues that contested provisions in the recently passed health-reform law, including the individual requirement to buy health insurance, are constitutional, based on longtime legal precedent.

The Next Step:

Additional Articles from Current Periodicals

Costs

Cowles, Robert, "Transparency Helps Keep Health-Care Costs Down," *Green Bay Press-Gazette*, Jan. 7, 2010, p. A7.
Patients often do not know the costs of certain procedures before they are performed, which doesn't allow them to make informed consumer decisions, says a Wisconsin state senator.

Ferry, Michael, "How Much Will Health Care Cost Us?" *Mobile Register*, Jan. 3, 2010, p. A17.
Americans are shielded from the true costs of health care because of employer-sponsored insurance.

Guy, Sandra, "Savings You Can Believe In," *Chicago Sun Times*, June 5, 2010, p. B15.
The Obama administration's health-care reform plan is structured to find novel, efficient and cost-effective treatments with fewer side effects.

Samuelson, Robert J., "Get Real on Health Costs," *Newsweek*, Dec. 21, 2009, p. 36.
The Obama administration says it can curb excessive health spending by tackling the waste in today's health-care system.

Medicaid

Herszenhorn, David M., "Spreading the Golden Corn," *The New York Times*, Jan. 8, 2010, p. A15.
Sen. Ben Nelson, D-Neb., is demanding that the federal government pay for a proposed Medicaid expansion in his state.

MacGillis, Alec, "Medicaid Growth Won't Cost States Much," *The Washington Post*, May 27, 2010, p. A25.
The federal government will bear virtually the entire cost of expanding Medicaid under the new health care law, according to the Kaiser Family Foundation.

Richert, Catharine, "Health Care Reform Bill Will Expand Medicaid, Increasing Demands on Doctors," *St. Petersburg Times*, March 1, 2010.
Medicaid expansion has proven controversial among state officials, who say local budgets are too tight to handle additional enrollees.

The States

Bisbee, Julie, "State GOP May Go to Court to Fight Health Care Measure," *The Oklahoman*, March 23, 2010, p. 3A.
Oklahoma Republicans have promised to fight the recent national health care reform bill in court.

Craig, Jon, "Legislation Would Bar Tax-Funded Abortion Coverage in Ohio," *Cincinnati Enquirer*, May 18, 2010.
Three Cincinnati-area lawmakers have introduced state legislation that would prohibit health insurance coverage for abortions if subsidized with tax money.

Rogers, Christina, "State Braces for Health Changes," *Detroit News*, March 27, 2010, p. B7.
Michigan insurers and health providers are readying themselves for an onslaught of changes amid the passage of federal health reform.

Sluss, Michael, "Cuccinelli to Sue Over Federal Health Care Bill," *Roanoke Times*, March 22, 2010.
Virginia's attorney general says Obama's health reform legislation is an unconstitutional overreach against his state's rights.

The Uninsured

Freyer, Felice J., "Number of Uninsured in R.I. Soars to Record 140,000," *Providence Journal-Bulletin*, March 16, 2010, p. 1.
The number of people in Rhode Island without health insurance has reached its highest level ever — 16 percent of the population — largely due to a soaring jobless rate.

Halladay, Doug, "It's Life or Death for State's Uninsured," *Detroit Free Press*, March 18, 2010, p. A20.
Access remains a challenge for the newly uninsured, especially those from smaller communities that lack community health centers and adequate facilities.

Templeton, David, "Middle Class Struggling With Health Care Costs, Report Finds," *Pittsburgh Post-Gazette*, March 18, 2010, p. A8.
More and more uninsured Americans are from the middle class, not just from poverty.

CITING *CQ RESEARCHER*

Sample formats for citing these reports in a bibliography include the ones listed below. Preferred styles and formats vary, so please check with your instructor or professor.

MLA STYLE

Jost, Kenneth. "Rethinking the Death Penalty." CQ Researcher 16 Nov. 2001: 945-68.

APA STYLE

Jost, K. (2001, November 16). Rethinking the death penalty. *CQ Researcher, 11*, 945-968.

CHICAGO STYLE

Jost, Kenneth. "Rethinking the Death Penalty." *CQ Researcher*, November 16, 2001, 945-968.

CHAPTER

2

Medication Abuse

By Marcia Clemmitt

Excerpted from the CQ Researcher. Marcia Clemmitt. (October 9, 2009). "Medication Abuse." *CQ Researcher*, 837-860.

Medication Abuse

BY MARCIA CLEMMITT

THE ISSUES

Michael Jackson's sudden death in June from an overdose of prescription sedatives and other drugs focused worldwide attention on prescription-drug abuse. Ultimately, manslaughter charges may be filed against the physician who injected the legendary entertainer with propofol, a hospital anesthetic given to Jackson as a sleep aid. [1]

Jackson's tragic story, while lurid, is far from unique. Prescription-drug abuse has become an increasingly large part of America's drug-abuse problem in recent decades, even as use of illegal narcotics has dropped. The most recent wave of increases began in the early 1990s, and abuse rates currently mirror the high levels reached in the early-to-mid 2000s.

Furthermore, with the introduction over the past few decades of new opiate painkillers chemically related to heroin, prescription-drug abuse may be more dangerous today than in the past.

Deaths from unintentional drug overdoses have increased steadily since the early 1970s, and "over the past 10 years they have reached historic highs," led by prescription opioids, * Leonard J. Paulozzi, a medical epidemiologist at the federal Centers for Disease Control and Prevention (CDC), told a Senate subcommittee last year. Rates of death from drug overdoses "are currently four to five times higher than . . . during the 'black tar' heroin epidemic in the mid-1970s and more than twice what they were during the peak years of crack cocaine in the early 1990s," said Paulozzi. "For the first time, more people in the 45-54 age group now die of drug overdoses than from traffic crashes." [2]

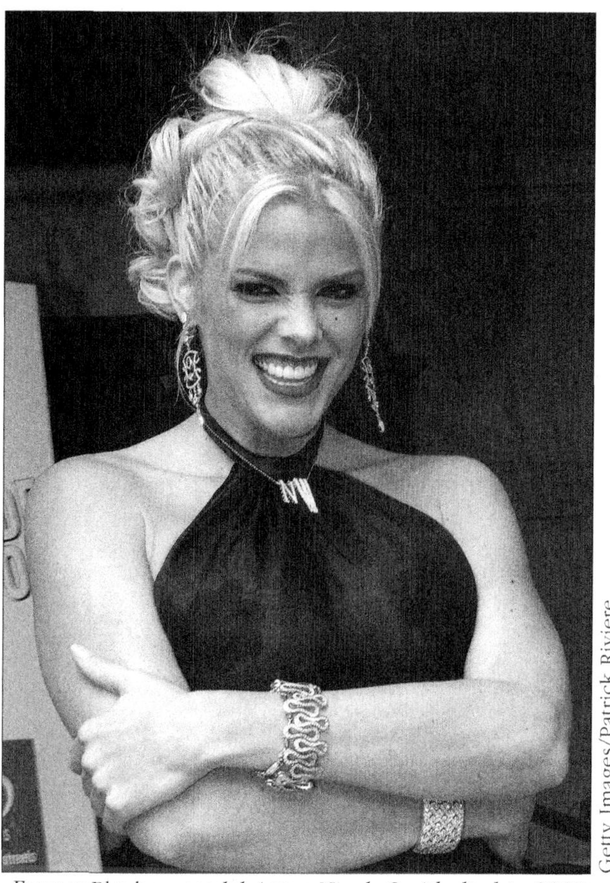

Getty Images/Patrick Riviere

Former Playboy *model Anna Nicole Smith died in 2007 from a lethal combination of drugs prescribed by her physicians. Deaths from unintentional drug overdoses have increased steadily since the early 1970s, with medications outpacing illegal drugs like heroin and cocaine as the cause. Often easier to obtain than illegal drugs, prescription drugs have become a powerful gateway to addiction and other drug-abuse problems.*

Celebrity entertainers have been prominent among the victims. In late September, the New York City medical examiner announced that the August death of 36-year-old club disc jockey and musician DJ AM — Adam Goldstein — resulted from an accidental overdose of cocaine and a large number of different prescription drugs, including anti-anxiety drugs that he reportedly was taking after surviving a plane crash in 2008. [3]

In February 2007, the death of Anna Nicole Smith dominated the gossip media for months after the model and sex symbol died from a lethal combination of drugs prescribed by her physicians. Last month, court documents revealed that at least one pharmacist refused to sell prescribed drugs to Smith, telling her doctor that the prescriptions amounted to "pharmaceutical suicide." [4]

"The stars — the problem is they have money," says Doug Thorburn, the author of *Drunks, Drugs & Debits: How to Recognize Addicts and Avoid Financial Abuse*. "Those who depend on a star for their livelihood have position, power and money at stake" if they refuse to give celebrities drugs or urge them to go into rehab. Michael Jackson's nanny "tried to do the right thing and lost her job several times because she said, 'Go to rehab,' " he adds.

Celebrity prescription-drug abuse might be expected to alert the public and the medical profession to the dangers of prescription-drug misuse, but it hasn't really had that effect, analysts say.

"We have a tendency to minimize" substance-abuse problems, says Kitty Harris-Wilkes, director of the Center for the Study of Addiction and Recovery at Texas Tech University in Lubbock. "If people really knew how much prescription-drug abuse happens, they'd freak out. There's a lot more going on than statistics show."

With many people finding prescription medications easier to procure

* Opioids are chemical compounds that have narcotic properties similar to opium-based drugs like heroin.

Monitoring Programs Target Abuse

Thirty-four states require the posting of patient prescription information online through prescription-drug monitoring programs (PDMPs), to allow investigators to obtain pharmacy data from multiple locations at once. Ten states and the District of Columbia have no legislation or programs.

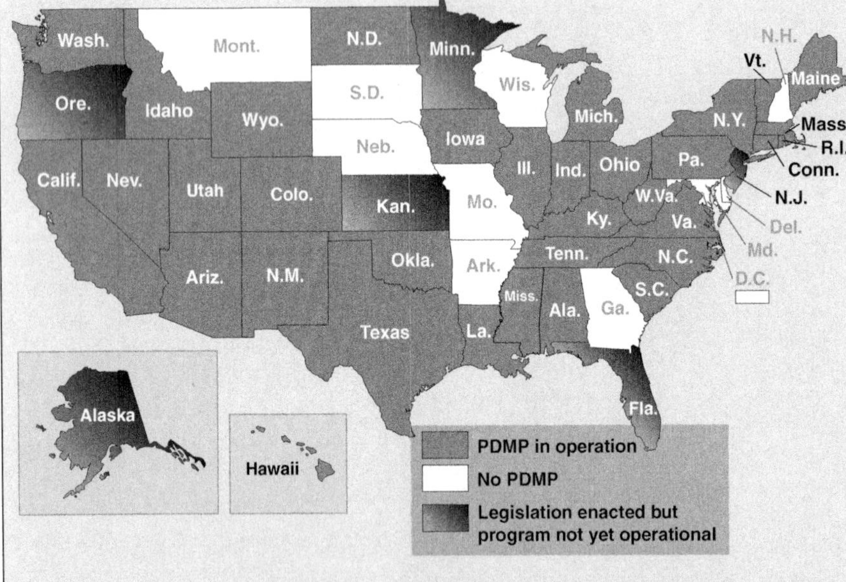

Source: "Status of State Prescription Drug Monitoring Programs (PDMPs)," National Alliance for Model State Drug Laws, July 2009

than illegal drugs, prescription drugs have become a powerful gateway to addiction and other drug-abuse problems, says Harris-Wilkes. "Drug availability often drives use. It's 'What am I willing to risk to buy dope off the street?' versus 'What am I willing to risk looking into somebody's medicine cabinet and nicking some Vicodin or other pills when I visit their house?' "

Nevertheless, since pharmaceutical companies, pharmacies and physicians are all regulated by the government, "you have many more places to intervene" to head off abuse of legal drugs compared to illegal ones, says Thomas R. Kosten, a professor of psychiatry and neuroscience at Baylor College of Medicine in Houston. For example, pharmaceutical companies can find ways to make potentially addictive products more tamper-resistant or less abusable by means such as "putting an opiate blocker into the drug," a tactic that's proven to "stop abuse very quickly."

Efforts are also under way to combat prescription abuse. For example, "Washington state and a number of others use information about the drug use of their Medicaid populations to identify high-volume users," sometimes " 'locking in' such users to a single physician and a single pharmacy to reduce the likelihood of 'doctor shopping' " to get multiple prescriptions, said Paulozzi. [5]

As of summer 2009, at least 40 state legislatures had authorized some kind of prescription-monitoring program, according to the National Alliance for Model State Drug Laws. (*See map, above.*) [6] Nevertheless, many analysts say current initiatives fall short.

"Doctors and nurses just turn off information" about the dangers of prescription-drug abuse, charges Bryan Liang, a professor of law at the California Western School of Law in San Diego. For example, when patients overdose, "doctors just treat them, give them the antidote for the acute problem" and "think they've done their job."

Not surprisingly, drug manufacturers haven't been proactive about developing drugs that are less easily abusable, says Marvin P. Seppala, chief medical officer of the Hazelden Foundation, an addiction treatment facility in Center City, Minn. "If I'm a pharmaceutical manufacturer, making remarkable sales partly because people are misusing the drugs, I don't have much motivation to change that."

Some patients and physicians argue that campaigns to limit prescription-drug abuse have severely hampered medical pain treatment.

The Drug Enforcement Administration (DEA) and the Justice Department consistently overreach on prescription-narcotics control, John P. Flannery, a federal drug prosecutor turned private-practice attorney, told a House subcommittee in 2007. The Supreme Court declared in 1975 that a "physician had to act 'outside the course of professional medical practice' and with the 'intent' to act as a drug pusher" to warrant prosecution under the Controlled Substances Act, he said. But "the Justice Department recently has been allowing these prosecutions to modify and restrict pain medicine in this nation to a dangerous degree." [7]

But while "there's been a lot of talk over the years about fear of DEA damaging pain prescriptions, only 40 percent of doctors say it's a problem, so it's not as big an issue as people think," says Susan Foster, director of policy research and analysis for the National Center on Addiction and Substance Abuse (CASA) at Columbia University in New York City.

As public health workers, addiction specialists and law-enforcement agencies seek ways to combat prescription-drug abuse, here are some of the questions being asked:

Is prescription-drug abuse as serious as illegal drug abuse?

The use of legitimate prescription drugs like opioid painkillers and stimulants to treat attention deficit hyperactivity disorder (ADHD) has soared in the United States over the past two decades. But along with increased legitimate use of opioids like Vicodin and OxyContin and stimulants like Ritalin and Adderall has come extensive abuse.

In recent years, prescription drugs have outpaced illegal drugs like heroin and cocaine as the cause of overdose deaths, according to both federal statistics and data from many states. "The number of deaths . . . that involved prescription opioid analgesics increased from 2,900 in 1999 to at least 7,500 in 2004," up "150 percent in just five years," with painkiller deaths more numerous than heroin- and cocaine-related deaths put together, said the CDC's Paulozzi. [8]

While the CDC has not analyzed data beyond 2004, the trend is likely to continue, said Paulozzi. The Substance Abuse and Mental Health Services Administration (SAMHSA), has found that "the number of emergency department visits for opioid overdoses increased steadily through 2007," so that "the mortality statistics through 2005 probably underestimate the present magnitude of the problem." [9]

Considering the high rate at which Americans consume prescription drugs, there should be little surprise in such numbers, some analysts say.

Indeed, frequently abused Vicodin is the most-prescribed drug in the United States, with 117 million prescriptions written in 2008, says David S. Kloth, a Danbury, Conn., anesthesiologist and past president of the American Society of Interventional Pain Physicians (ASIPP). By comparison, another heavily used drug, the cholesterol-lowering medicine Lipitor, was prescribed 61 million times last year, Kloth says.

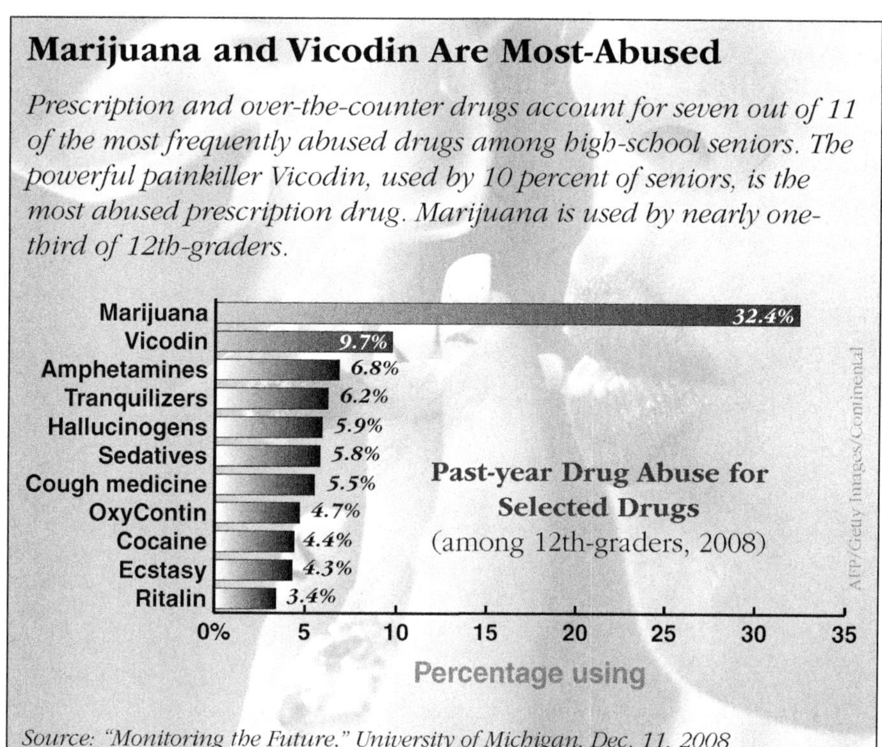

Ninety-nine percent of the world's hydrocodone — Vicodin's opioid component — and 80 percent of the world's supply of narcotics, generally, are consumed in the United States, he says. "The actual, indirect societal costs [of prescription-drug abuse] are so huge that the problem can no longer be ignored," says Kloth. "We have doctors assisting patients in abuse."

There also has been a dramatic increase in deaths from methadone — in the wafer form prescribed as a pain medication, not the liquid form used as maintenance for former heroin addicts, says Hazelden's Seppala. "The pill is a lethal drug because it's so slow going out of one's system," he says. But unwary people "take a whole bunch because it acts so slowly that they don't realize they're getting high," and they end up dying from the drug's toxicity, he explains.

Today there is more abuse of prescription opiates than marijuana, says Kosten of Baylor College of Medicine. "The average first-time user is 15 years old," and, unlike with most drug epidemics, females are as likely as males to abuse prescription medications. With illegal drugs, "boys are more likely to go out to find a dealer and get them," but boys and girls can get prescription opiates on their own, for free, from their families' medicine chests, he says.

"Illicit drugs come and go," but abuse of prescription drugs is likely to keep on expanding because of their availability, says Western Law School's Liang. "It's a growth industry for our kids, and addicted children become addicted adults."

Among his students, "it's a normal thing to buy on the Internet," Liang says. "This is the health-care system for kids today. And when you hear the justifications of college students — like, 'I'm using [Adderall] because I'm trying to get into med school,' followed by the admission that 'I couldn't really cope with the test because I was so buzzed from the drug' — you understand how serious substance-abuse-related problems can quickly grow," he says.

Furthermore, "there's a real synergy between opioids diverted to illegal use and heroin, since many people get hooked on the diverted opioids" and then shift to illegal drugs or add them to the mix, says Robert G. Carlson, director of the Center for Interventions, Treatment and Addictions Research at Wright State University's Boonshoft School of Medicine in Dayton, Ohio. Abuse of prescription drugs also likely brings sellers of illegal drugs like heroin into areas where illegal-drug pushers haven't previously operated. "Sellers follow the drugs," Carlson says.

Nevertheless, some observers say that facts on the ground may not warrant the alarms some substance-abuse specialists are sounding. "I haven't seen any communication from anyone indicating we're near a crisis mode or things have gotten a lot worse . . . in the recent past," said Ron Petrin, vice president of the Board of Pharmacy in New Hampshire, a state in which some analyses find a surging epidemic of prescription-drug addiction. [10]

Just as with illegal drugs, the number of people who initially abuse prescription drugs is far higher than those who actually become dependent, says Kosten. For both kinds of drugs, "eight people try opiates and one becomes dependent," he says. For that reason, "it's a good bet that a substantial proportion [of prescription-drug abusers] will outgrow" the habit. Nevertheless, Kosten adds, "a lot of damage can happen in the meantime," including education setbacks, such as poor grades, that take years to overcome, he says.

Abuse of prescription "opioids hit a peak in 2006, and it's still staying there, not really on the rise, but not dropping either," says Michael H. Lowenstein, co-director of the Waismann Institute, a detoxification center in Beverly Hills, Calif.

Still, an alarming story making the media rounds may be more legend than fact, says Hazelden's Seppala. Beginning in the early 2000s, some news reports described "pharm parties," in which teenagers scrounge up all the prescription drugs they can find, get together, toss all the drugs into a bowl, and grab and consume random handfuls of the medications. The story reached the mainstream with a *USA Today* account on June 13, 2006. [11] But while some "pharm parties" probably do occur, "I don't think it's a common phenomenon," says Seppala, who has researched them.

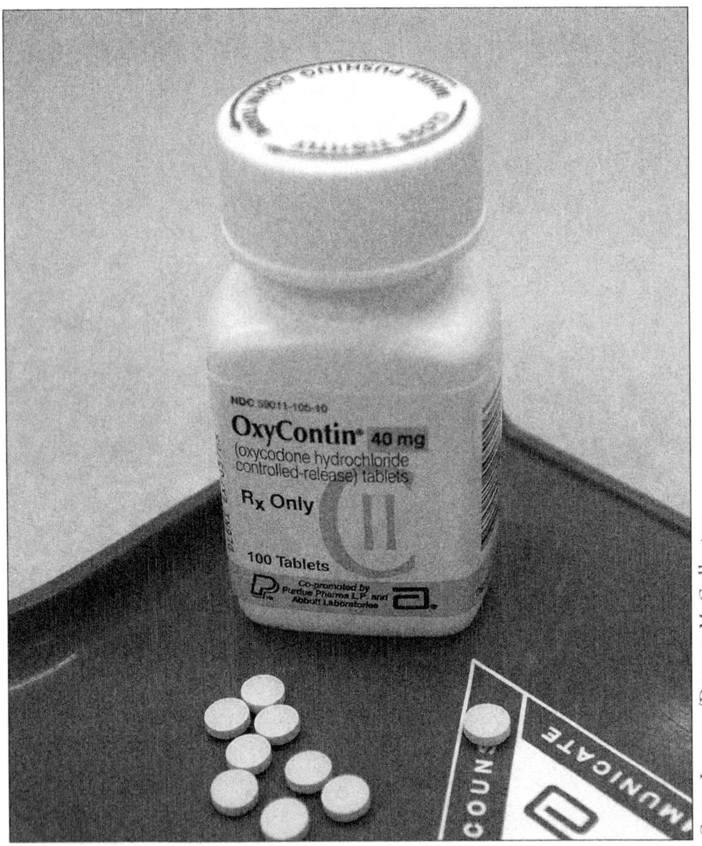

Getty Images/Darren McCollester

The increased legitimate use of powerful painkillers like OxyContin has been accompanied by extensive abuse. Heavy and somewhat deceptive marketing of OxyContin in the 1990s, when the drug was sold in a highly abusable form, has led to a backlash against it by some physicians and even some addicts. Nonetheless, OxyContin and the popular painkiller Vicodin remain at or near the peak levels of abuse they hit in the mid-2000s.

Similarly, while prescription sleeping pills are addictive, "the vast, vast majority of people never have a problem with them," says Leslie Lundt, a psychiatrist in Boise, Idaho, who is the author of *Think Like a Psychiatrist: Understanding Psychiatric Medicines*. "Nearly 100 percent of the people who have issues with the 'sleepers' have had another substance-abuse or gambling issue."

Some aspects of prescription drugs may ultimately make them easier for society to control than illegal drugs. As compared to alcoholics and heroin addicts, for example, "We see opioid pill addicts a lot earlier" in their substance-abusing lives, says Seppala. For all opioids, including heroin, "the addiction starts more quickly" than with most other substances, but pill addicts often find it harder to get a daily supply of their drug than street-drug addicts, and so fall into the pain of withdrawal sooner, which brings them to treatment, he says.

Unlike with illegal drugs, if abuse becomes a problem with a legal medication, "we can just make less of it, or make it a lot harder to get" by limiting the places at which the drug can be dispensed, requiring buyers to fill out certain forms, or the like, says Kosten.

Is enough being done to combat medication abuse?

Government and private efforts are under way to head off prescription-drug abuse and shut down enterprises — such as Internet pharmacies — that facilitate abuse, but some analysts say the problem dwarfs the programs that combat it.

The National Institute on Drug Abuse launched a prescription-drug-abuse program in 2001 and continuously monitors trends, said NIDA Director Nora Volkow. NIDA is "helping to develop a protocol doctors and others can use to screen patients for prescription abuse and conduct brief but effective interventions," she said. [12]

The institute also is developing new pain-treatment methods to sidestep addiction potential. For example, Volkow said, "compounds are being developed that act on a combination of two distinct opioid receptors," potentially giving them the ability "to induce strong analgesia without producing tolerance or dependence." [13]

The Food and Drug Administration is addressing the issue, too. For example, the FDA now orders pharmaceutical manufacturers to conduct post-marketing surveillance of drugs, including collecting data to answer the question, "Is our drug being abused?" says Baylor College's Kosten.

For its part, the federal Drug Enforcement Administration is making prescription-drug abuse a top priority, says Western Law School's Liang. "The DEA is going crazy over this," he says.

"Drug companies have become more responsible" about trying to quell abuse, says detox physician Lowenstein. For example, Vicodin maker Abbott Laboratories, in Abbott Park, Ill., is working with the Partnership for a Drug-Free America to develop an online educational program, "Not in My House," aimed at helping parents discourage prescription-drug abuse by teenagers.

Some Internet- and pharmacy-oversight groups say they've made significant efforts to control illicit prescriptions. The Go Daddy Group — a coalition of companies that host Web sites and register Internet domain names —"routinely investigates sites involving online drug sales" and works with law enforcement "in their attempts to remove such Web sites from our network," General Counsel Christine N. Jones told a House subcommittee last year. [14]

But many analysts say the response has not been up to the problem. "We in the U.S. are just naïve" about the seriousness of prescription-drug abuse, although "the rest of the world recognizes it," says Liang. The International Council of Nurses, for example, which represents some 12 million nurses worldwide, sponsored a "Counterfeits Kill" campaign to warn against the dangers of medication abuse. "The only country where they didn't get the nurses involved in this was the United States," Liang says.

After over a decade of rising abuse, "the states still aren't spending any money on prevention," says Liang. At the federal level, the CDC "is not really on it" either, he says.

Good information and education campaigns make a difference, as evidenced by the success of the Partnership for a Drug-Free America's anti-inhalant campaign, says Lloyd D. Johnston, a distinguished senior research scientist at the University of Michigan. Currently, though, the federal government is doing too little, says Johnston, who is the principal investigator for the ongoing Monitoring the Future study of teenagers' substance abuse. The Bush administration focused its anti-drug efforts on marijuana, "a very

Narcotic Pain Relievers Are Widely Abused

More than 5 million Americans were addicted to narcotic pain relievers in 2007, an increase of 800,000 from just three years earlier (top graph). By comparison, the number of heroin and methamphetamine users was well under 1 million (bottom).

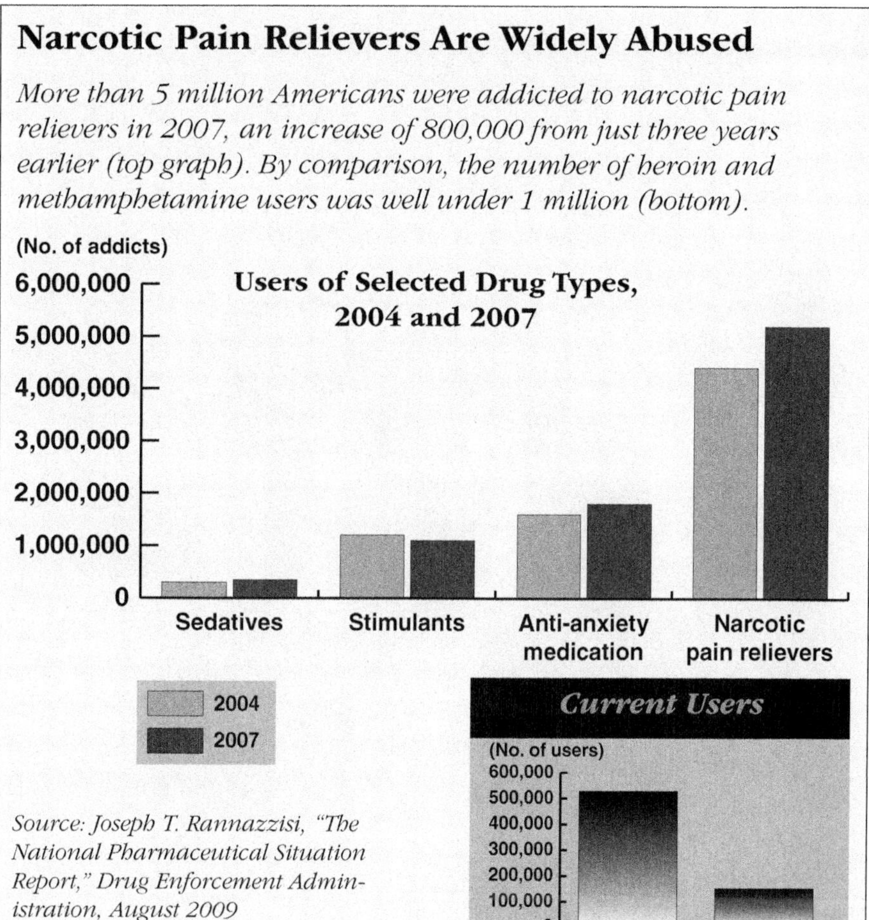

Source: Joseph T. Rannazzisi, "The National Pharmaceutical Situation Report," Drug Enforcement Administration, August 2009

Online Drug Sites Declined

The number of Internet sites that illegally sell or advertise prescription drugs decreased in 2008 to its second-lowest level in five years. The decline reflects efforts by law enforcement agencies, Internet service providers, package delivery services and credit card companies to stop illegal activities by "rogue" pharmacy operators.

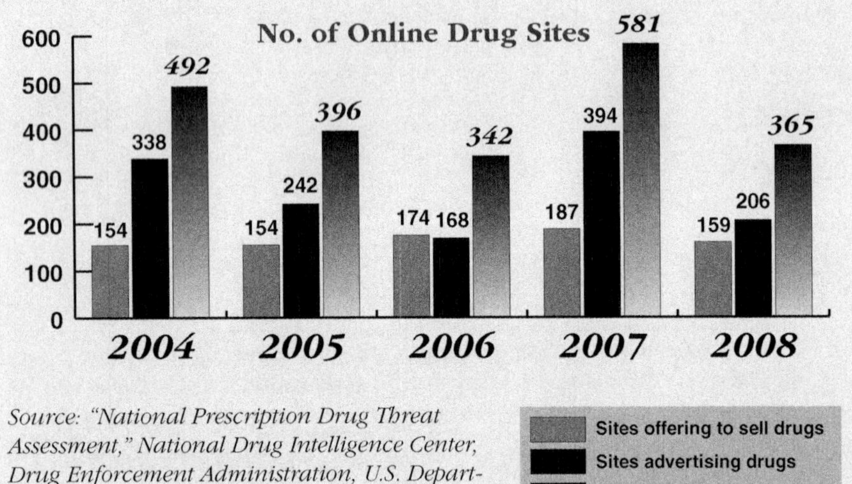

Source: "National Prescription Drug Threat Assessment," National Drug Intelligence Center, Drug Enforcement Administration, U.S. Department of Justice, April 2009

hard target," and the campaign showed "no effect or may even have caused a rebound" in use, Johnston explains. "Congress got mad about" the poor targeting and bad results and cut funding for federal anti-drug programs across the board, he says. "They threw the baby out with the bathwater."

When it comes to Internet pharmacies that operate illegally, the number and clout of other businesses — such as search engines — that profit from the stores' existence greatly limits the extent to which companies help rein them in, some analysts report. Microsoft's Bing.com search engine, for example, "enables 'rogue' Internet pharmacies that violate U.S. federal and state laws as well as Microsoft's stated policies," according to the Internet pharmacy-verification group LegitScript and the Internet-compliance company KnujOn. [15]

Search engines like Bing can't really control which Web pages show up in actual search results, but they earn ad revenue from the "sponsored links" — paid ads — that are generally posted on the right side of a search page. Since these are paid ads, Microsoft "has the ability to require that they meet certain criteria" and should decline ad dollars from companies that break laws, say the groups. However, "of the prescription drug and online pharmacy advertisements . . . that we reviewed, 89.7 percent led to 'rogue' Internet pharmacies that do not require a [written] prescription for prescription drugs, or are otherwise acting unlawfully or fraudulently," such as by selling counterfeit drugs manufactured outside the U.S. or Canada, LegitScript and KnujOn say. [16]

"About 40 percent of doctors have had some training on substance abuse and about 19 percent on diversion" of legal drugs to illicit purposes, says anesthesiologist Kloth. "But the real truth is that this amounts to one lecture in medical school, with most doctors having virtually no training" in these areas. Government agencies should work with professional groups to institute physician-certification programs for doctors authorized to prescribe abusable drugs, he says.

When it comes to blame for allowing prescription-drug abuse to worsen, "there's enormous responsibility to go around," says Foster, at the National Center on Addiction and Substance Abuse. For example, drug companies have known that they were producing addictive drugs in easy-to-abuse forms but produced and promoted the drugs anyway, such as when Purdue Pharma did "really extreme marketing of OxyContin," which was packaged in a very easy-to-abuse form in the early 2000s.

Are patients in pain suffering because doctors fear prosecution for medication abuse?

Pain drugs are the most likely to result in addiction when they are taken to get high rather than to ease pain — and some pain patients argue that anti-abuse efforts have gravely hampered pain treatments.

In the 19th century, narcotics like opium and the morphine-containing medicine laudanum, legally prescribed to treat pain and other medical conditions, got far out of hand in the United States, creating many addicts. By the 1940s the government had restricted legal use of opioids to medicines "prescribed by physicians according to strict regulatory controls," wrote Jane C. Ballantyne, professor of anesthesiology and critical care at the Hospital of the University of Pennsylvania, and Jianren Mao, director of the Massachusetts General Hospital Center for Translational Pain Research. "The immediate result of such strict regulatory control was that physicians became reluctant to prescribe opioids," fearing the loss of medical licenses and criminal prosecutions, and "as a result pain was woefully undertreated," Ballantyne and Mao explain. [17]

Similarly, the backlash against the painkiller OxyContin in the early 2000s "has caused physicians to treat pain less aggressively in many cases, to the detriment of their seriously ill patients," said John Shuster, a psychiatrist and palliative care specialist in Alabama. "The emphasis on managing pain is fairly new [in medicine], and I fear many patients will suffer needlessly as physicians rethink using any powerful painkillers in the wake of the adverse publicity" surrounding OxyContin. [18]

In 2002 alone, the DEA prosecuted 410 physicians "for recklessly prescribing opioids — an 800 percent increase in . . . prosecutions from 1999," wrote Steven P. Cohen, director of medical education in the pain management division at Johns Hopkins School of Medicine in Baltimore, and Srinivasa N. Raja, director of the division of pain medicine in the Department of Anesthesiology and Critical Care Medicine. [19]

Undertreatment of pain "is still a serious problem," said Brietta Clark, a professor of law at Loyola Law School in Los Angeles. Despite new state laws and professional guidelines stating that doctors must make pain treatment a priority and promising immunity from punishment if they follow treatment guidelines, "physicians report a continuing fear of scrutiny if they prescribe certain kinds of medications," said Clark. [20]

That's largely because doctors believe, correctly, that "liability for undertreatment" of pain is "difficult to prove, in part because there is no objective, verifiable measure of pain," Clark explained. Meanwhile, "physician over-prescribing remains easier to identify and punish."

Insurance plans also are adopting "fail first" medication policies, said Clark. "Plans make patients try cheaper, weaker pain medications to prove they do not work, before they will pay for stronger medication prescribed by the physician. They justify this ostensibly on safety and cost grounds," but pain treatment suffers as a result, she argued. [21]

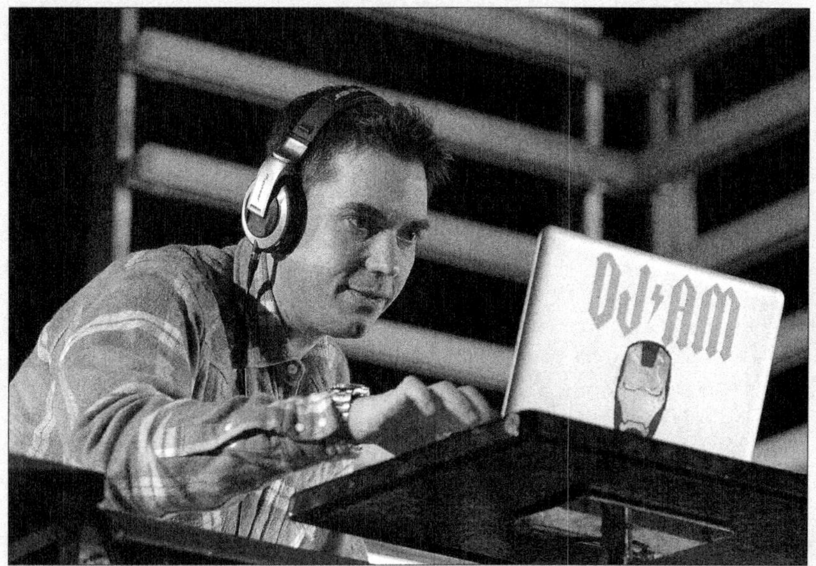

Getty Images/Noel Vasquez

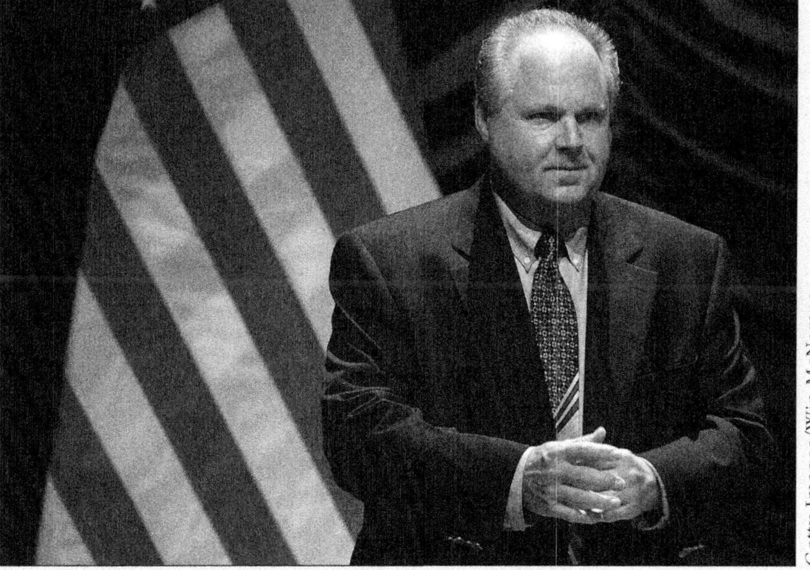

Getty Images/Win McNamee

Victims of Addiction

The death in August of 36-year-old New York City club disc jockey DJ AM — Adam Goldstein (top) — resulted from an accidental overdose of cocaine and a number of prescription drugs. Conservative radio host Rush Limbaugh (bottom) has admitted he became addicted to painkillers when suffering from back pain. In 2006 he pleaded "not guilty" to "doctor shopping" to obtain prescriptions and agreed to undergo random drug testing.

Siobhan Reynolds, founder of the advocacy group Pain Relief Network, said that "all the available evidence shows us that we are . . . living in an ongoing and worsening medical crisis as concerns the undertreatment of pain." The DEA made an agreement in the 1990s with the FDA and medical professional societies clearing the way for aggressive pain treatment and giving doctors and DEA agents clear, consistent guidelines on what was and was not allowable, Reynolds said. [22]

Since then, however DEA has "reneged on this agreement," Reynolds charged. As a result, "general searches of private patient records began to take place all over the country, physician's assets were seized prior to trial and physician after physician went down on drug trafficking convictions." In the end, Reynolds said, only a few tiny pain clinics were left around the country, while doctors were left in fear and patients in pain. [23]

But some pain experts note that advocacy by pain patients and physicians over the past two decades has convinced state governments and medical-oversight organizations, such as the Joint Commission on the Accreditation of Healthcare Organizations, to urge physicians to treat pain aggressively.

"The alleged undertreatment of pain as a major health problem in the United States has led to development of initiatives to address the multiple alleged barriers responsible," said Laxmaiah Manchikanti, founder and CEO of the American Society of Interventional Pain Physicians and an associate clinical professor of anesthesiology and perioperative medicine at the University of Louisville. [24]

"Patient advocacy groups and professional organizations have been formed with a focus on improving the management of pain, and numerous clinical guidelines also have been developed," although none have been "developed using evidence-based medicine," Manchikanti said. In addition, "over one-third of the state legislatures have instituted intractable-pain treatment acts that provide immunity from discipline" for doctors who follow the rules when prescribing opioids. [25]

In 1999, the U.S. Veteran's Health Administration announced that it would begin considering pain as a "fifth vital sign" — alongside temperature, pulse, respiratory rate and blood pressure — to encourage aggressive treatment. In 2000, the health care accrediting commission followed suit, says the Hazelden Foundation's Seppala.

Meanwhile, some analysts suggest that the best way out of the pain/addiction dilemma lies in a different direction: backing off the heavy reliance on opioids, which are proving to have some unsuspected downsides, while broadening the medical tools used to combat pain.

"Chronic non-cancer pain is undertreated in the United States for a variety of reasons," but fear of prosecution for overprescription isn't the key one, says Michael Ashburn, a professor of anesthesiology and director of the pain medicine and palliative care center at the University of Pennsylvania in Philadelphia. "Doctors are not well trained to diagnose and treat" pain, and pain specialists are scarce. In addition, interdisciplinary pain management teams were becoming the norm a few decades ago, but "few exist any more" because insurers were skeptical about their worth and stopped paying for them.

"I would argue that the most common error in pain treatment is the overreliance on a single drug class" — opioids — which can too easily slip into overuse and abuse, says Ashburn. In fact, "the scientific literature supporting opioids for non-cancer pain" is "pretty minimal," he says.

Furthermore, addiction doctors are now learning that, after a certain time, opiate painkillers may actually increase patients' sensitivity to pain, says Seppala. A young veterinarian he treated developed addiction to opioids after back surgery and, while her life had not yet spiraled out of control — as many addicts' lives do — she entered substance-abuse treatment because her drug habit had left her with no energy to work or live her life, says Seppala. "She was at unbelievably high doses of opioids, but after we got her off she was able to return to work basically pain free — a dramatic case but one that we're now finding is not that unusual," he says. "In at least some folks, these medications backfire, and they become more sensitive to pain." ■

BACKGROUND

Historic Highs

In the late 19th century, the average narcotics addict was a middle-class white woman addicted to medicinal drugs like morphine and laudanum, widely prescribed for depression, menopausal symptoms, menstrual cramps and other ills. [26]

An 1885 Iowa survey reported that repeat opiate users in the state were 63.8 percent female, and that opium addicts generally were middle-aged and middle-class, with the average user 46.5 years old and better educated than the average citizen. "The merchant, lawyer and physician are to be found among the host who sacrifice the choicest treasures of life at the shrine of Opium," said *Catholic World* magazine in 1881. [27]

Opiate medications — narcotic drugs extracted from seed capsules of the opium poppy or made from synthetic opium — may have provided a path to addiction for many who might not otherwise have encountered addictive drugs. "The extent to which alcohol-drinking by women was frowned upon may . . . have contributed to the excess of women among opiate users," observed a history of American drug use published by *Consumer Reports*. "Husbands drank alcohol in the saloon; wives took opium at home." [28]

Medications containing opiates were sold legally, at low, affordable prices, by groceries and general stores as

Continued on p. 849

Chronology

1800s-1909

Addiction to opium and cocaine-based medications swells across social classes.

1840
Less than one American in 1,000 is addicted to drugs.

1887
Oregon bans selling cocaine without a prescription.

1890
Five Americans in 1,000 are addicts.

1909
First International Opium Conference is held in Shanghai, China, amid growing worldwide concern.

1910s-1980s

Illegal drug use overtakes prescription-drug abuse as a cause of addiction.

1914
Congress passes Harrison Narcotics Tax Act, requiring all prescribers, sellers and handlers of opium and cocaine-based drugs to register and pay a tax.

1919
Supreme Court bans physicians from prescribing narcotics as "maintenance" drugs to help addicts avoid withdrawal pain.

1937
Prescription amphetamines in tablet form are sold to treat narcolepsy and attention problems.

1960
Doctors begin prescribing stimulant Ritalin for attention deficit disorder.

1970
Congress passes Controlled Substances Act, categorizing all drugs deemed dangerous and addictive into five "schedules" subject to various levels of regulation.

1990s

Substance abuse begins rising after a long decline. By decade's end, "no-prescription" Web sites selling controlled substances emerge.

1995
Prescription of stimulants like Ritalin soar, with 2 million American children taking the drug for attention deficit hyperactivity disorder (ADHD).

1996
Use of OxyContin, a time-release form of the opiate painkiller oxycodone that is easily abused, spreads among substance abusers, especially in rural areas.

1999
Veterans' Affairs health facilities begin monitoring patients for excessive pain following reports physicians aren't treating pain aggressively for fear of prosecution.

2000s

More overdose deaths involve prescription drugs than illegal drugs. Anti-drug programs focus on prescription abuse.

2001
National Institute on Drug Abuse launches research program on prescription drugs.

2003
Conservative radio host Rush Limbaugh admits he became addicted to painkillers when suffering from back pain and enters treatment.

2005
Congress passes National All Schedules Prescription Reporting Act (NASPER) to establish or improve prescription monitoring programs in all states but doesn't fund the effort until 2009.

2006
Limbaugh pleads "not guilty" to "doctor shopping" to obtain painkiller prescriptions and agrees to undergo random drug testing. . . . Up to 20 percent of college students may use ADHD stimulant drugs to get high or to stay awake while studying.

2007
Model and sex symbol Anna Nicole Smith, 39, dies of an overdose of multiple prescription drugs she obtained from her personal physicians.

2008
Australian actor Heath Ledger, 28, dies in New York after accidentally overdosing on prescription drugs, including sleeping pills. . . . Congress passes Ryan Haight Act, requiring online pharmacies to comply with state prescribing rules and post contact information online.

2009
Pop singer Michael Jackson, 50, dies from prescription-drug overdose. Officials label his death a homicide and begin investigating his personal physician. . . . Ryan Haight Act goes into effect. . . . Musician and disc jockey DJ AM (Adam Goldstein) dies of an overdose of multiple prescription drugs. . . . Washington state suspends its prescription-monitoring program due to budget cuts. . . . Court papers reveal a pharmacist refused to fill prescriptions for model Smith, dubbing it "pharmaceutical suicide."

Fickle Finger of Fate Can Make Painkillers Addictive

Biological factors cause some people to get "high."

Painkillers, when used responsibly, usually don't make the user "high" or lead to substance abuse. "People who take opiates because they're getting their teeth pulled generally don't" develop substance-abuse problems, says Thomas R. Kosten, a professor of psychiatry and neuroscience at Baylor College of Medicine in Houston. For most people, "if you're in significant pain, the drug takes the pain away," and "you feel a little sedated, a little nauseous."

"I've taken two Vicodin in my life, for dental procedures, and it just made me feel bad. I got nauseated," says Michael H. Lowenstein, co-director of the Waismann Institute, a detoxification center in Beverly Hills, Calif.

But about one-in-eight people "get high" from prescription painkillers, which can lead to drug abuse and addiction. Many prescription-drug abusers "start with a legitimate medical complaint," says Marvin P. Seppala, chief medical officer of the Hazelden Foundation, an addiction treatment facility in Center City, Minn.

Biological factors strongly influence who gets a rush from drugs and therefore has high risk of substance abuse, Kosten says.

For example, a person's genetic makeup may cause them to be both ultrasensitive to chemicals like opiates and to release more of the body's own stimulating chemicals in response to ingesting alcohol or an opiate drug. When people with that physical makeup take a powerful drug like Vicodin, their already supersensitive bodies actually receive an additional shot of chemicals, which creates an intense high, Kosten explains. "They're having an experience that's very, very different," and far more compelling, than what other people taking the same drug experience.

About 30 percent of Europeans and 50 percent of Chinese have a physical makeup that puts them at risk when they take prescription drugs with addiction potential, but most people at risk don't realize it, Kosten says.

Other factors also probably raise addiction risks, says Lowenstein. For example, "the majority of people we see" in detox "have some underlying issue" that's helped drive the drug abuse, "such as depression or anxiety."

Alcohol and drug abuse "are nothing but a desired altered state of consciousness," says Kitty Harris-Wilkes, director of the Center for the Study of Addiction and Recovery at Texas Tech University in Lubbock. "If I don't like the way I feel, I'll do something to change it." Such a desire can exist in anyone, "whether you're 13 or 83."

The urge to escape society's pressures and stress is at the root of much substance abuse today, she says. At schools like Texas Tech, for example, there is often a "higher level of chemicals" used in the Honors College, where more students feel they're under intense pressure, she says.

Nevertheless, people should not be afraid to take a drug for pain relief, especially if they keep their doctor informed and follow instructions, says Leslie Lundt, a Boise, Idaho, psychiatrist and author of *Think Like a Psychiatrist: Understanding Psychiatric Medicines*. If a patient is suffering from insomnia and has had no personal or family substance-abuse problems, "I say, 'So all of a sudden you're going to become a prostitute on a street corner just to get your sleeping pills?' "

Doctors, especially anesthesiologists, are at high risk for prescription-drug abuse. "The best estimate is that 20 percent of doctors are addicted" to some substance, says Doug Thorburn, author of *Drunks, Drugs & Debits: How to Recognize Addicts and Avoid Financial Abuse*.

Anesthesiologists' high rate of substance abuse shows the frightening power of addiction, says Seppala. "In spite of having the knowledge and awareness of addiction risks that they do, many anesthesiologists still get into it," he says. Anesthesiology residents are the most likely doctors to be addicted. "Some people who are already experimenting with substance abuse actually go into the field to get the drugs." Others apparently get involved out of "curiosity," Seppala says. Some anesthesia patients report that "it feels so good," and the doctors "start to wonder," he says.

Women may be at higher risk for abusing prescription drugs than illegal drugs, mainly because of ease of access. If one has both health insurance and a middle-class or higher income, it can be easy to get a legitimate prescription for an addictive drug and fill it at multiple pharmacies.

Seppala describes a 52-year-old stay-at-home mom who kept up an addiction for years because she had five doctors prescribing her the same amount of opioids repeatedly.

"She never showed up to get more pills before her prescription was scheduled to run out, and she never complained," so no doctor or pharmacist ever flagged her as a potential abuser, he says. The woman had a history of migraines and "knew what they were like, so she could give a good description" of her pain to justify her prescriptions, he says.

Because she was able to pay out of her own pocket for so many drugs, "she was kind of an exception" to the norm, he says. She only entered treatment when, finally, facing a divorce and foreclosure on her house, she was unable to pay for the drugs, he says.

"A group we're seeing more of is teens and young adults," often getting started on "their mothers' or grandmothers' medicine," says Christy Valentine, an internal-medicine and pediatrics physician in New Orleans. "The number of teens who've tried one of these narcotic medications or say they know someone who has is rampant," she says.

How do you know you're in trouble with a prescription drug? One strong indication is "that the drug becomes a central organizing pattern of your life" — you always know where it is, how much you have and where you can get more, says Harris-Wilkes.

Continued from p. 846

well as pharmacies and dispensed directly by physicians. For example, in 1885 in Iowa — a state with a population of under 2 million — 3,000 stores sold opiate drugs. Mail-order opiates were also sold. [29]

The pharmaceutical use of opiates — as well as stimulants like cocaine — went far beyond pain medication. Numerous "patent medicines" were advertised as treatment for ills ranging from consumption (tuberculosis) to coughs and diarrhea, and some narcotic medicines were even sold in the form of "soothing syrups," intended for teething babies, along with cocaine toothache drops for children and cocaine-containing lozenges for sore throats. [30]

"Careless prescription, incessant dispensation and hidden distribution of harmful drugs — the addictive effects of which were unknown until too late — fostered a large addict population which continued to increase in the early 20th century," wrote Richard J. Bonnie, a professor of law and medicine at the University of Virginia School of Law, and the late Charles H. Whitebread, II, a law professor at the University of Southern California's Gould School of Law. [31]

The rate of opiate addiction in the United States swelled from fewer than one addict per 1,000 people around 1840 to 4.59 per thousand in the 1890s, according to David T. Courtwright, a professor of history at the University of North Florida in Jacksonville. [32]

While many people disapproved of opium use, the earliest laws against the drugs were probably intended mainly to control the activities of Chinese immigrants — widely resented, especially on the West Coast, because they were perceived as taking jobs from Americans. In the 1870s and '80s, California and San Francisco prohibited opium smoking in commercial "opium dens," for example.

Soon, however, laws were enacted to tighten medical control of opiate drugs. For example, an 1887 Oregon statute barred the sale of cocaine without a doctor's prescription. By 1914, 46 states had similar cocaine bans, and 29 states had included non-prescription opiates in their sales bans. Only about six states had outlawed simple possession of restricted drugs, however. [33]

Few Doctors Receive Addiction Training

More than half of American physicians say they are primarily responsible for preventing prescription-drug abuse, but few received medical school training in its prevention and identification or the proper prescription methods for controlled drugs.

According to the National Center on Addiction and Substance Abuse, physicians say they . . .

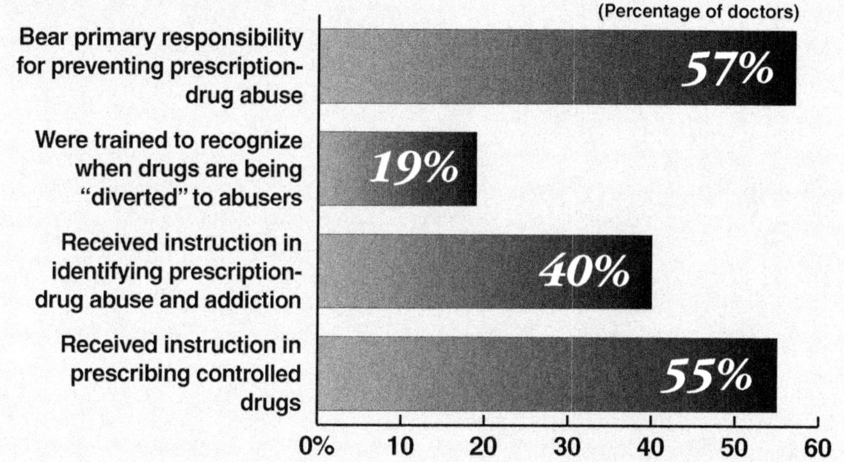

Source: "Under the Counter: The Diversion and Abuse of Controlled Prescription Drugs in the U.S.," National Center on Addiction and Substance Abuse, Columbia University, July 2005

Federal Action

With many states as well as foreign governments attempting crackdowns on non-medicinal drug use, and increased awareness that some drugs were highly addictive, pressure built for the U.S. to act. In 1909, the first federal legislation regulating narcotics distribution limited opium to a few entry ports and only for medicinal uses.

Major legislation soon followed that focused federal regulation of addictive drugs on pharmacies and prescribing physicians. The Harrison Narcotics Tax Act of 1914 required anyone who imported, produced, sold or otherwise dispensed opium, cocaine or drugs derived from them to register with the federal government and pay a special tax. In effect, the new law established a registered class of people authorized to possess the drugs and by extension outlawed their possession by unregistered sellers or users with no drug prescription.

"During the period of little or no regulation . . . innocent addicts were regarded as victims of an unfortunate sickness in need of treatment," and "usually they could find a friendly physician or druggist willing to sustain their habits," observed Bonnie and Whitebread. [34]

How to Avoid Problems With Medications

Don't underestimate drugs' addictive power, experts warn.

Prescription drugs play a major and positive role in the lives of millions of Americans, but the public's generally positive attitude about them may lead some people to underestimate medications' risks and treat them too casually. Here are some of the ways drug experts say medication users can stay out of trouble:

Don't share prescriptions. "Your specific attributes," such as weight, gender, age and medical history, "make it just Russian roulette" to assume that a drug prescribed for someone else would help you, too, says Jack E. Fincham, a professor of pharmacy practice and administration at the University of Missouri, Kansas City.

Sharing medications is rife in our society, says Richard Goldsworthy, CEO and director of research and development for The Academic Edge, a research firm in Bloomington, Ind. In studies with both adults and teenagers, Goldsworthy found that many people had extremely casual attitudes about sharing prescription drugs. Much of the activity is "altruistic sharing" — handing a drug to a friend because you think it might help them — and around 30 percent of adults and 20 percent of teenagers report they've been on one end or the other of such a transaction, often involving antibiotics, antihistamines and even birth-control pills.

The high numbers suggest there's very little understanding of drug side effects and rules for usage, such as the importance of taking the full course of some drugs, such as antibiotics, to make them work properly, he says. This also "indicates that our society is very laissez-faire about prescription drugs in general," which could increase comfort with taking dangerous drugs, he says.

ADHD drugs are more dangerous than you think. "If you look at Ritalin structurally, it's the closest relative to cocaine," but since the drug's been widely prescribed for youngsters with ADHD — Attention Deficit Hyperactivity Disorder — many people believe that it's quite safe, said Scott Teitelbaum, medical director of the Florida Recovery Center at the University of Florida, Gainesville.

Ritalin is also cheap and easy to procure. A friend with a prescription may sell it to you for just the price of their insurance co-pay, and "the modern student is . . . smart enough to go to a doctor and . . . tell them exactly what the [ADHD] symptoms are . . . to get stimulants," Teitelbaum said. [1]

But then the trouble begins. "Somebody might think if 10 milligrams keeps most people up, I need 20 or 30 or 40 to stay awake longer. I need more because I need to study, and I'm way behind." But that's not the way drug doses work, Teitelbaum said. "A higher dose might make them more likely to have an irregular heartbeat or get hyperthermia, or there could be another medicine that the person is on that could interact." [2]

Addicts are not who you think. If relatives and friends wait until someone actually shows signs of losing control over the abused substance, they'll be able to identify only very late-

In 1919, however, the Supreme Court cracked down on such "maintenance" prescriptions. [35] Although Memphis doctor W. S. Webb and pharmacist Jacob Goldbaum were registered as legitimate providers under the Harrison Act, they were convicted in Tennessee of "prescribing and selling narcotics not to cure but to keep the addicts comfortable," wrote historian R. Alton Lee. [36]

The pair appealed on the grounds that, since the Harrison Act was a revenue measure, the law could not rightly stipulate to whom drugs might be prescribed and sold. The Supreme Court upheld the conviction, effectively establishing the principle that maintenance of an addiction was not a legitimate medical reason to dispense drugs. As a result, doctors largely stopped prescribing drugs to people they believed were addicts, helping drive trade in opium, cocaine and similar drugs underground. [37]

As laws made addictive drugs harder to get, addiction rates waned. In 1970 Congress consolidated regulation of all federally restricted drugs under the Controlled Substances Act. The law classifies drugs as belonging to one of five "schedules" with decreasing levels of control and scrutiny applied to each successive category. Schedule I drugs, including marijuana and heroin, are deemed to have high abuse potential and no currently accepted medical use, and are essentially banned. Schedule V drugs, such as cough medicines that contain the low-level opiate codeine, which have accepted medical uses and a relatively low potential for physical or psychological dependence, are regulated but don't require a doctor's prescription. [38]

Nevertheless, prohibitions haven't stopped some addicts from getting their hands on addictive substances, including pharmaceuticals, over the years.

"Passing forged prescriptions was standard operating procedure" for obtaining drugs in small-town Arkansas in the 1960s and '70s, wrote addiction psychiatrist Martha A. Morrison, who became an addict as a teenager. "I could rip off prescription pads in a heartbeat; I'd just walk into a doctor's office, ask for an appointment, grab one of the pads that were always lying around, and slip it into my purse or down my pants." Later, Morrison would "write five or six prescriptions" and

stage addicts, says Doug Thorburn, author of *Drunks, Drugs & Debits: How to Recognize Addicts and Avoid Financial Abuse*. "Behavioral disorders" are a strong sign of addiction. "Whenever we shake our heads and say, 'What was he thinking?' about someone's behavior, the thought that 'This might be addiction' " should quickly follow, he argues.

So, intervene early, says Thorburn. "What are we waiting for? Just for more stuff to happen that they'll need to make amends for down the road?"

"Intervening early is one of the best things you can do," says Kitty Harris-Wilkes, director of the Center for the Study of Addiction and Recovery at Texas Tech University in Lubbock. For example, "you can hit young people with pretty specific consequences," like kicking them out of school on a second offense. It's vital to send signals loud enough for addicts to actually hear, she says.

Lock up or discard prescription meds. "If I pay for a prescription painkiller but don't use it all, I'm liable to wonder why I can't just save it in case I sprain my ankle a year from now," says Seppala. Use your judgment about that, but at the very least "you have to limit access to it — put it in a locked place," to avoid tempting others, especially teens looking to experiment.

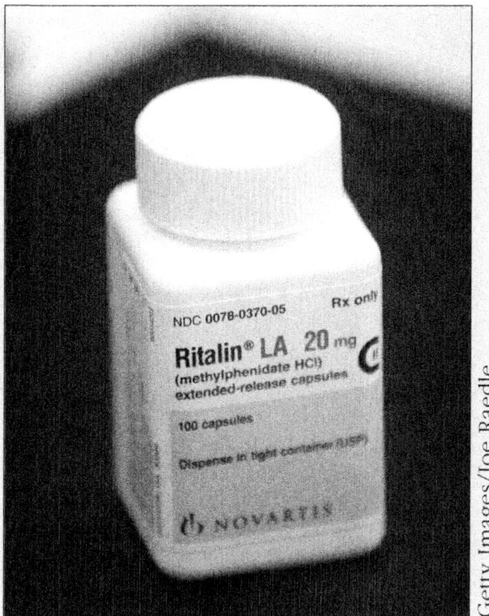

Getty Images/Joe Raedle

The ADHD drug Ritalin is easy to obtain and deceptively easy to misuse.

"I know plenty of adult addicts who go on open house tours and look in the medicine cabinets, too," he says.

Mixing meds can be substance abuse, too. So many medications are floating around today that it's easy to misuse them dangerously without even knowing it, says Fincham. For example, "many well-intentioned people take over-the-counter medications and herbal products," mixing them with prescription drugs without consulting a doctor or pharmacist.

"Every drug, prescription or not, can have a good effect, a bad effect and a null effect and if it's a null effect," the reaction of many people is to simply take more of the drug or take another drug on top of the first — both huge mistakes, Fincham says. The resulting overdoses and drug interactions are "a big and very understated problem in the United States."

---

[1] "Ritalin Abuse Poses Risks During College Exam Week," press release, University of Florida, May 10, 2007.

[2] *Ibid.*

"spend a day driving all over Arkansas" filling them at different stores.[39]

"The only time I was questioned was in a little drugstore in a city about 120 miles south of Fayetteville," where a pharmacist objected, saying, "I don't recognize this doctor's handwriting." After an "indignant" response from Morrison that she lived 120 miles away and was staying in town with relatives, "he filled it."

Internet and Beyond

Over the past two decades, several trends have converged to drive prescription-drug abuse upwards. Beginning in the 1940s so-called integrated pain-treatment teams, including physical therapists and psychologists, proliferated around the country, successfully treating severe chronic pain by a variety of means including drugs, says the University of Pennsylvania's Ashburn. But beginning in the early 1980s, insurers stopped paying for "integrated" treatment and the concept withered, leaving physicians and patients with "very few options" for pain management, he says. The decline of pain management, combined with the aggressive marketing of some pain medications in recent years, and an explosion in the use of opiates for chronic non-cancer pain, had dire consequences for increased drug abuse, Ashburn says.

On college campuses, meanwhile, stimulants are being used the most, notably drugs like Adderall that have been prescribed for attention deficit hyperactivity disorder (ADHD), says Harris-Wilkes of Texas Tech. Students believe, "If you don't have ADHD or a similar condition, these drugs will give you a huge buzz and you can stay up for days," she says.

Stimulant abuse has increased partly because the drugs are so widely available and well accepted, but societal stress also is a driver, Harris-Wilkes believes. "If you stand back and look at it, it's just an extension of the same thing we see with energy drinks like Red Bull and Rock Star. Hello, it's 10 o'clock in the morning, should you really be drinking this?" Nevertheless, she says, many teens are driven to stimulant abuse because they worry, "If I don't do well on my SAT, I'm not going to college."

Doctors Faulted for Prescribing Addictive Painkillers

Pain experts call for more awareness, holistic approaches.

"As a profession, we're not adequately treating pain," says Marvin P. Seppala, chief medical officer of the Hazelden Foundation, an addiction treatment organization in Center City, Minn. "At the same time, doctors have people coming in every day trying to scam them" to get addictive drugs for non-medical uses.

Both patients and doctors should be more aware of the abuse potential of pain medications, however, Seppala says. "These are really important medications, but if you're going to use them for an extended period you need to know that they can lead to addiction."

Addictive painkillers often are prescribed without much or any discussion, and even when they may not be necessary. "I went in with a broken foot and wasn't allowed to leave without a prescription for an addictive painkiller," even though "my foot didn't hurt unless I walked on it," says Susan Foster, director of policy research and analysis for the National Center on Addiction and Substance Abuse (CASA) at Columbia University in New York City.

All doctors who prescribe narcotic painkillers should query patients about any history of substance abuse, one of the biggest risk factors for running into trouble with the drugs, says Seppala.

Scheduled for a surgery of his own, Seppala, a recovering addict, told his physician about his substance-abuse history and asked for pain treatment that wouldn't trigger the addiction. "But as soon as I heard the surgeon say, 'Don't worry!' I knew he didn't get it," he says. After a relatively minor operation, he found himself in possession of 180 tablets of the opiate painkiller Vicodin. "I used only two the first night," he says.

Knowing the dangers, Seppala lined up his wife and an anesthesiologist friend to carefully oversee his painkiller use to keep him out of danger, but other at-risk people may not realize they should do this, he says.

Pain specialists are finding more downsides with pain treatment that relies heavily on opiates, says Michael Ashburn, a professor of anesthesiology and director of the pain medicine and palliative care center at the University of Pennsylvania. For example, "A fair amount of patients on very high opioids are seeing unforeseen problems," ranging from mental and other errors to criminal behavior. The university's pain center cares for about 75 patients at a time who have extremely serious chronic pain, "and every day I have to address drug-related behavior with a patient or two," he says.

"I have a love-hate relationship with opioids," he says. "In many people they can make a world of difference, but in some other patients the side effects" are extreme and very disturbing, he says.

As a result, more physicians are realizing that good pain treatment requires a more complex approach, Ashburn and others say. "We need to do more with cognitive behavioral therapy, acupuncture" and other non-opioid treatments for pain, says Michael H. Lowenstein, co-director of the Waismann Institute, a detoxification center in Beverly Hills, Calif.

But it's not always easy for patients to understand that the best way to treat pain often involves a pain specialist and other professionals like physical therapists, says Christy Valentine, an internal-medicine and pediatrics physician in New Orleans. That's where education and communication come in, she says.

"It's important to help patients recognize that there is a special process going on" to assemble the right multifaceted treatment for their pain, and that it's a different and more effective thing than "what they're used to, which is just going to the doctor and getting medications."

Changing the pain paradigm to a less opiate-focused, more holistic venture "is often easier when you get patients who haven't had a lot of pain before," says Valentine, because "the patient has to do the real work," engaging in exercise or cognitive behavioral therapy rather than just taking a pill.

But good pain treatment often is hard to find, many doctors say. "There are a lot of pain management doctors around the country and also a lot of wannabe" pain doctors who specialize in handing out pills, "and that's where the problem lies," says David S. Kloth, an anesthesiologist in Danbury, Conn., and past president of the American Society of Interventional Pain Physicians. Some so-called pain doctors in Miami, for example, are actually "pill mills" that "see hundreds of people a day," actually diagnosing and treating nothing but contributing hugely to the flow of prescription narcotics into society, he says.

The Internet also facilitates prescription abuse. Many Internet pharmacies dispense drugs without a prescription or even sell bogus prescriptions of their own that buyers can use at other drugstores. In 2006, for example, 34 Internet pharmacies known or suspected to be illicit operations dispensed 98.5 million doses of medicine containing the opiate hydrocodone, according to the DEA. The doses accounted for 95 percent of the stores' business and were enough to supply 410,000 patients with a month's dosage each. By contrast, controlled substances account for just 11 percent of the sales at "brick and mortar" pharmacies, according to the agency.[40]

Illegal Internet pharmacies are extremely difficult to stamp out, says Jack E. Fincham, a professor of pharmacy practice and administration at the University of Missouri, Kansas City. "One can be shut down by authorities and be back in business immediately" because enforcement agencies can't find its physical location.

Continued on p. 854

At Issue:

Can the Ryan Haight Act curb prescription-drug abuse?

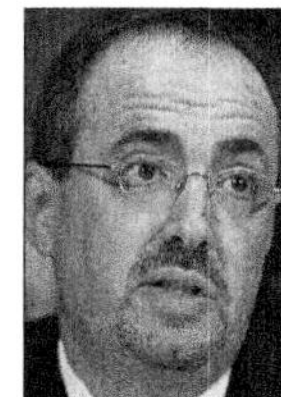

JOSEPH T. RANNAZZISI
DEPUTY ASSISTANT ADMINISTRATOR, DRUG ENFORCEMENT ADMINISTRATION

TESTIMONY BEFORE HOUSE JUDICIARY SUBCOMMITTEE ON CRIME, TERRORISM AND HOMELAND SECURITY, JUNE 24, 2008

yes

Prescription drugs can be illegally acquired through a variety of means. While the Drug Enforcement Administration and other law enforcement investigations have shown that OxyContin and other Schedule II drugs are most commonly obtained illegally through "doctor shopping" or other, more traditional methods of illegally acquiring controlled pharmaceutical substances, this has not been the case for Schedule III or Schedule IV substances (e.g., anti-anxiety medications, hydrocodone combination products and anabolic steroids). [They] are often illegally purchased through the Internet. Unlike someone stealing a few pills out of the medicine cabinet . . . illicit Internet sales commonly involve 100 or more high-potency pills; these sales occur hundreds of times every day.

The Internet has become one of the fastest-growing methods of diverting controlled pharmaceuticals. Certainly there are benefits to allowing individuals with a valid prescription to fill their prescriptions over the Internet, ranging from simple convenience to providing individuals in remote areas or with limited mobility with greater access to needed medications. Legitimate pharmacies operate every day providing services over the Internet and operate well within the bounds of the law and sound medical practice.

Unfortunately, other so-called "pharmacy" sites on the Internet illegally sell controlled pharmaceuticals. These rogue Internet sites are not there to benefit the public but to generate millions in illegal sales.

The controlled-substance laws and regulations were written before the advent of fax machines, let alone high-speed Internet service and the complexities associated with the advent of this technology. It should be noted that inter-agency engagement on how best to bring the laws that protect the American people from drug traffickers up to speed with the methods these traffickers now routinely employ has been ongoing for years. These discussions culminated with the Bush administration's formal endorsement of the Ryan Haight Online Pharmacy Consumer Protection Act.

The act updates the Controlled Substances Act to set forth both permissible and impermissible conduct for Internet Web site operators, medical practitioners and pharmacists involved in the distribution of controlled substances by means of the Internet. This legislation balances the legitimate benefits derived from using the Internet to provide consumers with controlled substances obtained through valid prescriptions with the need to combat the illegal online distribution of these same drugs.

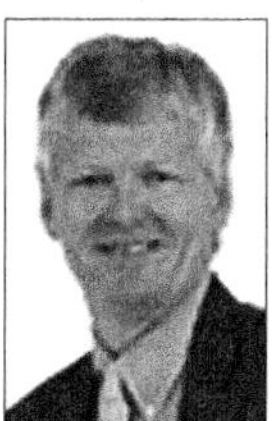

PATRICK J. EGAN
PARTNER, FOX ROTHSCHILD LLP, PHILADELPHIA

TESTIMONY BEFORE HOUSE JUDICIARY SUBCOMMITTEE ON CRIME TERRORISM AND HOMELAND SECURITY, JUNE 24, 2008

no

By criminalizing the sale of controlled substances without a valid prescription by online pharmacies, the Ryan Haight Online Pharmacy Consumer Protection Act fails to attack the source of addiction to prescription medication. Drug users have multiple, superior sources to acquire medication. Under the assumption that controlled substances used for medical purposes improve the lives of patients, the benefits of prescription medicine sold by online pharmacies without the need for a valid prescription significantly outweigh the risks of abuse of the drugs for non-medical purposes, especially in teens.

The benefit to low-income Americans and elderly Americans of having the ability to purchase prescription medicine from online pharmacies without a valid prescription grossly outweighs the risk to adults and teens purchasing pain medication from online pharmacies. For example, if the uninsured were forced to go to doctors to get a valid prescription, they would not go at all because these individuals cannot afford medical care. Thus, online pharmacies give uninsured Americans a unique benefit not offered elsewhere.

In 2006, 17.4 percent of the 17-year-old population had used pain relievers for non-medical use. In addition to pain medication, diet pills are commonly purchased through online pharmacies. But . . . the majority of these drugs are obtained from friends and relatives, not online pharmacies.

The Office of National Drug Control Policy reports that 70 percent of teens get the products from friends and relatives. More than three in five teens say they got prescription pain relievers from parents' medicine cabinets. The Ohio Prescription Monitoring Program attributes "doctor shopping" as a predominant factor and means of getting prescription medication for non-medical use. Additionally, the attorney general of Maryland cites stealing pills from the pharmacy as a means of obtaining prescription meds. Lastly, doctors individually contribute to the distribution of pain medication for non-medical purposes.

Therefore, the minor impact of requiring online pharmacies to only distribute controlled substances with a valid prescription would not be attacking the true and majority source of non-medical use of pain relievers. The most efficient means of attack are through parenting education and supervision. Moreover, those adolescents who are inclined to purchase controlled substances through online pharmacies will continue to do so. Only now the drugs they are purchasing will be from offshore pharmacies that the Ryan Haight Act cannot reach and will be more likely to be adulterated or counterfeit.

Continued from p. 852

Meanwhile, Internet "search engines are profiting off ads" from bogus pharmacies, giving them every reason to avoid cracking down on the stores, says Liang of Western Law School. "All the search engines" — such as Microsoft, Yahoo and Google — "say they use pharmacychecker.com, but that's a joke, because when you go to the sites they've ranked, many are not requiring prescriptions."

E-mailed "spam" can also bring controlled substances right to your door. "Most people who use e-mail have experienced sifting through unsolicited e-mails that offer controlled substances online," wrote Robert F. Forman, director of clinical resources and education for the biotech firm Alkermes, a maker of addiction treatments in Cambridge, Mass. "For individuals addicted to prescription drugs . . . those e-mails are equivalent to getting a phone call from a drug dealer." [41]

Researchers also find that many prescription drugs pass to abusers through informal networks of family and friends, networks that for young people, in particular, may be much larger than in the past because of Internet social networking, says Richard Goldsworthy, CEO and director of research and development for The Academic Edge, a research firm in Bloomington, Ind.

With so many people holding legitimate prescriptions to abusable drugs — young athletes who are prescribed opiates after injuries, for example — "access to these things is incredible through a clandestine network based on cellphones and texting," says Wright State's Carlson.

The increasingly positive view Americans generally have of prescriptions is also helping to drive abuse, analysts say, along with the proliferation of drug advertising.

"As a society, we have the idea that we shouldn't feel any discomfort," says the Waismann Institute's Lowenstein. "It got to the point where, if you had any ache or pain, you took Vicodin. . . . Sixty percent of Vicodin-using teens tried it before age 15, and most took it from grandparents' and parents' medicine cabinets."

For a health problem like insomnia, for example, "almost always there's a solution" that is not a pill, but pills are what doctors and patients usually opt for first, says psychiatrist Lundt. "People want to get the simplest solution, rather than putting money, time and energy into seeking out causes like sleep apnea," or prostrate or hormonal problems, or making lifestyle changes like "getting the dog or the TV out of the bedroom," she says. As a result, many physicians "just throw Ambien at people."

Today's physicians "were basically trained by drug companies," making doctors less likely to suggest non-drug treatments when drugs are available, says Lowenstein.

Direct-to-consumer (DTC) advertising of prescription medicines was first permitted in the late 1990s, and it's contributed to a cultural attitude that "Hey, it's acceptable to take drugs," says Western Law School's Liang.

"I don't know why DTC is accepted," says Fincham. "The U.S. stands alone in allowing it. It's not done in Canada, the U.K., or Western Europe." But Americans, bombarded by drug ads "with attractive people feeling absolutely great, are lulled into complacency" about potential risks of prescription drugs, he says.

States and the federal government have noted the prescription-abuse problem and devoted some attention to it, but with many competing priorities funding has lagged.

In 2005, for example, the American Society of Interventional Pain Physicians successfully advocated for the National All Schedules Prescription Electronic Reporting Act, says anesthesiologist Kloth, the society's immediate past president. The bill "was supposed to implement and improve prescription-monitoring programs" in all states but "was never funded," although Congress has provided $2 million in start-up funds in 2009.

That's especially ironic as Congress frets over how to pay for health-coverage expansion, says Kloth. About 15 percent of Medicare drugs — and about 38 percent of Medicaid drugs — are diverted to abusive purposes, along with hefty but unknown amounts of drugs for which privately insured people get prescriptions they fill at multiple pharmacies. The state of Missouri, for example, found that five drug-abusing patients alone ran up $400,000 in pharmacy bills. "We could potentially save millions of dollars" by beefing up monitoring efforts, he says. ■

CURRENT SITUATION

High, Not Rising

Prescription-drug abuse is no longer rising rapidly, as it was in the early 2000s, though levels are still high. "Among the general population, non-medical use of controlled prescription drugs was stable from 2003 to 2007, with 7 million Americans, age 12 and older, reporting past-month non-medical use," the White House Office of National Drug Control Policy (ONDCP) reported in May. [42]

As abuse of illegal drugs has declined, prescription-drug abuse has become a larger part of the nation's drug epidemic than it was in the past, even while it remains a relatively unrecognized issue, says University of Michigan research scientist Johnston.

"Prescription drugs have always been part of the problem" of drug abuse, with teenage abuse of amphetamines, tranquilizers, sedatives and other drugs reaching peaks in the 1970s and early '80s that have not been seen since, Johnston says. Beginning in the late 1970s, abuse of all drugs, including prescription drugs, dropped off for a decade or so, but began rising again in the early 1990s, he says.

Abuse of prescription drugs has generally leveled off after rising since about 1992, says Foster at the National Center on Addiction and Substance Abuse. But she says abuse still is rising for one group — 50- to 59-year-olds. "Baby boomers had higher drug use anyway, and they can get more prescriptions" than teenagers, she says. Boomers also may risk worse consequences from the drugs — a quicker path to addiction and health problems — than younger users, Foster says. "Older women don't realize that their bodies are more sensitive" to drugs as they age, for example.

Among teens, the Monitoring the Future survey reveals that use of the prescription amphetamine Ritalin — often prescribed for ADHD — continued to fall in 2008, having declined by about a third since 2001. Abuse of many other prescription medications, such as sedatives and tranquilizers, also has been modestly dropping among teens, says Johnston, the survey's principal investigator.

Some prescription narcotics, however, such as OxyContin and Vicodin, remain at or near the peak levels of abuse they hit in the mid-2000s. Unlike for most other prescription medications, the high abuse rates the two powerful drugs attained this decade were "new highs, at levels we hadn't seen before," says Johnston. "New drugs within that class [of prescription opioids] have helped to stimulate use."

Abuse of over-the-counter cough and cold medications also remains prevalent, Johnston says.

When abuse of any drug rises, it's mainly due to a decreased "perception of harm" connected with it in the public's mind, says Foster. For example, some prescription-drug abusers "won't touch OxyContin" because of the intense attention it received as a dangerous substance, says Carlson of Wright State. "They fear what they've heard," even though those fears don't translate into equivalent caution about other very similar opiate painkillers.

Thus, Johnston warns, even though prescription-drug abuse has generally plateaued or is currently dropping for most populations, it's no time to back off anti-abuse messages.

Ryan Haight Act

The nation "is in a period like the early 1990s," when policy makers and others let drug abuse slide from a public agenda crowded with other issues, raising the likelihood that drug abuse will rise again, Johnston says.

"This is the kind of problem that will recur and recur because all kids are susceptible to the same issues of curiosity" that draws people to try out substances, he says.

To counter that curiosity, education about the risks of drug addiction must be ongoing to reach each new cohort, Johnston says.

On Oct. 15, 2008, President Bush signed into law the federal government's most recent initiative to thwart prescription-drug abuse — the Ryan Haight Act. The Justice Department issued rules implementing the law in April 2009.

The law memorializes an 18-year-old high-school varsity tennis player and A student from La Mesa, Calif., who died in 2001 from an overdose of the painkiller Vicodin that he obtained over the Internet. The law officially prohibits anyone from selling or shipping "controlled substances" ordered over the Internet unless the customer has a "valid prescription" issued by a doctor during a live, in-person visit. [43] Haight had obtained his drugs after "consulting" with a physician online, a ploy that many online drug sellers use to get around state prescribing laws. [44]

The law also requires online pharmacies to comply with state laws for pharmacy licensure in all states in which they operate; post their address and telephone number, along with the qualifications of their lead pharmacist, on the Internet homepage; and notify states' attorneys general and pharmacy boards at least 30 days before offering to dispense any controlled drugs. The act also increases penalties for violations of prescribing laws. [45]

DEA Acting Administrator Michele M. Leonhart called it "landmark" legislation that "will bring rogue pharmacy operators out of the shadows by establishing a clear standard for legitimate online pharmaceutical sales." [46]

Other analysts say, however, that the law won't even touch the real culprits — actual "rogue" Internet pharmacies that already operate completely outside of the extensive state rules for pharmacy operation.

"It's an important thing, but they're just targeting legitimate Internet pharmacies" and totally missing the many rogue enterprises, says Liang of Western Law School. "Every state already requires a prescription anyway, so the legitimate sellers already do" what the Ryan Haight Act requires.

Meanwhile, many if not most of the bogus online pharmacies are operated by Chinese and Indian nationals, "Russian mafia guys," or others at mainly offshore sites, Liang says. "None of these people care" what U.S. law says. ■

OUTLOOK

'Unmet Needs'

With illegal drug use waning somewhat and legal prescriptions of addictive drugs rising, prescription-medication abuse has become a more important issue for substance-abuse and addiction treatment. Substance-abuse treatment capacity continues to lag behind need, however, and the medical profession is only beginning to recognize its potential role in heading off and treating prescription-drug abuse.

Currently, there are "enormous unmet needs" for better substance-abuse treatment as well as for education and prescription monitoring to prevent abuse, says Foster at the National Center on Addiction and Substance Abuse.

"The number of people needing care is overwhelming the treatment centers" in Ohio, for example, says Wright State University's Carlson.

Treatment efforts have lagged partly because of the blame long attached to drug abuse, but growing medical evidence that addiction is an illness may be gradually changing that, Foster says. "There have been a lot of examples of disease blamed on the patient," including tuberculosis and depression, and over time those views have shifted, as they are gradually shifting now for addiction, she says. "We still have a long way to go," however.

For one thing, the medical profession must recognize prescription-drug abuse and addiction generally as medical problems it must confront, and there are "signs of movement" in that direction, says Foster. For example, the Joint Commission on the Accreditation of Healthcare Organizations is proposing that all hospitals be required to screen for substance abuse, make treatment referrals and perform brief, evidence-based interventions for patients who show signs of abuse. [47]

Historically, however, addiction has not been viewed as a medical problem, Foster points out, even though the American Medical Association labeled it a disease as early as the 1950s. Consequently, she says, addicts of all kinds are "generally treated outside of medicine," in self-help groups like Narcotics Anonymous and at treatment centers run by non-physicians.

Despite studies demonstrating that addiction is a medical disease that "can become chronic" if untreated, "doctors are still uncomfortable" even talking about addiction with patients, let alone treating them, Foster says. In surveys, 47 percent of doctors "said they are uncomfortable discussing prescription-drug abuse" with patients.

Those barriers are gradually giving way, however, and "we're actually getting close to considering it malpractice" to prescribe addictive drugs without counseling about abuse risks and screening patients for any history of substance abuse in them or their families, she says.

It's also important to eliminate the easy availability of abusable prescription drugs, says University of Michigan research scientist Johnston. "Can we get physicians and dentists to give smaller prescriptions" of pain relievers, for example? "That would reduce the number of people who have leftover stuff in their medicine cabinets."

The Center on Addiction and Substance Abuse has "also petitioned the FDA to require abusable drugs to be made in less abusable forms," says Foster.

Nonetheless, drug-abuse battles will have to be refought in each new generation, says Carlson. "If we were able to solve the drug problem, we would have done so a long time ago." ■

About the Author

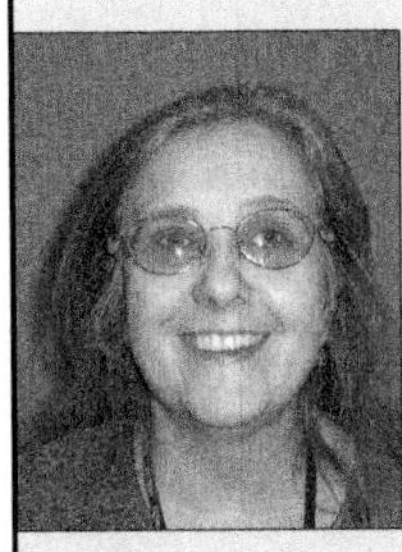

Staff writer **Marcia Clemmitt** is a veteran social-policy reporter who previously served as editor in chief of *Medicine & Health* and staff writer for *The Scientist*. She has also been a high-school math and physics teacher. She holds a liberal arts and sciences degree from St. John's College, Annapolis, and a master's degree in English from Georgetown University. Her recent reports include "Preventing Cancer" and "Treating Depression."

Notes

[1] For background, see "Coroner Rules Jackson's Death a Homicide," MSNBC.com, Aug. 24, 2009, www.msnbc.msn.com.

[2] Leonard J. Paulozzi, "Trends in Unintentional Drug Overdose Deaths," testimony before Senate Judiciary Subcommittee on Crime and Drugs, March 12, 2008.

[3] Gil Kaufman, "DJ AM's Death Caused by Accidental Overdose," Mtv.com, Sept. 29, 2009, www.mtv.com.

[4] Quoted in Harriet Ryan, "Pharmacist Refused to Fill Anna Nicole Smith's Prescription," *Los Angeles Times*, Sept. 22, 2009.

[5] Paulozzi, *op. cit.*

[6] "Prevention of Prescription Drug/Pharmaceutical Overdose and Abuse," National Conference of State Legislatures, June 2009, www.ncsl.org.

[7] Testimony before House Judiciary Subcommittee on Crime, Terrorism and Homeland Security, July 12, 2007.

[8] *Ibid.*

[9] *Ibid.*

[10] Quoted in Elaine Grant, "Pharmacy Board Stalls Drug Abuse Prevention Efforts, Advocates Say," New Hampshire Public Radio, July 27, 2009, www.Nhpr.org.

[11] Donna Leinwand, "Prescription Drugs Find Place in Teen Culture," *USA Today*, June 13, 2006, p. 1A. David Emery, "Are Pharm Parties for Real?" David Emery's Urban Legends Blog, About.com, March 24, 2009, http://urbanlegends.about.com/b/2009/03/24/are-pharm-parties-for-real.htm.

[12] Testimony before Senate Committee on the Judiciary, March 12, 2008, http://judiciary.authoring.senate.gove/hearings/testimony.cfm.
[13] *Ibid.*
[14] Testimony before House Judiciary Subcommittee on Crime, Terrorism, and Homeland Security, June 24, 2008.
[15] "No Prescription Required: Bing.com Prescription Drug Ads," LegitScript and KnujOn, Aug 3, 2009, www.legitscript.com/BingRx Report.pdf.
[16] *Ibid.*, p. 3.
[17] Jane C. Ballantyne and Jianren Mao, "Opioid Therapy for Chronic Pain," *New England Journal of Medicine*, Nov. 13, 2003, p. 1943, www.nejm.org.
[18] "OxyContin Backlash," press release, University of Alabama at Birmingham, About.com: Mental Health, http://mentalhealth.about.com/library/sci/0301/bloxycontin301.htm.
[19] Steven P. Cohen and Srinivasa N. Raja, "The Middle Way: A Practical Approach to Prescribing Opioids for Chronic Pain," Nature Clinical Practice, *Neurology*, Nov. 16, 2006, www.medscape.com.
[20] Brietta Clark, "A Painful Lesson," *Daily Journal*, Loyola Law School, July 22, 2009, http://media.lls.edu/DJclark072209.html.
[21] *Ibid.*
[22] Testimony before House Judiciary Subcommittee on Crime, Terrorism and Homeland Security, July 12, 2007.
[23] *Ibid.*
[24] Lakmaiah Manchikanti, "Prescription Drug Abuse: What Is Being Done to Address this New Drug Epidemic?" *Pain Physician*, October 2006, pp. 287-321, www.painphysician journal.com/2006/october/2006;9;287-321.pdf.
[25] *Ibid.*
[26] For background, see David T. Courtwright, *Dark Paradise: A History of Opiate Addiction in America* (2001).
[27] Quoted in Edward M. Brecher and editors of *Consumer Reports*, "The Consumers Union Report on Licit and Illicit Drugs," 1972, www.druglibrary.org/schaffer/Library/studies/cu/cu3.html.
[28] *Ibid.*
[29] *Ibid.*
[30] "Before Prohibition, Addiction Science Network," http://addictionscience.net/ASN preprohibition.htm.
[31] Richard J. Bonnie and Charles H. Whitebread, "The Forbidden Fruit and the Tree of Knowledge: An Inquiry Into the Legal History of American Marijuana Prohibition," *Virginia Law Review*, October 1970, www.drugtext.org/index.php/en/reports/229-the-forbidden-fruit-and-the-tree-of-knowledge-an-inquiry-into-the-legal-history-of-american-marijuana-prohibition.
[32] Courtwright, *op. cit.*, p. 9.
[33] Bonnie and Whitebread, *op. cit.*
[34] *Ibid.*
[35] R. Alton Lee, *A History of Regulatory Taxation* (1973), p. 122.
[36] *Ibid.*
[37] *Ibid.*
[38] "The Controlled Substances Act," U.S. Drug Enforcement Administration Web site, www.usdoj.gov/dea/pubs/abuse/1-csa.htm.
[39] Martha A. Morrison, *White Rabbit: A Doctor's Own Story of Addiction* (1991), p. 70.
[40] Testimony before Senate Committee on the Judiciary, May 16, 2007.
[41] Robert F. Forman, "Narcotics on the Net: The Availability of Web Sites Selling Controlled Substances," *Psychiatric Services*, January 2006, p. 24.
[42] "Prescription Opioid-related Deaths Increased 114 Percent from 2001 to 2005, Treatment Administration Up 74 Percent in Similar Period; Young Adults Hardest Hit," press release, Office of National Drug Control Policy, May 20, 2009, www.whitehousedrug policy.gov.
[43] Rhiannon Coppin, "What Is the Ryan Haight Act?" Behind Online Pharma Web site, Jan. 14, 2009, http://behindonlinepharma.com/2009011452/faqs/what-is-the-ryan-haight-act.
[44] Francine Haight, "Ryan Haight's Story," Get Smart About Drugs Web site, Drug Enforcement Administration, www.getsmartaboutdrugs.com/stories/ryan_haights_story.html.
[45] Coppin, *op. cit.*
[46] "Congress Passes Ryan Haight Online Pharmacy Consumer Protection Act," press release, Drug Enforcement Administration, Oct. 1, 2008, www.usdoj.gov/dea/pubs/pressrel/pr100108.html.
[47] Bob Curley, "Proposed Accreditation Standards Could Compel U.S. Hospitals to Screen Patients for Addictions," Join Together Web site, National Center on Addiction and Substance Abuse, Sept. 11, 2009, www.jointogether.org/news/features/2009/proposed-accreditation.html.

FOR MORE INFORMATION

Community Anti-Drug Coalitions of America (CADCA), 625 Slaters Ln., Suite 300, Alexandria, VA 22314; (800) 542-2322; www.cadca.org. National coalition of community-based groups that conducts anti-drug programs, including for medication abuse.

Drug Enforcement Administration, Mailstop: AES, 8701 Morrissette Dr., Springfield, VA 22152; (202) 307-1000; www.usdoj.gov/dea. Monitors and prosecutes unlawful prescribing and diversion of medications to illegal use.

LegitScript, (877) 534-4879; www.legitscript.com. A private company that disseminates information about online pharmacies and has formulated standards for recognizing legitimate pharmacies.

Monitoring the Future, www.monitoringthefuture.org. An annual National Institutes of Health-sponsored study that has surveyed teen substance use since 1975.

National Alliance for Model State Drug Laws, 1414 Prince St., Suite 312, Alexandria, VA 22314; (703) 836-6100; www.namsdl.org. A congressionally funded group that assists states in monitoring medication abuse.

National Center on Addiction and Substance Abuse at Columbia University (CASA), 633 Third Ave., 19th Floor, New York, NY 10017-6706; (212) 841-5200; www.casacolumbia.org. Conducts research and oversees information campaigns.

National Institute on Drug Abuse, 6001 Executive Blvd., Room 5213, Bethesda, MD 20892-9561; (301) 443-1124; www.nida.nih.gov. A branch of the National Institutes of Health that sponsors research on addiction-related health issues, including strategies for manufacturing medications like painkillers that are less susceptible to abuse.

White House Office of National Drug Control Policy, Drug Policy Information Clearinghouse, P.O. Box 6000, Rockville, MD 20849-6000; (800) 666-3332; www.whitehousedrugpolicy.gov. Establishes national drug-control policy and has declared prescription-drug abuse a priority.

Bibliography

Selected Sources

Books

Colvin, Rod, *Overcoming Prescription Drug Addiction: A Guide to Coping and Understanding*, 3rd edition, 2008.
The author, whose brother died at age 35 from abusing painkillers and tranquilizers, relates accounts of recovery from other prescription-drug abusers and describes in layman's terms the range of treatment options available.

Courtwright, David T., *Dark Paradise: A History of Opiate Addiction in America*, Harvard University Press, 2001.
A professor of history at the University of North Florida chronicles how opiate addiction shifted from a mostly middle-class problem in the 19th century to poor, urban communities in the 20th century and outlines the roles law and medicine may have played in the shift.

Hodgson, Barbara, *In the Arms of Morpheus: The Tragic History of Laudanum, Morphine and Patent Medicines*, Firefly Books, 2001.
A British novelist describes the widespread use of opiate medications in the 18th and 19th centuries, when physicians prescribed opium-containing drugs for conditions including tuberculosis and cholera, and habitual opium users included such cultural icons as Louisa May Alcott, George Washington and Florence Nightingale.

Musto, David F., *The American Disease: Origins of Narcotic Control*, 3rd edition, Oxford University Press, 1999.
A Yale University professor of child psychiatry and social historian describes how U.S. narcotics laws developed amid American society's repeatedly shifting, love-hate relationship with alcohol and drugs.

Articles

Grant, Elaine, "Prescription Drug Abuse a Serious, Growing Problem," New Hampshire Public Radio, June 9, 2009, www.nhpr.org/special/prescriptiondrugs.
The first story in a series on prescription-drug abuse in New Hampshire reports that state legislators have repeatedly failed to create a prescription-drug monitoring program to stem abuse, although overdose deaths quadrupled from 1995 to 2007, with much of the rise likely connected to prescription medications.

Tisch, Chris, and Abbie Vansickle, "Deadly Combinations," *St. Petersburg Times*, Feb. 17, 2008, www.tampabay.com/specials/2008/reports/drug-deaths.
The first article in a series on Florida's severe prescription-drug abuse problem reports that overdoses have increased rapidly and now kill about 500 people each year just in the Tampa Bay area — three times the number of deaths associated with illegal drugs such as cocaine and heroin.

Reports and Studies

"Children of the Mountains," ABC News Special Report, Feb. 13, 2009, http://abcnews.go.com/Video/playerIndex?id=6885766.
ABC News anchor Diane Sawyer spent two years researching this disturbing special report on the grim conditions faced by children growing up in the mountains of Eastern Kentucky, where poverty and prescription drug abuse are rampant.

"Monitoring the Future: National Survey Results on Drug Use, 1975-2008," National Institute on Drug Abuse, December 2008, http://monitoringthefuture.org/pubs/monographs/vol1_2008.pdf.
Prescription-drug abuse among teens is generally holding steady at or near the relatively high levels seen in the early-to-mid-2000s following a decade-long rise.

"National Prescription Drug Threat Assessment 2009," Drug Enforcement Administration, April 2009, www.usdoj.gov/ndic/pubs33/33775/index.htm.
In 2007 approximately 6.9 million Americans ages 12 or older reported they currently were non-medical users of prescription drugs.

"No Prescription Required: Bing.com Prescription Drug Ads," Legitscript and Knujon, August 2009, www.legitscript.com/BingRxReport.pdf.
Ninety percent of prescription drug and online pharmacy ads on the Bing.com search engine lead to "rogue" pharmacies, many of which don't require prescriptions to dispense controlled drugs, according to groups that accredit Internet pharmacies and monitor regulatory compliance of Web-based companies.

"Prescription Drug Overdose: State Health Agencies Respond," Centers for Disease Control and Prevention/Association of State and Territorial Health Officials, 2008, www.cdc.gov/HomeAndRecreationalSafety/Poisoning/prescription_overdose.html.
State public-health officials describe efforts to stem the rise in mortality from prescription drugs that has occurred since 1999, focusing on nine states, including several with the highest death rates.

"Under the Counter: The Diversion and Abuse of Controlled Prescription Drugs in the U.S.," National Center on Addiction and Substance Abuse at Columbia University, July 2005, www.casacolumbia.org.
Prescription-drug abuse has crept upward over the past two decades, even as abuse of other substances has dropped. Only 19 percent of physicians, however, say they've been educated about how to prevent diversion of prescription drugs to illegal use.

The Next Step:

Additional Articles from Current Periodicals

Abusers

Al-Husaini, Mudhafer, and Erica Goode, "Increasingly, Iraqi Soldiers Are Abusing Prescription Drugs to Endure Stress of War," *The New York Times*, Dec. 21, 2008, p. A28.
The stresses of war and lack of strict government regulation have led more Iraqi soldiers to abuse prescription drugs.

Mariano, Willoughby, "Prescription-Drug Overdoses on the Rise," *Orlando Sentinel*, July 2, 2009, p. B2.
Florida deaths caused by anti-anxiety drugs and painkillers surpassed those from cocaine in 2008, according to a commission of state medical examiners.

Newhouse, Eric, "Prescription Drugs 'Newest Monster' in Indian Country," *Great Falls Tribune*, July 10, 2009, p. 1A.
Prescription-drug abuse is continually increasing among American Indians across northern Montana.

Waters, TaMaryn, "Prescription Drug Abuse Among Teens Stays Steady," *Tallahassee Democrat*, Nov. 18, 2008, p. 10A.
About 5 percent of Florida high-school seniors have reported abusing prescription drugs, more or less the same percentage as in 2002.

Law Enforcement

Bush, Rudolph, "Doctor Faces Federal Charges in 14 Fatal Overdoses," *Chicago Tribune*, May 23, 2007, p. 7.
A Chicago doctor allegedly dispensed narcotic pain medication illegally, resulting in 14 overdose deaths.

Fausset, Richard, "The Nation; Sunshine State has Become a Magnet for Pain Pill Buyers; Florida's Regulation Void is Causing Drug Troubles in Appalachia," *Los Angeles Times*, April 25, 2009, p. 17.
Appalachian prescription-drug addicts take advantage of poorly regulated "pain clinics" in Florida, the largest state without a prescription-monitoring program.

"Painkiller Prescriptions Highest in Eastern Kentucky, Report Says," *Los Angeles Times*, Jan. 20, 2003, p. 18.
From 1998 to 2001, legal drug outlets in eastern Kentucky received the most prescription painkillers per capita in the nation, resulting in skyrocketing possession and trafficking charges and many more addicts in treatment.

Pain Treatment

Haskell, Meg, "Proposed Law Seeks to Limit Painkiller Abuse," *Bangor Daily News* (Maine), July 22, 2009, p. B1.
Doctors propose formal patient-physician contracts, random pill counts and urine tests to detect the abuse or diversion of prescription drugs.

Jamison, Michael, "Treating Pain Can be a Tricky Business," *Ventura County Star* (California), July 9, 2009.
Doctors call for a national narcotic data bank to prevent patients from "doctor shopping" to obtain multiple prescriptions.

Klein, Jeffrey S., "Chronic Pain Sufferers Deserve Treatment with Dignity," *Battle Creek Enquirer* (Michigan), June 22, 2008, p. 7A.
The Drug Enforcement Administration (DEA) has too much power to limit the amount and types of drugs, particularly narcotic drugs, that physicians prescribe, causing doctors to under-prescribe painkillers to avoid investigation.

Regulations

Boutselis, Kirk, "Lowell Unites to Combat Drug Abuse," *Lowell Sun*, April 16, 2009.
A Massachusetts state legislator is calling for increased regulation of prescription drugs to end fake prescriptions.

Del Marcus, Jonathan, "Resolution Takes Aim at Prescription Drug Abuse," *Sun-Sentinel*, April 30, 2009, p. 9.
The city of Oakland Park, Fla., has unanimously approved a resolution urging the state legislature to pass a bill curtailing the abuse of prescription drugs.

Pramik, Mike, "Pending Law Will Regulate Online Prescription-Drug Sales," *Columbus* (Ohio) *Dispatch*, Oct. 12, 2008, p. 14A.
Congress recently approved the Ryan Haight Online Pharmacy Consumer Protection Act, which curbs the illegal sale of prescription drugs over the Internet.

CITING *CQ RESEARCHER*

Sample formats for citing these reports in a bibliography include the ones listed below. Preferred styles and formats vary, so please check with your instructor or professor.

MLA STYLE

Jost, Kenneth. "Rethinking the Death Penalty." CQ Researcher 16 Nov. 2001: 945-68.

APA STYLE

Jost, K. (2001, November 16). Rethinking the death penalty. *CQ Researcher, 11*, 945-968.

CHICAGO STYLE

Jost, Kenneth. "Rethinking the Death Penalty." *CQ Researcher*, November 16, 2001, 945-968.

CHAPTER

3

Caring for Veterans

By Peter Katel

Excerpted from the CQ Researcher. Peter Katel. (April 23, 2010). "Caring for Veterans." *CQ Researcher*, 361-384.

Caring for Veterans

BY PETER KATEL

THE ISSUES

The car bomb exploded at dusk. Its target — a seven-ton U.S. Army personnel carrier — was blown about six feet by the force of the blast. Infantryman John Lamie came out alive, thanks to armor plating around his machine-gunner's cupola, but three of his buddies died in the Aug. 3, 2005, attack in Baghdad. Lamie went to Iraq a second time in 2007-2008, before the cumulative effects of combat eventually pushed him out of the Army.

Now he's fighting another kind of battle — with the Department of Veterans Affairs (VA). "I did two tours in Iraq and half my squad died," he says from his home in Cecil, Ga., only to "come home and get treated like a piece of crap in my own state."

Because of a series of complications over the validity of disability exams Lamie took for post-traumatic stress disorder (PTSD), traumatic brain injury (TBI) and other conditions, Lamie's most recent disability check amounted to $83.19. He and his wife have three children, and he's paying child support for a fourth child with his ex-wife.

Lamie says that when he tried to straighten out his case with staff of the VA's Veterans Benefits Administration (VBA), he ran into a wall of indifference. "The vet has no power, you are left to the wind," Lamie says. "You have to call and beg — I don't mean ask nicely, I mean beg — and I don't feel any vet should have to beg somebody to do their damn job."

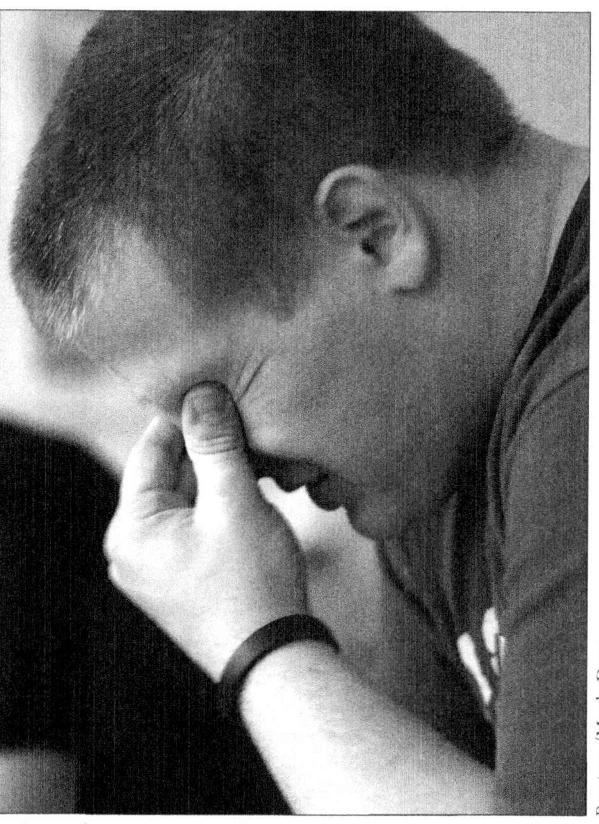

Reuters/Mark Dye

Eric Johnson, a scout from the 10th Mountain Division stationed at Fort Drum, near Watertown, N.Y., shares painful wartime experiences with friends at a coffeehouse catering to vets on April 16, 2008. Soldiers in Johnson's division have been deployed in Iraq and Afghanistan multiple times. Repeated deployments are creating an unprecedented number of cases of post-traumatic stress disorder, traumatic brain injury and associated mental-health conditions — overwhelming mental-health professionals in veterans' health care facilities.

However, by late April, Lamie had found a VA staffer who was trying to straighten out bureaucratic confusion involving multiple files shipped among multiple offices. "Fingers crossed," Lamie says. "Within another two months something might work itself out." He emphasizes "might."

Veterans' advocates, the Government Accountability Office (GAO) and the VA's own inspector general have all reported similar communications breakdowns and wildly varying standards for evaluating disability claims among VBA regional offices, even as a steady stream of new claims pours into the VA.

Soldiers wounded while serving their country "are waiting — and waiting — for the help they have been promised," said Rep. Bob Filner, D-Calif., chairman of the House Veterans' Affairs Committee, after meeting with agency officials and veterans' organizations in March. "Frankly, it's an insult to our veterans and their service." [1]

About 1 million claims of all kinds are backlogged at the VA, according to veterans' organizations, some of which help veterans on behalf of the VA, which says the backlog of initial claims alone totals 500,000, using a different calculation method.

While VA medical care, delivered through the Veterans Health Administration, tends to earn high marks from vets, the VBA presents a different picture. In 2007-2008, staff at VBA regional offices compiled an overall accuracy record on initial claims decisions of only 77 percent, Belinda J. Finn, VA deputy inspector general, told the House Veterans' Disability Assistance and Memorial Affairs Subcommittee in early March. "This equates to approximately . . . 203,000 total claims where veterans' monthly benefits may be incorrect," Finn told the subcommittee. [2]

The VA's scramble to meet mounting demand for its services is occurring amid continuing warfare on two fronts: Since U.S. forces entered Afghanistan in 2001, at least 5,190 service members have been wounded, 425 of them this year. Since the 2003 U.S. invasion of Iraq, 31,176 service members have been wounded there. [3]

Yet the VA's difficulties providing adequate care for veterans got only sporadic attention until 2007, when a

Brain Injuries Put Strain on VA Benefits

Nearly 91,000 U.S. soldiers have either died, been wounded or medically evacuated for noncombat-related reasons thus far in the Iraq and Afghanistan wars (top). The 760,000 veterans who suffer from either post-traumatic stress disorder (PTSD) or traumatic brain injury (TBI), or both, have put the Veterans Benefits Administration under increasing pressure to meet the needs of the country's injured veterans.

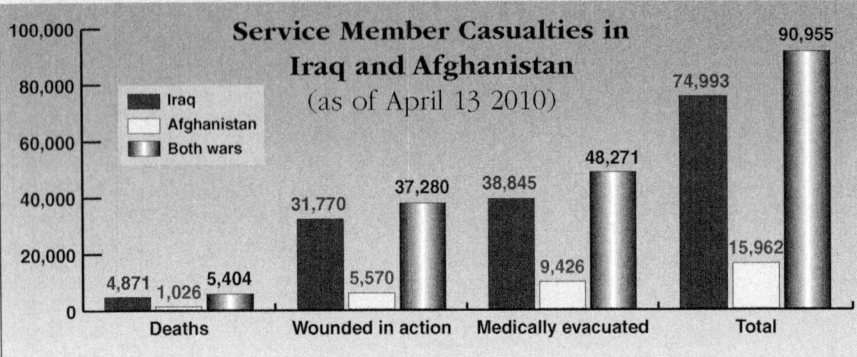

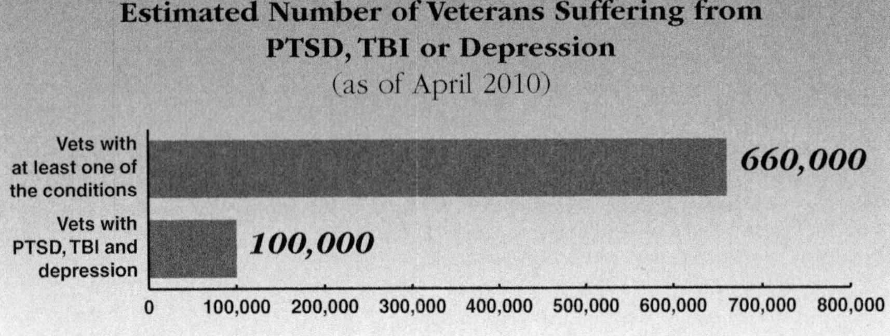

Sources: Veterans for Common Sense; RAND Center for Military Health Policy Research, 2008, www.rand.org/pubs/monographs/MG720

prize-winning *Washington Post* series pushed them to the top of the national agenda. (*See "Background," p. 375.*) With the issue in the spotlight, Congress in 2008 authorized free medical care for all Iraq and Afghanistan veterans for five years after leaving the military. And GI Bill educational benefits were expanded for veterans who entered the service after the Sept. 11, 2001, terrorist attacks.

Vets welcomed the new benefits, but questioned the VBA's ability to process all the new claims. The VA's new boss, retired Gen. Eric K. Shinseki, is vowing to shake up the agency. "2010 is my year to focus on finding and breaking the obstacles that deny us faster and better processing and higher quality outcomes," he told the Veterans of Foreign Wars in early March. To break the backlog while dealing with a rush of expected new claims, he proposes adding 4,000 claims examiners in the 2010-2011 fiscal year. [4]

His appointees aren't mincing words about what they found when they took over. "In my judgment, it cannot be fixed," Peter Levin, the VA's chief technology officer, said of the benefits claims system during a March meeting on Capitol Hill with veterans' organizations. (*See sidebar, p. 372.*) "We need to build a new system, and that is exactly what we are going to do." [5]

Veterans' advocates cheered Levin's comments and praise Shinseki's vision, but some wonder if he can put his stamp on the VA. A West Point graduate who lost most of a foot in Vietnam combat, Shinseki has earned a reputation for speaking out regardless of consequences. As Army chief of staff, he told the Senate Armed Services Committee in 2003 that securing Iraq after invading it would require "something on the order of several hundred thousand soldiers." Shinseki's civilian boss, Defense Secretary Donald Rumsfeld, contemptuously brushed that assessment aside and marginalized its author. But time proved Shinseki more accurate than Rumsfeld, who endorsed a forecast of 30,000-50,000 troops in Iraq after the invasion. By fiscal year 2008, U.S. troop strength had reached nearly 160,000. [6]

Now, Shinseki's leading an agency trying to adjust to the special demands created by 21st-century warfare. Vast advances in battlefield care are enabling thousands of vets to survive injuries that would have been fatal in the past. But those injuries, often caused by homemade bombs, or so-called improvised explosive devices (IEDs), can be crippling.

"IED blasts alone often cause multiple wounds, usually with severe injuries to extremities, and traumatic brain and other blast injuries, and they leave many . . . with serious physical, psychological and cognitive injuries," the government-funded Institute of Medicine (IOM) reported to Congress in a lengthy study published in March. [7]

Today's all-volunteer military is far smaller than past draftee-fed forces, requiring troops to be repeatedly recycled through combat zones. About a third of those who have been deployed to combat more than once have suffered from PTSD, TBI or major depression, and about 5 percent suffered from all three, according to the RAND Corp, a California think tank. Multiple deployments can double the risk of PTSD and other psychological problems, the Army surgeon general concluded in a 2008 report, which found mental health problems in 12 percent with one deployment and 27 percent with three or more deployments. [8]

Retired Army Capt. Anthony Kennedy, who attempted suicide after two tours in Iraq, described the nature of the fighting there and the psychological effects of the constant threat of being blown up by an IED. "One of my friends . . . had a friend whose arms and legs were blown off," Kennedy says. "All of us combat guys are thinking, 'Why do I want to go through life with no arms and no legs?' Our consensus: 'Can my battle buddy just put a bullet in me?' We talk about that."

Appeals Take Longer Than Claims

The average processing time to complete a veteran's compensation claim in 2008 was nearly 200 days, more or less the same since 2003. Finalizing appeals, however, took nearly four times longer — a constant trend since 2000.

Average Days to Complete Compensation Claims, FY 2000-2008

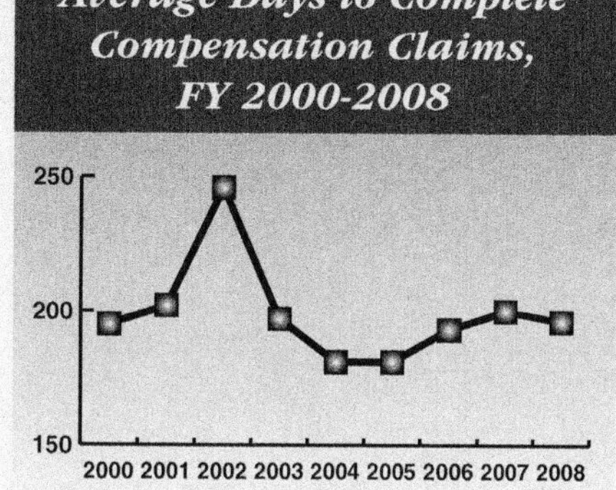

Average Days to Process Compensation Appeals, FY 2000-2008

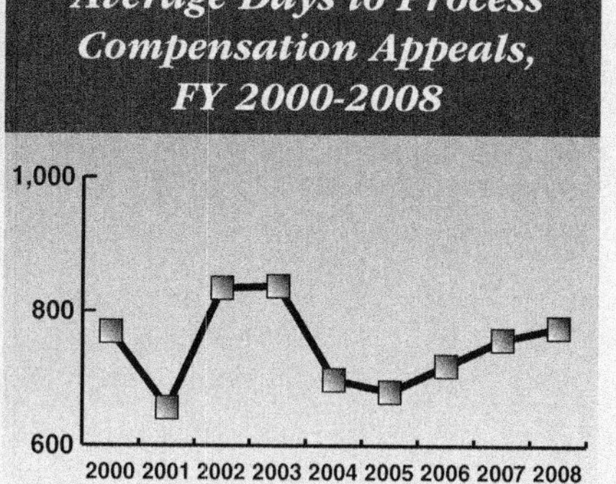

Source: "Veterans' Disability Benefits," Government Accountability Office, January 2010

Kennedy has had problems with the VA benefits system as well, but obtained a volunteer lawyer's help in pushing his PTSD rating from 30 percent to 70 percent disability. He says his 17 years in the service taught him how to deal with military-style bureaucracy. "I have the maturity and the knowledge to know that there's 100,000 applications out there, and I'm just one cog in the wheel," he says. "But I can imagine that if someone is completely disabled, and their father or mother comes in, the system can be a shock."

Even military reservists, accustomed to part-time service, can be taken aback by the VA system they encounter after active duty. Naval reservist Richard Sanchez of New York, a former paralegal for a Wall Street law firm, was discharged after his second deployment, which took him to Kuwait, where he was injured when an ammunition and weapons container fell on him in 2005.

After discharge, Sanchez began to suffer intense back pain, failing memory and depression. In his confused state, the VA system overcame him, he says. Eventually, he encountered a VA counselor who helped him straighten out a long series of bureaucratic complications, and in March received a letter from the VA apologizing for erroneous ratings and promising to reevaluate claims for PTSD, TBI and depression.

"I don't hate the VA," says Sanchez, who is attending college thanks to VA education benefits. "There are some faults there, but you can't blame the whole system."

That system is about to be tested even more forcefully. The VA is predicting that its claims workload will rise 30 percent next fiscal year, to about 1.3 million, in part because the department added three new ailments to the list of illnesses presumed to result from exposure to the Vietnam-era defoliant known as Agent Orange. And more "presumptive" illnesses associated with exposure to other battleground chemicals in more recent wars may be added later this year. (*See "Current Situation," p. 376.*) [9]

Still, it won't be easy to convince veterans that the VA has turned a new page. In Georgia, Iraq vet Lamie is trying to keep his family fed, his lights on and his car running on the small checks he receives now. "I've still got no faith in VA" — for now, he says.

As veterans' disablity claims mount, here are some of the questions being debated:

Is the VA benefits system broken beyond repair?

Vietnam vet Elmer A. Hawkins filed a claim for disability benefits in 1990. Repeated errors by Regional Office (RO) staffers kept his case — based on exposure to Agent Orange decades earlier while serving in Vietnam — bouncing between them and VA appeals boards.

Last year Hawkins tried to inject some urgency into the proceedings. He asked the Court of Appeals for the Federal Circuit to order the VA to finally decide his case. But the court rejected the request. After all, wrote Judge Haldane Robert Mayer, a decorated Vietnam combat veteran, "The RO may yet grant Hawkins VA benefits." [10]

However, the fact that the case has been pending for 20 years shocked U.S.

District Judge Claudia Wilken of Oakland, Calif. — a stranger to the VA benefits system and its slow-moving clock. Serving temporarily on the federal circuit, Judge Wilken wrote in a dissenting opinion that the VA had "made repeated errors which have prolonged the decision-making process." These errors "cannot be excused as products of a burdened system." [11]

Hawkins' wait was unusually long. But years-long battles over claims aren't at all unusual, say experts on the system. Barton Stichman, joint executive director of the nonprofit National Veterans Legal Services Program, testified last year that the first step alone in the appeal process took an average of 563 days in fiscal 2007-2008. "Frustrated veterans have to wait many years before receiving a final decision on their claims," Stichman told the House Veterans' Disability Assistance and Memorial Affairs Subcommittee. [12]

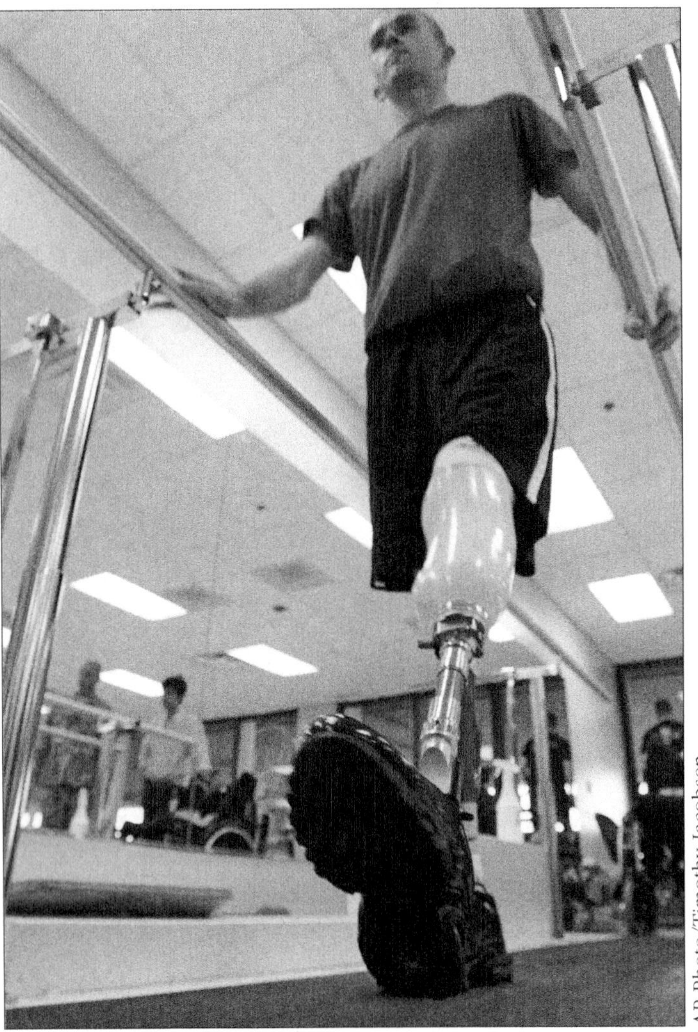

AP Photo/Timothy Jacobsen

Double amputee Bradley Walker practices walking on his new prosthetic legs, using a moving sidewalk at Walter Reed Army Medical Center in Washington, D.C., on April 4, 2007. Wounded veterans' benefit claims are projected to rise 30 percent next fiscal year, to about 1.3 million, in part because additional illnesses are being classified as caused by military service, including ailments linked to the Agent Orange defoliant used during the Vietnam War.

Meanwhile, claims pile up in the system. "This massive backlog has resulted in a six-month average wait for an initial rating decision, and a two-year average wait for an appeal decision," Thomas J. Tradwell, commander in chief of Veterans of Foreign Wars, testified in March to a joint hearing of the Senate and House Veterans' Affairs committees. "That is completely unacceptable." [13]

Finn of the VA inspector general's office cited the 22 percent error rate in regional office disability assessments when she testified that even VA staffers assigned to identify mistakes compiled an imperfect record. "They either did not thoroughly review available medical and non-medical evidence or identify the absence of necessary medical information," Finn told the Disability Assistance and Memorial Affairs Subcommittee. "Without an effective and reliable quality assurance program, VBA leadership cannot adequately monitor performance to make necessary program improvements and ensure veterans receive accurate and consistent ratings." [14]

Getting a disability rating is the key to the process. Veterans like Hawkins who claim their illnesses or conditions were "service-connected" must prove that connection. The VBA's staff then state their conclusions in the form of ratings — such as that a veteran is 50 percent disabled because of an event that occurred while in the military.

"A vet fills out a 23-page claim form, then VHA sends it to the VBA office and it takes six months to get an answer," says Paul Sullivan, executive director of Veterans for Common Sense, which has sued the VA over the workings of the benefit system. "And the appeals process takes four-five years. That's unconscionable. VBA leaders failed, and they crashed the agency. It has suffered catastrophic meltdown."

A Gulf War veteran who worked at VBA in the 1990s, Sullivan praises the VA's new leaders but says even they cannot save the VBA without replacing it with an entirely new agency. With a war ongoing in Afghanistan, 98,000 troops still deployed in Iraq, the recent expansion of benefits for victims of Agent Orange and the proposed addition of other chemical exposures to the "presumptives" list, he says, "VBA is overwhelmed. It's broken beyond repair." [15]

Other veterans' advocates agree but not on Sullivan's proposed solution. "I got an e-mail yesterday from a vet who's been fighting with the VA for six years," says Tom Tarantino, legislative associate for Iraq and Afghanistan Veterans of America (IAVA). The organization is pressing for greater efficiency and accuracy in the benefits process.

But Tarantino says the current VA leadership is making great strides. "The VA has in the last year been incredibly aggressive in trying to address this issue" of claims processing, he says. "They have put in place a very solid, ambitious plan to upgrade the workflow, management, technology and customer service. Our challenge in the veterans' community is making sure that what we push and what Congress introduces do not interfere with actual progress at VA."

That big-picture perspective may not reassure veterans who are dealing with the current system. "When you contact people at these ROs [regional offices], they don't want to hear they did something wrong," says injured Iraq veteran Lamie, who has been disputing his 50 percent disability rating since shortly after retiring from the Army late last year. "Instead of coming together with the vet and going through it page by page and seeing what went wrong, they blow you off, because you did something wrong — not them. You are left to the wind."

David E. Autry, deputy national communications director of Disabled American Veterans (DAV), agrees that some veterans encounter a lack of cooperation from some VA staffers. "It's clearly in the law that the VA has a 'duty to assist' the veteran," he says. "But in many cases we find that the VA is throwing up unnecessary roadblocks: 'You need to provide me with a documentary statement,' and you turn it in, and the VA loses it."

The VA benefits system, Autry says, "has been approaching critical mass for some time." Still, he says, "The good news is that the VA seems to be committed to making things work differently."

Is the VA adjusting to the needs of 21st-century combat and technology?

The wars in Afghanistan ("Operation Enduring Freedom") and Iraq ("Operation Iraqi Freedom") have already lasted longer than World War II, which for the United States ran from 1941 to 1945. The wars also are presenting the VA with a new constellation of disabilities, along with heightened veteran expectations of government efficiency and attention.

Today's veterans grew up with the Web and with speedy online shopping. These experiences don't prepare them for dealing with the VA. "FedEx can track where your package is," Rep. Phil Roe, R-Tenn., ranking Republican on the House Veterans Affairs Oversight and Investigations Subcommittee, told VA technology officials last February. "You can order your coat from L.L. Bean and you know exactly where it is before it gets to you. Will it be possible when a veteran puts in for their benefits to track where their claim is with this current system that we're setting up?" [16]

"Absolutely," said Roger Baker, the VA's assistant secretary for information and technology, citing work on a system for tracking education benefits planned for release this fiscal year. The VA will eventually have "a Web site to which veterans can come and see the exact status of their claim from the point where it's received by the VA . . . to the point where the check is cut and sent to the veteran, and it will tell them everywhere along the process where they sit." [17]

But the technology gap is only part of the problem. The nature and severity of today's injuries also complicate the VA's job. Most casualties are caused by IEDs, the favorite enemy weapon in both conflicts. Victims of these powerful bombs may lose limbs, which typically aren't protected by torso-covering body armor. And even troops who avoid penetrating wounds may suffer harder-to-detect brain injuries.

Thanks to recent advances in battlefield care, "more service members survive to return home with severe combat-related injuries that require additional care," the Institute of Medicine concludes in a new research report. [18]

And repeated deployments are causing a growing incidence of PTSD and associated mental-health conditions, including depression. Veterans' demand for psychological services is outpacing the availability of mental-health professionals in areas with large vet populations, according to the IOM. [19]

Furthermore, family members increasingly must care full time for the growing number of vets who survive injuries that would have killed soldiers in earlier wars. The Wounded Warrior Project, a Jacksonville, Fla.-based nonprofit, estimates that the families of 2,000 severely disabled Iraq and Afghanistan veterans are now caring for them full time. [20]

"But the department has no systematic Family Caregiver Program," Anna Frese, sister of a severely brain-injured survivor of an IED attack in Iraq, told the House Veterans Affairs' Health Subcommittee last year. (*See sidebar, p. 374.*) "It has mounted some pilot programs. But overall, our experience is that very little institutional attention is being paid to family caregivers even though they are a vital link in the veteran's lifelong rehabilitation process. Families are coping largely on their own." [21]

The VA doesn't support the comprehensive caregiver support program that Frese, the Wounded Warrior Project and other nonprofits advocate, which would provide financial support and health coverage for caregivers. One point of dispute is the agency's insistence that family care be overseen by a VA staff member or contractor, who, an official implied, would be more objective in dealing with the disabled patient. "Health-care providers maintain their relationships on a professional level," Dr. Madhulika Agarwal, chief of patient care services for the

Backlog Claims Increase After Afghanistan, Iraq

After the war in Afghanistan began in 2001, compensation claims to the Veterans Administration nearly doubled. The pace picked up again after the start of the war in Iraq. Claims pending for more than six months have remained relatively constant.

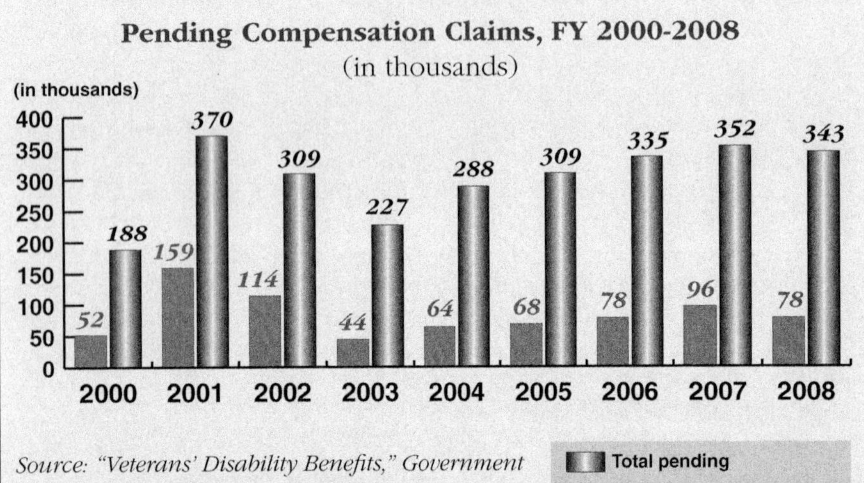

Source: "Veterans' Disability Benefits," Government Accountability Office, January 2010

VA's Veterans Health Administration, told the Health subcommittee. [22]

More recently, the VA has said it needs more information before proposing any policies and programs. "VA does not have adequate information on the number of caregivers, the number of family caregivers and the number of veterans receiving . . . services from family caregivers," says the agency's budget proposal for fiscal 2010-2011. [23]

The effects of intense combat during repeated deployments are showing up in another disturbing pattern. According to the most recent statistics available, suicides among young Iraq and Afghanistan veterans jumped 26 percent from 2005 to 2007, the VA reported early this year. [24]

Though the VA has strengthened its suicide-prevention programs, the agency's image among veterans lessens its effectiveness, according to M. David Rudd, dean of the University of Utah's College of Social and Behavioral Science. "It is important for the VA to recognize that they fight a longstanding image as an inflexible and unresponsive bureaucracy," Rudd told the Senate Veterans Affairs Committee in March. [25]

Seventy percent of veterans shun VA help, said Rudd, a specialist in military suicide. He urged the agency to establish partnerships with other mental-health providers. "Expansion of the existing VA system may not be the most effective expenditure of available funds," he testified. [26]

But, a top VA official countered at the same hearing, "Young veterans receiving VA care are significantly less likely to commit suicide than those not receiving VA care." Gerald M. Cross, acting principal deputy undersecretary for health, cited U.S. Centers for Disease Control and Prevention statistics showing a drop from 39 suicides per 100,000 in 2001 to 35 per 100,000 in 2007 among patients of VA health services, a decline equivalent to about 250 lives saved. [27]

Nevertheless, another VA mental health specialist said the VA is open to joining forces with other organizations, by contract or other arrangements. "We need to have partnerships," said Antoinette Zeiss, associate chief consultant for mental health. "We can't do it alone. If there is a level of care that VA is not able to provide in rural or in urban or suburban settings we should look for . . . well-tested programs." [28]

Before declaring that policy, Zeiss conceded that suicide-prevention programs have only recently been strengthened. For vets in danger of suicide, "We have instituted throughout the system far more intensive outpatient programs, so that instead of one, one-hour-a-week session," Zeiss said, "there are at least three hours a day, three days a week with an interdisciplinary team trying to deliver very complex and intensive services." [29]

Is the VA improving rapidly enough?

Debates about the quality of veterans' services are taking place amid a notable change in climate from the days of the Bush administration. Widespread agreement prevails that the VA's new leadership genuinely wants to make deep improvements and has the organizational competence to do so.

Under the Bush administration, even those who defended the VA against steadily increasing criticism from Iraq and Afghanistan vets didn't deliver more than pro-forma praise of top VA leaders. In October, 2007, under the pressure of months of revelations of substandard and inadequate care from the VA, VA Secretary James Nicholson, who had headed the agency since 2005, resigned. [30]

Shinseki's experience with the Bush-era Defense Department and his Vietnam service gave him considerable credibility in the veteran community. And he named as one of his assistant secretaries L. Tammy Duckworth, a former Illinois Veterans Affairs director and Illinois National Guard helicopter pilot who lost both legs in Iraq in 2004.

Measured by the size of his proposed new budget — an important gauge of intentions and administration support — Shinseki is planning to follow through on his modernization vows. He's asking for an increase of $9.4 billion in discretionary spending in fiscal 2011 — a 20 percent hike at a time of spending cutbacks and only modest increases elsewhere in government. [31]

Shinseki faced an early test in September, 2009, when the VA failed to send out scheduled checks to about 277,000 college-bound vets who had qualified for GI Bill education benefits. As the VA showed itself incapable of processing the payments on time, some vets were forced to borrow money or take other emergency measures. [32]

Shinseki ordered the agency to issue emergency checks of up to $3,000 and to distribute them to veterans at VA offices around the country. The fast action and acknowledgement of error struck many veterans' affairs specialists as a new approach. Shinseki explicitly endorsed that view. "We will change the [VA] culture," Shinseki told the House Veterans Affairs Committee three weeks later. "I assure you of that." [33]

Nevertheless, debate is still running strong on whether the agency's new leaders can transform the 300,000-employee department quickly enough to make a difference to the steadily growing ranks of veterans who depend on the VA.

Where benefits decision appeals are concerned, "The quality of decision-making hasn't improved," says Stichman of the National Veterans Legal Services Program. "It's in the same bad state."

Shinseki, he says, "does sound like he's intelligent and really wants to do something." But, the veterans-law expert says, "It's very difficult for a secretary to shake the bureaucracy. Can he get the lieutenants to follow orders?"

Autry of Disabled American Veterans acknowledges that giant institutions don't adapt to change easily or quickly. But the new leaders' determination is making a difference, he says. "The VA seems to be committed to making things work differently," he says.

To be sure, Autry, a Navy veteran of the Vietnam War, is also dissatisfied with the pace of transformation. "But this is an aircraft carrier," he says of the VA. "You don't just spin the wheel and turn it around."

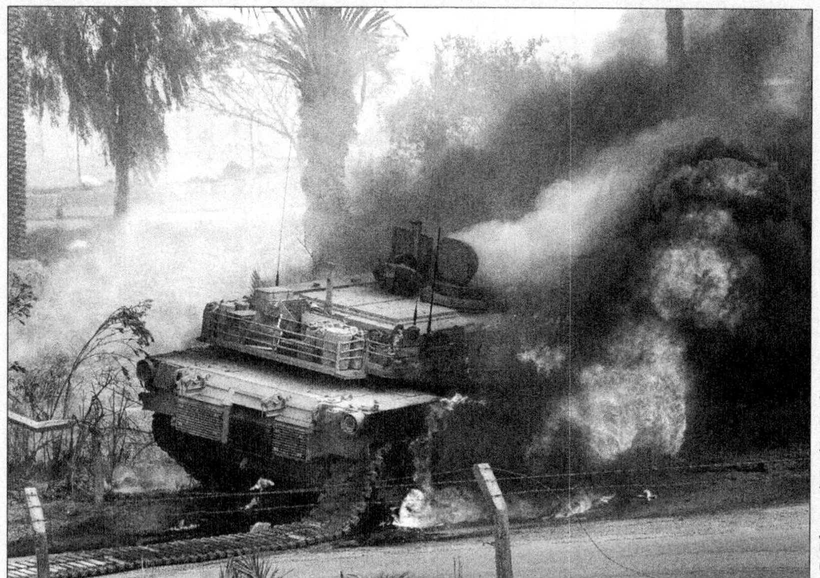

AP Photo/Hadi Mizban

AP Photo/Eric Gay

IED Aftermath

Flames engulf a U.S. Army tank in Baghdad, Iraq, after it was struck by a homemade roadside bomb known as an improvised explosive device (IED) (top). Its crew escaped unharmed from the March 10, 2006, explosion, but Marine Sgt. Merlin German (bottom left), being promoted by Lt. Gen. James F. Amos (right) on May 21, 2007, suffered burns on 97 percent of his body after his vehicle struck an IED in Iraq. Blasts from IEDs — widely used by insurgents in both Iraq and Afghanistan — often cause multiple wounds, usually with severe injuries to extremities.

But Sullivan of Veterans for Common Sense urges against accepting sluggishness as a given. "We're generally opposed to more layers of bureaucracy," he says. "But the agency has grown, and in order for Mr. Shinseki to leave his mark he is going to have to bring in new leaders."

Furthermore, growing pressures on the VA demand accelerated response, Sullivan says. The military is discharging a steady stream of combat veterans, at the same time as new data emerge that point to wartime conditions as causes of ailments suffered by Gulf War and Vietnam vets. "Right now is the pivotal moment," he says. "Will we repeat the mistakes of how horribly mistreated Vietnam and Gulf War veterans were when they came home?"

At least some of those veterans are still inclined to trust that Shinseki is moving as fast as possible, based on improvements already in place. "From my experience with the VA, from 2005 to now, there has been great change," says retired Capt. Kennedy, who served two tours in Iraq.

Kennedy won his fight to increase his PTSD disability rating to 70 percent, though he is still dealing with what he calls a VA error that cost him $13,000 in retirement pay — which he expects to recoup. He attributes part of his success to the free legal representation he received though the National Veterans Legal Services program.

However, he adds, "By hiring Gen. Shinseki as secretary, the Obama administration made a statement that they are committed to disabled veterans. People like me can see light at the end of the tunnel, but I know I'll never be part of it." ■

BACKGROUND

The Big Change

Victory in World War II, the biggest armed conflict by far in U.S. history, brought a monumental shift in veterans' care and compensation. For the first time, they were given a major opportunity to improve their lives, not just tend to their injuries or subsist on tiny pensions.

The new doctrine may have been inevitable. To achieve victory, the United States had mobilized more than 16 million men (and accepted 210,000 female volunteers) for military service — many of them for the entire four-year span of the war. More than 405,000 were killed, and more than 671,000 wounded. [34]

To be sure, veterans hadn't been ignored before World War II. Long before, Congress and the executive branch had established a series of institutions and systems designed to provide care and compensation. These included the Asylum for Disabled Volunteer Soldiers, created (under another name) in 1865, at the end of the Civil War, and the Consolidation Act of 1873, which set up a pension system based on the degree of disability, replacing a scale based on rank.

Of the 4.7 million men mobilized during World War I, 204,000 were wounded (and 116,000 were killed). But the veterans' system wasn't up to the challenge. In 1924, Congress made matters worse. Lawmakers created a bonus designed to make up the difference between military pay and the high wages earned by civilians who'd spent the war working in essential industries. But the money was granted in the form of a bond that would mature in 1945, and after the Great Depression began in 1929, vets needed their bonus immediately. Up to 40,000 veterans and their families — called the Bonus Marchers — set up an encampment in Washington in 1932, only to see it destroyed by Army troops, an event that shocked the nation. [35]

Fourteen years later, as World War II drew to a close, the Franklin D. Roosevelt administration and Congress were determined to prevent a repeat of the Bonus March disaster. Instead, the Servicemen's Readjustment Act of 1944 — known forever after as the "GI Bill of Rights" — created a broad range of opportunities for veterans. [36]

Under the bill, the Veterans Administration paid all or most of the costs of college or vocational training, provided guarantees for no-down-payment mortgages or business loans and granted unemployment compensation for up to a year. When the GI Bill expired in 1956, 7.8 million vets had received education or training, and the VA had guaranteed 5.9 million home mortgages worth a total of $50.1 billion.

The GI Bill, widely considered one of the most far-reaching pieces of social legislation ever enacted, "gave veterans from less-advantaged backgrounds chances they had never dreamed possible and a route toward the middle class," wrote Suzanne Metler, a political science professor at Syracuse University, author of a book about the law. [37]

In 1952, Congress passed a second version of the bill for veterans of the Korean War, which had begun in 1950. The new law was slightly less generous: For example, it covered only three years of college expenses instead of all four, and provided a smaller tuition subsidy.

Meanwhile, the magnitude of the veteran population created by World War II and the Korean conflict led to a vast expansion of the VA medical system, which by the early 1950s was caring for about 2.5 million vets.

Vietnam's Neglected Vets

The Vietnam War influenced veteran law and policy every bit as deeply as World War II, even though the conflict was much smaller than World War II. [38]

By the time the fighting ended with victory for the communist government

Continued on p. 372

Chronology

1944-1950s

GI Bill of Rights, enacted in final days of World War I, becomes the standard for all subsequent veteran care policy.

1944
As World War II nears an end, Congress passes GI Bill to provide for education, home mortgages and business loans; allows millions of vets to move into the middle class.

1952
Korean War vets get their own, slightly downsized version of GI Bill.

1958
Veterans' unemployment insurance extended to peacetime draftees.

1967-1980s

Vietnam War gives rise to complaints of shoddy VA medical care; scientists begin evaluating evidence of psychological trauma from combat and physical damage from radiation and chemical exposure.

1967
Six Vietnam veterans form Vietnam Veterans Against the War (VVAW), which grows into the thousands and directs much anger at VA.

1970
Life magazine reports on rat-infested VA hospital in the Bronx, N.Y.

1973
Paraplegic vet Ron Kovic leads takeover of Democratic Sen. Alan Cranston's office to call attention to deplorable conditions at VA hospitals.

1979
Accumulating evidence of psychological troubles among Vietnam vets leads Congress to authorize opening of 92 "Vet Centers" for counseling and other assistance. . . . Years-long debate among psychiatrists leads to inclusion of newly named post-traumatic stress disorder (PTSD) in *Diagnostic and Statistical Manual of Mental Disorders.*

1981
U.S. District Court in Washington throws out VA regulation that effectively excludes 400,000 radiation-exposed World War II and postwar vets from claiming benefits for cancer and other disabilities.

1982
General Accounting Office reports that VA offices give short shrift to vets reporting physical symptoms from Agent Orange defoliant exposure.

1988
President Ronald Reagan signs law granting disability benefits to "atomic veterans" suffering from 13 (later 16) specific cancers.

1990s-2000s

VA benefits system begins to buckle under strain of disability claims arising from wars in the Persian Gulf and Afghanistan, as well as recognition of disabilities arising from Vietnam War.

1991
VA recognizes two cancers are linked to Agent Orange.

1992
Persian Gulf War ends; reports emerge of physical and psychological symptoms among up to 100,000 veterans of the conflict.

1997
Medical researchers hypothesize that exposure to combinations of pesticide and nerve gas gave rise to "Gulf War syndrome." . . . VA begins providing benefits for Vietnam vets' children born with spina bifida.

2002
U.S. troops in Afghanistan report first enemy use of improvised explosive devices (IEDs).

2007
IEDs found to have caused two-thirds of 3,100 U.S. combat deaths in Iraq since U.S. invasion of 2003. . . . *Washington Post* publishes series on substandard conditions for outpatients at Walter Reed Army Medical Center in Washington.

2008
Congress authorizes free medical care for Iraq/Afghanistan veterans for five years after leaving military. . . . RAND Corp. reports that about one-third of service members deployed to combat suffered from PTSD, traumatic brain injury or major depression. . . . Delay in considering appeals of VA ratings rises to 563 days.

2009
VA issues emergency checks after agency fails to send education benefits to 277,000 college-bound vets. . . . IEDs reported to cause 55 percent of amputations among combat casualties.

2010
VA technology chief calls claims-management system "broken beyond repair." . . . Compromise reached on legislation to aid families caring for severely disabled vets. . . . Institute of Medicine reports shortage of mental health services for vets and "evidence of association" between Persian Gulf War service and multisymptom illness.

VA Benefits to Get High-Tech Overhaul

Current system is 'hopelessly broken.'

Members of today's tech-savvy military have grown up being able to buy virtually any product online and have it shipped overnight. Instantaneous communication by text, voice and video has been part of their everyday lives.

And it's now part of their military service as well. "I was battle captain for a unit that oversaw all the transportation into Iraq," says retired Army Capt. Anthony Kennedy about his second deployment there in 2007-2008. "Each night we had 3,000 trucks on the road. I needed to know where every truck was at every second."

Shortly thereafter, however, Kennedy retired from the military and encountered the VA benefits system. Suddenly, he was back in the mid-20th century, dealing with paper forms filled out by hand and sent by mail. His reaction: "Let's let Amazon run it," referring to the huge online retailer Amazon.com.

The VA recognizes the problem. "We have a manual, paper-bounded system; what we want is an automated electronic system," says Peter L. Levin, the VA's new chief technology officer. He has initiated several pilot projects designed to become the new system's backbone.

Levin became a "rock star" among veterans' organizations, says Tom Tarantino, legislative associate for Iraq and Afghanistan Veterans of America, by acknowledging at a March meeting organized by the House Veterans' Services Committee that the present system is hopelessly broken and must be replaced. "He said some of the gutsiest things I've ever heard a VA person say in front of Congress," Tarantino adds. [1]

But Levin makes clear that he isn't promising the new system will be up and running tomorrow, or even next year. The deadline, set by VA Secretary Eric K. Shinseki, is 2015 (though parts of the system are scheduled to be online before then). "I come from the private sector, and I think I got this job based on a good reputation for on-time, on-budget deliveries," he says. "That is a reputation I intend to keep. I don't want to give unrealistic dates. The instructions are clear that if it is going to move in any direction it is going to be earlier, not later."

Levin was hired last year away from DAFCA Inc., which he cofounded and where he was CEO. The Framingham, Mass.-based firm designs software to test the reliability of computer chips and block malicious circuitry. Levin, who has a doctorate in electrical and computer engineering from Carnegie Mellon University in Pittsburgh, served as a White House fellow and as expert consultant in the Office of Science and Technology Policy in the Clinton administration. [2]

Paper won't entirely disappear from the redesigned system. Some records, Levin says, are too important to exist in purely digital form — birth and marriage certificates in the civilian world, for example. But medical scans and lists of medications should be digitized, he says.

Still, the planned improvements won't make dealing with the benefits system like dealing with Amazon. Kennedy notes that Amazon's customers get invited to buy specific books, music and other merchandise based on their records of past purchases. A VA version, he says, could tell a user, "Your ac-

Continued from p. 370

of North Vietnam in 1975, 3.4 million service members had been deployed to Southeast Asia. [39]

U.S. society divided sharply over the war; so did the veterans' community. In 1967, six returnees founded Vietnam Veterans Against the War, which grew over the years and held a series of high-profile demonstrations, including one in 1971 in which several thousand veterans threw their service decorations over a fence at the U.S. Capitol. [40]

Debate over the rights and wrongs of the Vietnam War faded somewhat with its end, but anger and bitterness among veterans over shoddy VA services and treatment grew steadily. The discontent eventually transcended political views on the war itself, but challenges to the VA came at first from antiwar vets.

In 1973, paraplegic vet Ron Kovic (later portrayed by Tom Cruise in the 1989 film, "Born on the Fourth of July") [41] led other severely disabled vets in a 17-day hunger strike and occupation of the Los Angeles office of Sen. Alan Cranston, D-Calif. They were publicizing appalling conditions at VA hospitals in Southern California. A Senate hearing produced testimony about neglect of patients, brutal retaliation against those who complained and violations of basic hygiene. The testimony mirrored a 1970 *Life* magazine exposé about a VA hospital in the Bronx, N.Y., which was plagued by rats, filth and deficient medical care.

Meanwhile, with far less public attention, a group of psychiatrists with ties to antiwar veterans had started trying to describe and define a condition that they'd noticed in many Vietnam returnees. Symptoms included sleep disturbance, anxiety and depression. Eventually, the psychiatrists proposed that the American Psychiatric Association add the condition — which colleagues were also seeing in disaster survivors — to a new edition of the *Diagnostic and Statistical Manual of Mental Disorders*, the bible of the mental-health profession.

The fight to include what eventually became known as post-traumatic stress disorder went on for more than four years. Like the military and the VA, much of the psychiatric establishment initially dismissed the idea that intense

count shows you've been treated for this, this and this — you should apply for this disability."

But Levin, while acknowledging the appeal of the Amazon model, argues that it's not a precise fit. Amazon sells mass-produced goods, with one copy of a book or CD, for instance, indistinguishable from another. "It turns out that every vet is a little different," he says. Nevertheless, a VA variant could produce data that allow a records examiner to see how vets with similar characteristics were treated.

For a veteran with a given list of claims, "I want to know what guys who are about your age and who served about where you served, and did things like you did while serving — I want to know what they're talking about that maybe you forgot," Levin says. And at some point, an examiner might be able to instantly access information on specific health and environmental conditions in given areas of operation.

Meanwhile, even the basic system is complicated enough to design and install that Levin is trying to improve the present system pending its replacement. "We do not have the option of turning off the system for six months and building a new one really quickly."

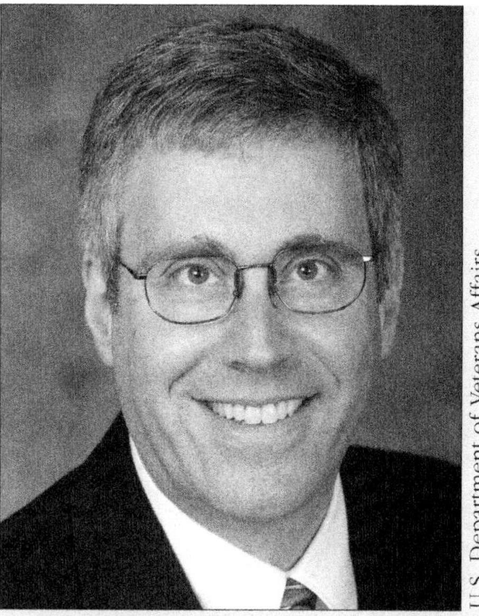

U.S. Department of Veterans Affairs

Peter L. Levin, the Department of Veterans Affairs' new chief technology officer, became an instant "rock star" among some veterans' organizations when he told Congress the VA benefits system is hopelessly broken and must be replaced.

For vets, the bottom line is that paper documents are still indispensable to dealing with the VA. Indeed, Richard Sanchez, a U.S. Navy veteran, says he's on his way to resolving four years of miscommunications with the VA, partly because he heeded an old sailor's advice.

"He said, 'Make copies of everything; doesn't matter if it's not important, it might be important later, it might have a date on it. And then make a copy, and then another copy.' I did that," says Sanchez, "and it was true. I have an archive at home, another with relatives and another one in a safe-deposit box."

— Peter Katel

[1] Rick Maze, "VA official: Disability claims system 'cannot be fixed,' " *Federal Times*, March 18, 2010, www.federaltimes.com/article/20100318/DEPARTMENTS04/3180302/1055/AGENCY.

[2] "Executive Biographies," U.S. Department of Veterans Affairs, undated, www1.va.gov/opa/bios; "Carnegie-Mellon Engineering Alumnus Peter L. Levin Named as Chief Technology Officer at U.S. Veterans Affairs," Carnegie Mellon University, press release, Aug. 3, 2009; John Markoff, "F.B.I. Says the Military Had Bogus Computer Gear," *The New York Times*, May 9, 2008, p. C4.

combat or other wartime experiences could produce serious disturbances in a well-adjusted individual. Troubled veterans suffered from conditions that afflicted them before they joined the military, the skeptics argued.

But mounting evidence weakened their position. In 1979, PTSD was added to the manual. The move marked the beginning of a change in outlook, eventually of global dimensions, about the deep effects of war and disaster.

In a more immediate sense, the PTSD debate influenced Congress to pass in 1979 (shortly before the definition was formally added to the manual) a bill to create 92 Vet Centers, where Vietnam returnees could obtain psychological counseling. In 1991, the centers were opened to all combat veterans of any conflict.

Chemicals and Radiation

Meanwhile, a major issue affecting Vietnam vets' physical health — and that of their children — was also emerging. In 1970, journalist Thomas Whiteside reported in *The New Yorker* that dioxin — the main ingredient of a defoliant nicknamed "Agent Orange" used in large quantities by U.S. forces to strip jungle cover in Vietnam — was a carcinogen. [42]

The article led the Pentagon to ban Agent Orange (the nickname came from the orange-banded barrels in which it was stored). But by then hundreds of thousands of vets already had been exposed. As the decade wore on, many developed diseases, including leukemia and other cancers, and were also reporting an unusual number of birth defects in their children.

Initially, the VA resisted vets' claims that Agent Orange was the cause of their symptoms. In 1982, a congressionally commissioned study by the General Accounting Office, now the Government Accountability Office (GAO), concluded that the VA had neglected the issue, for instance, taking medical histories from only 10 percent of the 90,000 vets who had filed Agent Orange-based claims.

Not until 1991 did the VA recognize links between two cancers — soft-tissue sarcoma and non-Hodgkin's lymphoma — and Agent Orange exposure. Several more were added in 1993, and still more in later years. And in 1997 — 22 years after the war

Full-time Caregiving Challenges Families

Families make huge sacrifices to deal with soldiers' catastrophic injuries.

For the Edmundsons of New Bern, N.C., veteran care is a family mission. On Oct. 2, 2005, Eric Edmundson, then a 25-year-old sergeant in the 172nd Stryker Brigade, took the impact of a roadside bomb, which sent shrapnel shooting into his brain and elsewhere in his body.

After emergency surgeries in Baghdad, the young soldier's heart stopped, depriving his brain of oxygen for a full 30 minutes. "Eric can't walk, talk; he has cognitive memory issues," says his father, Ed, from the family home, which used to house Eric, his wife Stephanie and their daughter, Gracie Rose, 5. Now Ed and his wife Beth live there as well.

"We downsized our lives to be here for Eric and Stephanie," says Ed, 52, who had worked as a warehouse supervisor at ConAgra Foods. "I took my retirement, burned down our debt load, basically got rid of all our possessions. We live in a bedroom in my son's house."

Eric returned to North Carolina after six months of intensive care and training at the Rehabilitation Institute of Chicago. His parents quickly realized that Eric would need full-time care, and that the load was too much for Stephanie to handle alone. [1] "There's a high rate of divorce among the injured," Eric's father says. "We don't want to allow that to happen. Eric has a beautiful family. What my wife and I do is take care of Eric, dealing with rehabilitation and his doctor visits. That allows Eric and Stephanie and Gracie to have as much of a life as possible."

Eric has been able to function more fully than initially expected. He is working as a greeter two days a week in a sporting-goods store. In January he attended the opening of a photo exhibit at the University of North Carolina, Wilmington, of images he took in Iraq before being wounded. He addressed the crowd using a computer voice-generating device. [2] The young family is expecting a second child.

As Eric napped on a recent afternoon, his father spoke by phone, recounting in a matter-of-fact tone the realities of life as a full-time caregiver. For one thing, Edmundson says, "We don't have any retirement or financial future."

Last year, after two bouts of pneumonia, he was able to see a doctor only because of financial help from Wounded Warriors Project, a Jacksonville, Fla.-based nonprofit. Another nonprofit, Homes For Our Troops, built a fully accessible house for the family. [3] "I can't imagine what we would be going through if we didn't have nonprofits," he says.

The Edmundsons' daughter, Anna Frese, has testified in support of legislation to provide financial support and health care to family caregivers (*see "Current Situation"*), and Edmundson too would welcome some help. "Some small compensation would allow us to get a change of clothes or service our vehicle," he says, "and health care insurance would keep me moving forward." Under the pending legislation, health care would be available only for him or his wife, not both of them.

Meanwhile, the Edmundsons are aware that they may represent only the first wave of families dealing with the aftereffects of catastrophic wounds "The war wasn't supposed to last this long," he says. "The system hadn't been tested. But if they're going to take these young men and women and send

ended — the VA began a program to provide medical benefits, vocational training and a monthly allowance for veterans' children born with spina bifida, one of the birth defects associated with exposure to the chemical.

But the long-running Agent Orange dispute was only one of several controversies surrounding service members' exposure to dangerous substances and atomic radiation.

World War II veterans, including thousands who had been assigned to clear rubble in Hiroshima and Nagasaki, Japan, after atomic bombs were dropped there, had filed about 1,500 claims for benefits, claiming adverse health consequences from the intense radiation they'd absorbed. Some survivors of deceased veterans also filed for death benefits. But the federal government long resisted paying for the claims; in 1979 the VA adopted a rule effectively rejecting 98 percent of claims by "atomic veterans." The group was substantial — 200,000 personnel who had been exposed to radiation in postwar Japan, and another 200,000 who had participated in atmospheric testing of atomic weapons. [43]

In 1981, U.S. District Judge June L. Green of Washington threw out that rule. Eventually, President Ronald W. Reagan signed a bill in 1988 establishing that atomic veterans suffering from 13 (later 16) specific kinds of cancers were automatically entitled to benefits. [44]

The Persian Gulf War of 1990-1991 prompted another wave of veteran medical concerns. About 100,000 of the 694,000 Gulf War veterans reported symptoms including fatigue, skin rash, headache, muscle and joint pain, memory loss, difficulty concentrating, shortness of breath, sleep disturbance, gastrointestinal problems and chest pain. Over the years, the number of vets reporting symptoms rose to 250,000.

Scientists and others advanced various hypotheses, including exposure to destroyed Iraqi stocks of sarin nerve gas, smoke from oil well fires or pesticides. Government-sponsored and private medical and environmental studies offered contradictory conclusions on whether an identifiable "Gulf War Syndrome" existed.

them to war, they'd better be able to take care of them. They need to ramp up post-trauma care and rehabilitation."

Though the family is relying on Eric's VA benefit payments and on his VA-financed health care, the entire care mission otherwise has been independent of the VA. Edmundson says he's found the agency peopled with dedicated staff but somewhat snarled in its own procedures.

"For the first three years I spent almost 100 percent of my time dealing with VA red tape," Edmundson says. "We did a lot of self-education. We'd get up in the morning, take care of Eric and get on the computer and research and talk to people: Why were you able to do this or that? Why are we not able?"

Dealing with the VA isn't for the passive, Edmundson has concluded. "If you don't plead your case, you fall through the cracks." The Edmundsons located the Chicago Rehabilitation Institute on their own, for instance, and found it superior to the VA hospital where Edmundson had been previously. The VA did, however, finance the cost of the private rehab program.

The deeper issue, Edmundson says he's come to believe, is that the VA — and the government in general — are only now starting to adjust to advances in rehabilitative medicine. "For years, the answer was to institutionalize the soldier," he says. "But the soldiers of today don't want to be taken care of, they want to be rehabilitated, they want to go home."

— Peter Katel

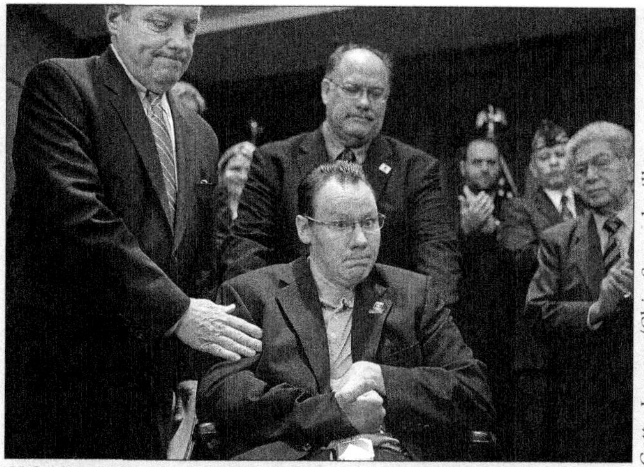

Getty Images/Chip Somodevilla

U.S. Army Specialist Eric Edmondson (center), who suffered a severe traumatic brain injury in Iraq in 2005, and his father Ed (top) appear at a Nov. 10, 2009, news conference in Washington, D.C., to discuss legislation to provide financial support and health care for family members caring for wounded vets full time. The Edmondsons, who sold their house and moved in with their son and his family in order to care for him, may represent the first wave of families dealing with the after-effects of catastrophic wounds. Senate Majority Whip Dick Durbin (D-Ill.) (left) thanks Edmondson for his sacrifice.

1 For a detailed account of Eric's stay at the Rehabilitation Institute, see "Eric Edmundson's Patient Story," Rehabilitation Institute of Chicago, undated, www.ric.org/aboutus/stories/EricEdmundson.aspx.

2 Ashley White, "Photo collection at UNCW illustrates life as a soldier," News14 Carolina, Jan. 10, 2010, http://news14.com/triad-news-94-content/military/620344/photo-collection-at-uncw-illustrates-life-as-a-soldier.

3 "Severely Wounded Army SGT Eric Edmundson Receives Specially Adapted Home from Homes for Our Troops," *Homes for Our Troops*, Nov. 5, 2007, www.homesforourtroops.org/site/News2?page=NewsArticle&id=5743.

Nevertheless, Gulf War veterans continued to report ailments, some of them serious. And after President George W. Bush ordered troops into Afghanistan in 2001, and into Iraq, in 2003, veterans of both wars began reporting similar ailments, leading the VA and Defense Department to focus more closely on the possible effects of chemical exposure from "burn pits" on military bases, where plastics, electronics, lubricants and medical waste were incinerated, among other things. *(See "Current Situation," p. 376.)* [45]

21st-Century Wounds

The nature of the wars in Afghanistan and Iraq, coupled with tremendous advances in battlefield medicine, produced significant increases in the numbers of severely disabled veterans. But some six years into the fighting, many began to question whether the military and VA were prepared for the consequences of the century's first two wars.

Initially, the focus was on the military. In 2007, *The Washington Post* published a devastating series of articles about conditions for injured service members recovering at Walter Reed Army Medical Center outpatient facilities in Washington, D.C. The exposé led to the firings of Army Secretary Francis Harvey and of the Walter Reed commander, Lt. Gen. George W. Weightman. Lt. Gen. Kevin Kiley, Army surgeon general and a former Walter Reed commander who initially had minimized *The Post*'s accounts, was also forced to resign. [46]

The Walter Reed scandal focused media and political attention on the treatment of veterans in general. President George W. Bush appointed former Sen. Robert Dole, R-Kan., a disabled World War II vet, and former Health and Human Services Secretary Donna Shalala to co-chair a commission to examine the entire veterans' health care system. The commission recommended simplifying the ratings system and improving care for TBI and PTSD, among other steps.

The commission blamed much of the problem on the kind of war U.S.

troops were fighting. Enemies in Iraq and Afghanistan were using IEDs as their major weapon. The bombs produce devastating effects without exposing the anti-American guerrillas to battlefield confrontations, in which U.S. forces held the advantage. Deployed as mines, packed into cars and trucks as well as bicycles and motorcycles, the bombs first appeared in Afghanistan in 2002 as radio-controlled roadside devices. But military officials planning the following year's invasion of Iraq didn't foresee the use of IEDs there, despite plentiful supplies of explosives.

By late 2007, IEDs were causing two-thirds of the 3,100 U.S. combat deaths registered through September of that year in Iraq. By then, IEDs had killed or wounded more than 21,000 Americans in Iraq. And by late 2009, the Pentagon calculated that the bombs accounted for up to 80 percent of U.S. and NATO casualties in Afghanistan. [47]

Aside from their appalling efficiency as killing machines, IEDs wrought damages on survivors that would have ended their lives in any previous war. Dramatic advancements in both the protective gear worn by soldiers and in military urgent care made the difference.

"This is the first war in which troops are very unlikely to die if they're still alive when a medic arrives," Dr. Ronald Glasser, who had treated troops wounded in Vietnam in 1968-1970, pointed out in *The Washington Post* in 2007. [48]

At that point, about 1,800 troops had survived brain injuries caused by penetrating wounds. But nearly a third of military personnel involved in heavy combat in Iraq or Afghanistan for at least four months were at risk of brain disorders from IED and mortar blasts. Symptoms of such shock-wave neurological disorders include memory loss, confusion, anxiety and depression, Glasser wrote. [49]

But the IEDs produced other types of injuries as well: As of mid-January, 2009, 1,184 U.S. personnel had suffered amputations, 55 percent of them the result of IED injuries. [50] ■

CURRENT SITUATION

'Presumptive' Diseases

In veterans' jargon, they're "presumptives" — certain diseases or conditions presumed by the VA to arise from military service in a certain time or place. In addition to having recently added to the list of ailments associated with exposure to Agent Orange in Vietnam, the agency is proposing to add nine new conditions that have developed among veterans of the 1990-91 Gulf War and the Afghan and Iraq conflicts.

Vets suffering from the following diseases or their after-effects would be presumed to have contracted them while serving: brucellosis, campylobacter jejuni, coxiella burnetii (Q fever), malaria, mycobacterium, tuberculosis, nontyphoid salmonella, shigella, visceral leishmaniasis and West Nile virus.

"We recognize the frustrations that many Gulf War and Afghanistan veterans and their families experience on a daily basis as they look for answers to health questions and seek benefits from VA," Shinseki said in announcing the proposed rule. [51]

In addition, the VA is proposing to add a presumption of service connection for Gulf-Iraq-Afghanistan vets suffering from "medically unexplained chronic multisymptom illness." Characteristics include fatigue, pain and inconsistent laboratory reports. That definition would cover Gulf War Syndrome, noted Sullivan of Veterans for Common Sense. "The proposed new VA rules may finally, after nearly two decades, open the door to a lifetime of free VA medical care for tens of thousands or more sick Gulf War veterans," he told *Military Times*. [52]

On the heels of the VA announcement, the Institute of Medicine issued the latest volume in its long study of Gulf War symptoms, finding that "sufficient evidence of association" exists between deployment to the Persian Gulf operations area and "multisymptom illness." That conclusion falls one step short of establishing a causal relationship between the illness and Gulf War service. "There is some doubt as to the influence of chance, bias and confounding," the report said, using a statistical term for an element of an issue that mistakenly leads to associating exposure with outcome. [53]

Still, given the long and contentious history of Gulf War veterans' attempts to obtain scientific confirmation that they were suffering from something other than random, imagined or exaggerated symptoms, the institute's report marked an important milestone.

"The multisymptom illness that affects so many Gulf War veterans is a terrible, distinct illness," James E. Finn, chairman of a VA-appointed advisory committee on Gulf War illnesses, told *The Washington Post*, "and . . . this nation can and should launch a Manhattan Project-style research program to identify treatments and prevent this from happening again." [54]

Meanwhile, the VA is trying to pinpoint specific causes of Gulf War illness, including exposure to substances including "smoke and particles from military installation burn-pit fires that incinerated a wide range of toxic-waste materials," Bradley Mayes, director of the VBA Compensation and Pension Service, wrote in a February letter to VA medical personnel and claims examiners. *The Military Times*, which has no ties to the Defense Department, had reported on growing suspicions of burn-pit exposure as a cause of disease. [55]

Continued on p. 378

At Issue:

Should the VA's Veterans Benefits Administration be scrapped and rebuilt?

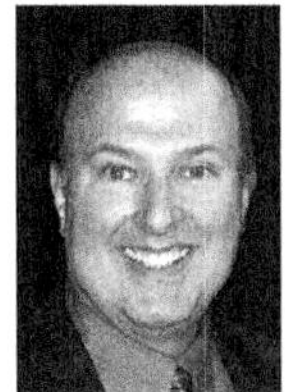

PAUL SULLIVAN
EXECUTIVE DIRECTOR, VETERANS FOR COMMON SENSE

WRITTEN FOR *CQ RESEARCHER*, APRIL 2010

VA's top leaders and auditors have confirmed that benefit claim processing at the Veterans Benefits Administration (VBA) cannot be fixed, as it represents an obsolete and unsustainable model. VBA leaders have no permanent solution for the 60-year-old system, and VBA should eventually be replaced using a careful plan.

This year, VA Secretary Eric Shinseki has a rare window of opportunity to build a new, high-tech, veteran-friendly VBA when he names a new under secretary for benefits. Fixing VBA is vital because an approved disability claim usually opens the door for both disability payments and health care. VBA's current woes include:

- 500,000 veterans now waiting an average of six months for a disability claim decision, plus 200,000 more veterans waiting five more years for an appealed decision.
- 70,000 new pages of paper clog up VBA every day.
- VBA makes an error in nearly one-in-four decisions.
- VBA improperly shredded claims, lost claims and backdated records.
- VBA leaders paid themselves millions in cash bonuses while rank-and-file employees struggled.
- Distraught veterans call VA's suicide prevention hotline out of frustration with endless VBA delays.

We urge the VA to begin a series of public meetings with Congress, veteran advocates and academic experts to pass new laws to design, build and deploy a new VBA with the shortest path possible between the veteran and VA benefits, including health care. Here are practical solutions for a new, high-quality VBA:

- Use a one-page claim form, a single, automated computer system and decide each claim within 30 days.
- Use easy-to-understand rules that presume more medical conditions are linked to military service.
- Use the new, robust lifetime military medical record.
- Move claims staff, currently isolated in a single office in each state, into medical facilities to help veterans set up claim exams as well as quickly and accurately decide claims.
- Allow veterans to hire an attorney before they file a claim, especially veterans with brain injuries or mental health conditions.

When these common sense solutions are adopted, then more of our veterans are welcomed home with the VA benefits and health care they need and earned after defending our freedom. Learn more at: www.FixVA.org.

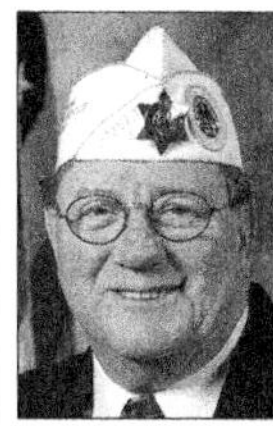

JAMES B. KING
NATIONAL EXECUTIVE DIRECTOR, AMVETS; MARINE CORPS VETERAN OF VIETNAM

WRITTEN FOR *CQ RESEARCHER*, APRIL 2010

Since 2001, the Department of Veterans Affairs disability claims backlog has grown precipitously because of the ongoing conflicts in Iraq and Afghanistan and the establishment of new presumptive health conditions.

Thankfully, through constructive dialogue with the nation's top veterans' service organizations, the VA has implemented significant changes over the last few months that should help to alleviate strains on the system.

AMVETS is encouraged by the VA's recent steps to streamline the process, making a proposed scrapping of the current Veterans Benefits Administration (VBA) system duplicative and unnecessary. Today, VA has launched pilot programs at regional offices around the country, investigating ways to modernize the claims process, building on opinions and suggestions from leading veterans' groups. These pilot programs include the paperless claims process in Providence, the virtual regional office in Baltimore, team-based workload management in Little Rock and tiered case-management teams in Pittsburgh. AMVETS and other groups have had access to each of these programs, offering opinions and recommendations where necessary, based on decades of experience in the VA claims process. VA also recently implemented eight system-wide solutions to transform the mindset of all involved in the claims process — from the individual veteran to the VA adjudicator.

AMVETS will continue to monitor the progress of these initiatives to help find the best solutions to the daunting backlog. We encourage Congress to do the same before taking hasty legislative action. In AMVETS' opinion, plans to scrap the VBA would only exacerbate current benefits-delivery issues. Today, millions of veterans are entitled to care and compensation through their VBA ratings. By scrapping VBA, VA would need to develop a new corollary to deliver care and benefits to the millions of veterans already enrolled, dating back to World War II.

Plus, would veterans rated under the old system be entitled to reopen their claims? AMVETS believes that they must, which only creates more roadblocks to benefits. Forget the current 400,000-claim backlog — VA would be facing more than 3 million reopened claims and appeals.

AMVETS believes we are on the cusp of developing a modern VA claims process through constructive collaboration among VA and the veterans' groups that have helped our heroes navigate the system for decades. The proposed solutions could finally provide veterans with the timely and accurate claims processing they deserve. Thus, it's critical that the VBA be preserved.

Continued from p. 376

Legal Benefits

The VA pipeline may be clogged for health and education claims, but vets facing criminal charges are getting a new form of assistance from federal and state court systems around the country.

At least 21 states, cities and counties have set up "veterans' courts." Modeled on "drug courts," which provide a chance at supervised addiction treatment — and in some cases a clean record — instead of jail time, the veterans' versions are designed to take into account the repercussions of military service, especially combat tours in Iraq and Afghanistan. PTSD, TBI and other after-effects have become widely acknowledged and, in the view of many in the criminal-justice system, deserve to be weighed when a vet is being prosecuted or sentenced.

In Buffalo, N.Y., where Judge Robert T. Russell Jr. pioneered the concept in 2008, the vets' court takes only those accused of nonviolent felonies and misdemeanors. But the Santa Ana, Calif., court is open to those charged with any offense. Judge Wendy Lindley, who established the program, told the *National Law Journal* that California criminal law specifically allows treatment instead of incarceration for a convicted veteran who has served in a combat zone and developed psychological or substance-abuse problems. Veterans' courts are also in session in Anchorage, Chicago, Pittsburgh and Tulsa. [56]

The VA started a program last year to work with veterans' courts, and VA Secretary Shinseki visited the Buffalo court in April to underline his support. "The secretary's purpose was to receive first-hand knowledge about how the program works in order to integrate and develop similar endeavors in other communities," the Erie County Veterans Service Agency said on its Web site. [57]

The VA formed its own Veterans' Justice Outreach Initiative last year. The program is designed in part to provide detailed reports to judges on a vet's medical history and on VA benefits and programs that might help him if he were sentenced to probation instead of jail. Staffers are also trained to work with vets serving jail time. [58]

As support grows, dissenters are making themselves heard. In Nevada, which along with Illinois and New York enacted statewide veterans' courts last year, the general counsel for the American Civil Liberties Union of Nevada argued that they represent a dangerous trend of creating different avenues of justice for certain kinds of people. Veterans' courts amount to establishing special courts for "police officers, teachers or politicians," Allen Lichtenstein told the Stateline.org news service. [59]

He also rejected the analogy to drug courts, which are open to defendants suffering from a condition. But all veterans are eligible for veterans' court, Lichtenstein pointed out. [60]

Nevertheless, federal judges are starting to take veterans' wartime experiences into account in sentencing. In Denver, Senior U.S. District Judge John Kane sentenced a federal prison guard to five years' probation, with mental-health treatment required, because of his Air Force service in Afghanistan and Iraq, where he dealt with seriously injured and dead service members and civilians. John Brownfield Jr. had pleaded guilty to accepting at least $3,000 in bribes for smuggling contraband to inmates. [61]

"It would be a grave injustice," Kane said in a written decision, "to turn a blind eye to the potential effects of multiple deployments to war zones on Brownfield's subsequent behavior." [62]

Sentencing guidelines aside, Kane's move seemed consistent with a U.S. Supreme Court decision in November, 2009, to throw out a death sentence for a Korean War veteran convicted of murdering his ex-girlfriend and her boyfriend. Ordering a new sentencing hearing, the justices cited "the intense stress and emotional toll that combat took" on George Porter Jr. [63]

Aiding Caregivers

Legislation is pending in Congress to channel aid to families and others who have become full time caregivers for catastrophically disabled Iraq and Afghanistan veterans.

In a unanimous vote in November, the Senate passed the Caregivers and Veterans Omnibus Health Services Act, sponsored by Senate Veterans Chairman Daniel Akaka, D-Hawaii. House action was held up while Akaka's staff negotiated changes with his counterparts. The resulting compromise is ready for action, which is expected some time in April or May.

The legislation represents the first comprehensive attempt to assist those suddenly thrust into the 24-hour-a-day caregiver role. Approximately $3.7 billion would be spent on stipends — amount unspecified — for caregivers, on temporary alternative care ("respite care") arrangements to give caregivers a breather, on training caregivers and on other forms of support, including expense reimbursement to accompany disabled vets to distant hospitals. [64]

Only those caring for veterans from Operation Enduring Freedom (OEF) — the Afghanistan war — and Operation Iraqi Freedom (OIF) would be covered by the bill. Yet, as veterans of other wars age, issues of round-the-clock care for them are beginning to weigh on families. "Veterans' service organizations would like to see the legislation open to all," says Barbara Cohoon, deputy director of government relations for the National Military Families Association. "But we recognize that OIF and OEF caregivers are experiencing the biggest hardship right now and that resources are limited. But this needs to be done for all at some point." ■

OUTLOOK

National Priority?

Researchers have been trying for the past several years to forecast the medium-term effects of the Iraq and Afghanistan wars on veterans and, by extension, on the government agency that deals with them most closely.

Trend lines are exceptionally difficult to forecast, in part because fighting is still under way and may be for some time. Meanwhile, the VA "does not have the personnel, the funding, or the mandate from Congress to produce broad forecasts of service needs," the Institute of Medicine concluded in its recent report. [65]

The after-effects of past wars are of only limited usefulness, the institute noted, because so many more severely wounded service members are surviving combat now. The entire picture of the wounded veteran population has changed. "These survivors of very severe injuries need more intensive care than the most severely wounded service members from prior wars," the report said. "Extrapolating from past conflicts might result in an underestimation of the overall burden of need for persons impacted by OEF and OIF." [66]

What is clear, the institute reported, is that the needs of these veterans will be extensive. "The burden borne by wounded service members and their families, and thus the public responsibility to treat or compensate them, is large and probably will persist for the rest of their lives." [67]

Moreover, "peak demand for compensation" is likely to increase as veterans age, the institute said. "So the maximum stress on support systems for OEF and OIF veterans and their families might not be felt until 2040 or later." [68]

In the veterans' community, some express confidence in the VA's ability to keep up with an already growing demand for its services. "It has the potential to be as great as it needs to be," says Autry of Disabled American Veterans. "There are an awful lot of very dedicated people in the VA."

Their dedication is already being tested, and is certain to be tested even further, by the high incidence of PTSD, TBI and depression among Afghanistan and Iraq vets. "The prevalence of those injuries is relatively high and may grow as the conflicts continue," RAND has reported. Yet, both the Defense Department and the VA "have had difficulty in recruiting and retaining appropriately trained mental health professionals to fill existing or new slots." [69]

The RAND report urges that dealing with the trio of conditions be elevated to a "national priority." But even some relatively optimistic veterans say raising public concern to that level requires some heavy lifting. "We're less than 1 percent of the population," says Kennedy, the retired Army captain.

For his own part, Kennedy is still "pretty sure" the VA will be "a lot better than it is" now, but he's not sure how it will have improved.

Sullivan of Veterans for Common Sense is a bit more skeptical. The VA is still trying to protect its reputation, he says, similar to shipping company officials who "were saying everything was fine while the *Titanic* was sinking."

But the potential exists to transform VA's benefits service into a smooth-running operation in which veterans have confidence. "A tremendous amount of effort must be invested in this moment of opportunity," Sullivan says. "We have a new administration, a Congress eager to help, veterans' groups who want to help and public understanding of an urgent need. We have a golden moment of opportunity now."

Sullivan's outlook is considerably sunnier than that of Lamie, the IED attack survivor. In 10 years, he says, "I think the situation will be worse. In 10 years, everybody is going to forget all about the Iraq war. If there's a war in 2020, those guys will probably be treated great. But if there's nobody dying on the TV screen nobody will care."

An outsider might say that Lamie's combat scars are still raw; his brother Gene, an Army sergeant, died in an IED attack in Iraq in 2007. [70] But dismissing his bleak outlook could be a mistake. The searing experiences that inform his forecast are shared by a growing number of young veterans. ■

Notes

[1] "Radical Change Needed for Veterans Disability Claims Process," House Committee on Veterans Affairs, press statement, March 18, 2010, http://veterans.house.gov/news/PRArticle.aspx?NewsID=559.

[2] "Statement of Belinda J. Finn, Assistant Inspector General for Audits and Evaluations, Office of Inspector General, Department of Veterans Affairs," VA Office of Inspector General, March 24, 2010, www4.va.gov/OIG/pubs/VAOIG-statement-20100324-Finn.pdf.

[3] Icasualties.org, updated regularly, http://icasualties.org/OEF/Index.aspx.

[4] "Remarks by Secretary Eric K. Shinseki," Veterans of Foreign Wars National Legislative Conference, March 8, 2010, www1.va.gov/opa/speeches/2010/10_0308.asp; "Fiscal 2011 Budget: VA," Committee Testimony, Senate Veterans' Affairs Committee, Feb. 26, 2010; "FY 2011 Budget Submission," Department of Veterans Affairs, pp. 2B-4, 2C-2, www4.va.gov/budget/docs/summary/Fy2011_Volume_1-Summary_Volume.pdf.

[5] Quoted in Rick Maze, "VA official: Disability claims system 'cannot be fixed,' " *Federal Times*, March 18, 2010, www.federaltimes.com/article/20100318/DEPARTMENTS04/3180302/1055/AGENCY.

[6] Quoted in Philip Rucker, "Obama Picks Shinseki to Lead Veterans Affairs," *The Washington*

Post, Dec. 7, 2008, www.washingtonpost.com/wp-dyn/content/article/2008/12/07/AR2008120701487.html; Bernard Weinraub and Thom Shanker, "Rumsfeld's Design for War Criticized on the Battlefield," *The New York Times*, April 1, 2003, p. A1; Amy Belaso, "Troop Levels in the Afghan and Iraq Wars," Congressional Research Service, July 2, 2009, Summary page, www.fas.org/sgp/crs/natsec/R40682.pdf; "US Forces Order of Battle," GlobalSecurity.org, undated, www.globalsecurity.org/military/ops/iraq_orbat.htm.

[7] "Returning Home from Iraq and Afghanistan: Preliminary Assessment of Readjustment Needs of Veterans, Service Members, and Their Families," Institute of Medicine of the National Academies (2010), p. 52, http://books.nap.edu/openbook.php?record_id=12812&page=R1.

[8] Terri Tanielian and Lisa H. Jaycox, eds., "Invisible Wounds of War: Psychological and Cognitive Injuries, Their Consequences, and Services to Assist Recovery," RAND Center for Military Health Policy Research, 2008, p. xxi, www.rand.org/pubs/monographs/MG720; U.S. Army Surgeon General study cited in Kline, Anna, *et al.*, "Effects of Repeated Deployment to Iraq and Afghanistan on the Health of New Jersey Army National Guard Troops: Implications for Military Readiness," *American Journal of Public Health*, February 2010, http://ajph.aphapublications.org/cgi/content/abstract/100/2/276.

[9] The three are Parkinson's Disease, ischemic heart disease and B-cell leukemias. "FY 2011 Budget Submission," *op. cit.*, p. 1A-3; Gregg Zoroya, "VA to automate its Agent Orange claims process," *USA Today*, March 9, 2010, p. 4A.

[10] *Hawkins v. Shinseki*, U.S. Court of Appeals for the Federal Circuit, 2009-7068, Dec. 7, 2009, www.cafc.uscourts.gov/opinions/09-7068.pdf.

[11] *Ibid.*

[12] "VA Appellate Processes," Committee Testimony, House Veterans' Affairs Committee, Subcommittee on Disability Assistance and Memorial Affairs, May 24, 2009.

[13] "Legislative Presentations of Veterans' Organizations," House Veterans' Affairs Committee, Senate Veterans' Affairs Committee, March 9, 2010. For VA backlog figure, see "2010 Monday Morning Workload Reports," Department of Veterans Affairs, March 29, 2010, www.vba.va.gov/REPORTS/mmwr/index.asp.

[14] Finn, *op. cit.*

[15] "Iraq Index: Tracking Variables of Reconstruction and Security in Post-Saddam Iraq," Brookings Institution, updated March 30, 2010, p. 19, www.brookings.edu/~/media/Files/Centers/Saban/Iraq Index/index.pdf.

[16] "The House Veterans' Affairs Subcommittee on Oversight and Investigations," *op. cit.*

[17] *Ibid.*

[18] "Returning Home from Iraq and Afghanistan . . . ," *op. cit.*, pp. 29, 69.

[19] *Ibid.*, p. 69.

[20] *Ibid.*, p. 32.

[21] "Needs of Family Caregivers," House Veterans' Affairs Committee, June 4, 2009.

[22] *Ibid.*

[23] "FY 2011 Budget Submission," Department of Veterans Affairs, p. 3A-7, www4.va.gov/budget/docs/summary/Fy2011_Volume_1-Summary_Volume.pdf.

[24] Kimberly Hefling, "Increase in suicide rate of veterans noted," The Associated Press (*Army Times*), Jan. 12, 2010, www.armytimes.com/news/2010/01/ap_vet_suicide_011110.

[25] "Veterans Suicide Prevention," Senate Veterans' Affairs Committee, March 3, 2010.

[26] *Ibid.*

[27] *Ibid.*

[28] "Veterans Suicide Prevention," Senate Veterans' Affairs Committee, March 3, 2010, (Web video), http://veterans.senate.gov/hearings.cfm?action=release.display&release_id=d1a8548c-de2c-49a8-b7f9-d0855265d435.

[29] *Ibid.*

[30] Walter F. Roche Jr., and James Gerstenzang, "Doctor picked to head VA," *Los Angeles Times*, Oct. 31, 2007, p. A11.

[31] "FY 2011 Budget Submission," *op. cit.*, p. 1A-1; Jackie Calmes, "In $3.8 Trillion Budget, Obama Pivots to Trim Future Deficits," *The New York Times*, Feb. 1, 2010, www.nytimes.com/2010/02/02/us/politics/02budget.html?pagewanted=all.

[32] James Dao, "Late Benefit Checks Causing Problems for Veterans Attending College On New G.I. Bill," *The New York Times*, Sept. 25, 2009, p. A16.

[33] "House Veterans' Affairs Committee Holds Hearing on the State of the Department of Veterans Affairs," CQ Congressional Transcripts, Oct. 14, 2009.

[34] Except where otherwise indicated, this subsection is drawn from "VA History in Brief," Department of Veterans Affairs, undated, www1.va.gov/opa/publications/archives/docs/history_in_brief.pdf. For number serving in the World War II military, male and female, "Facts for Features," U.S. Census Bureau, April 29, 2004, www.census.gov/Press-Release/www/2004/cb04-ffse07.pdf.

[35] For background, see P. Webbink, "Veteran-aid Policies of the United States," *Editorial Research Reports*, Vol. IV, Oct. 6, 1930; and B. W. Patch, "The Bonus and Veterans' Pensions," *Editorial Research Reports*, Vol. I, Jan. 10, 1936, both available at *CQ Researcher Plus Archive*, www.library.cqpress.com.

[36] For background, see R. McNickle, "Service Pensions for War Veterans," *Editorial Research Reports*, May 4, 1949, available at *CQ Researcher Plus Archive*, www.library.cqpress.com.

[37] Suzanne Metler, "Why Skimp on GI Bill?" Military.com, Nov. 18, 2005, www.military.com/opinion/0,15202,80830,00.html. The book is Suzanne Metler, *Soldiers and Citizens: The GI Bill and the Making of the Greatest Generation* (2005).

[38] Except where otherwise indicated, this subsection is drawn from Gerald Nicosia, *Home to War: A History of the Vietnam Veterans Movement* (2001), and "VA History in Brief," *op. cit.*

[39] Neil Sheehan, *A Bright Shining Lie: John Paul Vann and America in Vietnam* (1988), p. 39; "Vietnam War," GlobalSecurity.org, undated, www.globalsecurity.org/military/ops/vietnam.htm; "America's Wars," Department of Veterans Affairs, updated November, 2009, www1.va.gov/opa/publications/factsheets/fs_americas_wars.pdf.

[40] "VVAW: Where We Came From, Who We Are," Vietnam Veterans Against the War, un-

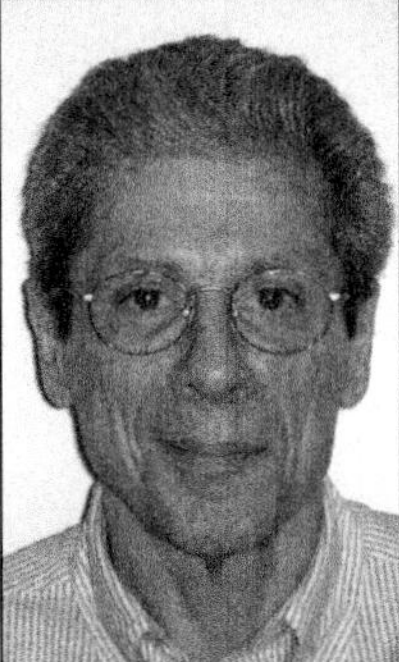

About the Author

Peter Katel is a *CQ Researcher* staff writer who previously reported on Haiti and Latin America for *Time* and *Newsweek* and covered the Southwest for newspapers in New Mexico. He has received several journalism awards, including the Bartolomé Mitre Award for coverage of drug trafficking, from the Inter-American Press Association. He holds an A.B. in university studies from the University of New Mexico. His recent reports include "New Strategy in Iraq," "Rise in Counterinsurgency" and "Wounded Veterans."

dated, www.vvaw.org/about/; Jason Zengerle, "The Vet Wars," *The New York Times Magazine*, May 23, 2004, p. 30.

[41] "Born on the Fourth of July," Internet Movie Database, www.imdb.com/title/tt0096969/.

[42] Except as otherwise indicated, material in this section is drawn from "VA History in Brief," *op. cit.* For background, see Peter Katel, "Wounded Veterans," *CQ Researcher*, Aug. 31, 2007, pp. 697-720.

[43] "Independent Review Could Improve Credibility of Radiation Exposure Estimates," GAO, January, 2000, p. 2, www.gao.gov/archive/2000/he00032.pdf; "Rules for Veterans' Radiation Benefits Voided," The Associated Press (*The New York Times*), Oct. 8, 1981, www.nytimes.com/1981/10/08/us/rules-for-veterans-radiation-benefits-voided.html.

[44] "House Votes Bill Giving Benefits to Veterans Exposed to Radiation," The Associated Press (*The New York Times*), May 3, 1988, p. A26; "Independent Review . . . ," *op. cit.*, p. 6; "Statement on Signing the Radiation-Exposed Veterans Compensation Act of 1988," Ronald Reagan, May 20, 1988 the American Presidency Project, www.presidency.ucsb.edu/ws/index.php?pid=35855.

[45] David Zucchino, "Veterans speak out against burn pits," *Los Angeles Times*, Feb. 18, 2010, http://articles.latimes.com/2010/feb/18/nation/la-na-burn-pits18-2010feb18.

[46] Thom Shanker and David Stout, "Chief Army Medical Officer Ousted in Walter Reed Furor," *The New York Times*, March 13, 2007, p. A5.

[47] Rick Atkinson, " 'The single most effective weapon against our deployed forces,' " *The Washington Post*, Sept. 30, 2008, p. A1; Ann Scott Tyson, "U.S. combat injuries rise sharply," *The Washington Post*, Oct. 31, 2009, p. A1.

[48] Ronald Glasser, "A Shock Wave of Brain Injuries," *The Washington Post*, April 8, 2007, Outlook, p. B1.

[49] *Ibid.*

[50] "Returning Home from Iraq and Afghanistan . . . ," *op. cit.*

[51] Quoted in "VA recognizes 'presumptive' illnesses in Iraq, Afghanistan," Veterans Administration, March 24, 2010, www.army.mil/-news/2010/03/24/36272-va-recognizes-presumptive-illnesses-in-iraq-afghanistan.

[52] Quoted in Kelly Kennedy, "VA may designate 9 infectious diseases as service-connected," *Military Times*, April 5, 2010, p. A12; "Proposed Rule," Department of Veterans Affairs, *Federal Register*, Vol. 75, No. 52, March 18, 2010, www1.va.gov/ORPM/docs/20100318_AN24_PresumptionsPersianGulfService.pdf.

[53] "Gulf War and Health, Vol. 8: Update of Health Effects of Serving in the Gulf War," Institute of Medicine, April 9, 2010, pp. 5-7, 25, www.iom.edu/Reports/2010/Gulf-War-and-Health-Volume-8-Health-Effects-of-Serving-in-the-Gulf-War.aspx.

[54] David Brown, "Up to 250,000 Gulf War veterans have 'unexplained medical symptoms,' " *The Washington Post*, April 10, 2010, www.washingtonpost.com/wp-dyn/content/article/2010/04/09/AR2010040904712.html.

[55] Quoted in Kennedy, *op. cit.*

[56] Lynne Marek, "Courts for veterans spreading across U.S.," *National Law Journal*, Dec. 22, 2008, www.law.com/jsp/nlj/PubArticlePrinterFriendlyNLJ.jsp?id=1202426915992&hbxlogin=1; Carolyn Thompson, "Special court for veterans addresses more than crime," The Associated Press (*Boston Globe*), July 7, 2008, www.boston.com/news/nation/articles/2008/07/07/special_court_for_veterans_addresses_more_than_crime; John Gramlich, "New courts tailored to war veterans," Stateline.org, June, 18, 2009, www.stateline.org/live/details/story?contentId=407573.

[57] Sergio R. Rodriguez, "VA Secretary Eric K. Shinseki visits the Buffalo Veterans Treatment Court," Veterans Service Agency, April 6, 2010, www.erie.gov/veterans/veterans_court.asp.

[58] P. Solomon Banda, "Troubled Veterans Get a Hand," The Associated Press (*The Washington Post*), Aug. 7, 2009, p. A19.

[59] Quoted in John Gramlich, *op. cit.*

[60] *Ibid.*

[61] Robert Boczkiewicz, "Veteran of Afghanistan, Iraq gets probation," *Pueblo Chieftain*, Dec. 19, 2009, www.chieftain.com/news/local/article_d2d823fb-19ee-5eb4-ac54-dca372dd75d4.html.

[62] Quoted in *ibid.*

[63] Quoted in John Schwartz, "Defendants Fresh From War Find Service Counts in Court," *The New York Times*, March 16, 2010, p. A14.

[64] Leah Nylen and Jennifer Scholtes, "Senate Passes Vets' Package Despite Coburn's Concerns," *CQ Today*, Nov. 19, 2009; "S 1963 CRS Bill Digest Summary," March 10, 2010.

[65] "Returning Home from Iraq and Afghanistan," *op. cit.*, p. 98.

[66] *Ibid.*, p. 97.

[67] *Ibid.*, p. 98.

[68] *Ibid.*

[69] "Invisible Wounds of War," *op. cit.*, pp. 452, 446.

[70] "Sgt. Gene L. Lamie, United States Army, KIA 06 July 2007," www.ourfallensoldier.com/LamieGeneL_MemorialPage.html.

FOR MORE INFORMATION

Amvets, 4647 Forbes Blvd., Lanham, MD 20706; (301) 459-9600; www.amvets.org. Originally formed for World War II vets; specializes in public policy and legislative work and aids vets with claims to the U.S. Department of Veterans' Affairs (VA).

Disabled American Veterans, P.O. Box 14301, Cincinnati, OH 45250; (859) 441-7300; www.dav.org. Specializes in VA claims work and other services for severely wounded vets.

Lawyers Serving Warriors, P.O. Box 65762, Washington, DC 20035; (202) 265-8305; www.lawyersservingwarriors.com. Provides free lawyers to veterans in disability and other cases, but is not accepting new clients; Web site remains a valuable source of information.

U.S. Department of Veterans Affairs, 810 Vermont Ave., N.W., Washington, DC 20420; (800) 827-1000; www.va.gov. Maintains a Web site that is a rich source of information on benefits and policy.

Veterans for Common Sense, 900 2nd St., S.E., Suite 216, Washington, DC 20003; (202) 558-4553; www.veteransforcommonsense.org. Advocacy organization focuses on VA reform.

Wounded Warriors Project, 7020 AC Skinner Pkwy., Suite 100, Jacksonville, FL 32256; (877) 832-6997; www.woundedwarriorproject.org. Provides aid to severely disabled veterans and their families.

Bibliography

Selected Sources

Books

Glantz, Aaron, *The War Comes Home: Washington's Battle Against America's Veterans*, University of California Press, 2009.
A journalist who covered the Iraq war reports critically on the state of VA services.

Nicosia, Gerald, *Home to War: A History of the Vietnam Veterans' Movement*, Crown, 2001.
The influence of the groundbreaking movement still resonates today, having helped to get post-traumatic stress disorder classified as a disability caused by military service.

Schram, Martin, *Vets Under Siege*, St. Martin's Press, 2008.
A veteran Washington reporter examines the VA's efforts to meet the demands placed on it by the Iraq and Afghanistan wars.

Articles

Cave, Damien, "A Combat Role, and Anguish, Too," *The New York Times*, Nov. 1, 2009, p. A1.
Women vets suffering from PTSD are more isolated than their male counterparts, because they are fewer in number and are expected to immediately jump back into household duties.

Chong, Jia-Rui, "Veterans' long-term ills linked to brain injuries," *Los Angeles Times*, Dec. 5, 2008, p. A25.
The first comprehensive report links TBI to long-term conditions including seizures and aggression.

Cullison, Alan, "On Battlefields, Survival Odds Rise," *The Wall Street Journal*, April 3, 2010, online.wsj.com/article/SB20001424052748704655004575114623837930294.html.
A journalist experienced in covering warfare in Afghanistan provides a close-in look at advances in battlefield medicine.

Dao, James, and Thom Shanker, "No Longer a Soldier, Shinseki Has a New Mission," *The New York Times*, Nov. 11, 2009, p. A21.
The VA's new boss as profiled by correspondents on the Pentagon and veterans' affairs beats.

Hefling, Kimberly, "The veterans hall is growing — online," The Associated Press, Dec. 7, 2008, p. A15.
The newest veterans are taking their postwar bonding to the Internet.

Kennedy, Kelly, "DoD concedes rise in burn-pit ailments," *Military Times*, Feb. 8, 2010, p. 10.
The Defense Department admits there are possible connections between waste-burning emissions and health problems.

Marcus, Mary Brophy, "Military families cry for help," *USA Today*, Jan. 27, 2010, p. 8B.
Families taking care of catastrophically wounded veterans struggle financially and emotionally, a medical correspondent reports.

Ungar, Laura, "Suicide takes growing toll among military, veterans," *The Courier-Journal* (Ky.), Sept. 13, 2009.
The health-affairs specialist for a newspaper situated near a big military base (Fort Knox) covers the rising tide of suicide.

Whitlock, Craig, "IED attacks soaring in Afghanistan," *The Washington Post*, March 18, 2010, p. A10.
A war correspondent for *The Post* charts the Taliban's growing use of the explosive devices.

Zoroya, Gregg, "Repeated deployments weigh heavily on troops," *USA Today*, Jan. 13, 2010, p. A1.
As repeat deployments continue, the newspaper's veterans-beat reporter covers the toll on service members.

Reports and Studies

"Gulf War and Health: Vol. 8: Update of Health Effects of Serving in the Gulf War," Institute of Medicine, 2009, www.nap.edu/catalog/12835.html.
The federally funded institute is finding evidence of a link between service in the Gulf and multisymptom illness.

"Returning Home from Iraq and Afghanistan: Preliminary Assessment of Readjustment Needs of Veterans, Service Members, and Their Families," Institute of Medicine, 2010, www.nap.edu/catalog/12812.html.
A massive examination and analysis of research data that attempts to portray the effects of the present wars on service members and society at large.

"Veterans' Disability Benefits: Further Evaluation of Ongoing Initiatives Could Help Identify Effective Approaches for Improving Claims Processing," Government Accountability Office, January 2010, www.gao.gov/new.items/d10213.pdf.
In the most recent of its reports on the VA claims system, Congress' investigative arm concludes that the backlog problem remains serious.

Mulhall, Erin, and Vanessa Williamson, "Red Tape: Veterans Fight New Battles for Care and Benefits," Iraq and Afghanistan Veterans of America, February 2010, media.iava.org/reports/redtape_2010.pdf.
The advocacy organization reports on delays and complicated procedures that still characterize the VA's disability claims system.

The Next Step:

Additional Articles from Current Periodicals

Backlogs

Dao, James, "Veterans Affairs, Already Struggling With Backlog, Faces Surge of Disability Claims," *The New York Times*, July 13, 2009, p. A10.

The backlog of unprocessed claims for veterans' benefits is now more than 400,000, up from 253,000 in 2003.

Neal, Rebecca, "Obama Seeks Employees' Ideas on Cutting VA Backlogs," *Federal Times*, Aug. 24, 2009, p. 4.

President Obama is asking employees of the Veterans' Benefits Administration on how to reduce its backlogs and get benefits to veterans quicker.

Vogel, Steve, "Groups Urge VA to Reform Disability Claim Procedures," *The Washington Post*, June 25, 2009, p. A17.

Veterans' groups and members of Congress are calling for an overhaul of the Department of Veterans Affairs' procedures for handling a backlog of unresolved claims.

Brain Injuries

Cevallos, Marissa, "Santa Clara Valley Medical Begins Study on Traumatic Brain Injuries," *San Jose* (California) *Mercury News*, March 16, 2010.

Several hospitals in California are teaming up to conduct trials that will hopefully develop a drug to treat traumatic brain injury.

Channick, Robert, "Virtual Iraq Targets Combat Disorders," *Chicago Tribune*, July 8, 2009, p. A4.

Virtual Iraq, a combat-like video game, is being used by several medical centers to treat veterans suffering from post-traumatic stress disorder.

Kenning, Chris, "Brain Injuries Prompt More Epilepsy Problems Among Veterans," *Courier-Journal* (Kentucky), Nov. 10, 2009.

Brain-injury induced epilepsy is a growing nationwide trend among veterans, according to medical experts.

Stobbe, Mike, "Army Officials Say War Concussions Overdiagnosed," The Associated Press, April 16, 2009.

Mild brain injuries among returning military troops are being overdiagnosed because the government is using soft criteria instead of hard medical evidence, according to several Army officials.

Caregivers

Maze, Rick, "Caretaker Bill Faces Opposition From VA," *Air Force Times*, May 4, 2009, p. 11.

The Obama administration supports the idea of providing more assistance to families caring for wounded veterans, but critics say a bill must apply to veterans of previous wars and not just those in Iraq and Afghanistan.

Miller, Barbara, "VA Seeks Private Homes for Care," *Patriot-News* (Pennsylvania), June 12, 2009.

The Veterans Administration is pushing for a new foster program in Pennsylvania that would allow more veterans to live in a homelike setting.

Wise, Lindsey, "Caring for Disabled Veterans, Loved Ones Face Own Battles," *Houston Chronicle*, April 12, 2010, p. A1.

Many family members have to quit their jobs or even relocate in order to care for wounded veterans.

Legislation

Capriccioso, Rob, "Housing Bill Introduced to Assist Native Veterans," *Indian Country Today* (New York), Sept. 30, 2009.

A new bill in Congress is aiming to help disabled Native American veterans maintain housing assistance.

Lee, Eunice, "Proposed Legislation May Up Veterans' College Tuition Aid," *Victorville* (California) *Daily Press*, May 25, 2009.

The Veterans Education Equity Act aims to increase the reimbursements recent veterans who enroll in private universities would receive under provisions set forth by the Post-9/11 GI Bill.

Schaffer, Tim, "Ohio Senate Working on Legislation That Honors Veterans, Military Families," *Newark* (Ohio) *Advocate*, May 25, 2009.

An Ohio state senator talks about how the Ohio senate authorized monetary bonuses to residents returning from military service.

CITING *CQ RESEARCHER*

Sample formats for citing these reports in a bibliography include the ones listed below. Preferred styles and formats vary, so please check with your instructor or professor.

MLA STYLE

Jost, Kenneth. "Rethinking the Death Penalty." CQ Researcher 16 Nov. 2001: 945-68.

APA STYLE

Jost, K. (2001, November 16). Rethinking the death penalty. *CQ Researcher, 11*, 945-968.

CHICAGO STYLE

Jost, Kenneth. "Rethinking the Death Penalty." *CQ Researcher*, November 16, 2001, 945-968.

CHAPTER

4

Legalizing Marijuana

By Peter Katel

Excerpted from the CQ Researcher. Peter Katel. (June 12, 2009). "Legalizing Marijuana." *CQ Researcher*, 525-548.

Legalizing Marijuana

BY PETER KATEL

THE ISSUES

Cmdr. Marc Alcantara of the San Mateo County Narcotics Task Force has his priorities, and they don't include pot-smokers toking on a joint at home or growing a couple of cannabis plants in the backyard or under a basement grow light.

"If people are truly growing it for personal consumption," he says, "it's not an issue with us."

Instead, Alcantara and his 22-officer unit focus on commercial marijuana-growing. It's a booming industry in the affluent coastal county between Silicon Valley and San Francisco. From 2006 to 2008, task force seizures of marijuana grown indoors rose 265 percent, to more than 36,000 plants from 39 sites.

"Indoor grow operations are capable of turning out three crops a year," he says, "typically grossing $250,000 per crop."

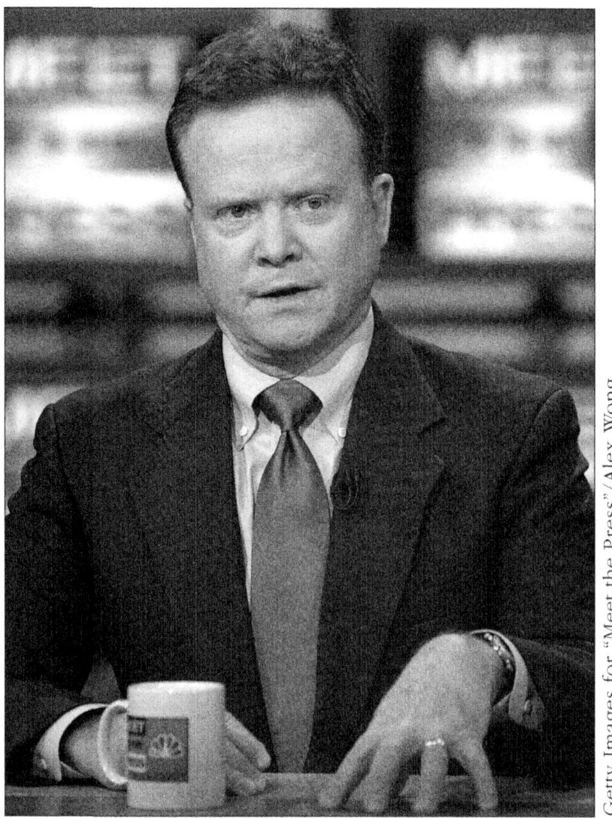

Getty Images for "Meet the Press"/Alex Wong

Democratic Sen. Jim Webb of Virginia is proposing a national commission to study the nation's drug laws and prison policies. "We are not protecting our citizens from the increasing danger of criminals who perpetrate violence and intimidation as a way of life, and we are locking up too many people who do not belong in jail," he said.

That's $250,000 in untaxed revenue per crop — or a potential total of more than $25 million just for those 39 sites in San Mateo County. In a state where desperate politicians are wrestling with a bankruptcy-threatening $24 billion budget deficit, the prospect of adding any kind of business to the tax rolls can start to sound like a plan.

Enter Tom Ammiano, a freshman Democratic state assemblyman from San Francisco. With marijuana already a lucrative California crop, with the state's medical-marijuana system now 13 years old and with personal use effectively decriminalized, the 68-year-old Ammiano says California ought to go all the way: legalize the entire cannabis industry and tax the product.

"Our drug policies have failed; the state of California is in dire economic need," he says. "We're looking at a perfect storm."

Ammiano's proposal has major support. A legalize-and-tax plan is favored by 56 percent of Californians, according to the Field Poll. Tax boss Betty T. Yee, chairwoman of the State Board of Equalization, backs the plan and says it could produce annual tax revenues of $1.4 billion. "I think the tide is starting to turn in terms of marijuana being part of the mainstream," she said." [1]

Marijuana-reform advocates point to signs of a national climate change as well. In Massachusetts, a pot-decriminalization law took effect this year that calls for no jail time for the first-time possession of a small amount of pot. And though the Food and Drug Administration doesn't classify marijuana as medication, 14 states permit it to be used by cancer patients and others to control pain. Several other states are considering medical-pot bills as well, though some proposals have died. National polls register a trend in favor of decriminalization — though falling short of a majority.

"I do sense a change in the discussion, a willingness of mainstream politicians, Republican and Democrat, maybe not to come out in favor of ending prohibition, but at least to talk about it," says Bruce Mirken, national spokesman for the pro-legalization Marijuana Policy Project. "For a long time, it was only people on the relatively far left and libertarian right."

But moderate Republican Gov. Arnold Schwarzenegger, carefully avoiding condemning the idea, is more cautious. "I think it's not time for that, but it's time for debate," he said in response to Ammiano's proposal. [2]

Scott Burns, deputy drug czar during most of the vehemently anti-marijuana George W. Bush administration, argues that changes in rhetorical tone here and there shouldn't be confused with a genuine political trend, even on the less politically charged issue of medical marijuana.

"If they have that much support, either in science or the will of people, they should call their local senators or congressmen," says Burns, now executive director of the National District Attorneys Association. "But right now nobody can convince the U.S. Congress that smoking weed is medicine."

Still, the Obama administration is getting only token pushback after reversing many Bush administration policies.

Ten States Ease Penalties on Pot Possession

Possession of a small quantity of marijuana is a misdemeanor for the first offense in all the states, with penalties varying widely, including jail time. In 10 states, however, there is no jail time in such cases. So-called medical marijuana is permitted in 14 states.

State Marijuana Laws

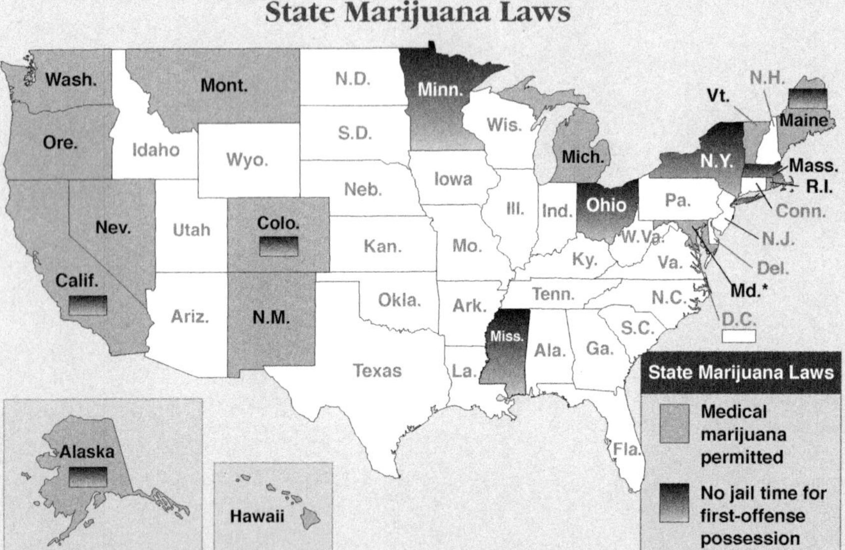

** No program, but allows courts to consider marijuana for medical use as a mitigating factor in marijuana-related prosecution. If a defendant is successful in proving medical necessity, the maximum fine is $100.*

Source: National Organization for the Reform of Marijuana Laws

In March, Attorney General Eric H. Holder Jr. announced that federal authorities would de-escalate the Bush campaign against California's state-authorized medical-marijuana dispensaries and, by extension, medical-pot distributors in the other 13 states that have legalized medical-marijuana, targeting only drug traffickers who "use medical-marijuana laws as a shield." [3]

The reversal of the Bush policy of declaring all the state's hundreds of pot outlets vulnerable to federal raids prompted only gentle criticism from Sen. Charles Grassley, R-Iowa, and Los Angeles Police Chief Howard Bratton, who called the new policy "unfortunate." [4]

Obama drug czar Gil Kerlikowske himself rejected the doctrine that most presidents have adopted — or at least not repudiated — ever since President Richard M. Nixon declared a "war on drugs" in the early 1970s.

"Regardless of how you try to explain to people [that] it's a war on drugs or a war on a product, people see a war as a war on them," Kerlikowske told *The Wall Street Journal*. "We're not at war with people in this country." [5]

But later, in a speech to law-enforcement officials in Nashville in May, Kerlikowske made clear that the Obama administration has placed a limit on its drug-policy objectives. "Legalization isn't in the president's vocabulary, and it certainly isn't in mine," he told a gathering of law-enforcement officials. [6]

Still, the drug czar also made clear that his top priority for now is prescription-drug abuse. [7] And in another sign of changing times, some of the toughest critics in the marijuana debates include drug policy experts, who also question the effectiveness of prohibition. "I deny that prohibiting drugs causes a drug-free America, and that not prohibiting drugs ends the drug problem," says Mark A. R. Kleiman, director of the drug policy analysis program at the University of California, Los Angeles (UCLA) and author of a forthcoming book on criminal-justice policy. [8]

Kleiman and others argue, however, that the solution to the nation's drug problem must inevitably include a law-enforcement dimension regardless of marijuana's legal status.

"The general public's view is that marijuana use is harmless, and in one's own home I think it is the case," says Rosalie Liccardo Pacula, co-director of the Drug Policy Center at the RAND Corp., a California think tank. "The problem is, it's not only used alone. Youths using it are also using alcohol, and alcohol used with cannabis increases risk more than alcohol alone."

Indeed, marijuana arrests figure prominently in the nation's overall crime statistics. Roughly 14 million people a year are arrested nationwide on all charges. In a 2007 study of 10 U.S. counties, 40 percent of the arrestees tested positive for marijuana. At that rate, when extrapolated for the nation as a whole, about 5.6 million of the 14 million would recently have smoked pot. Overall, the federal government's annual survey of drug, alcohol and tobacco use estimates that about 14.4 million people a year smoke marijuana monthly in the United States and about 25 million at least once a year. [9]

Americans hardly have a monopoly on cannabis use. But of 17 countries studied by the World Health Organization, the United States leads the list, with 42 percent of the entire U.S. population estimated to have used marijuana at some point in their lives.

"Drug use is not . . . simply related to drug policy," the study said, "since countries with stringent user-level illegal-drug policies did not have lower levels of use than countries with more liberal ones." [10]

The high level of marijuana use is even raising questions in Congress, which long has resisted following the states in softening marijuana laws. Conservative Democratic Sen. Jim Webb of Virginia is proposing a national commission to study the law-enforcement system, including marijuana policies. "I saw more drug use at Georgetown Law School than anywhere else I've been," the much-decorated Vietnam War veteran told columnist Neal Peirce. "A lot of those people went on to be judges." [11]

And in the House, veteran Rep. Charles Rangel, D-N.Y., powerful chairman of the tax-writing Ways and Means Committee, has endorsed ending federal marijuana prohibition.

"There's no question that with the limited resources . . . that we put on law enforcement, that we ought to decriminalize it," he told the House Judiciary Subcommittee on Crime, Terrorism and Homeland Security on May 21. [12]

Subcommittee member Dan Lungren, R-Calif., posed the only counterargument, noting that today's marijuana is more dangerous because of its higher content of THC (tetrahydrocannabinol, the main active compound in cannabis). And marijuana crops are "devastating wilderness areas, national parks . . . controlled by foreign nationals armed with assault weapons in some cases, a far more serious situation today than it was 10 years ago, 20 years ago." [13]

Last summer, the Bush administration launched a campaign against large-scale growing operations in California's Sequoia National Forest thought to be run by Mexican drug cartels; 420,000 plants were destroyed. [14]

And yet, across the border from Ciudad Juárez, which has been devastated by warring Mexican drug gangs, the El Paso City Council voted in January to open a debate on whether to end marijuana prohibition, as a way to deprive cartels of at least some of their revenue. The resolution's author, council member Beto O'Rourke, said news coverage of the proposal "did confirm that we're part of much larger national and hemispheric conversation about the failure of our drug policies."

California Is Nation's Marijuana Heartland

According to one of many estimates, California growers produced nearly 9 million pounds of marijuana in 2006 worth nearly $14 billion — or more than the value of the next-three biggest producers.

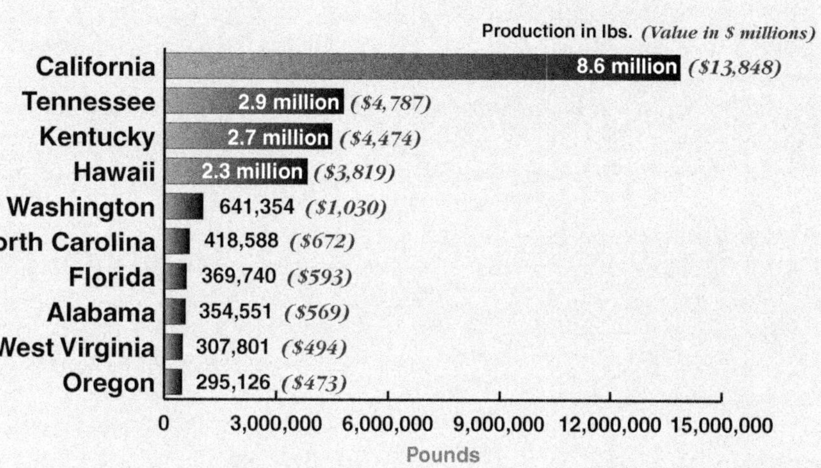

Source: Jon Gettman, "Marijuana Production in the United States (2006)," Bulletin of Cannabis Reform, December 2006

Mayor John Cook vetoed the resolution, however, and O'Rourke's colleagues backed off overturning Cook after Rep. Silvestre Reyes, D-Texas, and the county's delegation to the state House said the resolution would obstruct their efforts to secure aid for the city. [15]

Judging by public opinion on marijuana, those politicians are still on safe ground. Nationwide surveys show a majority still opposing legalization, though results vary sharply between surveys — from 46 percent opposed (the Rasmussen Poll) to 63 percent (CBS News). [16]

Still, Gallup reports a decades-long trend of growing support for legalization — from 12 percent in 1969 to 36 percent in 2005, the most recent Gallup survey data available. [17]

Decades of news reports crediting marijuana with relieving pain and suffering may have softened resistance to marijuana liberalization. But political analyst Nate Silver argues that the key to the outcome may be the nation's changing demographics.

"As members of the Silent Generation are replaced in the electorate by younger voters, who are more likely to have either smoked marijuana themselves or been around those that have, support for legalization is likely to continue to gain momentum," Silver wrote recently. [18]

As policy advocates, politicians and citizens debate decriminalization, here are some of the questions being asked:

Should marijuana be legalized and taxed?

California legislator Ammiano has put the big marijuana question squarely on the table.

The interest his bill has drawn owes as much to his taxation plan as to the legalization aspect. But evaluating marijuana as a revenue source requires solid estimates of the size of marijuana crops, and the figures vary widely.

California tax chief Yee's $1.4 billion tax revenue estimate was itself derived from an estimate of a California crop worth $14 billion, a figure that traces back to a nationwide cannabis crop estimate of 10 million metric tons — worth $35.8 billion — by the White House drug-policy office in 2003. [19]

Some experts dismiss the 10 million metric ton figure. "To accept [that], it would be necessary to assume that the United States produces 4 to 10 times more cannabis than it needs to cover domestic consumption," said Martin Bouchard, a criminology professor at Simon Fraser University in Vancouver, British Columbia. "This is highly implausible." He estimates U.S. consumption at probably only around 1,000-2,500 metric tons. [20]

"Discussing it in terms of the California budget crisis — that's a joke," says Kleiman of UCLA, arguing that California's cannabis crop is far smaller than the $14 billion wholesale price estimate. He notes that a nationwide estimate of drug prices in 2000 concluded that Americans paid about $11 billion a year for marijuana at the retail level. [21]

The costs of enforcing marijuana prohibition are difficult to calculate because there are many variables, such as determining how many arrested for marijuana possession are charged with other crimes. Jeffrey A. Miron, a senior economics lecturer at Harvard University, took that factor into account when he came up with the most recent prohibition cost estimate: about $13 billion in federal and state enforcement-related expenses. Miron estimated that 50 percent of possession arrests are for possession alone. But he did not include estimates of drug-treatment and other health system costs that some legalization opponents argue would increase if marijuana became a legal product. [22]

Estimates aside, legalizing and taxing marijuana wouldn't work fiscally, argues Kleiman, who opposes marijuana prohibition. "If you made it licit, and taxed it, the price would collapse," he says, arguing that marijuana's illegality accounts for its relatively high price.

"The commercial product I can think of that's closest to fancy pot is fancy tea. Really, really, really fancy tea can go for up to $100 a pound."

Narcotic News, a Web site for the law-enforcement community, cites wholesale prices of up to $3,500 a pound for high-grade cannabis — consistent with a price average of $3,572 a pound calculated by the pro-legalization online *Bulletin of Cannabis Reform*. [23]

Some prohibition critics, however, call the possible economic benefits of legalization a secondary issue. "The moral and human cost of the drug war is the most compelling reason to change the law," says El Paso City Council member O'Rourke. One of those costs, he says, is measured in bodies. "Because it's a black market that does not have access to our judicial system, any business conflict has to be resolved outside of it — often very violently."

O'Rourke now advocates marijuana decriminalization — not merely a debate. If pot consumption were legal, he says, the high drug prices created by prohibition would decline, taking economic support away from the violent Mexican cartels now ravaging Ciudád Juárez and other communities in Mexico.

"Our drug policy is directly responsible for the murder and violence that people are experiencing in our sister community," he says, arguing that legalization would create economic benefits as well. Decriminalization would "relieve a lot of the costs related to interdiction and imprisonment and enforcement and tap new revenues we're missing out on."

Meanwhile, law-enforcement experts say Mexican drug gangs have opened pot-growing and sales operations in the United States, including in national forests. [24]

But Burns at the National District Attorneys Association says taxation won't work. "I doubt that Mexican cartels are going to want to be regulated or taxed — that's a pipe dream," he said. [25]

Burns also opposes legalization in principle, citing the frequent comparisons of marijuana to alcohol — with its obvious links to drunken driving and alcoholism. "Should we legalize marijuana for the sake of the argument that alcohol is as bad or worse, that it's become the social norm?" he asks. "That amounts to — if you've smashed your thumb with a hammer, smash the other one."

Yet a comparison between marijuana and legally available — but unhealthy — substances can serve a pro-legalization argument as well. Bill Piper, national affairs director of the Drug Policy Alliance Network, notes that cigarette smoking has declined drastically in recent decades as publicity campaigns have driven home the message of its harmful effects. In 2005, for example, the 378 billion cigarettes sold in the United States was the lowest number since 1951, when the nation's population was about half its present size. [26]

"The number of people who smoke cigarettes has plummeted, and you didn't have to arrest a single person," Piper says. "That suggests that regulation is far superior to prohibition."

Would pot legalization spur a big increase in consumption?

The nature of marijuana's effects lie at the heart of the legalization debate. In fact, that is where the entire subject of marijuana and the law began. When politicians and law-enforcement officials began campaigning in the early-20th century for national marijuana prohibition, the effect of cannabis on the mind and body had been hotly debated, and exaggerated. The lurid hyping of marijuana as a catalyst for violent crime that was a popular mass-media storyline in the 1920s and '30s is now valued for its comic effect.

In an era in which millions of people are personally familiar with marijuana's effects, prohibition advocates have downplayed such descriptions. Instead, the debate centers on the dangers of chronic use and on whether more people will develop dependence on marijuana if the number of marijuana users booms as a result of legalization.

The National Institute on Drug Abuse (NIDA) now focuses almost entirely on chronic use in discussing marijuana's dangers.

"Long-term marijuana use can be addictive for some people," NIDA says. "A study of 129 college students found that among heavy users of marijuana — those who smoked the drug at least 27 of the preceding 30 days — critical skills related to attention, memory and learning were significantly impaired, even after they had not used the drug for at least 24 hours."

NIDA also cites scientific evidence that frequent marijuana use in early adolescence can increase the likelihood of drug problems later in life. [27]

For their part, those campaigning for legalization or decriminalization accept that heavy, long-term use — as well as use by the very young — can be problematic. But they emphasize the relatively small percentage of marijuana users who develop dependence.

"A small minority of Americans — less than 1 percent — smoke marijuana on a daily basis," the Drug Policy Alliance Network says. "An even smaller minority develop a dependence on marijuana." [28]

That conclusion is consistent with the judgment of the Institute of Medicine, which published a major study of marijuana in 1999. "Compared to most other drugs . . . dependence among marijuana users is relatively rare," the institute said, adding that daily use of marijuana is rare. "Dependence appears to be less severe among people who use only marijuana than those who abuse cocaine, or those who abuse marijuana with other drugs (including alcohol)." [29]

Support for Marijuana Legalization Growing

Forty percent of Americans polled in 2009 said marijuana use should be legalized — more than three times the percentage from 1969. Opposition to legalization dropped by 35 percentage points — from 84 percent to 49 — over the same period.

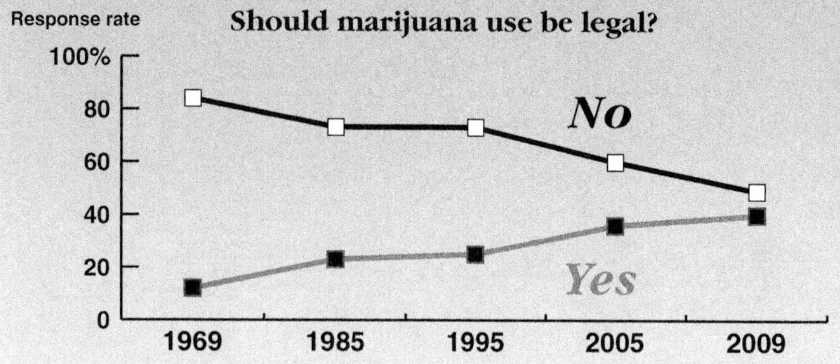

Sources: Joseph Carroll, "Who Supports Marijuana Legalization?" Gallup, November 2005; "40 Percent Say Marijuana Should Be Legalized," Rasmussen Reports, February 2009.

The institute cited studies showing that marijuana is much less addictive, for instance, than alcohol. Marijuana dependence ranges from 4.4 percent to 9 percent of the adult population at one time or another, compared to 13.8 percent for alcohol. [30]

As varied as the survey data can be, all of it was gathered about a drug that remains largely illegal. Kleiman of UCLA argues that if marijuana were legalized under the same conditions as alcohol or cigarettes, the laws of the marketplace would push sellers into massive promotion in order to increase consumption. "If you set it up as a system where a number of peoples' wealth depends on creating pot addicts, they will do so," he says. "Selling cannabis or any other intoxicant to people who use it moderately gets you no money."

In a new book on reducing crime and punishment, Kleiman argues for permitting homegrown marijuana, as well as marijuana grown by consumer cooperatives, but prohibiting advertising and commercial production. That policy, he says, would remove commercial incentives for cannabis producers and sellers to expand their market, thereby adding to the drug-dependent population. [31]

Drug-war advocates argue that the best policy is to continue prohibition. "When you push back [with tough laws], use gets reduced," says Burns of the district attorneys association, citing National Survey on Drug Use and Health data. They show a decline in adolescent marijuana use from 8.2 percent in 2002 to 7.6 percent in 2007 under the Bush administration's stringent anti-marijuana policies. [32]

"Fewer young people are smoking" marijuana today, Burns says. "But if you say that it's legal, you reduce the perception of risk — and clearly it would become much more available — that use is going to go up."

Among adults ages 50-59, however, rates of illicit drug use rose during the same period, from 2.7 percent to 5 percent. The pattern was similar for those even older. "This is the generation that used and abused drugs at

Pot Smoking in U.S. Tops the Charts

An estimated 42 percent of Americans and New Zealanders have smoked marijuana at least once, significantly more than most nations and more than twice the percentage of European countries.

Estimated Cannabis Use Among Population
(at least one usage)

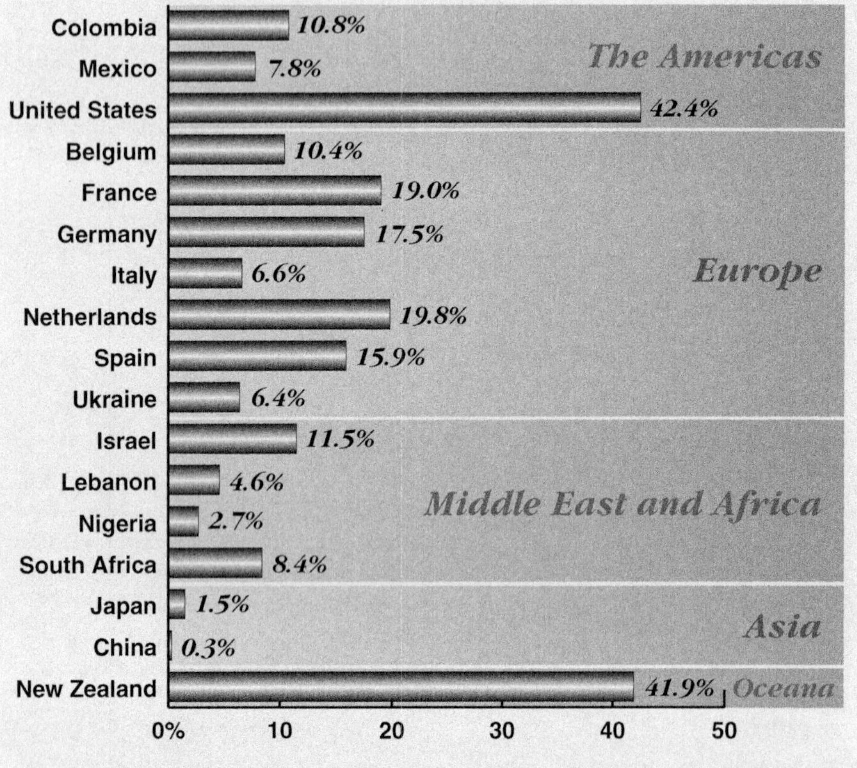

Source: Louisa Degenhardt, et al., *"Toward a Global View of Alcohol, Tobacco, Cannabis, and Cocaine Use: Findings from the WHO World Mental Health Surveys,"* PloS Medicine, *July 2008*

a much higher level when they were younger," Burns says. "For many people, it's for life."

In El Paso, Councilman O'Rourke concedes that the possibility of a spike in use is a "very valid concern." But he argues that decriminalizing or legalizing marijuana is the first step toward creating an effective regulatory system.

"When it's criminalized and underground, the criminals decide what the market is," he says. "They're selling to 10-year-olds and 12-year-olds."

Would legalizing marijuana help the criminal-justice system?

Advocates of legalization or decriminalization argue that law-enforcement time and resources shouldn't be spent on arresting marijuana users. Those who want to keep marijuana illegal say that whatever negative effects may exist are negligible compared with the advantages of allowing police and prosecutors to keep a crime-control tool that proves useful.

The context of the debate is a law-enforcement climate in which marijuana use and small-quantity possession is a low priority, at least in much of the country.

With the vast majority of marijuana users — as opposed to dealers — spending no more than a night behind bars, the criminal-justice argument has shifted to the issue of whether police and courts should spend any time or resources on low-level pot busts.

Considerable — if anecdotal — evidence can be found of police tolerance of low-level drug use. A recent *Washington Post* review of a concert by The Dead (formerly the Grateful Dead) described seeing in the audience a "50-something with a tucked-in, button-down shirt and a BlackBerry holster on his hip slyly taking a hit off a joint." [33]

In commentator Andrew Sullivan's popular blog the Daily Dish, the "Cannabis Closet" series features reports from readers that provide further anecdotal indications of police tolerance. "I live in Boulder, CO and there is no closet here," a reader e-mailed. "People just assume that you smoke pot. And the police don't care about it unless you are a big-time grower. . . . We smoke joints openly in public, and the cops usually won't even ask us to put it out if they see us doing it. I've smoked pot with a cop. In public." [34]

New York City, however, appears to be an exception to no-bust policies. The New York Civil Liberties Union in a 2008 report documented a 10-fold increase in street marijuana arrests over the previous 10 years. According to city statistics, the report said, arrests began to soar during the 1994-2001 administration of Mayor Rudolph Giuliani and continued under Michael Bloomberg. The number rose from 3,200 in 1987 to 39,700 in 2007. [35]

In the New York system, arrestees spend no more than a night in jail on a first or second offense, and then serve a version of probation for six months to a year, when the case is dismissed if no other infractions have occurred. [36]

Elsewhere in the country as well, even marijuana-prohibition critics acknowledge that most people serving time for marijuana are dealers. "By and large, it's not the case that you're going to go to prison for smoking a joint these days," says Marc Mauer, executive director of the Sentencing Project, which advocates reduced use of incarceration.

Still, says Mauer, who co-authored a study on the subject, 40 percent of the country's annual 1.8 million drug arrests are for marijuana — mostly low-level dealers, with higher-level dealers being the ones who end up doing time. [37] Though most of those arrested don't go to prison, "Law-enforcement resources go into arresting, processing, the court system parceling out cases," he says. "Clearly we're talking about tens of millions of dollars in police processing time. And for every hour police spend on making and processing marijuana arrests, that's an hour not responding to domestic violence or conducting community policing."

Burns of the district attorneys association counters that the vast majority of pot cases soak up relatively little in law-enforcement resources. "Low-level possession cases are already diverted — citation, dismissal, maybe a day or two in jail after multiple offenses — and by the time a court invests time and money in an offender via drug court or an intense diversion program, the offender has engaged in felony activity on multiple occasions," he says.

Nor do pot busts divert police from other duties, argues Burns, once a prosecutor in Zion, Utah. "The citation usually occurs when someone is being stopped or investigated for something else — traffic offense, assault, petty theft — so an officer is going to be there anyway. And there is a fine associated with the marijuana violation that more than pays for the officer's time."

Some prohibition opponents downplay the issue of criminal-justice resources. "The budget issue is very important, but we should not lose sight of the moral component — 700,000 Americans are being arrested every year for nothing more than marijuana possession," says Piper of the Drug Policy Alliance.

He adds that those arrested face consequences even if they don't go to jail or prison. "Those arrested are separated from their loved ones, branded criminals, denied jobs and in many cases prohibited from accessing public assistance for life."

Pacula at the RAND Corp. argues that questions of morality aren't a government province and shouldn't play a part in the debate.

Pacula argues that data on prohibition's law-enforcement costs should be weighed against projected costs to the system of legalizing or decriminalizing. "All of the literature suggests to me that harms will go up," she says. "And the cost of those harms is not zero."

She points to a 2004 study she co-authored that found a statistical association between increased marijuana use — because of lower pot prices — and income-producing crimes such as robbery, burglary, vehicle theft, forgery and prostitution. [38]

But Pacula acknowledges that the study isn't absolutely definitive, because it's based on data from crime in general, and from marijuana arrests — that is, not from the entire population of marijuana users, but from those who get charged with crimes. The conclusion she draws would be familiar to anyone who has seen a "Cheech and Chong" film: "It may be that people are more likely to get caught if they're using marijuana." ■

BACKGROUND

'The Poisonous Weed'

In the late 19th century, the use of opium and its derivatives — morphine and heroin — as well as cocaine, began emerging as an issue for state and federal governments. By the early 20th century, states were starting to regulate medical prescriptions more rigorously. And in 1914, the Harrison Narcotics Act strictly limited access to opiates, cocaine and other drugs. [39]

Meanwhile, marijuana — often incorrectly demonized as a narcotic — was making its way into the United States. Mexican immigrants and Caribbean sailors had introduced the drug, which soon became popular in big cities, especially in the black community, and, in the West and Southwest, among Mexican-Americans.

By 1930, 24 states had prohibited marijuana, though the public at large still had little awareness of it. That changed with the 1930 formation of the Federal Bureau of Narcotics within the Treasury Department. Its fabled director — Harry J. Anslinger, who held the job until 1962 — was widely considered the father of marijuana prohibition.

Many authors attribute to him the wildly sensationalized tales of marijuana-induced crimes that became staple fare in tabloids, true-crime magazines and movies in the 1930s. The blizzard of lurid tales made for entertaining reading and viewing decades later, including the 1936 film "Tell Your Children" — known as "Reefer Madness" — which became a cult classic among college students in the 1970s and went on to inspire an off-Broadway musical. [40]

However, David F. Musto, who teaches the history of medicine at Yale University and is considered the leading historian of U.S. drug use and drug policy, debunks the popular view of Anslinger as an anti-marijuana crusader. In the early and mid-1930s, he writes, Anslinger's main priority was heroin; he wanted to keep marijuana a state matter. [41]

But pressure for a federal law, especially from law enforcement agencies in the Southwest, proved irresistible. That pressure included breathless newspaper headlines, such as this one in a newspaper published by the then-powerful Hearst chain: "MARIJUANA MAKES FIENDS OF BOYS IN 30 DAYS; HASHISH GOADS USERS TO BLOOD LUST." [42]

Even the relatively staid *New York Times* joined the campaign to make marijuana illegal nationwide. "The poisonous weed . . . maddens the senses and emaciates the body of the user," said a 1934 story from Denver about marijuana's wide availability in the West. "Most crimes of violence in this section, especially in the country districts, are laid to users of the drug." [43]

The Times also noted that marijuana was "particularly popular with Latin Americans." Such scare stories aimed to drive home the point that no federal law against marijuana existed, and that state laws often weren't rigorously enforced.

In 1937, Congress passed the Marihuana Tax Act, which, despite its name, was effectively a prohibition measure. And by that year, all states had enacted marijuana prohibition laws of their own. [44]

In the wake of the new law, Anslinger promoted anti-marijuana campaigns, but Musto says he didn't push scare stories that gave the impression of an out-of-control problem.

Drug Culture

For about 20 years after the Marihuana Tax Act, marijuana remained in the cultural and legal shadows. Alcohol and tobacco were the only socially approved drugs, said a 1972 report from the National Commission on Marihuana and Drug Abuse, a panel appointed by President Nixon and headed by former Pennsylvania Gov. Raymond P. Shafer. [45]

But by the time the Shafer commission began its work, the tables had turned. "While marihuana is perceived as less harmful than before, alcohol and tobacco are regarded as more harmful," the panel reported. [46]

The commission also noted that Americans had been using alcohol and tobacco since colonial times (and, in the case of American Indians and tobacco, since before European settlers arrived). But marijuana, the opiates and cocaine had all arrived relatively recently. "And the users of these drugs were either aliens, like the Chinese opium smokers, or perceived to be marginal members of society," the commission noted. [47]

But the social revolution of the 1960s and '70s blurred the boundaries between mainstream and marginal. Sowers of the seeds of change included the poets and novelists who became known as "the Beats," notably poet Allen Ginsberg. He won respectful attention in some cultural institutions for his argument that marijuana and psychedelics had benign uses. "Marijuana is a useful catalyst for specific optical and aural aesthetic perceptions," he wrote in *The Atlantic* in 1966. [48]

Ginsberg had by then cofounded the New York chapter of the country's first anti-prohibition organization, LeMar (Legalize Marijuana), which had been formed in San Francisco in 1964. The poet's role drew law-enforcement attention. "From what I have read and heard, it would appear that the reported increased and widespread use of marihuana by college students could be attributed in part to the influence of Allen Ginsberg and persons of his ilk," a Federal Bureau of Narcotics agent reported in 1965. [49]

As the war in Vietnam escalated during the late 1960s, in turn strengthening the antiwar movement, pot smoking took on a political character, representing rejection of laws and social codes seen as unjust — like the war itself — and antiquated.

U.S. forces in Vietnam embraced the rebelliousness. In 1970, a *New York Times* correspondent reported how soldiers returning from a 10-day jungle mission shared a joint on the helicopter with the door gunner. Another soldier told the reporter he smoked marijuana constantly while on patrol. [50]

In fact, the *Times* said that in some areas 20-40 percent of soldiers used the drug. But a Vietnam vet, John Steinbeck IV, son of the Nobel Prize-winning novelist, told a Senate subcommittee in 1968 that 60 percent of the troops ages 19 to 27 smoked marijuana. [51]

On the home front, too, news media and popular culture began to acknowledge widespread marijuana use. In music, a number of songs depicted or praised drug use — the Jefferson Airplane's "White Rabbit," with its exhortation to "feed your head," heads the list. In films, the iconic "Easy Rider" (1969) and "Woodstock" (1970) started the trend. By the 1970s, any number of films contained matter-of-fact scenes or references to drug use.

The major annual national survey on drug use among young people confirmed the impression that use of marijuana and other drugs climbed during the 1970s. "Monitoring the Future," a federally funded project of the University of Michigan's Institute for Social Research, shows that marijuana use by 12th-graders climbed during the '70s in all regions and among all racial and ethnic groups, and social classes, peaking for most of them in 1979. By then an all-time high of 50.8 percent of all high-school seniors had used marijuana. [52]

Drug War

As drug use mounted, a succession of presidential administrations searched for ways to respond. The enduring "war on drugs" metaphor is attributed to President Nixon, who took office in 1969, though he favored emphasizing treatment for those addicted to drugs. [53]

Nixon's administration funded programs that treated heroin addicts with methadone, a policy that some hardliners opposed because it replaced one drug with another. And under Nixon, the federal government focused on narcotics addicts, not marijuana users.

Continued on p. 536

Chronology

1930s *Marijuana is prohibited nationwide.*

1930
Federal Bureau of Narcotics is established in the Treasury Department.

1937
Congress passes the Marihuana Tax Act, which effectively bans the drug.

1960s-1970s
During political upheavals, drug culture spreads from artists and writers to universities and broader society, prompting conflicting government responses.

1968
Novelist's son and Vietnam veteran John Steinbeck IV testifies in Congress that 60 percent of young troops in Southeast Asia are smoking pot.

1969
Film "Easy Rider" starts a cinematic trend of depicting pot smoking.

1970
Comprehensive Drug Abuse Treatment Act combines tough measures such as no-knock searches with low penalty for first-time marijuana offenders; classifies marijuana as a Schedule 1 drug with no medical uses and high abuse potential.

1975
Half of all high-school seniors have smoked marijuana — an all-time peak.

1977
President Jimmy Carter endorses decriminalization of marijuana possession of one ounce or less, but the plan dies after a scandal involving his drug-policy adviser.

1978
New Mexico lawmakers pass the nation's first medical-marijuana law.

1980s-1990s
Drug policy reverts to hard-line enforcement, partly in response to epidemic of crack cocaine use in inner cities; marijuana-liberalization forces gather strength.

1982
U.S. Food and Drug Administration (FDA) shuts down a tiny program that supplied medical marijuana.

1983
First lady Nancy Reagan launches "Just Say No" anti-drug campaign.

1985
Reagan administration adopts U.S. Navy's "zero tolerance" doctrine.

1986
Drug Abuse Act strengthens drug law, imposes heavy mandatory-minimum sentences.

1990
Opposition to mandatory sentences includes some federal judges, including a Reagan appointee who resigns from the bench in protest. . . . President George H. W. Bush says drug convicts deserve no sympathy.

1996
California voters pass a medical-marijuana law, opening a new era of medical-pot legislation. . . . Arizona voters also approve medical-pot law, but legislature kills it.

1999
In exhaustive scientific study of marijuana, Institute of Medicine recommends clinical trials of therapeutic uses of the drug.

2000s *Medical marijuana moves to center of debate as public opinion appears to shift toward legalization.*

2000
Hawaii's legislature creates first medical-marijuana law promoted by lawmakers rather than citizens.

2001
Drug Enforcement Administration refuses to remove marijuana from Schedule 1 classification, based on Department of Health and Human Services recommendation.

2005
Gallup Poll shows one-third of Americans support legalizing marijuana, up from 25 percent in 1995.

2006
FDA says marijuana has no medical use and that smoking it is harmful.

2007
Gov. M. Jodi Rell, R-Conn., vetoes medical-marijuana law.

2008
Sen. Jim Webb, D-Va., advocates creation of a commission to review the criminal-justice system, including drug laws.

2009
Attorney General Eric H. Holder Jr. says Obama administration will defer to state medical-marijuana laws. . . . U.S. Supreme Court declines to hear two California counties' challenge to state medical-marijuana law. . . . Minnesota medical-marijuana law and Massachusetts marijuana decriminalization take effect. . . . California Assemblyman Tom Ammiano proposes legalizing and taxing marijuana. . . . Senate Judiciary Crime and Drugs Subcommittee schedules June 11 hearing on Webb's commission bill.

California Pot Dispensaries Are Flourishing

"And the state hasn't gone to hell."

Some states are cautious about medical marijuana. They limit the number of marijuana "prescriptions" that one doctor can write, prohibit the opening of supply outlets, and permit only sufferers from certain specific illnesses to qualify. [1]

Seen from California, such precautions can look a little timid. In the Golden State, where the modern medical-marijuana era began with a law passed by voter initiative in 1996, medical marijuana is available from hundreds of storefront "dispensaries" and has spawned a large market in cannabis grown for these outlets.

At least 200,000 Californians are authorized medical-marijuana users, according to Americans for Safe Access, an Oakland-based medical-marijuana advocacy organization. [2] "Certainly in Northern California, well over 1 percent of the adult population are medical-marijuana users, in some places 2 percent," says Dale Gieringer, veteran state coordinator for California NORML (National Organization for the Reform of Marijuana Laws).

Law-enforcement officials concede that Californians on the whole support the system as it's developed. Yet that system and the state laws that underpin it fly in the face of federal law prohibiting sale, possession and use of cannabis, law-enforcement authorities argue. But the Obama administration's new policy of deferring to state medical-marijuana laws was followed by a California law-enforcement defeat on medical marijuana in the U.S. Supreme Court.

In May, the high court declined to consider a challenge to California's law that was based on its inconsistency with federal law. San Diego and San Bernardino counties had pursued that argument unsuccessfully through California state courts. The U.S. Supreme Court turned down without comment the counties' appeal of a California Supreme Court decision. [3]

But an attorney representing the California Police Chiefs Association maintains that city governments are still prohibited from violating federal law. "Since distribution of marijuana violates federal law," Martin J. Mayer wrote in a May memo to all police chiefs and sheriffs, "passing a zoning ordinance which, for example, only allows such operations to be conducted in the industrial or commercial zone of a city, would still be in violation of the laws of the United States and, therefore, prohibited." [4]

So far, that argument hasn't carried much weight with California's cities and counties. "The limited legal protections afforded to pot growers and dispensary owners have turned marijuana cultivation and distribution in California into a classic 'gray area' business, like gambling or strip clubs, which are tolerated or not, to varying degrees, depending on where you live and on how aggressive your local sheriff is feeling that afternoon," David Samuels of *The New Yorker* reported last year in a long, from-the-inside look at the state's marijuana industry. [5]

Since then, the "gray area" has expanded. In June, the *Los Angeles Times* reported that at least 600 medical-marijuana "dispensaries" — many if not most of them storefronts — are operating in Los Angeles County alone. They've proliferated because of a loophole in a city moratorium on new dispensaries. A hardship exemption allows outlets that opened after the moratorium began to keep running while the City Council prepares a comprehensive ordinance. That project has been under way for more than a year. [6]

Some in law enforcement argue that dispensaries are illegal even under the state medical-marijuana law. Storefront outlets aren't mentioned either in the 1996 law that voters passed nor in the 2004 law designed to provide further specifications of how the medical-marijuana system would operate, medical-marijuana advocates acknowledge. [7]

The law does mention that nonprofit cooperatives can supply marijuana. California Attorney General Edmund G. Brown Jr. concluded in formal guidelines issued last year that dispensaries could meet legal requirements as long as they could prove they weren't making profits, nor allowing any pot to enter the non-medical market. [8]

The guidelines also said that cooperatives shouldn't buy cannabis from non-members. California NORML, which has played an active

Continued from p. 534

The Comprehensive Drug Abuse Treatment Act of 1970 — the Nixon administration's milestone in drug-law history — represented a compromise between the treatment and law-enforcement approaches to drug policy. For example, the penalty for a first offense for possessing a small amount of marijuana would be probation. But police also were authorized to mount surprise, "no-knock" searches. And the law created a drug-categorization scheme that defined marijuana as a Schedule 1 drug — that is, a substance with "a high potential for abuse" and "no currently accepted medical use." [54]

The Watergate scandal coincided with growing acceptance of marijuana. President Gerald R. Ford, who became president when Nixon resigned in disgrace, had little effect on drug policy. But President Jimmy Carter attempted to revamp federal marijuana policy. In 1977, he endorsed legislation to remove criminal penalties for possession of an ounce or less of marijuana. [55]

Carter also advocated some hard-line steps, including an order to the Justice Department to consider removing restrictions on government access to personal financial information on known drug traffickers — in effect drawing a line between personal use and participation in the illegal trade in drugs. [56]

Moreover, the administration agreed to pay for the Mexican government to spray a herbicide, paraquat, on marijuana and opium-poppy plantations. That created a scandal that sank the

role in the evolution of the medical-marijuana system, challenges that conclusion. But, NORML adds, "In practice, this restriction can be easily avoided by simply enrolling all outside vendors as members of the collective." [9]

But that approach doesn't look so kosher to police.

"Too often 'medical marijuana' has been used as a smokescreen for those who want to legalize it and profit off it, and storefront dispensaries established as cover for selling an illegal substance for a lucrative return," the California Police Chiefs Association says in a 2009 "white paper" on dispensaries. [10]

The paper also concedes that protests haven't erupted, which in turn influences city and county officials. "Because the majority of their citizens have been sympathetic and projected a favorable attitude toward medical-marijuana patients, and have been tolerant of the cultivation and use of marijuana, public officials . . . have taken a hands-off attitude."

The public acceptance may reflect the fact that marijuana use hasn't exploded in the state's high schools — though, to be sure, the level is relatively high. The California attorney general's most recent annual survey of high-school students reported that since 2003, the share of students who have smoked pot in the previous six months has remained stable, at about 20 percent for ninth-graders and 31 percent for 11th-graders. [11]

"One of the most disturbing findings of the current survey is, among older students, recreational use of diverted (not prescribed by physicians) prescription painkillers ranks highest in illegal use behind marijuana," the report said.

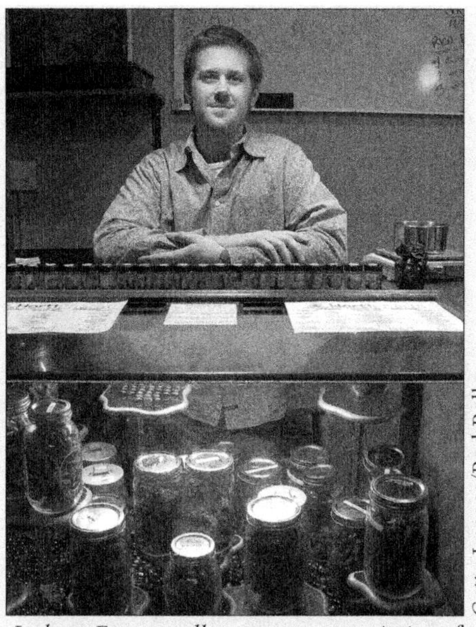

Getty Images/Rod Rolle

Joshua Braun sells numerous varieties of marijuana at his HortiPharm Caregivers dispensary in Santa Barbara, Calif.

In short, says Ellen Komp, a spokeswoman for California NORML, the medical-marijuana system is providing cannabis to patients without causing social disruption.

"Dispensaries are operating in neighborhoods," she says, "and the state hasn't gone to hell."

---

1 "Active State Medical Marijuana Programs," National Organization for the Reform of Marijuana Laws, http://norml.org/index.cfm?Group_ID=3391#top.

2 "Activist Newsletter," Americans for Safe Access, March 2009, p. 2, www.safeaccessnow.org/downloads/ASA_mar09_newsletter.pdf.

3 David G. Savage, "Justices reject California appeals on medical pot," *Los Angeles Times*, May 19, 2009, p. 19.

4 Martin J. Mayer, "Client Alert Memorandum," California Police Chiefs Association, May 19, 2009, www.californiapolicechiefs.org/nav_files/marijuana_files/vol_24_no_14_may_09.pdf.

5 David Samuels, "Dr. Kush: How Medical Marijuana Is Transforming the Pot Industry," *The New Yorker*, July 28, 2008.

6 John Hoeffel, "L.A.'s medical pot dispensary moratorium led to a boom instead," *Los Angeles Times*, June 3, 2009, www.latimes.com/news/local/la-me-medical-marijuana3-2009jun03,0,6866563,full.story.

7 "California NORML Advice for Medical Marijuana Providers," California NORML, April 2009, www.canorml.org/prop/collectivetips.html.

8 "Guidelines for the Security and Non-Diversion of Marijuana Grown for Medical Use," California Department of Justice, August 2008, http://ag.ca.gov/cms_attachments/press/pdfs/n1601_medicalmarijuanaguidelines.pdf.

9 "New AG Guidelines Don't Substantially Conflict With Previous Guidelines," California NORML, Aug. 27, 2008, www.canorml.org/news/AGguides.html.

10 "White Paper on Marijuana Dispensaries,' California Police Chiefs Association, April 2009, p. vi, www.californiapolicechiefs.org/nav_files/marijuana_files/MarijuanaDispensariesWhitePaper_042209.pdf.

11 Gregory Austin and Rodney Skager, "Highlights, 12th Biennial California Student Survey, Drug, Alcohol and Tobacco Use, 2007-2008," California Attorney General's Office, winter 2008, pp. 10, 24, http://safestate.org/documents/CSS_12th_Highlights_Report.pdf.

---

marijuana-decriminalization proposal.

Keith Stroup, founder of the country's first Washington-based, pro-legalization lobbying group — the National Organization for the Reform of Marijuana Laws (NORML) — had been friendly with Peter Bourne, a physician who was Carter's drug-policy adviser. But after Bourne endorsed the spraying, a furious Stroup gave a reporter the names of witnesses to Bourne's presence at a party where some guests — possibly including Bourne — snorted cocaine. [57]

The ensuing scandal not only ended Bourne's government career but also the prospects of drug-decriminalization legislation, linked as it was to the disgraced ex-drug adviser. [58]

President Ronald W. Reagan, who succeeded Carter, came to embody the drug war more than any other president before or since. Politically, drug use and drug tolerance had become linked with Democrats and the left. Moreover, Reagan's two terms (1981-1989) coincided with a boom in cocaine trafficking from South America and the beginnings of what became the crack cocaine boom.

Cocaine got most of the attention. But the Reagan administration made clear its hard-line approach applied to all drugs — a policy embodied in the "Zero Tolerance" and "Just Say No" slogans. First lady Nancy Reagan debuted the latter line in 1983. The administration apparently borrowed "zero tolerance" from the U.S. Navy. [59]

More substantively, the Reagan administration won passage of the tough

Would Legalizing Pot Hurt the Mexican Cartels?

Former President Vicente Fox: "It's time to open the debate."

The bloody war raging in Mexico among drug cartels is fueling arguments on both sides in the marijuana-decriminalization debate heating up in the United States. The gangs, which are fighting the government as well as each other, get most of their revenue from U.S. drug consumers, including marijuana smokers. [1]

"Legalizing drugs is the worst thing we could do for President Felipe Calderón and our Mexican allies," the George W. Bush administration's drug czar, John P. Walters, wrote in *The Wall Street Journal* in April. "It would weaken the moral authority of his fight, and the Mexicans would immediately realize that we have no intention of reducing consumption. Who do we think would take the profits from a legal drug trade? U.S. suppliers would certainly spring up, but that wouldn't preclude Mexican suppliers as well." [2] Walters is now executive vice president of the Hudson Institute, a nonpartisan think tank.

But how much the cartels make from marijuana alone is uncertain. The Justice Department's National Drug Intelligence Center (NDIC) says marijuana seizures on the U.S. side of the border increased in recent years, to about 1.4 million kilograms (about 3 million pounds) in 2007, but with a projected falloff for 2008 to 1.1 million kilos. U.S. domestic production was seen as increasing, but the center said no estimates were considered reliable enough to cite. [3]

Amid the uncertainty, Mark A. R. Kleiman, director of the drug policy analysis program at the University of California, Los Angeles, noted in a blog posting that marijuana couldn't account for most cartel revenues "since most of our cocaine still comes through Mexico, and the cocaine market is 250 percent the size of the pot market." [4]

Still, says the NDIC — reflecting a law-enforcement community consensus — Mexican gangs, known in Justice Department lingo as Drug-Trafficking Organizations (DTOs), also run large outdoor marijuana-growing operations in the West, which have been hit hard by drought and stepped-up police operations; drug agents eradicated a total of 6.6 million plants in 2007, some 2.6 million of them on public lands. [5]

In principle, legalizing marijuana would lower prices by removing the risk of arrest and by allowing more participants to enter the field. The extent to which Mexican gangs would be hit in the pocketbook, though, is as uncertain as crop estimates.

Scott Burns, executive director of the National District Attorneys Association, ridicules the idea that outlaw gangs would meekly join the legal business world, or give way to new competitors. It would be naïve to think, he says, "That cartels would file for tax status, that they'd somehow stop and say, 'We don't have a business license, so we won't grow those 20,000 plants in Yosemite this year.' "

Legalization advocates say law-enforcement agencies, unburdened by the duty to take on the entire drug industry, could focus their efforts on DTOs operating illegally.

"If we could take tens of millions of dollars away from the Mexican DTOs, are they still going to be making money?" asks Bill Piper, national affairs director of the Drug Policy Alliance. "Yes, but they may not still have $20 million a year for bribery and buying machine guns. It would be a crime issue but not a national security issue for Mexico and the United States."

Similar views are now being heard from Mexico and elsewhere in Latin America, where drug-producing countries have been a centerpiece of U.S. anti-drug policy for three decades.

Indeed, ex-drug czar Walters wrote his anti-legalization column in response to a call for decriminalization throughout the region from a commission headed by the former president of Mexico,

Anti-Drug Abuse Acts of 1986 and 1988. The laws' provisions included life sentences — and the death penalty in some circumstances — for top figures in major drug organizations. But the two statutes would become better known for a 100-to-1 disparity between mandatory-minimum sentences for crack cocaine and cocaine powder. The minimum for just five grams of crack (mainly used by blacks) was five years — the same penalty as for 500 grams of powder (used mainly by whites). [60]

Mandatory minimums also applied to marijuana. A conviction in a case involving at least 100 kilograms (220 pounds) of marijuana, or 100 plants, requires a five-year sentence. [61]

The sentencing scheme soon generated opposition — by judges, among others — who argued that low-level drug runners were getting longer terms than higher-ups with information to trade for lesser charges. "I can't continue to do it — I can't continue to give out sentences that I feel in some instances are unconscionable," U.S. District Judge J. Lawrence Irving of San Diego, a Reagan appointee, said in announcing he was quitting the bench. [62]

Prosecutors and other drug-war advocates told the critics to save their sympathies for victims of the drug trade, not traffickers, even low-level ones. Then President George H. W. Bush, asked about a 19-year-old sentenced to 10 years for selling crack within 1,000 feet of a school, said: "I can't feel sorry for this fellow." [63]

Decriminalization Push

Tough sentencing laws re-energized decriminalization campaigns. State legislatures didn't abolish marijuana laws, but most did reduce first-offense possession cases involving small

Ernesto Zedillo, together with the ex-presidents of Colombia, César Gaviria, and Brazil, Henrique Cardoso. "The available empirical evidence shows that the harm caused by this drug [marijuana] is similar to the harm caused by alcohol or tobacco," the Latin American Commission on Drugs and Democracy said in a policy proposal issued in April. "Most of the damage associated with cannabis use — from the indiscriminate arrest and incarceration of consumers to the violence and corruption that affect all of society — is the result of the current prohibitionist policies." [6]

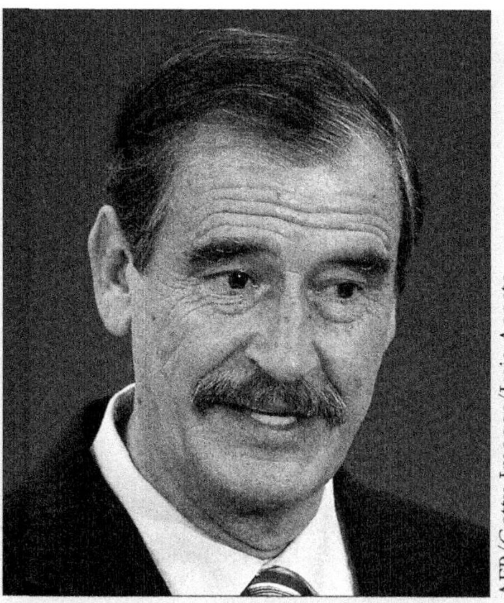
AFP/Getty Images/Luis Acosta

Former Mexican President Vicente Fox.

Another former Mexican president, Vicente Fox, is largely in agreement. "I believe it's time to open the debate over legalizing drugs," he told CNN in May. "It must be done in conjunction with the United States, but it is time to open the debate." [7]

As president, Fox vetoed legislation from the Mexican Congress to decriminalize small quantities of cocaine and marijuana. [8] But he made that move under U.S. pressure, and before Mexico's drug violence skyrocketed after his successor, Calderón, mounted a major offensive against the drug gangs. An estimated 6,300 Mexicans were killed last year alone, though Mexican authorities reported in April that the toll had fallen by 25 percent during the first three months of this year, to about 1,600, compared to the final quarter of 2008. [9]

Most of the killing results from turf battles along the border between rival gangs, though police and journalists have also been targeted, and associated violence has also claimed the lives of uninvolved civilians.

In El Paso, Texas, whose twin city of Ciudad Juárez, Mexico, is connected by a bridge over the Rio Grande, City Councilman Beto O'Rourke acknowledges that the marijuana decriminalization he favors likely wouldn't play a major role in reducing the violence. he says, "because until you get to a holistic solution that gets to the production and distribution supply chain, you're not going to end the situation with the cartels."

[1] For background, see Peter Katel, "Mexico's Drug War," *CQ Researcher*, Dec. 12, 2008, pp. 1009-1032.

[2] John P. Walters, "Drugs: To Legalize or Not," *The Wall Street Journal*, April 25, 2009, accessible at www.hudson.org/index.cfm?fuseaction=publication_details&id=6198.

[3] "National Drug Threat Assessment, 2009," National Drug Intelligence Center, December 2008, pp. 21-22, www.usdoj.gov/ndic/pubs31/31379/31379p.pdf.

[4] Mark A.R. Kleiman, "Joe Klein on drug legalization: same old, same old," The Reality-Based Community (blog), April 3, 2009, www.samefacts.com/archives/drug_policy_/2009/04/joe_klein_on_drug_legalization_same_old_same_old.php.

[5] "National Drug Threat Assessment," *op. cit.*, p. 20.

[6] "Drugs and Democracy: Toward a Paradigm Shift," Latin American Commission on Drugs and Democracy, April 2009, pp. 8-9, http://drugsanddemocracy.org/files/2009/02/declaracao_ingles_site.pdf.

[7] Arthur Brice, "Former Mexican president calls for legalizing marijuana," CNN, May 13, 2009, http://edition.cnn.com/2009/WORLD/americas/05/13/mexico.fox.marijuana/index.html.

[8] Marc Lacey, "In an Escalating Drug War, Mexico Fights the Cartels, and Itself," *The New York Times*, March 30, 2009, p. A1.

[9] Michael O'Boyle, "Mexico says death toll from drug war is falling," Reuters, April 3, 2009, http://uk.reuters.com/article/worldNews/idUKTRE5320CG20090403.

amounts to misdemeanors, in some cases eliminating the requirement that offenders serve jail time. [64]

Support for legalizing marijuana also drew strength from the growing "medical-marijuana" movement. Efforts to authorize use of the drug for medicinal purposes had begun in the 1970s among sufferers from chronic diseases such as glaucoma and multiple sclerosis, as well as cancer patients receiving chemotherapy. Speaking to state legislatures, journalists and anyone else who would listen, they said that smoking marijuana relieved their symptoms. A sizable number of doctors agreed. [65]

The first state to take action was New Mexico. In 1978, the legislature authorized medical marijuana in response to a campaign waged nearly single-handedly by a 26-year-old Vietnam veteran, Lynn Pierson, who'd been left painfully thin by testicular cancer and chemotherapy. Only marijuana (smoked on a doctor's recommendation) allowed him to endure the therapy, he said. [66]

But Pierson didn't live to see the result of his work. Only after he died, in August 1978, did the state medical-marijuana program receive any marijuana from its required supplier, the federal government. [67]

Following New Mexico's lead, other states passed similar laws, all permitting use of marijuana or THC, its psychoactive ingredient, supplied by the federal government. By 1980, 24 states had such laws, but only five or six had received either drug, according to the National Institute on Drug Abuse. [68]

The government's slowness in providing medical marijuana discouraged the activists, as did its preference for THC capsules, which many patients said did not provide the relief they received from smoking. The push for medical marijuana gained strength as the HIV/AIDS crisis worsened, and some sufferers said that only marijuana restored their appetites, enabling them to survive.

But the Food and Drug Administration didn't classify marijuana as medication, and in 1992 the U.S. Public Health Service stopped providing marijuana to certified medical users. [69]

In 1996, California voters approved a more radical approach authorizing anyone, including caregivers, to grow or possess marijuana if recommended by a physician for medical reasons. The referendum passed by a 56 percent-44 percent vote.

Other states began to follow California's lead, but with uneven results. Arizona voters in 1996 approved a medical-pot law by referendum, but the legislature overturned the measure, and another referendum failed in 2002. Hawaii in 2000 became the first state to act by legislative action rather than referendum. [70] Republican Connecticut Gov. M. Jodi Rell vetoed in 2007 a medical-marijuana bill that the legislature had passed. [71] By then, the Bush administration had been waging its own campaign against the "medical-marijuana" trend.

In 2001, the Drug Enforcement Administration refused a request to remove marijuana from the Schedule 1 category, citing a Health and Human Services Department assessment. In 2006, the U.S. Food and Drug Administration, in an apparent rebuttal of the 1999 Institute of Medicine report, issued an opinion that no scientific basis existed for use of marijuana as medicine. [72] ■

CURRENT SITUATION

Action in the States

California may get the headlines on marijuana-law issues, but other states are grappling with a variety of marijuana-decriminalization measures.

Massachusetts cities and towns are coming to terms with a law approved by 65 percent of voters last year that defines possession of one ounce or less of pot as a civil offense. That law makes the state among the most liberal of even the other 10 states that have abolished jail time for first-offense, small-quantity possession. [73]

The Massachusetts law imposed a $100 fine for the offense — significantly less than the $300 fine for drinking in public — and didn't mention smoking in public. So, police argue, the new law effectively favors public pot-smokers.

"I just see this as a problem that wasn't addressed in the law that was passed," Lt. Joseph Aiello of the Gloucester Police Department said. "What does that say to kids? It says: Don't drink beer — smoke pot, because if you drink a beer you're going to get arrested; if you smoke pot you're only going to get a citation for $100." [74]

Aiello advocated a $300 fine for public pot-smoking — but the Gloucester City Council rejected the proposal, which had mixed results elsewhere in the state. Marijuana-legalization advocates say police are looking for problems with a new law that rubs them the wrong way. "This seems to be much more about people who never liked the law to begin with looking for an end run around the will of the voters," said Dan Bernath, a spokesman for the Marijuana Policy Project. [75]

In other states, the focus of marijuana-law debates remains medical pot. Michigan is making history this year, becoming the first — so far, the only — Midwestern state to put a medical-marijuana law into effect. In 2008, Michigan voters approved cannabis use for people with cancer, HIV/AIDS, glaucoma and other chronic diseases whose symptoms marijuana has long been said to ease.

The new Michigan law refrains from authorizing California-style dispensaries. Medical users, or their caregivers, can grow their own. If they buy it on the black market, they won't be charged, but the sellers would be. And the law doesn't protect medical-pot users who are fired for failing job drug tests. [76] Majorie Russell, a professor at Thomas M. Cooley Law School in Lansing, said the voter initiative that passed the law succeeded because many citizens have experienced chemotherapy or chronic pain, or know people who've suffered those conditions. "That changed a lot of attitudes," she said. [77]

Elsewhere in the Midwest, though, the prospects for medical-marijuana laws are mixed. Republican Minnesota Gov. Tim Pawlenty vetoed legislation in May that would have authorized cannabis use solely for terminally ill patients. "While I am very sympathetic to those dealing with end-of-life illnesses and accompanying pain, I stand with law enforcement in opposition to this legislation," the governor said. Police and prosecutors had said that even the restricted approach would expand the general availability of marijuana. The bill had passed by votes of 36-28 in the Senate, and 70-64 in the House. [78]

Medical-marijuana backers immediately vowed to mount a ballot initiative next year to put the issue directly before voters. "Our basic approach is, we would spend what's needed," said Mirken at the Marijuana Policy Project. [79]

In Illinois, the state Senate passed a medical-marijuana bill on May 27 on a close 30-28 vote; the bill's House sponsor was considering delaying action until the fall in order to build more support. [80]

Political support for medical marijuana runs far stronger in other states. In New Mexico for example, a law that took effect in 2007 authorizes patients or caregivers — upon individual application — to cultivate cannabis to relieve symptoms of 15 specific conditions or illnesses, including cancer, Lou Gehrig's disease and HIV/AIDS. [81]

Continued on p. 542

At Issue:

Does permitting medical marijuana amount to "back-door legalization" of pot?

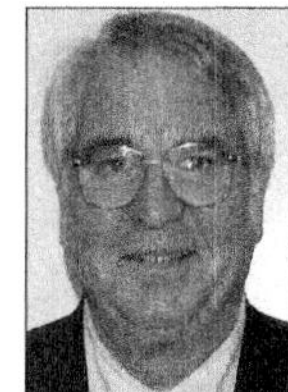

JOHN LOVELL
LEGISLATIVE COUNSEL, CALIFORNIA NARCOTIC OFFICERS ASSOCIATION

WRITTEN FOR *CQ RESEARCHER*, JUNE 8, 2009

Although presented to voters as providing relief to the terminally ill, medical-marijuana laws have become a subterfuge for recreational use of the drug. California is a pointed example of the evasion of the stated intent of the law.

Under California law, a physician is not required to issue a prescription for medical marijuana — that would invite professional inquiry into the appropriateness of that prescription. Instead, physicians are permitted to "recommend" marijuana to patients who think they require it. There are no medical standards governing that recommendation — as with prescription drugs — nor is there any serious medical oversight in determining whether a "recommendation" should be issued.

Thus, California has seen recommendations for the use of medical marijuana given to males for *their* menstrual cramps, to females for the discomfort high heels may cause them, to slackers to "ease the stress of life." Still another received "caregiver" status to provide marijuana for his dog! These are all specific examples of recommendations that have been given by compliant physicians. Such frivolous reasons should not be confused with the practice of medicine.

In other words, medical marijuana has virtually nothing to do with medicine and everything to do with attempting to evade controlled-substance laws. To allege that there are medical benefits to smoking marijuana is analogous to arguing for a medical benefit to the smoking of opium.

In addition to a law that permits easy evasion, medical-marijuana laws have spawned so-called medical-marijuana dispensaries. These large, retail outlets are not authorized under California law (which only permits co-ops for distribution where no profit is earned from distribution) and have become magnets for criminal activity. The fact that they are magnets for crime and have a corrosive impact on neighborhoods should not be a surprise — they have dope and large amounts of cash and have caused genuine alarm in the communities where the dispensaries are located. California crime reports are replete with incidences of violence in and around these locations.

California's medical-marijuana laws have been manipulated to evade California's controlled-substance laws. A true "medical" statute would have provided strict guidelines for prescribing the drug, would have fairly informed patients of the side-effects of the drug and would have imposed strict distribution controls.

The fact that the drafters of California's medical-marijuana law chose not to replicate standard medical practices speaks volumes about their true intent.

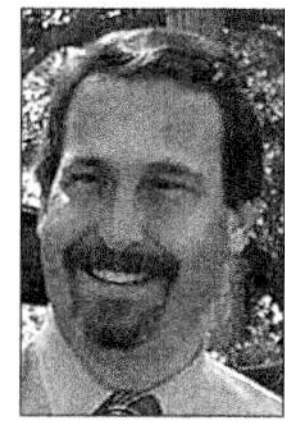

BRUCE MIRKEN
DIRECTOR OF COMMUNICATIONS MARIJUANA POLICY PROJECT

WRITTEN FOR *CQ RESEARCHER*, JUNE 6, 2009

One of the oldest and lamest arguments against laws allowing medical use of marijuana is that they somehow constitute "back-door legalization." The notion is absurd but continues to be stated with a straight face by those who oppose medical marijuana.

I say this as representative of an organization that believes marijuana should be treated like alcoholic beverages: Legal for adults but subject to sensible regulations and taxes.

But that's an entirely separate question. We can and do allow lots of drugs for medical use — morphine, OxyContin, even methamphetamine — that are not legal as toys. Personally, I got involved in this issue because I have friends with AIDS who are literally alive today because of medical marijuana.

The question here is not, "Might someone who isn't in legitimate medical need manage to possess marijuana under the guise of medicine?" Of course, a few manage to do so, just as about 7 million Americans illegally use prescription drugs in a given month, according to federal surveys. There has never been a system devised by humans that someone won't manage to cheat.

But even in California, whose loosely written medical-marijuana law has led to often-hysterical media reports of alleged abuse, marijuana arrests have increased — not declined — since the law went into effect in 1996. In 2007, 74,000 Californians were busted on marijuana charges, 80 percent of them for possession. If that's legalization, it's sure come in an odd form.

Other state medical-marijuana laws are much more tightly controlled than California's. Most require patients to register with the state, keep a copy of their doctor's recommendation on file and carry an ID card identifying them as a legal patient. Only specific conditions enumerated in the statute qualify for legal protection. These restrictions are not applied to any prescription drug, not even morphine or OxyContin.

That may surprise some, but it's true. A physician can legally prescribe any approved drug for any purpose, regardless of whether or not the FDA OK'd it for that use. About half of all prescriptions are written "off-label" — i.e. for uses not approved by the FDA. And you don't have to apply to the state or get an ID card to have your morphine prescription filled.

If anyone wants to talk about whether marijuana should be legal for adults, we're happy to have that discussion. But muddying the waters by claiming that limited, highly restricted laws aimed at protecting the sick and suffering are "back-door legalization" is simply dishonest.

Continued from p. 540

Rhode Island, however, may follow the California model in expanding its 2006 medical-marijuana law. Under the law, about 600 residents currently are authorized to use cannabis, but they and their political backers are arguing that without state-authorized dispensaries the only sources of supply are dope dealers. [82]

In early June the legislature passed a dispensary bill and sent it to Republican Gov. Donald L. Carcieri, who was expected to veto it. But members said they had the votes to override. [83]

Elsewhere in the Northeast, medical-cannabis bills are pending in New York, New Jersey and New Hampshire, where Democratic Gov. John Lynch is expected to veto the measure, which Attorney General Kelly Ayotte and county prosecutors have aggressively opposed.

Among other objections, Ayotte called marijuana a gateway to harder drugs, a traditional argument against any moves to soften marijuana laws. "Studies have shown that very few young people turn to illegal drugs such as cocaine or heroin without first experimenting with marijuana," Ayotte said in a letter to lawmakers.

But Sen. Kathy Sgambati, a Democrat, called Ayotte's point irrelevant to the medical-marijuana legislation and the patients who would benefit. "Ninety percent at least of the people who testified have medicine chests full of opiates," she said, adding that they weren't seeking "a stronger drug," but an effective one. [84]

In New York and New Jersey, medical-pot bills were given good chances in late May of reaching the floors of both houses, but the legislative sessions had only one month left to run. Both David A. Paterson, the New York governor, and New Jersey Gov. Jon Corzine, both Democrats, are expected to sign the bills if they pass. [85]

In New Jersey, where Attorney General Anne Milgram has also backed the bill, legislation has passed the Senate and is pending in the lower house. [86]

The Webb Approach

Freshman Sen. Jim Webb, D-Va. argues that the criminal-justice system demands urgent attention. "Justice statistics . . . show that 47.5 percent of all the drug arrests in our country in 2007 were for marijuana offenses," Webb wrote in *Parade* in March. "Additionally, nearly 60 percent of the people in state prisons serving time for a drug offense had no history of violence or of any significant selling activity." [87]

Yet mounting drug arrests in general, and marijuana arrests in particular, have simply flooded prisons with new convicts without making a dent in the market for drugs, including hard drugs, Webb insists. "We are not protecting our citizens from the increasing danger of criminals who perpetrate violence and intimidation as a way of life, and we are locking up too many people who do not belong in jail," Webb argued. [88]

Webb has introduced legislation calling for a National Criminal Justice Commission to examine all aspects of the system, including drug laws. Webb hasn't rejected pot legalization, but he hasn't advocated it either.

"It's true, we have way too many people in prison," Tom Riley, a spokesman for the Bush administration's drug czar, told *The Washington Post* in late 2008. "But it's not because the laws are unjust, but because there are too many people who are causing havoc and misery in the community." [89]

And J. Scott Leake, a Republican strategist in Virginia, told *The Post* that Webb was making a mistake in tackling laws that, Leake said, brought crime rates down. "If Sen. Webb were to try to roll some of that back, I think he would have a fight on his hands." [90]

The metaphor is apt. A decorated Marine and Vietnam veteran, Webb served as Navy secretary in the Reagan administration, long before he changed his party affiliation to Democrat. Webb has taught pistol marksmanship, and in his 2006 Senate campaign he displayed his concealed-weapon permit. [91]

In short, Webb is about as far from the stereotypical bleeding-heart liberal as one can get. "With Jim's personality, he's never going to strike somebody as being soft on crime or any other issue," said Virginia state Sen. J. Chapman Petersen, a Democrat. [92]

Toughness aside, Webb isn't proposing immediate changes to the system. But he minces no words in arguing that drug policy is a failed part of a failed system. "In 1980, we had 41,000 drug offenders in prison," he said on the Senate floor, when formally introducing his bill. "Today we have more than 500,000, an increase of 1,200 percent . . . and a significant percentage of those are incarcerated for possession or nonviolent offenses stemming from drug addiction." [93]

OUTLOOK

Congress' Move

Some newcomers to the long-running marijuana debate argue that the present state of affairs can't continue past another decade. "In 10 years, certainly, marijuana will be decriminalized," says El Paso City Council member O'Rourke, likening the present day to the last years of alcohol prohibition. "We're like we were in the early '30s. Our leaders are going to say, 'We can't afford to spend on this any more.' The country will come to that conclusion soon."

Veteran criminal-justice system analysts tend to make more nuanced forecasts. "I think we're likely to see a number of jurisdictions in effect decriminalizing marijuana," says Mauer at The Sentencing Project. "I don't know how many legislative bodies will take the step to do it in a formal way. I think there is still a reluctance to put their names on bottom lines."

Mainstream politicians approach marijuana prohibition in much the same way as they do the death penalty, Mauer says. "A couple of states have abolished capital punishment, but in practice prosecutors in many places have lost enthusiasm for it; it's a cost and a burden. That's a likely scenario for marijuana: 'Let's not get too worked up about it.' Enforcing it as a criminal-justice issue will decline in popularity."

Burns at the National District Attorneys Association is on the other side of the criminal-justice debate. But to some extent he shares Mauer's view on politicians' reluctance to dive into changing marijuana law. The Obama administration, Burns says, has no interest in turning up the heat on the debate, which would focus attention on its hands-off approach to state medical-marijuana laws.

In general, there's no reason to think that the marijuana-prohibition fight is anywhere near over, Burns says. "Debates go on in opinion pages of large and small papers; it's interesting for radio talk shows or late-night TV, in bars," he says. "But until the U.S. Congress says it's legal, or the FDA says it's a medicine, I don't know what the debate is about."

Still, further state actions to decriminalize cannabis are possible, says Pacula at the RAND Corp. think tank. But full-scale legalization — putting the entire cannabis business within the law — would require Congress to act. "The federal government doesn't have a strong reason to legalize marijuana right now," she says. "In 10 years, this issue will have been determined by the federal government, or we'll still be having this discussion."

Piper at the Drug Policy Alliance makes a similar forecast. A decade from now, he says, "I think we'll be at a point where several states have passed legalization, and we may very well be in a position on legalization that we are in medical marijuana right now. Federal law is still in the way, and the conflict will have to be resolved."

But another possibility is a continuing erosion of marijuana prohibition that leads to de facto legalization, says Kleiman of UCLA. The mechanism could easily be medical-marijuana authorization. "I don't think I know anybody who has a medical recommendation for cannabis; I can easily imagine that changing over the next five years," he says. "If it became non-weird to have that [authorization] card, you really have legalized pot. And without any sharp demarcation line, you could go from a situation where cannabis is illegal to where it's medical and it's sort of legal."

Kleiman adds, "I used to laugh at people who said medical marijuana is legalization. I don't laugh any more." ■

Notes

[1] Quoted in Karl Vick, "In Calif., Medical Marijuana Laws Are Moving Pot Into the Mainstream," *The Washington Post*, April 12, 2009, p. A3, www.washingtonpost.com/wp-dyn/content/article/2009/04/11/AR2009041100767_pf.html. Schwarzenegger quoted in Jonathan Lloyd, "Schwarzenegger: High Time for Marijuana Debate," NBC Los Angeles, May 5, 2009, www.nbclosangeles.com/news/local/Arnold-Ready-to-Look-into-Legalization.html. See also "The Field Poll," April 30, 2009, http://field.com/fieldpollonline/subscribers/Rls2306.pdf.

[2] Quoted in Lloyd, *op. cit.*

[3] Quoted in David Johnston and Neil A. Lewis, "Ending Raids of Dispensers of Marijuana for Patients," *The New York Times*, March 19, 2009, p. A20.

[4] Quoted in "LA chief calls state marijuana laws 'Looney Tunes,' " MercuryNews.com (The Associated Press), April 2, 2009, www.mercurynews.com/news/ci_12056082?nclick_check=1.

[5] Quoted in Gary Fields, "White House Czar Calls For an End to 'War on Drugs,' " *The Wall Street Journal*, May 14, 2009, http://online.wsj.com/article/SB124225891527617397.html.

[6] Donna Leinwand, "U.S.' new drug czar targets prescription abuse as priority," Freep.com, May 21, 2009, http://content.usatoday.net/dist/custom/gci/InsidePage.aspx?cId=freep&sParam=35111116.story.

[7] *Ibid.*

[8] Mark A. R. Kleiman, *When Brute Force Fails: How to Have Less Crime and Less Punishment* (2009).

[9] "Estimated Number of Arrests, United States, 2005," FBI, September 2006, www.fbi.gov/ucr/05cius/data/table_29.html; "Results from the 2007 National Survey on Drug Use and Health: National Findings," Sept. 4, 2008, www.oas.samhsa.gov/NSDUH/2k7NSDUH/2k7results.cfm#Ch2.

[10] Louisa Degenhardt, *et al.*, "Toward a Global View of Alcohol, Tobacco, Cannabis, and Cocaine Use: Findings from the WHO World Mental Health Surveys," *PloS Medicine*, July 2008, www.plosmedicine.org/article/info:doi/10.1371/journal.pmed.0050141.

[11] Quoted in Neal Peirce, "Webb Leads the Charge in Much-Needed Drug, Prison Reform," *Richmond Times-Dispatch*, April 5, 2009, www.timesdispatch.com/rtd/news/opinion/commentary/article/webb_leads_the_charge_for_much-needed_drug_prison_reform/249095/.

[12] "House Judiciary Subcommittee on Crime, Terrorism and Homeland Security Holds Hearing on Unfairness in Federal Cocaine Sentencing," CQ Congressional Transcripts, May 21, 2009.

[13] *Ibid.* For background see Peter Katel, "Mexico's Drug War," *CQ Researcher*, Dec. 12, 2008, pp. 1009-1032.

[14] Dan Simon, "Mexican cartels running pot farms in U.S. national forest," CNN, Aug. 8, 2008, www.cnn.com/2008/CRIME/08/08/pot.eradication/.

[15] Letter, state Reps. Joe C. Pickett, Chente Quintanilla, Joseph E. Moody, Norma Chávez, Marisa Marquez, Jan. 12, 2009; letter, Rep. Silvestre Reyes, Jan. 13, 2009.

[16] "Washington Post-ABC News Poll," April 21-24, 2009, www.washingtonpost.com/wp-srv/politics/polls/postpoll_042609.html; "Possible Law Changes," CBS News Poll, March 19, 2009, www.cbsnews.com/htdocs/pdf/poll_031909_marijuana.pdf; "40 Percent Say Marijuana Should Be Legalized," Rasmussen Reports, Feb. 19, 2009, www.rasmussenreports.com/public_content/lifestyle/general_lifestyle/february_2009/40_say_marijuana_should_be_legalized.

[17] Joseph Carroll, "Who Supports Marijuana Legalization?" Gallup, Nov. 1, 2005, www.gallup.com/poll/19561/Who-Supports-Marijuana-Legalization.aspxLegalization.aspx.

[18] Nate Silver, "Why Marijuana Legalization is Gaining Momentum," FiveThirtyEight, April 5, 2009, www.fivethirtyeight.com/2009/04/why-marijuana-legalization-is-gaining.html.

[19] Jon Gettman, "Marijuana Production in the United States (2006)," *Bulletin of Cannabis Reform*, December 2006, www.drugscience.org/Archive/bcr2/MJCropReport_2006.pdf.

[20] Martin Bouchard, "A capture-recapture-derived method to estimate cannabis production in industrialized countries," School of Criminology, Simon Fraser University, 2007, www.issdp.org/conferences/oslo2007/Martin_Bouchard.pdf.

[21] "What America's Users Spend on Illegal Drugs," Abt Associates, December 2001, pp. 32-33, www.whitehousedrugpolicy.gov/publications/pdf/american_users_spend_2002.pdf. Abt is a Cambridge, Mass.-based consulting firm working under contract for the ONCDP.

[22] Jeffrey A. Miron, "The Budgetary Implications of Drug Prohibition," Department of Economics, Harvard University, December 2008, www.economics.harvard.edu/faculty/directory/faculty/M/O.

[23] "Wholesale Marijuana Prices," *Narcotic News*, undated, www.narcoticnews.com/Marijuana/Prices/USA/Marijuana_Prices_USA.html; "Price Index for the Years 2003 to 2006 Converted to 2007 Constant Dollars," DrugScience.org, 2007, www.drugscience.org/Archive/bcr4/Table11.html.

[24] Solomon Moore, "Tougher Border Can't Stop Mexican Marijuana Cartels," *The New York Times*, Feb. 1, 2009, www.nytimes.com/2009/02/02/us/02pot.html?sq=mexicancartels-marijuanau.s.&st=cse&scp=1&pagewanted=all.

[25] *Ibid.*

[26] Marc Kaufman, "Smoking in U.S. Declines Sharply," *The Washington Post*, March 9, 2006, p. A1.

[27] "Marijuana Abuse," National Institute on Drug Abuse, July 22, 2008, www.nida.nih.gov/researchreports/marijuana/Marijuana3.html.

[28] "Marijuana: The Facts," Drug Policy Alliance, undated, www.drugpolicy.org/marijuana/factsmyths/.

[29] Janet E. Joy, *et al.*, *Marijuana and Medicine: Assessing the Science Base* (1999), Institute of Medicine, pp. 94-97, www.nap.edu/openbook.php?record_id=6376&page=94.

[30] *Ibid.*

[31] Kleiman, *op. cit.*

[32] "Results from the 2007 National Survey on Drug Use and Health: National Findings," *op. cit.*

[33] David Malitz, "One Night With the Dead Turns Into Eternal Jamnation," *The Washington Post*, April 16, 2009, p. C3.

[34] Chris Bodenner, "The Daily Dish," May 24, 2009, http://andrewsullivan.theatlantic.com/the_daily_dish/2009/05/the-cannabis-closet-safe-havens.html.

[35] Harry G. Levine and Deborah Peterson Small, "Marijuana Arrest Crusade: Racial Bias and Police Policy in New York City 1997-2007," New York Civil Liberties Union, April 2008, p. 7, www.nyclu.org/files/MARIJUANA-ARREST-CRUSADE_Final.pdf.

[36] *Ibid.*

[37] Ryan S. King and Marc Mauer, "The War on Marijuana: The Transformation of the War on Drugs in the 1990s," The Sentencing Project, May 2005, www.sentencingproject.org/Admin\Documents\publications\dp_waronmarijuana.pdf.

[38] Rosalie Liccardo Pacula and Beau Kilmer, "Marijuana and Crime: Is There a Connection Beyond Prohibition?" RAND, January 2004, www.rand.org/pubs/working_papers/2004/RAND_WR125.pdf.

[39] Except where otherwise noted, this subsection is drawn from Martin Booth, *Cannabis: A History* (2004); Rudolph J. Gerber, *Legalizing Marijuana: Drug policy Reform and Prohibition Politics* (2004); and David F. Musto, *The American Disease: Origins of Narcotic Control* (1999).

[40] "Reefer Madness: The Movie Musical (2005)," Internet Movie Database, www.imdb.com/title/tt0404364/.

[41] Musto, *op. cit.*, pp. 221-225.

[42] Quoted in Gerber, *op. cit.*, p. 7.

[43] "Use of Marijuana Spreading in West," *The New York Times*, Sept. 16, 1934.

[44] "Marihuana: A Signal of Misunderstanding," The National Commission on Marihuana and Drug Abuse, 1972, www.druglibrary.org/Schaffer/Library/studies/nc/mis2_6.htm. For background, see Peter Katel, "War on Drugs," *CQ Researcher*, June 2, 2006, pp. 481-504.

[45] Unless otherwise noted, this subsection draws on "Marihuana: A Signal . . .," *op. cit.*; and Musto, *op. cit.*

[46] "Marihuana: A Signal . . .," *op. cit.*

[47] *Ibid.*

[48] Quoted in Booth, *op. cit.*, pp. 210-211.

[49] *Ibid.*, p. 210.

[50] Quoted in James P. Sterba, "G.I.'s Find Marijuana Is Plentiful," *The New York Times*, Sept. 2, 1970.

[51] "U.S. Troops in Vietnam Are Said to Get Pep Pills," *The New York Times*, March 6, 1968.

[52] Lloyd D. Johnston, *et al.*, "Demographic Subgroup Trends for Various Licit and Illicit Drugs, 1975-2007," *Monitoring the Future*, 2008, p. 274, www.monitoringthefuture.org/pubs/occpapers/occ69.pdf.

[53] Unless otherwise indicated, this subsection draws on Musto, *op. cit.* Also see Michael Massing, *The Fix* (2000). For additional background, see Mary H. Cooper, "Drug-Policy Debate," *CQ Researcher*, July 28, 2000, pp. 595-620.

[54] Mark Eddy, "Medical Marijuana: Review and Analysis of Federal and State Policies," Congressional Research Service, March 31 2009, p. 3, www.fas.org/sgp/crs/misc/RL33211.pdf.

[55] Edward Walsh, "Carter Endorses Decriminalization of Marijuana," *The Washington Post*, Aug. 3, 1977, p. A1.

[56] *Ibid.*

[57] Patrick Anderson, *High in America: The True Story Behind NORML and the Politics of Marijuana* (1981), pp. 274-284.

[58] Kenneth J. Meier, *The Politics of Sin: Drugs, Alcohol, and Public Policy* (1994), pp. 48-49.

[59] Paul Houston, "Bumper Stickers Would Brand Offenders," *Los Angeles Times*, May 28, 1988, A1; Peter Kerr, "Anatomy of the Drug Issue," *The New York Times*, Nov. 17, 1986, p. A1; Donnie Radcliffe, "Seafarer Nancy Reagan," *The Washington Post*, July 2, 1985, p. C2; Philip H. Dougherty, "Drug Drive Outlined to First Lady," *The New York Times*, Oct. 12, 1983, p. D22.

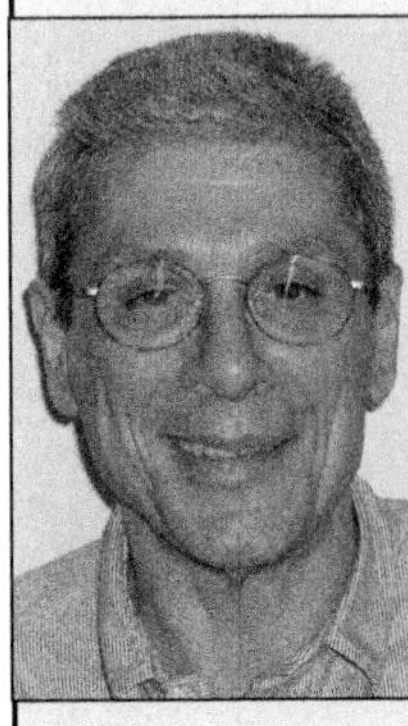

About the Author

Peter Katel is a *CQ Researcher* staff writer who previously reported on Haiti and Latin America for *Time* and *Newsweek* and covered the Southwest for newspapers in New Mexico. He has received several journalism awards, including the Bartolomé Mitre Award for coverage of drug trafficking, from the Inter-American Press Association. He holds an A.B. in university studies from the University of New Mexico. His recent reports include "Mexico's Drug War," "Hate Groups" and "Vanishing Jobs."

[60] Gerald M. Boyd, "Reagan Signs Anti-Drug Measure," *The New York Times*, Oct. 28, 1986; Deborah J. Vagins and Jesselyn McCurdy, "Cracks in the System: Twenty Years of the Unjust Federal Crack Cocaine Law," ACLU, October 2006, www.aclu.org/pdfs/drugpolicy/cracksinsystem_20061025.pdf.
[61] David Risley, "Mandatory Minimum Sentences: An Overview," Drug Watch International, May 2000, www.drugwatch.org/MandatoryMinimumSentences.htm.
[62] Quoted in Michael Isikoff and Tracy Thompson, "Getting Too Tough on Drugs," *The Washington Post*, Nov. 4, 1990, p. C1.
[63] Quoted in *ibid.*
[64] For a state-by-state list of marijuana penalties, see "State By State Laws," National Organization for Reform of Marijuana Laws, Aug. 5, 2006, www.norml.org/index.cfm?Group_ID=4516.
[65] For background, see Kathy Koch, "Medical Marijuana," *CQ Researcher*, Aug. 20, 1999, pp. 705-728.
[66] Anderson, *op. cit.*, pp. 245-248.
[67] Larry Calloway, "New Mexico's Been There, California," *Albuquerque Journal*, Dec. 1, 1996, p. B1. Eugene L. Meyer, "Uncle Sam's Aunt Mary," *The Washington Post*, Oct. 22, 1995, p. F1.
[68] Susan Okie, "Cancer Victims to Get Marijuana Ingredient," *The Washington Post*, Nov. 11, 1980, p. A1.
[69] Dianne Klein, "The Empty Pot," *Los Angeles Times*, April 1, 1992, p. A3.
[70] "Hawaii Becomes First State to Approve Medical Marijuana Bill," *The New York Times*, June 15, 2000, www.nytimes.com/2000/06/15/us/hawaii-becomes-first-state-to-approve-medical-marijuana-bill.html.
[71] Anjanette Riley and Amanda Crawford, "Arizona voters might get another shot at medical marijuana," *Arizona Capitol Times*, April 24, 2009; Matthew J. Malone, "Medical Marijuana Measure Falls With Connecticut Governor's Veto," *The New York Times*, June 20, 2007.
[72] Eddy, *op. cit.*, p. 11. For additional details on the 1999 IOM report, see Koch, *op. cit.*
[73] "State By State Laws," *op. cit.*
[74] Quoted in Steven Rosenberg, "Drug use in public targeted," *The Boston Globe*, April 9, 2009, p. B1.
[75] Quoted in Jonathan Saltzman, "Towns try to punish public marijuana use," *The Boston Globe*, March 25, 2009, p. B1. See also Patrick Anderson, "Council nixes hike in pot fines," *Gloucester Daily Times*, May 7, 2009, www.gloucestertimes.com/archivesearch/local_story_126224820.html.

FOR MORE INFORMATION

Drug Free America Foundation, 5999 Central Ave., Suite 301, St. Petersburg, FL 33710; (727) 828-0211; www.dfaf.org. Advocates drug prohibition and serves as a clearinghouse for information on marijuana's adverse effects.

Drug Policy Alliance Network, 70 West 36th St., 16th Floor, New York, NY 10018; (212) 613-8020; www.drugpolicy.org. Advocates an end to law-enforcement-oriented policies for substances including marijuana.

Marijuana Policy Project, P.O. Box 77492, Capitol Hill, Washington, DC 20013; (202) 462-5747; www.mpp.org. Seeks to liberalize laws on marijuana.

National Institute on Drug Abuse, 6001 Executive Blvd., Room 5213, Bethesda, MD 20892; (301) 443-1124; www.nida.nih.gov. The government's lead agency on addiction makes available data and studies on addiction and drug dependency.

National Organization for the Reform of Marijuana Laws, 1600 K St., N.W., Suite 501, Washington DC 20006; (202) 483-5500; http://norml.org. Spearheaded the marijuana-decriminalization campaign of the early 1970s.

Office of National Drug Control Policy/Drug Policy Information Clearinghouse, P.O. Box 6000, Rockville, MD 20849; (800) 666-3332; whitehousedrugpolicy.gov. Provides information on government strategy and priorities.

The Sentencing Project, 514 10th St., N.W., Suite 1000, Washington, DC 20004; (202) 628-0871; www.sentencingproject.org. Advocates less use of incarceration in criminal-justice drug policies.

[76] Tim Jones, "Legal pot debuts in Midwest," *Chicago Tribune*, March 20, 2009, p. A4.
[77] Quoted in *ibid.*
[78] Quoted in Jason Hoppin, "Pot fight on ballot? That's their plan," *St. Paul Pioneer Press*, May 27, 2009; Mark Brunswick, "Minnesota Senate approves medical marijuana," *StarTribune.com*, April 30, 2009, www.startribune.com/politics/state/44005777.html.
[79] *Ibid.*
[80] Kevin McDermott, "As deadline nears, Illinois House dawdles on tax hike," *St. Louis Post-Dispatch*, May 30, 2009, p. A1.
[81] "Severe chronic pain added to medical marijuana," The Associated Press, May 7, 2009; Sue Major Holmes, "First medical marijuana producer in NM approved," The Associated Press, March 19, 2009.
[82] Cynthia Needham, "House OKs plan to establish up to 3 marijuana dispensaries," *Providence Journal-Bulletin*, May 21, 2009, p. A6.
[83] *Ibid.*
[84] Quoted in Lauren R. Dorgan, "Marijuana debate sharpens," *Concord Monitor*, May 14, 2009.
[85] "Medical Marijuana: New York Bill Wins Senate Committee Vote," *Drug War Chronicle*, May 29, 2009, http://stopthedrugwar.org/chronicle/587/new_york_medical_marijuana_bill_wins_senate_committee_vote; Tom Precious, "Approval predicted for medical marijuana," *Buffalo News*, April 22, 2009, p. A1.
[86] Adrienne Lu, "Backers of medical marijuana hopeful in N.J.," *The Philadelphia Inquirer*, March 9, 2009, p. A1.
[87] Sen. Jim Webb, "Why We Must Fix Our Prisons," *Parade*, March 29, 2009, www.parade.com/news/2009/03/why-we-must-fix-our-prisons.html.
[88] *Ibid.*
[89] Quoted in Sandhya Somashekhar, "Webb Sets His Sights on Prison Reform," *The Washington Post*, Dec. 29, 2008, p. B1.
[90] Quoted in *ibid.*
[91] Allison Klein, "Webb Aide Tried to Take Gun Into Senate Building, Capitol Police Say," *The Washington Post*, March 27, 2007, www.washingtonpost.com/wp-dyn/content/article/2007/03/26/AR2007032602102.html.
[92] Quoted in Somashekhar, *op. cit.*
[93] "Sen. Jim Webb's Floor Speech to Introduce 'The National Criminal Justice Commission Act of 2009,'" March 26, 2009, http://webb.senate.gov/email/incardocs/FS_CrimJust_3-26-09.pdf.

Bibliography

Selected Sources

Books

Anderson, Patrick, *High in America: The True Story Behind NORML and the Politics of Marijuana*, Viking, 1981.
A veteran journalist tells the inside story of the rise and fall of decriminalization attempts during the Carter administration.

Booth, Martin, *Cannabis: A History*, St. Martin's Press, 2004.
The late British novelist and biographer entertainingly chronicles marijuana back to its earliest known use in China.

Gerber, Rudolph J., *Legalizing Marijuana*, Praeger, 2004.
A retired Arizona Court of Appeals judge attacks drug laws as an unjust exercise of government power backed by hyped scientific evidence.

Kleiman, Mark A. R., *When Brute Force Fails: How to Have Less Crime and Less Punishment*, Princeton University Press, 2009.
Proposed new approaches to drug use, including marijuana, form a major part of the plans advocated by a veteran criminal-justice policy expert, now at UCLA.

Musto, David F., *The American Disease*, Oxford University Press, 1999 (revised).
A Yale University medical historian and psychiatrist has written what many consider the definitive history of U.S. drug policy.

Articles

Dubner, Stephen J., "What Would Happen if Marijuana Were Legalized?" Freakonomics blog, *The New York Times*, May 22, 2009, http://freakonomics.blogs.nytimes.com/2009/05/22/pot-quorum/.
Several experts debate the question, including an ex-marijuana smuggler and a former Drug Enforcement Administration official.

Egelko, Bob, "Impact of pot proposal depends on federal law," *San Francisco Chronicle*, May 11, 2009, p. A1.
The hometown daily of California's major pro-legalization legislator examines his proposal.

Meeks, Torrey, "El Paso 'dialogue' on drugs leaves some speechless," *The Washington Times*, Feb. 2, 2009, p. A1.
Meeks reports on a controversial decriminalization proposal in a major Texas border city.

Padgett, Tim, "On the Bloody Border," *Time*, April 23, 2009, www.time.com/time/magazine/article/0,9171,1893512,00.html.
Mexico's vicious drug-cartel wars are pushing some Americans to reconsider drug decriminalization.

Rosenberg, Steven, "Drug use in public targeted," *The Boston Globe*, April 9, 2009, p. B1.
Massachusetts' major decriminalization law has some police chiefs worrying that it could encourage pot smoking in public.

Samuels, David, "Dr. Kush: How medical marijuana is transforming the pot industry," *The New Yorker*, July 28, 2008, www.newyorker.com/reporting/2008/07/28/080728fa_fact_samuels.
A journalist with an inside track to the California cannabis industry paints a detailed picture of its members.

Vick, Karl, "In Calif., Medical Marijuana Laws Are Moving Pot Into the Mainstream," *The Washington Post*, April 12, 2009, p. A3.
A veteran correspondent reports from ground zero of the medical-marijuana trend.

Reports

"White Paper on Marijuana Dispensaries," California Police Chiefs Association, April 2009, www.californiapolicechiefs.org/nav_files/marijuana_files/MarijuanaDispensariesWhitePaper_042209.pdf.
The association concludes that, as enforced in much of the state, the medical-marijuana law functions as legal cover for profit-making enterprises that provide cannabis to virtually anyone.

Eddy, Mark, "Medical Marijuana: Review and Analysis of Federal and State Policies," Congressional Research Service, March 31, 2009, www.fas.org/sgp/crs/misc/RL33211.pdf.
A criminal-justice policy expert for Congress' research arm provides an up-to-date assessment of state and national trends.

Gettman, Jon, "Marijuana Production in the United States," *Bulletin of Cannabis Reform*, 2006, www.drugscience.org/Archive/bcr2/MJCropReport_2006.pdf.
In a widely cited paper that some dispute, a marijuana-legalization advocate analyzes a variety of data to conclude that marijuana is the nation's No. 1 cash crop.

Joy, Janet E., *et al.*, "Marijuana and Medicine: Assessing the Science Base," Institute of Medicine, 1999, www.nap.edu/openbook.php?record_id=6376.
The institute attempts to present a balanced, academically sound examination of marijuana as intoxicant and potential medication.

Paluca, Rosalie Liccardo, and Beau Kilmer, "Marijuana and Crime: Is There a Connection Beyond Prohibition?," RAND Corp., January 2004, www.rand.org/pubs/working_papers/2004/RAND_WR125.pdf.
Researchers find data that point to marijuana-crime connections, though not necessarily to crime-causing effects of cannabis.

The Next Step:

Additional Articles from Current Periodicals

Consumption

Plumb, Taryn, "Changes Sought in Marijuana Laws," *The Boston Globe*, Feb. 10, 2008, p. Reg1.
An increase in marijuana use will also increase crime and various accidents stemming from the use of the drug.

Roetlin, J. J., "Legalizing Drugs Would Cause More Harm Than Good," *Iowa City Press-Citizen*, Feb. 15, 2008, p. 13A.
Drug use and drug-related deaths will inevitably increase if recreational use of marijuana is permitted.

Sabet, Kevin A., "California Can't Afford to Legalize Marijuana," *San Jose Mercury News*, March 8, 2009.
Legalizing marijuana in California would increase the drug's consumption and enormous social costs.

Medical Marijuana

"Critics Denounce Proposed Medical Marijuana Ban for Parolees," The Associated Press, March 6, 2008.
Critics in Montana have denounced a proposed rule that would bar anyone on parole or probation from obtaining marijuana as a prescription drug.

Bailey, Eric, "Doctors Urge Easing of Marijuana Ban," *Los Angeles Times*, Feb. 15, 2008, p. A14.
The American College of Physicians wants the United States to drop marijuana from the list of drugs that have no medicinal value.

Davis, Scott, "Acquiring Medical Marijuana Remains a Challenge," *Lansing State Journal*, April 20, 2009, p. 1A.
Michigan's medical-marijuana law makes no provisions for patients to obtain the drug at pharmacies or retail sources.

Ostrom, Carol M., "Medical Marijuana: How Much Is Enough?" *Seattle Times*, May 21, 2008, p. A1.
A Washington Health Department proposal that medical-marijuana patients be allowed more than two pounds of pot every month prompted Democratic Gov. Christine Gregoire to tell health officials to start over.

Schirripa, Nick, "Medicinal Marijuana OK, But the Critics Persist," *Battle Creek Enquirer*, Nov. 23, 2008, p. 1A.
Supporters say the medical value of pot justifies legalization, but opponents say it would only lead to more abuse.

Public Opinion

Saltzman, Jonathan, "Towns Try to Punish Public Marijuana Use," *The Boston Globe*, March 25, 2009, p. A1.
Dozens of Massachusetts cities and towns are taking steps to impose fines for smoking marijuana in public, but critics say such initiatives undermine the state ballot question that voters approved to decriminalize possession of small amounts of the drug.

Simerman, John, "Legalize Pot? Advocates Thrilled With Change in Polls, Governor's Call for Debate," *Contra Costa Times*, May 12, 2009.
A shift in California public opinion is apparently leaning toward the legalization, possession and taxation of marijuana.

Vitiello, Michael, "Should Marijuana Be Legal?" *Sacramento Bee*, April 5, 2009, p. E1.
Critics of decriminalization in California say it would not decrease prison overcrowding because not many prisoners are incarcerated for marijuana possession.

Taxation

Buchanan, Wyatt, "Effort to Ease Pot Laws Gets a Boost," *The San Francisco Chronicle*, May 6, 2009, p. A1.
California Gov. Arnold Schwarzenegger has called for a public debate regarding the legalization and taxation of marijuana.

Sanders, Jim, "Legal Pot: A Cash Harvest for State?" *Sacramento Bee*, Feb. 24, 2009, p. A1.
A proposed bill in California would allow recreational use of marijuana for adults 21 and older and would tax both users and distributors of the drug.

Woo, Stu, "Oakland Council Backs a Tax on Marijuana," *The Wall Street Journal*, April 30, 2009, p. A4.
The City Council of Oakland, Calif., has approved a 1.8-percent tax on medical marijuana in an effort to help close the city's budget shortfall.

CITING *CQ RESEARCHER*

Sample formats for citing these reports in a bibliography include the ones listed below. Preferred styles and formats vary, so please check with your instructor or professor.

MLA STYLE

Jost, Kenneth. "Rethinking the Death Penalty." CQ Researcher 16 Nov. 2001: 945-68.

APA STYLE

Jost, K. (2001, November 16). Rethinking the death penalty. *CQ Researcher, 11*, 945-968.

CHICAGO STYLE

Jost, Kenneth. "Rethinking the Death Penalty." *CQ Researcher*, November 16, 2001, 945-968.

CHAPTER

5

Prison Health Care

By Marcia Clemmitt

Excerpted from the CQ Researcher. Marcia Clemmitt. (January 5, 2007). "Prison Health Care." *CQ Researcher*, 1-24.

Prison Health Care

BY MARCIA CLEMMITT

THE ISSUES

Jail officials knew Bridgett Fogell was pregnant when she began serving a prison sentence in Delaware for traffic violations and driving under the influence. When she began having severe cramps and vaginal discharge, contract health-care workers checked on Fogell and deemed her healthy. [1]

When Fogell's water broke, a nurse told her that she'd simply urinated in her clothes. After nine hours in the prison infirmary, Fogell was finally taken to a hospital. She gave birth the next day, but her baby, Anna Lee, lived only a few hours.

As a prisoner, "you're helpless," said Fogell. She had called for help when Anna Lee's breathing became shallow and her heartbeat slowed, but it never came. "It's not like you can get in your car and leave, looking for competent medical care." [2]

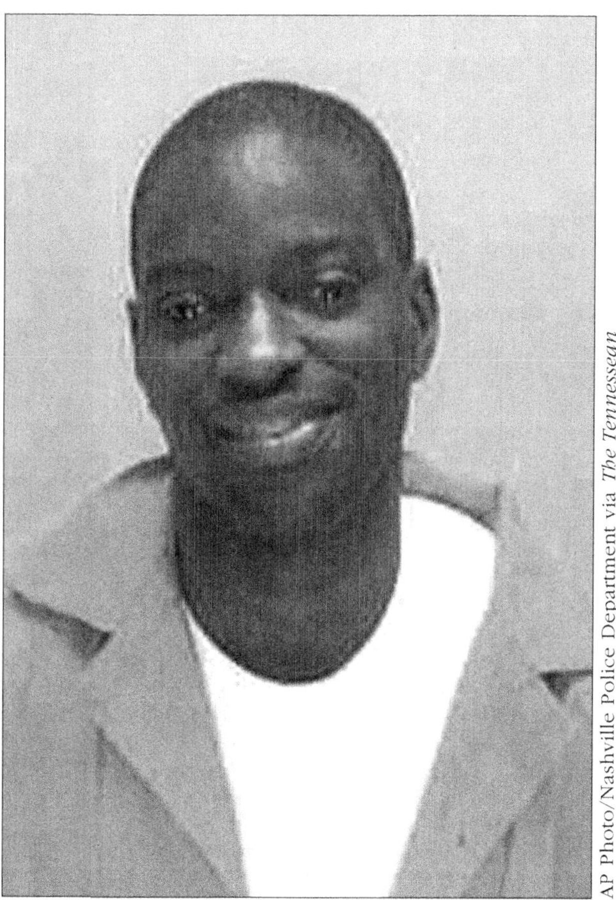

AP Photo/Nashville Police Department via *The Tennessean*

Diabetic inmate Ricky Douglas died in a Nashville jail after failing to receive his medication. Poor prison health care has prompted the courts to order reforms in several states.

St. Louis-based Correctional Medical Services Inc. (CMS) — one of the country's two largest prison health contractors — lost its Delaware contract in 2002, shortly after Fogell's baby died, but regained it in 2005.

Health-care horror stories like Fogell's are common throughout the nation's jails and prisons. For example, in November 2006, a federal judge ordered Michigan to implement massive reforms in its prison mental health-care programs after the deaths of several mentally ill prisoners, including a 21-year-old man who died after being strapped naked to a concrete table for four days. [3]

America's prisons have become a dumping ground for the mentally ill and those with drug and alcohol addiction, in part because non-prison treatment facilities are unavailable or unaffordable. More than half of all prison and jail inmates in 2005 had mental-health problems, according to the U.S. Department of Justice — a problem some experts attribute to the decision beginning in the 1950s to replace mental hospitals with community-based facilities, which remain understaffed and underfunded. [4]

Moreover, because of a serious shortage of drug-treatment programs, a disproportionate percentage of the nation's inmates are addicts. In a 2004 survey, 56 percent of state and half of all federal prisoners said they had used illegal drugs in the month before they committed their offenses, and up to a third were using drugs when they broke the law. [5]

Prisoners also are sicker, in general, than the population as a whole. More than a third of jail inmates had medical problems in 2002, including 13 percent with arthritis, 11 percent with hypertension and 10 percent with asthma. [6]

The health problems are compounded by the stratospheric HIV/AIDS rate among prisoners — more than triple the rate in the overall population. [7] And other common inmate diseases — such as Hepatitis C — are expensive and not always able to be treated.

"That creates a quandary for systems on a tight budget," says William J. Winslade, a professor of the philosophy of medicine at the University of Texas Medical Branch at Galveston.

Caring for the nation's 2.3 million state, federal and jail prisoners costs the cash-strapped federal, state and local governments about $7 billion a year — and the price tag is expected to rise as prisoners age and develop age-related diseases. [8]

Aside from serious budget shortfalls, two of the biggest obstacles to delivering quality health care to inmates are the huge size of the nation's prison population and the high percentage of mentally ill inmates, which makes it difficult to hire enough trained staff. [9]

"Many mentally ill people are in prison who should not be there," says Jeffrey L. Metzner, a psychiatrist and clinical professor at the University of Colorado School of Medicine. Unless the country develops a good community mental-health system, "this will continue."

The problem extends to mentally ill children and teens, who often are "parked" in juvenile corrections facilities — even when they haven't committed any offense, said Carol Carothers, executive director of the Maine chapter of the National Alliance for the Mentally Ill. Such "parking" typically happens when mental-health care is unavailable locally or exasperated parents can't cope with their child's behavior.

And incarceration can aggravate mental illness, as Maine officials found out in the case of a suicidal 13-year-old. During one of several stays in juvenile detention, Carothers said, "he was held in isolation for 152 of his first 240 days," which led him to mutilate himself, "spiraling deeper and deeper into his illness." The state settled a lawsuit on the child's behalf in 2004, said Carothers. [10]

Two-thirds of prisoners are merely serving life sentences "on the installment plan," says V. Morgan Moss, co-founder of the Center for Therapeutic Justice, which promotes inmate-run therapeutic communities in correctional institutions. "Inmates have substance-abuse problems, mental illness and few job skills" but get no help either inside or outside of the institutions, Moss says.

"With a 67-percent failure rate, people just go right back in," he laments. "We need to do something different. Instead, we just continue to build more jails and more prisons. It's a joke."

But resources and training to help ill prisoners are sparse, says M. Douglas Anglin, associate director of the Integrated Substance Abuse Programs at the University of California, Los Angeles (UCLA). For example, "you have correctional officers with no training in this area dealing with people with both mental illness and substance abuse."

There has been some improvement, however, in drug treatment, says Anglin. In the early 1990s, only about 5 percent of inmates received substance-abuse treatment, he says, compared to about 15 percent today. But "that's still a drop in the bucket."

Prison Health Costs Nearly Doubled

States' per-capita spending on health care for prisoners almost doubled between 1986 and 2001, according to the latest available data. Experts estimate that the figures have probably doubled again since 2001, based on the general rate of increase in health costs.

State Health Expenditures Per Prisoner
(for selected expenditures)

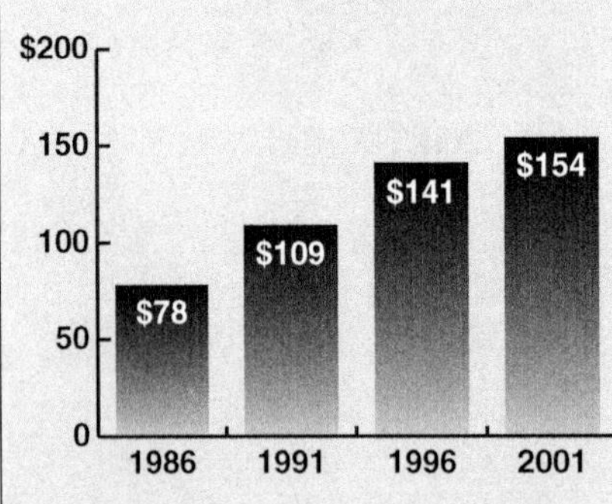

Source: "State Prison Expenditures, 2001," Bureau of Justice Statistics Special Report, 2004

As bad as prison health care usually is, it's often better than what inmates were getting in their communities. A large proportion of prisoners have no access to health care before being incarcerated, usually because they are uninsured and cannot afford health care.

"The average male in the New York prison system has 12 or 13 bad teeth, and the average woman two or three more," says Lester Wright, chief medical officer of the New York State Department of Correctional Services. "Most have never seen a dentist."

Yet, ironically, once people are incarcerated, they acquire the constitutional right to receive free health care — unlike other U.S. citizens. The Supreme Court in 1976 ruled that "deliberate indifference" to an inmate's medical needs is "cruel and unusual punishment" prohibited by the Eighth Amendment. [11]

Some Americans object to lawbreakers being entitled to free health care while more than 40 million Americans do not have health insurance. [12] Resentment over inmate health care erupted into a nationwide debate in 2002, after a California inmate received a $1 million heart transplant.

"The average Joe, who's getting squeezed by his chintzy HMO, has palpitations when he opens the paper to see that he just bought a Stanford [University] heart transplant for a con," wrote *Los Angeles Times* columnist Steve Lopez. The incident raised several ethical questions, Lopez noted, including, "What moral imperative says we should care more about the health of 160,000 inmates than of uninsured people, one-quarter of whom are children?" [13]

The case also sparked a nationwide debate over who should get scarce organs. At the time, 500 Californians and more than 4,000 people nationwide were waiting for heart transplants. "You have to wonder if a law-abiding, tax-paying citizen drew one last breath while Jailhouse Joe was getting a second wind," Lopez wrote. [14]

California officials said the 1976 Supreme Court decision compelled them to provide quality care for the prisoner. Indeed, lawsuits have been a driving force behind improvements in correctional health care. As recently as 2005, a federal judge in California placed jurisdiction over prison health care in the hands of a court-appointed administrator. [15]

The lack of adequate prison health care ultimately can lead officials to ignore even glaring matters of public health, says Dori Lewis, senior supervising attorney at the New York City-based Legal Aid Society's Prisoners' Rights Project. "The Department of Corrections is likely to say, 'What do we care about TB [tuberculosis] testing?' "

But as inmates cycle in and out of the community, they put correctional health care center stage in the fight against infectious disease and untreated chronic illnesses like diabetes. "The prisoner today is my neighbor tomorrow," says Timothy P. Flanigan, director of the division of infectious diseases at Brown Medical School in Providence, R.I.

Despite some court victories and the efforts of dedicated health-care workers, "prison health care is, by and large, abysmal in this country," says David C. Fathi, senior staff counsel at the American Civil Liberties Union's (ACLU) National Prison Project. "When you cast somebody outside the human family, you don't care what happens to them."

As growing numbers of aging and mentally ill prisoners swell jail and prison populations, here are some of the questions being asked:

Inmate Mental Problems Are Widespread

More than half of all state prison and jail inmates had a mental-health problem in 2005. More than half of all jail inmates met the criteria for mania and 30 percent had major depression.

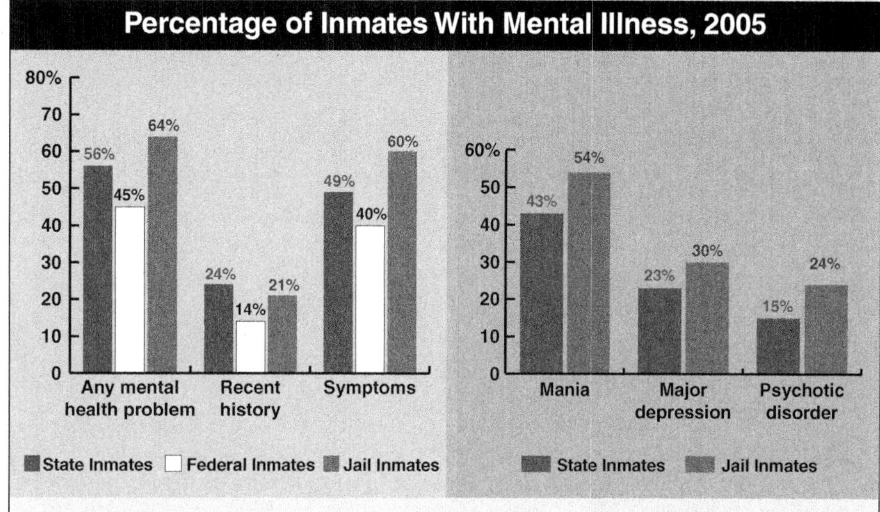

Source: U.S. Department of Justice, Bureau of Justice Statistics, September 2006

Do correctional institutions provide decent health care?

Inmate populations suffer from high rates of mental illness, substance abuse and below-average physical health. Critics say prisoner care remains substandard because too few health professionals will work in prisons, and negative public attitudes toward prisoners keep public resources lean. Some corrections officials say, however, that institutions in recent years have beefed up mental-health staffs, launched health screenings and hired better-trained staff — albeit largely as a result of court orders.

"There are still some people who think nobody in prison gets any decent care, but that isn't true," says chief medical officer Wright, in New York state. While the quality of correctional health care varies widely, Wright acknowledges, at least some systems are making progress. For example, more than 90 percent of prison doctors in New York now are either board certified or eligible for certification — "a big difference from 15 years ago, when many were unlicensed," he says.

And prisons are getting a better handle on some infectious diseases, such as tuberculosis, which once ran rampant, says Wright. In New York, for example, the TB rate in prisons has dropped from 220 new infections for every 100,000 prisoners in 1991 to around 10 per 100,000 in the last several years — a rate comparable to New York City's general population, he says.

Lawsuits have helped improve mental-health services in Ohio, according to Gary E. Beven, a psychiatrist at the maximum-security prison in Lucasville. In the mid-1990s, Beven was the only psychiatrist at the facility, working part time, with one psychiatric nurse. "There was a psychology staff, but they were beleaguered and overburdened . . . no group [mental health] programs, no individual counseling," he said. [16]

In 1993, following a riot at the prison, a federal lawsuit alleged that Ohio prisons didn't provide adequate mental-health care. A court-imposed monitoring system triggered big changes, said Beven. Today "we have the staffing, we have the support from central office," as well as the training and the budget to provide "care that really is effective." [17]

"There were six psychiatrists for the entire Ohio penal system when the [*Dunn v. Voinovich*] lawsuit was filed," Fred Cohen, professor emeritus at the State University of New York at Albany and the prisons' court-appointed monitor, told "Frontline." By the time the case had ended, however, there were more than 40 psychiatrists. [18]

Other health-care experts point out that even the most basic prison health care is better than the low quality — or total lack — of mental and physical health care available in the low-income communities many prisoners came from. "It's sad to say, but if a jail has a decent mental-health system, people are getting better treatment than they do in the community," says Metzner, at the University of Colorado. "Correctional people almost always want to do the right thing" by mentally ill prisoners, he

Keeping Substance Abusers Out of Jail

By the time Altamese McIntosh faced Judge Jeri Cohen in Miami's drug court, she had been cycling in and out of the justice system for years, and five of her eight children had been born drug-dependent.

That was in 1999. Today, McIntosh, 44, has been clean for seven years. "I realized that [the judge] was . . . no-nonsense. You either did what she said or she would terminate your parental rights. She wanted me to live in society drug-free so that I could be a good parent." [1]

That's the kind of story substance-abuse experts — and a growing number of lawmakers and corrections officials — would like to hear more. Although American corrections officials have generally resisted drug therapy, the high cost of recidivism among abusers is forcing a re-evaluation.

About 85 percent of all incarcerated people have had substance-abuse problems at some point, says M. Douglas Anglin, associate director of the Integrated Substance Abuse Program (ISAP) at the University of California, Los Angeles (UCLA). And, with two-thirds of all inmates re-entering the criminal-justice system a few years after release, say many experts, it's time for new strategies.

"For the past 10 years or so, the consensus has generally been that prison-based treatment with after-care is effective," says Michael Prendergast, director of ISAP's criminal justice research group.

But ISAP researcher Betsy Hall says that little phrase "after-care" is awfully important, because to be effective, substance-abuse programs must stretch over time. Unfortunately, few people persist, either because after-care isn't available or because they drop out.

Moreover, despite general agreement that the right treatment can work, only a limited number of therapeutic options exist — either in correctional facilities or in communities. Nationwide, Anglin estimates, about 15 percent of prisoners (including those in local jails and juvenile facilities) who need assistance get it while incarcerated. Although that's up from a decade or so ago, it's still "a drop in the bucket," he says.

Corrections officials often balk at having their budgets siphoned off to therapeutic programs they don't control, Anglin says. And in the name of accountability, states may dump programs before they can be tweaked into shape, he says. Generally, it "takes about five years of cyclical improvements" to get a program working properly, he says.

Even interventions that prove effective in the community suffer from a "dilution of effect" when launched inside an institution, in part because the staff do not have an affinity for the work or don't believe they are worthwhile, Anglin says.

Strong staff commitment is crucial, agrees ISAP research assistant Jerry Cartier. "People in the program are being asked for commitment strong enough to change their lives," he says, but if the staff appears uncommitted, it can drain inmates' own will to change.

Some wardens "pay lip service" to substance-abuse therapy, but the real test of support is in the behavior of prison staff with direct contact with inmates, says ISAP Principal Investigator William Burdon. "I've seen people go back to the housing unit

says, "but unless they're in a very rich or liberal state, they have a hard time making the case" to legislators and the public.

Lawsuits have triggered important improvements in prison health care as well, Metzner says. For example, he says, "up-front health-care screening is now pretty standard. Most systems these days are pretty good at determining health-care needs," although "not all are good at meeting them."

Some institutions "are making significant progress" on HIV/AIDS, says Flanigan, at Brown Medical School. For example, in a longstanding collaboration with the local health department, the jail in Hampden County, Mass., delivers timely primary care and HIV education to detainees. "That model should be applied for other diseases, like severe hypertension and diabetes," he says.

But critics say the overall health-care picture is bleak. With a few exceptions, correctional health systems are "like the HMO from hell," says Fathi, at the National Prison Project.

Mental-health care is often "poorly understood, not paid for or treated," says Daniel P. Mears, an associate professor of criminology at Florida State University.

Many correctional staff are unfamiliar with the mental illnesses that afflict inmates, and "even those who are aware of the issues are massively hamstrung," says Mears. Low resources and tension between correctional imperatives and health imperatives leave most facilities without the ability to provide needed care, he says.

"The difference between theory and practice is just monumental," says Mears. "Prisoners weren't getting care 20 years ago, and when you quadruple the size of the systems that gets worse."

For example, all detainees are supposed to be screened for mental-health problems when they enter institutions, says Mears, but there is "extreme variation" across the country.

State and local bureaucracies don't effectively cooperate, he says. When jail health staff diagnose an offender with a disorder like serious depression, "it would be good to be able to call up a local mental-health agency and say, 'Please send somebody over,' since most jails can't afford an in-house

in the pouring rain" after a substance-abuse treatment "and have the guards not open the door for them," he says. "Some guards call treatment 'hug-a-thug' programs."

Moreover, even though a very high percentage of prisoners have both mental illness and substance abuse, mental-health programs "are not well integrated with substance-abuse programs, and they should be," says Hall.

But even if institutions develop better substance-abuse efforts inside the walls, the need for longer-term after-care — plus the hope of keeping some substance abusers and potential abusers out of jail altogether — means more and better community-based programs are needed. In California prisons, for example, most studies show that those who just get prison treatment without after-care "don't do any better than those who get nothing," says ISAP Principal Investigator David Farabee. "That's led to a reluctant consensus that we ought to be spending more on the re-entry phase" — after inmates are released, he says.

In addition, more and more experts believe that diverting substance abusers from prison altogether is more effective, says Anglin. The country now has more than 1,200 drug courts that require drug offenders to get — and persist in — treatment rather than go to jail. Both Arizona and California overwhelmingly passed ballot initiatives directing that substance abusers who commit minor offenses be diverted from incarceration.

Diversion programs are more effective than throwing abusers in jail, says Anglin. Such programs give people time to change, "acknowledging that there are inevitable slips" as people try to kick habits, says Anglin. ISAP research also shows that diverting substance abusers from incarceration saves money, beyond what is saved in pure incarceration costs, Anglin says. "I'm an advocate of things that give people doors out of their lifestyle," he says.

Treatment programs both within institutions and in community-based programs are getting a boost from a new idea about substance abuse: that people can be successfully pressured into treatment. "The old idea is that people had to be ready to accept change," says John Roman, a senior research associate at the liberal-leaning Urban Institute. But, "the evidence is pretty overwhelming that you can intervene with people with substance abuse," he says. "The criminal-justice system can push them to stay in treatment."

When substance abusers are diverted to drug courts, for example, "there's magic in those judicial robes," says Bruce J. Winick, a professor of law and psychiatry at the University of Miami and an originator of the "therapeutic courts" concept. Having someone as august as a judge personally involved with them, for the first time, "helps propel people through the inevitable difficulties" of overcoming addiction, he says.

Nevertheless, if people are to kick substance abuse for good, many more services must be available, in jails and prisons and in the community, experts say. But "accessible, evidence-based substance-abuse treatment is just plain hard to find," says Anglin.

[1] Arles Carballo, "A Juvenile Court Judge Is Helping Drug-Addicted Women Get a New Lease on Life Through an Innovative Approach to Administering the Law," *The Miami Herald*, www.herald.com, Sept. 3, 2006.

counselor." But local mental-health officials don't want to spend their money on patients who are the jails' responsibility, or they believe — rightly or wrongly — that they don't have the legal right to assist, he says.

Most university medical centers try to combat health disparities — such as the poor health of African-American men — by offering health care to low-income residents in their communities, says Flanigan. But colleges and universities ignore corrections health, he says: "Correctional health care has been removed from the mainstream of medicine, and particularly academia."

In fact, says T. Howard Stone, an associate professor of bioethics at the University of Texas Health Center at Tyler, there are no longer any academic programs to train health workers to deal with prison populations.

Low salaries, remote locations and lack of prestige make hiring staff difficult. "Recruiters try to keep salaries competitive with local government pay, but even for states and cities that try to keep up, it's very hard," says Edward Harrison, president of the Chicago-based National Commission on Correctional Health Care.

And correctional facilities constantly "deal with financial cutbacks," says Alvin Cohn, a Rockville, Md.-based consultant on conditions in correctional facilities. "Many were built long ago. They're outmoded and in disrepair." An ailing boiler or roof "takes precedence over hiring a psychiatrist."

To save money, some states and localities use private health-care companies, but critics say oversight is often lax. Tennessee-based Prison Health Services (PHS), for example, often skimps on staff training, said a former PHS nurse. "When they hire someone, they don't even orient them but put them right on the floor," she says. "That is really scary for someone who's never been in a prison before." [19]

Should prisoners get the same quality of care as law-abiding citizens?

When a California court ruled in 2002 that a prison inmate could receive a publicly funded heart transplant, many people questioned whether prisoners should receive cutting-edge

U.S. Inmate Population Topped 2 Million

The number of federal, state and local prisoners topped 2.3 million in 2005 for the first time. The number of federal prisoners nearly doubled in the decade from 1995 to 2005 while the state inmate population grew by more than 25 percent.

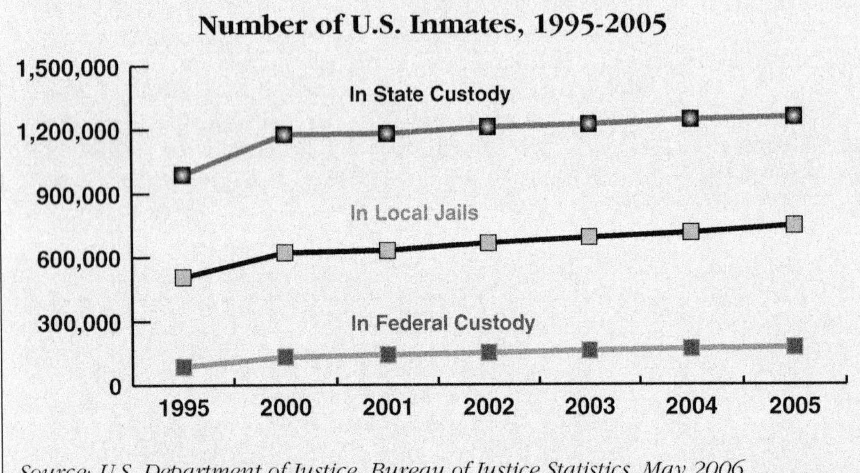

Source: U.S. Department of Justice, Bureau of Justice Statistics, May 2006

care at taxpayers' expense — especially when many of those taxpayers cannot afford health insurance. Prison health officials say the government is obligated to provide health care for prisoners because incarceration prevents them from obtaining care on their own. Moreover, they say, it is shortsighted to allow the mental and physical health of prisoners to deteriorate.

But giving prisoners access to scarce resources like organ transplants is unwarranted, wrote David L. Perry, now a professor of ethics at the U.S. Army War College in Carlisle, Pa. "Imagine watching a loved one die for lack of a heart, then reading in the paper the story about our fortunate felon," wrote Perry, who formerly directed the ethics program at California's Santa Clara University. [20]

The 31-year-old prisoner who received the heart had been convicted of robbery, Perry pointed out, a crime that "implies at least the threat of injury or death to its victims. . . . In my view, those who deliberately threaten the lives of innocent persons thereby forfeit whatever moral claim they otherwise might have had to an organ transplant." [21]

The Supreme Court's 1976 ruling, in *Estelle v. Gamble*, that all prisoners must be given adequate health care does not require governments to give prisoners sophisticated treatments like heart transplants, argued George Mason University Law School student Carrie S. Frank in a 2005 law journal paper. To be unconstitutional, denial of medical treatment to prisoners "must be so egregious that it offends the evolving standards of decency and is repugnant to the conscience of mankind," said Frank. [22]

Because of the high cost and the scarcity of organs, transplants are only provided to "a select few" patients, she pointed out. So denying a transplant to a prisoner does not qualify as the kind of "deliberate indifference" the Supreme Court banned, she wrote. "There is no reason why criminals living inside prison walls should be given a financial advantage over law-abiding citizens." [23]

The outrage triggered by the prisoner's heart transplant highlighted the irony that in the U.S. health system prisoners are the only citizens guaranteed a constitutional right to health care, while many law-abiding Americans can't afford health care. "Medical care is better in jail than on the street," lamented a corrections medical director surveyed by Stone of Texas in a nationwide study. [24]

Some bioethicists analyze the transplant situation differently. "At first glance, one thinks, 'Why should they get transplants?' " says Winslade, at the University of Texas Medical Branch at Galveston. "But what if a guy's going to prison for three years, and he's the most medically suitable for an available heart? He hasn't been condemned to death, and yet depriving him of the heart could have that effect.

"I don't think people on death row should get a heart transplanted," he continues. "But it would be discriminatory not to give a medically eligible short-termer a transplant. If it's a lifetime prisoner, though, I can see how the cost and burden of the immunosuppressive drugs raises issues." Transplant recipients must receive costly drugs for the rest of their lives to prevent organ rejection.

"In a society in which we haven't decided that health care is a human right, I can see how prison health care becomes a more difficult decision," says Felicia G. Cohn, director of medical ethics at the University of California's Irvine School of Medicine and a daughter of criminologist Alvin Cohn.

Americans have decided to punish millions of people, not just violent criminals, by locking them away and making it impossible for them to get care for themselves, she says. The inability of prisoners, including the many non-violent prisoners, to procure care for themselves is what makes providing health care for incarcerated people a government responsibility, she says. 'There are alternative ways of punishment that wouldn't require us to provide health care."

Despite what many think, prisoners have not been granted a right to health-care frills, the University of Colorado's Metzner says: The Supreme Court has said only that prisoners have a right to care for "serious medical needs, including mental illness."

Since the *Estelle v. Gamble* decision, lower courts and correctional systems have struggled to define "serious medical needs," but the definition remains fuzzy, many analysts say.

For example, while some prisoners do receive organ transplants, especially kidneys, in most cases "where prisoners have tried to sue for things like transplants, they've lost," says Brietta R. Clark, a professor at Loyola Law School in Los Angeles. "Cost is playing a role" in the medical decisions, "and courts have said that it's reasonable to look at the cost of alternatives. They aren't getting the best and the most expensive care."

To put inmates on a par with other Americans, some jurisdictions require them to make co-payments in order to receive care.

However, "no studies show that it saves money," says New York City internist Robert L. Cohen, who directed a health-care program for city jail inmates and has been a court-appointed monitor of correctional health-care settlement agreements in Connecticut, New York, Ohio and Michigan.

Kidney transplants usually are cost-effective, compared to the alternative — dialysis — with a transplant recouping its additional cost in three years, Cohen says.

The case for providing incarcerated people with decent health care is hard to make to the public, in part because most are "minorities that are despised," says Lewis, at the Prisoners' Rights Project.

"Most people don't think it through," says Lewis. "Most everyone knows somebody who has done drugs at sometime in their lives," and it's drug users who currently swell the incarcerated population, she says. "Prisons are the dumping grounds for poor people." Some 80 percent of the women in state prisons were convicted of non-violent offenses, and they are not "the horrible people who should languish and die," Lewis notes.

"If you don't want to provide care for humanitarian reasons, do it to ensure that your neighbors" don't suffer from untreated infectious disease or mental illness, says Brown Medical School's Flanigan.

"Society benefits" if incarcerated people get treatment "and suffers if they don't," says Florida State's Mears. Untreated mental and physical diseases end up costing everyone more years down the line, he says. "So why wouldn't society demand that they get these things?"

Should correctional facilities require HIV tests?

The deadly HIV/AIDS infection can be spread within correctional facilities through sex and shared needles used for illicit drug use or tattooing. And infected prisoners can spread the disease in communities after their release. Thus, some analysts say, prisoners should be required to undergo HIV testing, either at entry or before release. Critics of mandated testing, how-

Many Jail Inmates Have Medical Problems

Nearly 40 percent of jail inmates had a current medical problem in 2002 (graph at top, left), and 22 percent reported a learning impairment (bottom graph). Arthritis was the most common medical problem reported (top right).

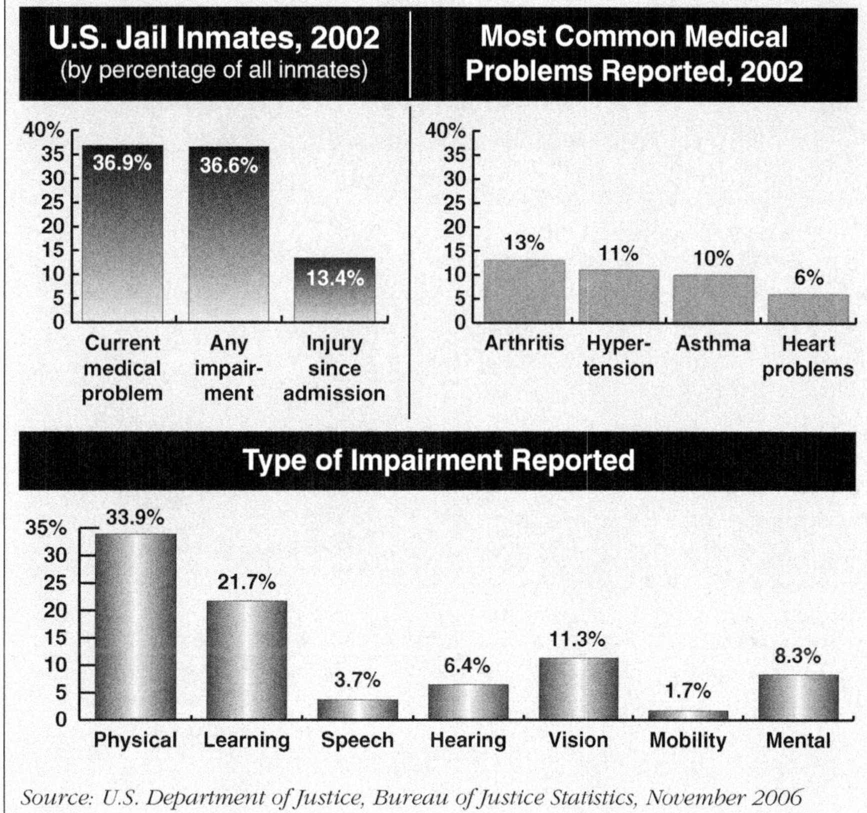

Source: U.S. Department of Justice, Bureau of Justice Statistics, November 2006

ever, argue that HIV education and optional testing can stop the spread of AIDS just as effectively without violating inmates' privacy or human rights.

"There's no question in my mind" that prisoners should be screened for HIV, says the University of Texas' Winslade. "Sex occurs in prison, and we should do everything we can to prevent the spread of HIV," he says. "Testing everybody in the free world would be silly, but prisoners are a much higher-risk population with drug users and high-risk sex."

"Public-health issues far outweigh the privacy issues" of individual inmates when it comes to HIV/AIDS, said Louisiana Democratic state Rep. Austin Badon Jr. in September, while introducing legislation to require testing for HIV and hepatitis for everyone who passes through the state prison system. [25]

Some states already require pre-release screening to keep HIV/AIDS from spreading in the community. But Barry Zack, an assistant clinical professor at the University of California, San Francisco, and executive director of Centerforce, a nonprofit agency serving California prisoners and their families, says that's too late. Released inmates who are HIV-positive are likely to find themselves without any access to health-care services, he says, adding, "Yet, you just had an opportunity to treat them and wasted it."

One of the first things a released inmate does is return to a wife or girlfriend and have sex, often unprotected, said Badon. "It's a no-brainer to do what we can." [26]

Optional testing, on the other hand, leaves "a substantial proportion of infected inmates . . . undetected," according to researchers at the University of North Carolina at Chapel Hill. [27]

Studies in Maryland and Wisconsin found that infection rates among inmates overall were twice as high as infection rates among inmates who volunteered to be tested. For instance, two-thirds of the HIV-infected inmates in Maryland — and 31 percent in Wisconsin — declined testing. [28]

Inmate Drug Abuse Is Widespread

More than half of all state prisoners were drug dependent in 2004, and 49 percent of federal inmates received drug treatment or participated in a therapy program.

Percentage of Prisoners Who Abused Drugs, Got Treatment
(in 2004)

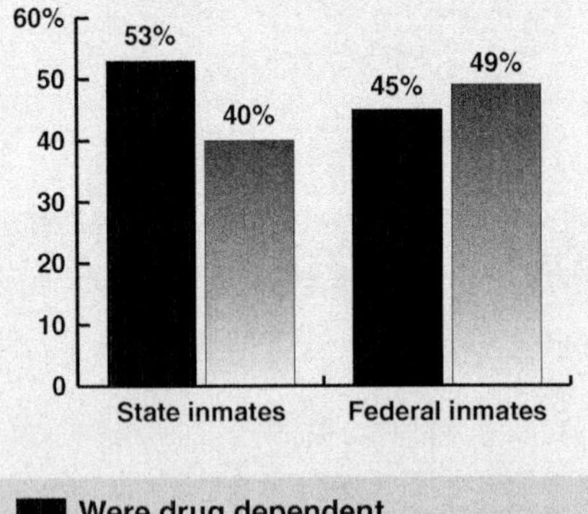

Source: U.S. Department of Justice, Bureau of Justice Statistics, Oct. 2006

The American Medical Association recommended mandatory HIV testing of prison inmates as early as 1987. The federal Bureau of Prisons advocates mandatory testing only of prisoners with clear risk factors, such as a history of injection-drug use. Many AIDS advocacy and human-rights groups oppose mandatory testing. [29]

Compulsory HIV testing of prisoners is "unethical and ineffective, and should be prohibited," according to the World Health Organization. Likewise, AIDS Action calls mandatory testing "unethical, ineffective and an invasion of privacy." [30]

Compulsory universal HIV testing is "based on the paranoid position that prisoners are responsible for spreading HIV to a chaste public," wrote *Prison Legal News* contributing writer Gary Hunter. [31]

Correctional institutions should facilitate HIV prevention, not mandate intrusive testing, says internist and correctional-health monitor Cohen. Prison systems "should give out condoms, and prisoners should be offered testing when they want to be tested." ■

BACKGROUND

Population Explosion

Two very large trends underlie the nation's prison health-care problems. One is the steady increase in the prison population, resulting in often-overcrowded facilities and the incarceration of high numbers of mentally ill and addicted inmates. [32]

The national inmate population is now more than six times the approximately 330,000 people incarcerated in 1972 — far outpacing overall population growth, which has not even doubled. [33]

At the same time, U.S. health care overall faces unprecedented challenges. Care has grown astronomically more expensive, hitherto undreamed of diseases like HIV/AIDS and antibiotic-resistant tuberculosis have developed, the incidence of chronic ills like diabetes has increased as the population has aged, and health care for mentally ill and lower-income people has continued to decline in quality and availability. [34]

All those trends are reflected, and magnified, in corrections, says Harrison of the National Commission on

Continued on p. 12

Chronology

1950s-1970s

More mentally ill people drift into jails and prisons as psychiatric hospitals are closed.

1955
Introduction of the first effective antipsychotic drug, Thorazine, begins the deinstitutionalization of the mentally ill.

1969
California becomes the first state to make it more difficult to involuntarily hospitalize the mentally ill.

1976
The Supreme Court's *Estelle v. Gamble* ruling declares it unconstitutional for prisons to show "deliberate indifference" to a prisoner's serious medical needs.

1977
At the first World Congress of Prison Medicine, corrections health officers pledge to keep inmates' medical information confidential, abstain from authorizing any physical punishment and give medical judgments priority over other concerns, like security.

1980s-2000s

Continued dismantling of residential mental-health facilities and get-tough policies on crime increase U.S. prison and jail populations. Infectious disease increases behind bars.

1980
Just over 500,000 Americans are incarcerated.

1981
First AIDS case is reported.

1987
American Correctional Health Services Association opposes mandatory AIDS testing for prisoners.

1989
Supreme Court's *Mistretta v. the United States* ruling upholds federal sentencing guidelines, barring judges from considering prisoners' amenability to treatment and rehabilitation during sentencing. . . . Dade County (Miami) experiments with a drug court to divert substance abusers from prison.

1994
Supreme Court's *Farmer v. Brennan* ruling defines its "deliberate indifference" standard for health care that violates prisoners' constitutional rights: Simple negligence isn't bad enough but prisons can violate the Constitution even if they don't knowingly do a prisoner harm.

1995
Federal government begins funding demonstration drug courts to steer substance abusers toward treatment rather than prison. . . . Nearly 1.6 million Americans are incarcerated. . . . In Ohio, a court-appointed monitor oversees a complete overhaul of mental-health care in state prisons.

1997
Broward County (Fort Lauderdale) opens the nation's first mental-health court to direct mentally ill offenders into treatment instead of prison.

1999
New York City jail inmates challenge the practice of releasing mentally ill detainees without helping them to continue treatment.

2001
Federal Bureau of Prisons says it will pay for some organ transplants.

2002
California court allows a convicted felon to get a heart transplant at Stanford Medical Center. . . . Erie County (Buffalo), N.Y., models the nation's first gambling-addiction court after drug courts.

2003
Federal Centers for Disease Control and Prevention recommends screening all at-risk prisoners for hepatitis C.

2004
Alabama settles lawsuit stemming from the death of 42 state prisoners from AIDS between 1999 and 2004 with an agreement to provide HIV- and AIDS-specific care and better nutrition to infected inmates.

2005
Federal judge places California's entire $1.1-billion-a-year prison health system under a court-appointed receiver, deeming the care it delivers "deplorable." . . . More than 2.3 million Americans are incarcerated. . . . Texas prisoners are required to get HIV testing before release. . . . Colorado prison audit finds that health contractor ignores inmates' cancers and prescribes medication without patient exams.

2006
Landmark Department of Justice report finds that more than half of jail and prison inmates have mental illness, a much higher rate than previously believed. . . . California bans shackling of women inmates during labor and delivery. . . . Delaware lawmakers reject $30 million bill requiring special care for pregnant inmates, infectious-disease screening and health training for guards.

Prisons Replace Hospitals for the Mentally Ill

When Catharine Harrold was arrested last summer, police wouldn't allow her to bring her best friends — two stuffed bunnies — to jail with her. "What I've been worried about is that they would send me to the hospital before Little and Big get here, she said." [1]

Harrold has had seizures, mood disorders and dementia — and has been arrested 24 times, mostly on drug and driving charges — since suffering severe head injuries in a car crash in the early 1990s.

Nearly six months later, Harrold is still being held in a Florida jail, even though state law requires that mentally ill inmates be moved to psychiatric facilities within 15 days of their arrest. She is only one of about 250 mentally ill prisoners in Florida who have been held for more than two weeks. In 2006, the average wait for a transfer was three months; some inmates waited more than five months. [2]

Now, some angry Florida judges are threatening to jail state officials themselves over the delays. "This type of arrogant activity cannot be tolerated in an orderly society," Circuit Judge Crocket Farnell wrote in an October ruling. [3]

Treatment of mentally ill inmates is not just an issue in Florida. An angry federal judge ordered Michigan officials in November to make sure state prisons are adequately staffed with psychologists and psychiatrists and that mental-health staff make daily rounds. [4]

"Here is the basic message," an angry U.S. District Judge Richard A. Enslen told state corrections officials, suggesting they say prayers for mentally ill inmates who have died in custody. "You are valuable providers of life-saving services and medicines. You are not coat racks who collect government paychecks while your work is taken to the sexton for burial." [5]

A recent U.S. Department of Justice study found that in 2005 more than half of all prison and jail inmates in the United States had a mental-health problem. Various analyses have traced some of the overall rise in the numbers of incarcerated mentally ill Americans to the closing of mental hospitals beginning in the 1950s.

For example, a 1972 California study found that the local jail population in Santa Clara County rose 300 percent in the four years after a local psychiatric hospital closed. And a 1992 survey by the advocacy group Public Citizen found that 29 percent of jails were holding people who had no charges against them but were waiting for mental-health services. [6]

"Jails and prisons have been viewed as the easiest place to park the severely mentally ill," says Morgan Moss, co-founder of the Center for Therapeutic Justice, which promotes development of therapeutic, inmate-run communities inside correctional institutions. "Jailing people helps us avoid the problems society needs to deal with. Instead, we just stick you there. And if we build 500 new prison beds, we never have to bite the bullet."

Jails and prisons are the worst possible places for the mentally ill, who often unwittingly break institution rules and end up in isolation. "The mentally ill in isolation . . . simply fall

Continued from p. 10

Correctional Health Care. "It's not that prisons or jails are a breeding ground for disease," he says. "They're a catch basin for poor people in the community with poor health histories." While prisoners are in poorer health than average Americans, prisoners' health status reflects conditions in the low-income communities from which many inmates come, he says.

"The only solution to the medical problem in California prisons [now under federal control] is to build fewer prisons," says health-monitor Cohen. That's because "they can't find the doctors to run them," he says.

To cut back on incarceration, more mental-health and substance-abuse treatment and prevention would have to be available inside current correctional institutions and in the community, many analysts say.

"Prior to the 1980s, rehab was a strong component in correctional health thinking," says Anglin, at the University of California's Integrated Substance Abuse Programs. "Then you had a huge philosophical shift. Rehab had shown only marginal results, and the thinking became, 'Let's throw a sentence at people,' " he says. [35]

"Various epidemics of drugs" over the years — from LSD and heroin to cocaine, crack cocaine and methamphetamines — combined with increased emphasis on penalizing drug use, "effectively criminalized whole generations of black people and now, increasingly, Hispanics," Anglin says.

Add this to "three-strikes-and-you're-out" laws and a trend toward longer prison sentences, "and you get a huge proportion of people who are growing old" behind bars, Anglin says.

In 2003, more than 20 percent of sentenced inmates were imprisoned for drug offenses. Offense rates varied by race, however, with 24 percent of black inmates and 23 percent of Hispanics serving time for drug offenses, compared to 14 percent of white inmates. [36]

The deinstitutionalization of mentally ill people, which began in the 1950s with the development of antipsychotic medication and accelerated through the 1980s, also has swollen prison populations. [37] Between 1955 and 1994, the proportion of the population living in public psychiatric hospitals dropped by more than 90 percent. [38]

apart," said Fred Cohen, professor emeritus at the State University of New York at Albany and a court-appointed monitor for mental health in Ohio prisons. "They have no support, they have no sensory stimulus, their hallucinations get worse." [7]

Some courts have required state and local corrections departments to improve care for mentally ill inmates. In Ohio, for example, prisons were ordered in 1995 to beef up their mental-health capacity. "There just wasn't enough staff," said Debbie Nixon-Hughes, chief of the Bureau of Mental Health Services in Ohio. "We had approximately 12 doctors, and now we have 67." [8]

Keeping as many mentally ill people as possible out of correctional institutions is a key goal, some experts say. "Jails simply cannot deal with these people," says Bruce J. Winick, professor of law and psychiatry at the University of Miami. Winick originated the concept of therapeutic courts, which offer a small but growing option, similar to drug courts, he says. Instead of jailing the mentally ill, judges refer them to treatment and exert continuing pressure to help them stay on their medications and out of trouble. More than 100 mental-health courts now operate nationwide, including a handful that handle felony offenders as well as people charged with misdemeanors. [9]

Creating more humane and socially oriented environments within correctional facilities also can provide options for mentally ill offenders, Moss says. He's helped set up special, inmate-directed living units in correctional facilities, where like-minded detainees agree to help each other improve their lives. "We set up a community inside the jail built on pro-social values like honesty and respect," says Moss. "Behind the walls, inmates mostly run things anyway."

Once a community is running, "the jail itself often will put mentally ill prisoners in there and have the other inmates look after them," reducing suicides and the isolation that often worsens the condition of mentally ill prisoners, says Moss.

Cohen cautioned that while jail and prison environments can be made more helpful for the mentally ill, the real support work is needed in the community. "The prison is simply not a place of first choice in which to provide mental-health care," he said. "We should be devoting ourselves to . . . keeping people out."

---

[1] Quoted in Sarah Lundy, " 'Humanity' " Put to Test as Mentally Ill Languish in Jails," *Orlando Sentinel*, Dec. 12, 2006, p. A1.

[2] *Ibid.*

[3] Quoted in Abby Goodnough, "Officials Clash Over Mentally Ill in Florida Jails," *The New York Times*, Nov. 15, 2006, p. A1.

[4] David Ashenfelter, "Fix Prison Health Care Now, Judge Says," *Detroit Free Press*, Nov. 14, 2006, p. 1.

[5] Quoted in *ibid.*

[6] E. Fuller Torrey, *Out of the Shadows: Confronting America's Mental Illness Crisis* (1997), quoted in "Deinstitutionalization: A Psychiatric Titanic," "The New Asylums," PBS "Frontline."

[7] Quoted in "The New Asylums," *ibid.*

[8] *Ibid.*

[9] For background on drug courts, see Mary H. Cooper, "Drug-Policy Debates," *CQ Researcher*, July 28, 2000, pp. 593-624.

Many have ended up in jails and prisons, says Harrison. "When people get picked up for a crime, there's often an underlying mental illness that led to it. Correctional facilities have in a sense become the dumping ground for the mentally ill."

"Many are being punished for behavior that could be prevented," says Loyola Law School's Clark.

But "no one likes to spend money on preventive care," says Florida State's Mears. "It's hard to sell politically" when the monetary and social payoffs occur years down the line.

Legal Aid

Actually, it's a step forward in human rights for anyone to worry at all about prisoners getting health care. Throughout history, prison conditions have been atrocious, with inmates facing health-threatening conditions such as rotten food, no heat and cells flooded with raw sewage. As late as the 1970s, prisoner lawsuits complained about "health-care" incidents in which unsupervised prisoners were allowed to perform "medical" procedures like tooth pulling and suturing on their fellow inmates. [39]

In the landmark 1976 case that established prisoners' constitutional right to health care — *Estelle v. Gamble* — a falling bale of hay injured inmate J. W. Gamble while he worked on a prison farm in Texas. Gamble — who claimed that prison staff failed to adequately diagnose and treat his injury — lost his case. In its ruling, however, the U.S. Supreme Court did establish the fundamental principle that corrections facilities must not show "deliberate indifference to serious medical needs" of inmates. [40]

"The Supreme Court made it very clear that people on the outside and people locked up are in very different positions with regard to their entitlements," says the ACLU's Fathi. "When the state disables you from acting on your own behalf," as it does with prisoners, then there's a presumption that the state must provide you with health care.

In fact, all major initiatives to improve correctional health care have come from the courts, not from legislators or the public. "This is a population that nobody wants to interact with, that nobody feels a connection

HIV-Positive Inmate Population Declines

The number of HIV-positive prison inmates dropped to less than 2 percent of the nation's overall prison population in 2001 and dropped again in 2004.

HIV-Positive Prison Inmates

Year	Number	Percentage of State and Federal Inmates
1998	25,680	2.2%
1999	25,807	2.1
2000	25,333	2.0
2001	24,147	1.9
2002	23,866	1.9
2003	23,663	1.9
2004	23,046	1.8

Source: U.S. Department of Justice, Bureau of Justice Statistics, November 2006

with," says Centerforce Executive Director Zack. "That's why the court has to make these decisions."

Since 1976, the courts have struggled to define "deliberate indifference" and "serious" medical need. The broadest outlines are clear, says Fathi. Mental-health care and physical-health care both are covered, but substance-abuse and addiction treatment are not — except for treating withdrawal. "Once you're done withdrawing and just want help to get off opioids, no one's required to give you that," he says.

Lower-court decisions have clarified that it is not enough to prove that a correctional system was "negligent" with regard to a prisoner's care, says Fathi. One must prove "deliberate indifference" on the part of corrections officials who knew but ignored the fact that a prisoner was at serious risk due to a medical condition. "They're not entitled to care for a hang nail; they are entitled to care for a heart attack," Fathi says. Questions arise when a prisoner has a condition somewhere between those two extremes, he explains, "with something like a hernia being a prime example of a gray area."

The major role of lawsuits has been to ensure that prisoners get access to at least some health care, says Lewis of the Legal Aid Society. "One of the first goals of lawsuits has been to ensure sufficient staff," and most litigation has played out over many years, she says.

"Litigating quality of care is one of the hardest parts," says Lewis. "You can say you have to have a person who's a board-certified internist [on staff]. But this doesn't mean he's competent or cares or hasn't had his license suspended in three other states." Using legal means to improve care quality is "where we have a bad time."

Many cases are too narrow to offer much guidance, says the University of Texas' Stone. Most "are limited to a specific fact pattern — like certain levels of HIV care," he says. A ruling in such a case does nothing to help set care standards for other diseases like cancer or diabetes, or even for future HIV cases, as medical research and standards of care keep advancing, he says. So, despite the fact that lawsuits have been by far the strongest instrument for improving correctional health care, "litigation has only limited usefulness when it comes to setting real standards and broader goals for health care," Stone says.

In cases involving access to care, "the two most common themes are lack of resources and security interfering with medical treatment," says Fathi. When a federal judge ordered the court takeover of California's prisons last year, for example, a key issue cited was that health-staff salaries were too low, says Fathi.

"If lawsuits are done right, they can demonstrate problems [occurring] on a massive scale," says Loyola's Clark. "You have to be able to amass enough evidence and show that the problems aren't rare."

In addition, lawsuit allegations are not necessarily valid, said Martha Harbin, a spokeswoman for Prison Health Services (PHS), which provides contract correctional health care. "Inmates are one of the most litigious groups in society, and a vast majority of the suits filed against PHS are dismissed as baseless," she said. [41]

Meanwhile, correctional health professionals and researchers also work from within to improve correctional health care. Two main organizations — the National Commission on Correctional Health Care and the American Correctional Association — certify facilities and workers and offer training on care improvement.

For example, the commission accredits about 500 facilities, including prisons, jails and juvenile facilities, says Harrison. Its most important role is training and educating correctional health staff, through consultations, conferences and care guidelines, he says. The group issues care guidelines for many conditions, customizing diabetes-care guidelines created by the American Diabetes Association, for instance, by "adding a description of the barriers to meeting those guidelines in correctional institutions and how they might be handled."

Population Health

Delivering health care in correctional institutions is difficult because funding is low, and prison bureaucracies focus primarily on providing security and punishment — not health care. And, inmates show a higher incidence of all types of illness, making prisons the "crucibles" for all the nation's health-care problems, says Florida State University's Mears.

In 2005, around 23 percent of state prisoners and 30 percent of jail inmates reported symptoms of major depression, while 15 percent of state prisoners and 24 percent of jail inmates had symptoms of psychotic disorders. [42]

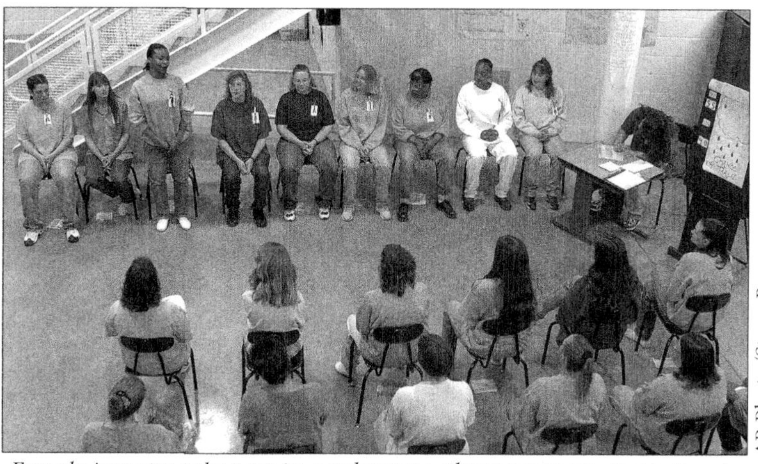

AP Photo/Steve Pope

Female inmates take part in a substance-abuse program at a prison in Mitchellville, Iowa. About 15 percent of the nation's inmates participate in such programs, but many experts say more programs are needed in both correctional facilities and local communities.

Beyond the overall rate of mental illness, "at any given time, from 5 to 15 percent of inmates will need some kind of crisis intervention," says the University of Colorado's Metzner.

Some studies show that improving community mental-health treatment can keep people out of jail and save money. For example, an Arkansas program decreased patients' mean number of annual jail days to between 46 and 83 from well over 100. An Illinois program decreased both jail days and hospital days for a group of 30 patients, saving $157,000 in jail costs and $917,000 in hospital costs. [43]

Helping prisoners get off addictive drugs isn't part of prisoners' constitutional guarantee of health care, but with substance abuse being the reason many people end up behind bars in the first place, it's an inescapable feature of the correctional health landscape.

Twenty-one percent of state prisoners and 55 percent of federal inmates were being held for drug-law violations in 2004. Among state inmates who had been dependent on or had abused drugs, 53 percent had at least three prior sentences to either probation or incarceration, compared to 32 percent of other prisoners. [44]

That makes it important to try addressing prisoners' substance-abuse issues while they're inside, says Wright of the New York state system. "If 80 or 90 percent had these issues in the past, why not take advantage" of the fact that, while incarcerated, "they have time" to work on a substance-abuse program? "Once they're on the outside, they'll have the same problems as everybody else, going to work, trying to make ends meet. We have committed to giving it to everybody who needs it, at least before they get out," he says.

Prisoners and jail inmates also have high rates of infectious diseases, including AIDS.

In 2003, nearly 1-in-13 prisoner deaths was from AIDS-related causes. [45]

The percentage of HIV-positive prisoners varies by prior involvement with illegal drugs. Of prisoners who had never used drugs, 1.3 percent are HIV-positive compared to 2.8 percent who have used a needle to inject drugs and 5.1 percent of those who say they have shared a needle. [46]

Chronic diseases like diabetes and hypertension also are more prevalent in prisons, especially in their most serious forms.

"If you're 50 years old [and in prison], your condition probably makes you geriatric," says Metzner.

"The biggest problem is that they didn't have care before we got them," says Wright. "They come in with undiagnosed hypertension and pulmonary disease," often coupled with a history of unhealthy substance abuse, "and we see advanced cases of diseases like diabetes that we don't see in the community."

The high proportion of racial minorities among inmates increases the rate of some serious chronic diseases. For example, the prevalence of diabetes in African-Americans is 70 percent higher than in the white population, and the diabetes rate in Hispanics is nearly twice that in whites. [47]

The growing number of incarcerated women adds another burden to correctional health care, says Wright. "About 5 to 6 percent come in pregnant," he says.

Multiple Systems

Beyond the poor health of entering inmates, many aspects of institutionalized life make providing health care difficult. There's a constant and probably unavoidable culture clash between security concerns and health concerns.

For example, "In many jails and prisons mentally ill people, because of their illness, don't follow rules," says Metzner. "So they get put into lockdown, which makes their illness worse, and where they again don't follow rules," ending up in more and more stringent segregation, which can greatly worsen their illness. "That's a tragedy.'

Pre-incarceration health-care regimens get disrupted because "offenders can't bring their own medication into a facility," says correctional-care consultant Cohn. "Often, they don't know what they were taking. It was 'a blue pill and a green pill.' "

And "offenders know how to manipulate," says Cohn. "They want to get out of their cells, and a significant number come to the infirmary when there's nothing wrong."

"Many problems are fundamentally structural," says the ACLU's Fathi. For example, often a serious medical problem requires a time-and-resource-consuming trip outside the prison to see a specialist, and "sometimes the security staff will keep this from happening."

In addition, as people move through different parts of the corrections system — juvenile-detention centers, jails, prisons, probation and parole — the health care they receive, if any, is completely disjointed.

"One of the biggest problems is the criminal-justice system is *not* a system," says Moss, of the Center for Therapeutic Justice. "Nobody talks to anybody else. Judges rarely ever talk to anybody. Most have never been inside a jail to look at what goes on in there. You'll find almost no one who'll tell you that this system is working."

Since jails are the first stage in the criminal-justice process, typically 80 to 90 percent of their inmates "are pretrial," explains Cohn. Many small-town jails are small and have no on-site health staff.

There are 3,360 jails nationwide, and well under 10 percent "have any significant program of any kind" to assist inmates, such as education, therapy or substance-abuse treatment, says Moss.

"The smaller the jail, the less likely . . . you're going to have any kind of medical and mental-health care," said court-appointed prison monitor Cohen.

"In many jails and prisons mentally ill people, because of their illness, don't follow rules. So they get put into lockdown, which makes their illness worse, and they again don't follow rules."

—Jeffrey L. Metzner, M.D., University of Colorado School of Medicine

"Yet, if prisons have become the hospitals, the jails are the emergency rooms," Cohen said. [48]

Nevertheless, jails must cope with serious health issues. Many detainees are in acute phases of mental illness and have committed relatively minor offenses like urinating on someone's lawn or leaving a restaurant without paying. In addition, "people in jails are withdrawing [from drug addiction], they get taken off their meds and they're dealing with the situational stress of just being arrested," says Fathi.

So-called supermax prisons or units keep presumably the most violent and dangerous inmates isolated and deprived of sensory stimulation. But supermax imprisonment carries special dangers for mentally ill people, who often end up there because their illness leads them to inadvertently break prison rules.

In one such unit in Indiana, "at least half the inmates were mentally ill," says Fathi. "They do therapy by locking the prisoner and therapist into adjacent cells." The prisoner bends down and talks through the floor-level slit through which food trays are passed, "The therapist sits on a milk crate on the other side. . . . It's been well established that mentally ill people break down" in such conditions, he says. The ACLU has worked with several states to keep mentally ill prisoners out of supermax, Fathi says.

"We've got to stop spending money to build [supermax] prisons," says Stone at the University of Texas. Building the prisons, then staffing and maintaining them over the facilities' lifetime drains money from other priorities, like health care, he says.

In recent years, juvenile facilities frequently have housed mentally ill children as they wait for mental-health services to become available.

Continued on p. 18

At Issue:

Are drug courts a good alternative to imprisonment for substance abusers?

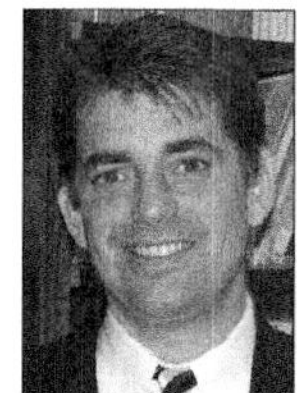

JOHN ROMAN
SENIOR RESEARCH ASSOCIATE
JUSTICE POLICY CENTER
THE URBAN INSTITUTE

WRITTEN FOR *CQ RESEARCHER*, DECEMBER 2006

Drug-fueled crime is hard to conquer, but drug courts are a strategy that has been shown to work. For the past 15 years, judges have used a new approach to penalizing drug-involved offenders: requiring treatment under criminal-justice supervision, incarcerating those who fail and letting those who succeed return to the community for a new chance. The operating principle is that chronic criminal behavior — such as street crime, prostitution and domestic violence — results from drug dependence that can be addressed therapeutically, thus preventing future offending.

According to the best available research, drug courts not only work but also represent a solid investment. In a review of published drug-court evaluations, University of Maryland researchers found that future offending dropped an average of 20 percent. Reviewing 27 drug-court studies, the Washington State Institute of Public Policy found drug courts yield at least $2.83 in benefits for every dollar spent.

Despite complaints that drug courts are "soft on crime," analysis shows no reduction in jail time. Instead, jail beds are simply used more effectively, as those who continue to use drugs stay behind bars and those who do not are released. More important, addicts who succeed in drug treatment will commit fewer crimes, on average, while addicts sent to prison without treatment are likely to resume criminal activity after release. The effect of this approach on crime rates could be substantial because drug-involved offenders commit voluminous crimes.

Drug courts have evolved from a small, grassroots movement to business as usual in some — but not nearly enough — jurisdictions. The Urban Institute estimates that each year fewer than 5 percent of drug-dependent arrestees receive drug-court services. If drug courts reduce crime but serve only a small percentage of offenders, the effect on crime will be negligible and a great opportunity wasted.

The bottom line? We recommend a dramatic expansion in the number of drug courts, and, even more important, in the number of drug-involved offenders being served by drug courts. Experiences in New York City provide important insight. In the last decade, crime has declined there and — reversing the trend elsewhere in the United States — so has the number of people incarcerated. Not coincidentally, during this time more than 9,000 offenders — including almost 7,000 felony offenders — have been treated in a drug court in New York.

If policymakers expand access to drug courts, the level of crime in the United States can be expected to fall measurably.

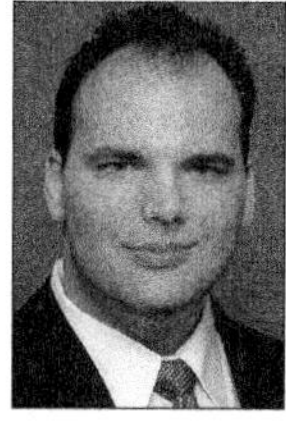

STEVEN K. ERICKSON, J.D., LL.M., PH.D.
MENTAL ILLNESS RESEARCH, EDUCATION AND CLINICAL CENTER FELLOW
YALE UNIVERSITY

WRITTEN FOR *CQ RESEARCHER*, DECEMBER 2006

Implementing alternative punishments to drug offenders is a noble attempt to stem the tide of recidivism that plagues our criminal-justice system. So, too, is the wish to provide leveraged, integrated treatment in the hope that our fellow citizens will quit abusing drugs. But in the zeal to do both the drug-court movement has become more of a dogmatic belief in therapeutic courts than an effective intervention program supported by science. Numerous taxpayer-funded studies about the effectiveness of drug courts leave much to be desired and do not answer many questions about the proper role of our court system.

While proponents frequently claim a large body of studies demonstrates the effectiveness of drug courts, a careful review of those studies reveals many troubling aspects. Most prominently, many fail to use "intent-to-treat" analysis. Simply put, defendants who leave the program before completion are routinely excluded from drug-court analysis. Thus, claims about the courts' effectiveness are highly questionable.

It is hardly beyond imagination that many drug-court defendants will leave the program for a number of reasons — chief among these is to use more drugs — and thus choose to suffer the traditional punishment of incarceration. Excluding these participants not only confounds the analysis of effectiveness but also is dishonest, since intent-to-treat analysis is the gold standard in outcomes research and mandatory in most published studies that appear in science journals.

The claims of effectiveness are plagued by other shortcomings as well. In addiction research, sustained sobriety is the benchmark of treatment success. Yet, few drug-court studies follow participants for any length of time, and none follow participants beyond the term of drug-court monitoring. Since research has consistently shown that internal motivation is largely responsible for sobriety success, the elephant-in-the-room question is whether drug-court defendants maintain their sobriety beyond their participation in the drug courts themselves.

More crucial, though, is the question of whether transforming courts into mental-health providers is wise and proper. Therapeutic courts, like drug courts, fundamentally alter the criminal-justice system in a manner that is at odds with our Constitution and traditions. Defense attorneys are relegated to passive-treatment advocates, judges are presumed behavioral experts and the judicial process becomes less about justice than about engineering social change. The good intentions of the therapeutic courts are not enough to overcome these troubling aspects.

Continued from p. 16

"On any given night, nearly 2,000 children and youth — some as young as 7 — languish in juvenile-detention facilities across the country because they cannot access needed mental-health services," Tammy Seltzer, senior staff attorney at the Washington-based Bazelon Center for Mental Health Law, told a Senate panel. [49]

According to a 2003 study, nearly 15,000 young people — around 8 percent of those in juvenile detention during a six-month period — were detained while they awaited mental-health services, said Seltzer. "Many had no criminal charges pending, while others were arrested for minor offenses, such as truancy or trespassing, generally traced to their mental-health problems."

The study authors believe their survey probably understated the extent of the problem, said Seltzer. Juveniles with mental disorders also stay in detention 36 percent longer than other detainees and have four times the rate of suicide or other self-harm, Seltzer said.

In addition, thousands of people in the criminal-justice system are on probation or parole every day, or are nearing their release date and a period that criminologists call community "re-entry." But few prisoners have access to adequate health care in the communities they return to, and even fewer get help finding and obtaining what services there are.

"I can't remember a parole officer calling me up and saying, " 'What do you recommend for this guy when he gets out?' " says Moss. "Parole people talk to jail people? It could happen, but hell could also freeze over."

So-called discharge planning isn't easy, says Flanigan, at Brown Medical School. To ensure that discharged inmates continue to get care for serious diseases, "people need a personal contact, not just the name of a clinic," and an initial appointment, he says. That's available to few inmates, however, because both institutional discharge planning and community services are scarce.

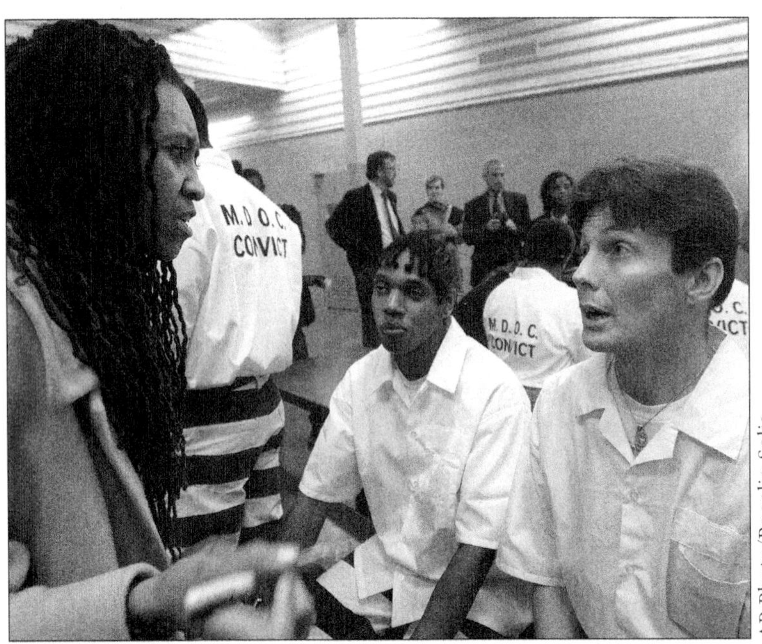

AP Photo/Rogelio Solis

Prison inmates in Mississippi talk with AIDS counselor Jackie Walker, of the American Civil Liberties Union. Civil liberties advocates argue that HIV education and optional testing can stop AIDS just as effectively as mandatory testing without violating inmates' privacy or human rights.

Increasingly, corrections officials want to provide those opportunities, says Colorado's Metzner. "A decade ago, you could talk to wardens about mental health, and they would say we're a prison not a hospital," he says. "They don't say that now. Sheriffs and wardens are in favor of adequate discharge planning." One big reason, says Metzner: "When mentally ill prisoners get it, they come back slower — or not at all." ■

CURRENT SITUATION

Prisoners and Research

Correctional health remains low on the political agenda, although a few initiatives may be bubbling up in state legislatures and Congress. However, lawsuits seeking better care are ongoing, and some corrections health systems are being overhauled under court supervision.

For example, in 2005 a federal judge placed California's entire $1.2-billion-a-year health system under a court-appointed receiver empowered to order new medical facilities built, charging it to the state treasury, and waive any law, regulation, contract provision, or labor agreement in order to bring care up to snuff. [50]

Also in 2005, Ohio settled a prisoner class-action suit, agreeing to hire 321 new medical personnel, add $7 billion to the annual health-care budget and overhaul prison medical facilities. [51] In July 2006 a Missouri court ordered all of that state's prisons to transport women prisoners to abortion facilities at their request. [52]

Also in 2006, an expert panel at the Institute of Medicine recommended changes to 30-year-old federal guidelines on research involving prisoners.

As late as the 1960s and '70s, "some very bad things" were done to prisoners recruited for research studies, mainly because prisoners are powerless, says Harrison, of the National Commission on Correctional Health Care.

In a Pennsylvania prison, for example, a dermatologist reportedly gloated over the "acres of skin" the prison would provide for experimentation with cosmetics, Harrison says.

Such cases have spurred federal rules strictly limiting most research involving prisoners. But prisoners themselves eventually questioned those restrictions, says Harrison. Early in the AIDS crisis, many treatments were available only to people participating in research, and "prisoners were coming to us, saying that it's unfair we can't be in trials," he says.

Under the new guidelines, prisoners can be subjects in a much broader range of studies. Instead of strictly excluding prisoners from some kinds of research, the new rules stipulate that risks and benefits of each proposed study must be weighed, just as they are when the subjects are non-prisoners.

That change "is a major step forward," says the University of Texas' Stone. However, he says the new rules won't accomplish what ought to have been their most important goal: stimulating research to improve prisoners' health, decrease recidivism and find ways to keep the mentally ill, substance abusers, sex offenders and others out of prison in the first place. "The panel missed a big opportunity by not naming research priorities" related to criminal justice, he says.

Prison Politics

Politically, prisoners' health gets little attention and few resources, although some observers think that as lawsuits continue and prison populations and budgets keep rising, the lack of attention to health care will have to change.

Health care for this sicker-than-average population "is a big-ticket item at a time when legislatures are continually asking, 'Do we cut prisons, or something else?' " says ACLU's Fathi. "You often see the prison system just not get the money for health care, despite their sincere pleas to the legislature."

But it may be high costs that finally drive lawmakers to action on prison-related health care, such as community mental-health and substance-abuse services that could keep some people from being incarcerated.

"State legislators that have to deal with prison health are overwhelmed by the costs," says Winslade, the professor of the philosophy of medicine at the University of Texas.

Several Texas lawmakers currently are saying, "Rather than build two more prisons, divert that money to substance-abuse" treatment, says Stone.

While in recent years substance abuse has received little legislative attention, research on treating it has been piling up, says UCLA's Anglin. "We have a vast store of knowledge." Meanwhile, the public and lawmakers are becoming somewhat "more receptive" toward the idea of treatment rather than long incarceration, he says. "That shift will only be enhanced with the Democratic takeover" of Congress.

In the past few years, Congress has discussed but not acted on bipartisan legislative proposals to assist released prisoners with community re-entry, to help prevent recidivism.

In 2007, Congress also may move legislation to improve mentally ill detainees' access to Medicaid upon release. Without such insurance, mentally ill people can't get needed services and are likely to wind up right back in jail or juvenile detention, mental-health advocates say.

"Keeping detainees with severe mental illness on Medicaid can benefit the criminal-justice system as well as the mental-health system," said Joseph P. Morrissey, a professor of health policy and psychiatry at the University of North Carolina, Chapel Hill. [53] ■

OUTLOOK

Aging Behind Bars

As the incarcerated population ages, health costs will rise. But it's not clear where the money will come from.

Over the past several decades, longer and longer prison sentences have been handed out, and people have been required to serve more of their sentences. Couple that with the huge size of the baby-boom generation and the frail health of many prisoners over age 50, and you have a cost nightmare.

"The geriatric problem is going to be huge," says Florida State University's Mears. "When someone's on tubes with five different diseases, it sucks up a lot of money."

One wave of the future is already beginning, as some prisons erect units for dementia patients, train inmates to work as hospice volunteers and plan for assisted-living sections. In October 2006, New York state's corrections department "opened its first 30-bed unit for people who've developed dementia," says Deputy Commissioner Wright. An assisted-living center is in the planning stages.

Many jurisdictions are struggling with how to care for a coming generation of older prisoners. The average cost of housing an elderly inmate is estimated at $70,000 per year, three times the cost of a younger inmate. [54]

For example, California has a "compassionate early release" program for sick inmates who are expected to die within six months and are low risks to the community; about a dozen people per year are released under the program. But California, like most other jurisdictions, is reluctant to commute sentences or risk being accused of "dumping" sick released prisoners on the community. [55]

Other options being discussed by corrections experts include shifting aging prisoners into hospices and other medical facilities in the community. In recent years, some analysts have recommended that large states like California build special geriatric prisons. However, except for a few small facilities, such as the dementia ward in New York, corrections systems haven't gone that far. [56]

Hospice care or the "early release of terminally ill prisoners" also are in corrections systems' future, says medical ethicist Cohn at the University of California, Irvine.

Wright, of New York's Department of Correctional Services, would like to see public-health agencies set up branches in jails and prisons to treat inmates for chronic and infectious diseases so that prisoners will be healthier when they return home, reducing disease in the general population. "My [prison] patients are all insured, and I can find them," he points out.

But the prison-building boom of the last three decades is siphoning off a lot of cash that otherwise might go to health care, says Mears. Texas, for example, "quadrupled its system in just over a decade, from 40,000 to 160,000" inmates.

Besides paying to erect the buildings, their staffing and upkeep "is a substantial expense — billions of dollars you can't spend on other needs," Mears says. Thus, while some prisoner advocates would like to see drug-addicted and mentally ill prisoners diverted into a more therapeutic system, Mears says that's not likely now, because states are so invested in the current prison system. "We can't close the beds."

Analysts point to better preventive health care and a rethinking of long sentences as potential solutions, but there's no easy way out, they concede.

"To change things, there has to be real leadership," says prisoner-advocate Zack, "and this is not a constituency that people care about." ■

Notes

[1] David M. Reutter, "Privatized Medical Services in Delaware Kill and Maim," *Prison Legal News*, December 2005, p. 1.
[2] Quoted in *Ibid.*, p. 3.
[3] David Ashenfelter, "Judge Orders State Prisons to Clean Up Act," *Detroit Free Press*, Nov. 13, 2006.
[4] Doris J. James and Lauren E. Glaze, "Mental Health Problems of Prison and Jail Inmates," Bureau of Justice Statistics Special Report, U.S. Department of Justice, September 2006.
[5] Christopher J. Mumola and Jennifer C. Karberg, "Drug Use and Dependence, State and Federal Prisoners, 2004," Bureau of Justice Statistics Special Report, October 2006.
[6] Laura M. Maruschak, "Medical Problems of Jail Inmates," Bureau of Justice Statistics Special Report, U.S. Department of Justice, November 2006.
[7] Laura M. Maruschak, "HIV in Prisons, 2004," *Bureau of Justice Statistics Bulletin*, U.S. Department of Justice, November 2006, p. 5.
[8] Maureen Milford, "Inmates grow old, health costs rise," *The* [Wilmington, Del.] *News Journal*, March 26, 2006.
[9] That figure includes those in state and federal prisons, jails, juvenile detention centers and other facilities, such as Bureau of Immigration facilities and jails on Indian reservations.
[10] Testimony before Senate Governmental Affairs Committee, July 7, 2004, www.nami.org.
[11] The case is *Estelle v. Gamble*, 429 U.S. 97 (1976).
[12] Keith Epstein, "Covering the Uninsured," *CQ Researcher*, June 14, 2002, pp. 521-544.
[13] Steve Lopez, "The Prisoner With the Million-Dollar Heart," *Los Angeles Times*, Feb. 13, 2002.
[14] Steve Lopez, "Doin' Time With a New Ticker," *Los Angeles Times*, Jan. 28, 2002, p. 1.
[15] For background, see James Stemgold, "U.S. Seizes State Prison Health Care," *San Francisco Chronicle*, July 1, 2005, http://sfgate.com/cgi-bin/article.cgi?file=/c/a/2005/07/01/MNGOCDHPP71.DTL.
[16] "Frontline" interview with Gary Beven, "The New Asylums," October 2004, www.pbs.org.
[17] *Ibid.* The case is *Dunn v. Voinovich*.
[18] "Frontline" interview with Fred Cohen, *ibid.*
[19] Quoted in John E. Dannenberg, "PHS Redux: Sued in a Dozen States, Contract Losses, Stock Plummets, Business Continues," *Prison Legal News*, November 2006.
[20] David L. Perry, "Should Violent Felons Receive Organ Transplants," Markkula Center for Applied Ethics, www.scu.edu.
[21] *Ibid.*
[22] Carrie S. Frank, "Must Inmates Be Provided Free Organ Transplants? Revisiting the Deliberate Indifference Standard," *George Mason University Civil Rights Law Journal*, spring 2005.
[23] *Ibid.*
[24] T. Howard Stone and William J. Winslade, "Report on a National Survey of Correctional Health Facilities: A Needs Assessment of Health Issues," *Journal of Correctional Health Care*, spring 1998.
[25] Quoted in Ed Anderson, "Badon Presses for HIV Tests in Prisons," *Times Picayune* [New Orleans] and *Nola.com*, Sept. 15, 2006; www.nola.com.
[26] *Ibid.*
[27] David L. Rosen, Victor J. Schoenback and Andrew H. Kaplan, "HIV Testing in State Prisons; Balancing Human Rights and Public Health, Infectious Diseases in Corrections Report," April 2006, www.IDCRonline.org.
[28] *Ibid.*
[29] *Ibid.*
[30] Quoted in Jeffrey Young, "Waters Seeks to Sway AIDS Groups on Prisoner Testing," *The Hill*, Nov. 27, 2006, http://thehill.com.
[31] Gary Hunter, "Texas Legislature Requires

About the Author

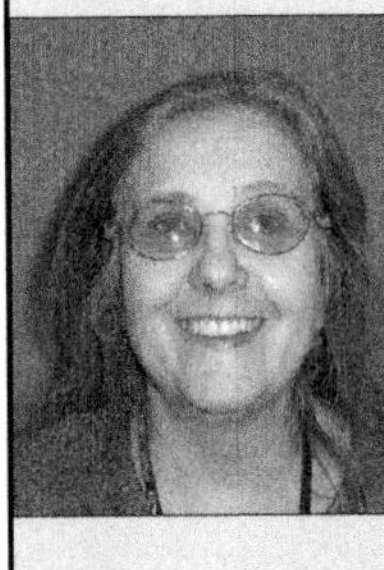

Staff writer **Marcia Clemmitt** is a veteran social-policy reporter who previously served as editor in chief of *Medicine and Health* and staff writer for *The Scientist*. She has also been a high-school math and physics teacher. She holds a liberal arts and sciences degree from St. John's College, Annapolis, and a master's degree in English from Georgetown University. Her recent reports include "Climate Change," "Controlling the Internet," "Pork Barrel Politics" and "Cyber Socializing."

HIV Testing for Prisoners," *Prison Legal News*, www.prisonlegalnews.org.

[32] For background, see David Masci, "Prison-Building Boom," *CQ Researcher*, Sept. 17, 1999, pp. 801-824.

[33] Marc Mauer, "Comparative International Rates of Incarceration: An Examination of Causes and Trends," The Sentencing Project, paper presented to the U.S. Commission on Civil Rights, June 20, 2003.

[34] For background, see Marcia Clemmitt, "Rising Health Costs," *CQ Researcher*, April 7, 2006, pp. 289-312.

[35] For background, see Peter Katel, "War on Drugs," *CQ Researcher*, June 2, 2006, pp. 481-504.

[36] Harrison and Beck, *op. cit.*, p. 9.

[37] For background, see "The New Asylums," PBS "Frontline," *op. cit.*

[38] *Ibid.*

[39] William J. Rold, "30 Years After *Estelle v. Gamble:* A Legal Retrospective," *CorrectCare*, National Commission on Correctional Health Care, summer 2006, www.ncchc.org.

[40] *Ibid.*

[41] Quoted in Dannenberg, *op. cit.*

[42] James and Glaze, *op. cit.*

[43] J. Steven Lamberti, Robert Weisman and Dara I. Faden, "Forensic Assertive Community Treatment: Preventing Incarceration of Adults With Severe Mental Illness," *Psychiatric Services*, November 2004, p. 1285.

[44] Mumola and Karberg, *op. cit.*

[45] Maruschak, *op. cit.*, p. 8 ("HIV in Prisons, 2006").

[46] *Ibid.*, p. 10.

[47] Lois M. Davis and Sharon Pacchiana, "Health Profile of the State Prison Population and Returning Offenders: Public Health Challenges," *Journal of Correctional Health Care*, fall 2003, p. 303.

[48] "Frontline" interview with Fred Cohen, *op. cit.*

[49] Testimony before Senate Committee on Governmental Affairs, July 7, 2004, http://hsgac.senate.gov.

[50] Marvin Mento, "Federal Court Seizes California Prisons' Medical Care; Appoints Receiver With Unprecedented Powers," *Prison Legal News*, www.prisonlegalnews.org.

[51] John E. Dannenberg, "Ohio DOC Stipulates to Vastly Improved Medical Care," *Prison Legal News*, www.prisonlegalnews.

[52] "ACLU Applauds Decision Allowing Women Prisoners in Missouri to Access Abortion Care," American Civil Liberties Union, July 18, 2006, www.aclu.org.

[53] Joseph P. Morrissey, "Medicaid Benefits and Recidivism of Mentally Ill People Released From Jail," National Institute of Justice, Dec. 8, 2004, www.ncjrs.gov/pdffiles1/nij/grants/214169.pdf.

[54] Jonathan Turley, testimony on "California's Aging Prisoner: Demographics, Costs, and Recommendations," before California Senate Subcommittee on Aging and Long-Term Care, February 2003, www.sen.ca.gov/ftp/SEN/COMMITTEE/SUB/HHS_AGE/_home/AGING_PRISONERS_TRANSCRIPT.DOC.

[55] Sandra Kobrin, "Dying on Our Dime — California's Prisons Are Teeming With Older Inmates Who Run Up Staggering Medical Costs," *Los Angeles Times*, June 26, 2005.

[56] Turley, *op. cit.*

FOR MORE INFORMATION

American Civil Liberties Union National Prison Project, 915 15th St., N.W., 7th Floor, Washington, DC 20005; (202) 393-4930; www.aclu.org/prison/gen/14759res20010131.html. Founded in 1972; litigates to secure prisoners' constitutional rights, including adequate health care.

American Correctional Association, 206 N. Washington St., Suite 200, Alexandria, VA 22314; (703) 224-0000; www.aca.org. Sets standards for corrections health care and advocates for corrections professionals.

American Correctional Health Services Association, 250 Gatsby Place, Alpharetta, GA 30022-6161; (877) 918-1842; www.achsa.org/index.cfm. Trains corrections staff and informs other health-care workers and the public about corrections health issues.

Bureau of Justice Statistics, U.S. Department of Justice, 810 Seventh St., N.W., Washington, DC 20531; (202) 307-0765; www.ojp.usdoj.gov/bjs/welcome.html. Federal agency that compiles and publishes statistics on U.S. correctional systems.

Human Rights Watch, 350 Fifth Ave., 34th Floor, New York, NY 10118-3299; (212) 290-4700; www.hrw.org/prisons. Nonprofit advocacy group that monitors treatment of prisoners in the United States and internationally, including prison health care.

Integrated Substance Abuse Programs, University of California, Los Angeles, 11075 Santa Monica Blvd., Suite 200, Los Angeles, CA 90025; www.uclaisap.org/index.html. Conducts research and training on substance abuse and substance-abuse treatment, including in corrections facilities.

Legal Aid Society of New York Prisoners' Rights Project, 199 Water St., New York, NY 10038; (212) 577-3300; www.legal-aid.org/supportDocumentIndex.htm?docID=19&catid=45. Lawyers' group that litigates and advocates for better conditions in New York correctional facilities.

National Commission on Correctional Health Care, 1145 W. Diversey Pkwy., Chicago, IL 60614; (773) 880-1460; www.ncchc.org. Sets standards for correctional health care and trains correctional staff.

The New Asylums, Frontline, PBS, http://149.48.228.121/wgbh/pages/frontline/shows/asylums. Web site of PBS documentary; contains interviews with corrections mental-health experts and data on mentally ill prisoners.

The Real Cost of Prisons Project, The Sentencing Project, 514 10th St., N.W., Suite 1000, Washington, DC 20004; (202) 628-0871; www.realcostofprisons.org/blog. Activist group that educates and provides news about prison issues, especially through its news weblog.

Understanding Prison Health Care, http://movementbuilding.org/prisonhealth/barriers.html. Education and advocacy Web site that archives audio and video interviews with physicians, activists and correctional health experts.

Bibliography

Selected Sources

Books

Anderson, Lloyd C., *Voices From a Southern Prison*, University of Georgia Press, 2000.
A professor of law at the University of Akron who led a legal team representing inmates at the Kentucky State Reformatory recounts the prisoners' decades-long fight for better conditions.

Hornblum, Allen, *Acres of Skin*, Routledge, 1999.
An instructor in urban studies at Temple University recounts the history of medical experiments carried out on prisoners at Philadelphia's Holmesburg Prison.

Jacobson, Michael, *Downsizing Prisons: How to Reduce Crime and End Mass Incarceration*, New York University Press, 2005.
A former chief of the New York City Department of Corrections — who argues that mass incarceration fails to reduce crime and has created a permanent criminal underclass — suggests political strategies to develop an alternative system.

Kupers, Terry, *Prison Madness: The Mental Health Crisis Behind Bars and What We Must Do About It*, Jossey-Bass, 1999.
A psychiatrist and professor at the Wright Institute in Berkeley, Calif., describes the lives of mentally ill inmates in overcrowded prisons.

Latessa, Edward J., and Alexander M. Holsinger, eds., *Correctional Contexts: Contemporary and Classical Readings*, Roxbury Publishing Co., August 2005 (3rd edition).
Criminal-justice professors at the universities of Cincinnati and Missouri assemble readings on the history of corrections, including sections on treatment programs, prison conditions and community re-entry.

Petersilia, Joan, *When Prisoners Come Home: Parole and Prisoner Reentry*, Oxford University Press, 2003.
A professor of criminology at the University of California, Irvine, describes the plight of the more than half a million prisoners released each year after receiving little treatment or training while incarcerated.

Articles

Lundy, Sarah, " 'Humanity' Put to Test as Mentally Ill Languish in Jails," *Orlando Sentinel*, Dec. 12, 2006, p. A1.
A mentally ill woman spends weeks in jail because beds in local mental hospitals are filled.

Von Zeilbauer, Paul, "A Spotty Record of Health Care for Children in City Detention," *The New York Times*, March 1, 2005, p. A1.
A for-profit company makes questionable health decisions for mentally ill children in New York City juvenile facilities.

Reports and Studies

"Adult Drug Courts: Evidence Indicates Recidivism Reductions and Mixed Results for Other Outcomes," Government Accountability Office, February 2005.
Congress' nonpartisan research and analysis agency found that drug courts that divert adults from prison into substance-abuse treatment prevent many from committing subsequent offenses.

"Confronting Confinement," Commission on Safety and Abuse in America's Prisons, June 2006.
A national expert panel reports on dangerous cultures inside prisons, including poor health and bad health care, and argues that prison health deficiencies harm communities as well.

"The Health Status of Soon-to-be-Released Inmates: A Report to Congress," National Commission on Correctional Health Care, 2002.
The main accrediting and training organization for correctional health care details the prevalence of infectious, chronic and mental disease among inmates.

"Mental Health in the House of Corrections: A Study of Mental Health Care in New York State Prisons," Correctional Association of New York, June 2004, www.correctionalassociation.org.
An independent advocacy group found that New York state prisons have too little space and provide too little treatment for their many mentally ill inmates, whose numbers increased by 71 percent between 1991 and 2004.

"The Public Health Dimensions of Prisoner Reentry: Addressing the Health Needs and Risks of Returning Prisoners and Their Families," Urban Institute Justice Policy Center, December 2002.
Criminal-justice and health-care analysts summarize the presentations and discussions from a national symposium on health concerns related to prisoner re-entry.

Mears, Daniel P., Laura Winterfeld, John Hunsaker, Gretchen E. Moore and Ruth M. White, "Drug Treatment in the Criminal Justice System: The Current State of Knowledge," Urban Institute Justice Policy Center, January 2003.
Analysts affiliated with a liberal-leaning think tank describe the recent history of substance-abuse treatment in prisons, including a decline in treatment-program enrollment through the late-1990s, after which participation began to increase.

The Next Step:

Additional Articles from Current Periodicals

Drug Courts

Brulliard, Karin, "Uncertain Future For County's Drug Court," *The Washington Post*, June 19, 2005, p. T1.
Commonwealth's Attorney James E. Plowman (R) has been vocal about his lack of support for Loudoun County's pilot drug program in Virginia.

Hahn, Valerie Schremp, "Drug Court Marks Success," *St. Louis Post-Dispatch*, June 5, 2006, p. B1.
A young, former cocaine addict charged with marijuana possession successfully graduated from a drug court in Lincoln County, Mo.

Tilghman, Andrew, "Alternate Offender Program Growing," *The Houston Chronicle*, March 27, 2005, p. B1.
The drug court in Harris County, Texas, is getting a boost from President Bush's faith-based initiatives, which include money to expand drug courts by giving addicts the option of treatment with church-based groups.

Elderly Prisoners

Ove, Torsten, "Growing Old in Prison," *Pittsburgh Post-Gazette*, March 6, 2005, p. A1.
Because a growing number of baby-boomer prisoners are getting older, policymakers are debating whether to continue keeping so many older prisoners incarcerated.

Sterngold, James, "California Bracing For A Flood of Elderly Inmates," *The San Francisco Chronicle*, Dec. 25, 2005, p. A21.
California's legislative analyst's office projects that by 2022 there will be at least 30,200 inmates 55 and older, compared with 7,580 now.

Wright, Gary L., "As Inmates Age, Cost of Health Care Climbs," *Charlotte Observer*, April 17, 2005, p. A1.
The cost of providing health care to prison inmates in North Carolina has nearly doubled in less than 10 years because of a growing elderly population and rising medical costs.

Yamaguchi, Mari, "Japan's Prisons Adapting to Rapidly Graying Populations," *The Houston Chronicle*, Feb. 12, 2006, p. A28.
Japan's 67 prisons are being forced to adapt to a new trend of an aging population — with the number of inmates 60 years old or older tripling in the past decade.

Infectious Diseases and Prisons

Fox, Maggie, "Prisoner Medical Research Lacks Oversight, Group Says," *The Houston Chronicle*, Aug. 6, 2006, p. A15.
The U.S. prison population needs more protection from potential medical-research abuses, according to a panel of experts from the Institute of Medicine.

von Zielbauer, Paul, "A Company's Troubled Answer for Prisoners With H.I.V.," *The New York Times*, Aug. 1, 2005, p. A1.
Prison Health Services, the nation's largest commercial provider of prison health care, has a turbulent record in many of the 33 states where it has provided jail medicine.

Mentally Ill Prisoners

Lopez, Steve, "Mentally Ill in the Jail? It's a Crime," *Los Angeles Times*, Dec. 11, 2005, p. B1.
Lopez says jails have become dumping grounds for the mentally ill because there is often nowhere else to put them.

Puente, Mark, "Care of Mentally Ill Prisoners Costly For Jails," *Plain Dealer* (Cleveland), Jan. 20, 2006, p. B1.
Jails across Northeast Ohio say mentally ill inmates who used to be sent to psychiatric institutions are filling up prison cells needed for more traditional criminals.

Scott, Rebekah, "Three-Year-Old Program For Mentally Challenged Prisoners To Be Reviewed," *Pittsburgh Post-Gazette*, June 2, 2005, p. EZ-7.
Two mental-health caseworkers at Pennsylvania's Westmoreland County Prison have helped about 60 prisoners connect to services and get out of jail sooner.

Wachtler, Sol, "A Cell of One's Own," *The New York Times*, Sept. 24, 2006, p. 15.
A former judge with bipolar disorder writes about why he supports alternative confinement for disruptive mentally ill prisoners.

Citing *CQ Researcher*

Sample formats for citing these reports in a bibliography include the ones listed below. Preferred styles and formats vary, so please check with your instructor or professor.

MLA Style

Jost, Kenneth. "Rethinking the Death Penalty." CQ Researcher 16 Nov. 2001: 945-68.

APA Style

Jost, K. (2001, November 16). Rethinking the death penalty. *CQ Researcher, 11*, 945-968.

Chicago Style

Jost, Kenneth. "Rethinking the Death Penalty." *CQ Researcher*, November 16, 2001, 945-968.

CHAPTER

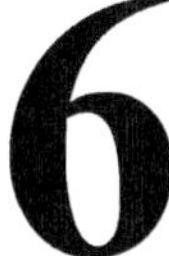

Reproductive Ethics

By Marcia Clemmitt

Excerpted from the CQ Researcher. Marcia Clemmitt. (May 15, 2009). "Reproductive Ethics." *CQ Researcher*, 449-472.

Reproductive Ethics

BY MARCIA CLEMMITT

THE ISSUES

After 33-year-old Nadya Suleman, a mother of six, gave birth to octuplets on Jan. 26, the California fertility specialist who treated her was summoned to appear before the Medical Board of California. The board — which can revoke physicians' licenses for egregious misconduct — is investigating whether Michael Kamrava, head of the West Coast IVF Clinic in Beverly Hills, violated accepted standards of medical practice when he implanted at least six embryos in Suleman during in vitro fertilization (IVF) treatment in 2008, leading to the multiple birth. [1]

Suleman has told reporters that all 14 of her children were conceived using IVF — a high-tech treatment in which eggs are fertilized in the laboratory, then implanted into a woman's uterus for gestation — and that six embryos were implanted in each of her six pregnancies, although she's had only two multiple births: the octuplets and a set of twins. But professional guidelines from the American Society for Reproductive Medicine recommend implanting only one or two embryos in younger women, such as Suleman, because of the high risk multiple births pose to children and mothers.

Multiple-birth babies, including twins, have a significantly higher risk for developing severe, debilitating disabilities such as chronic lung diseases or cerebral palsy, which occurs six times more often among twins and 20 times more often in triplets than it does in single babies. [2]

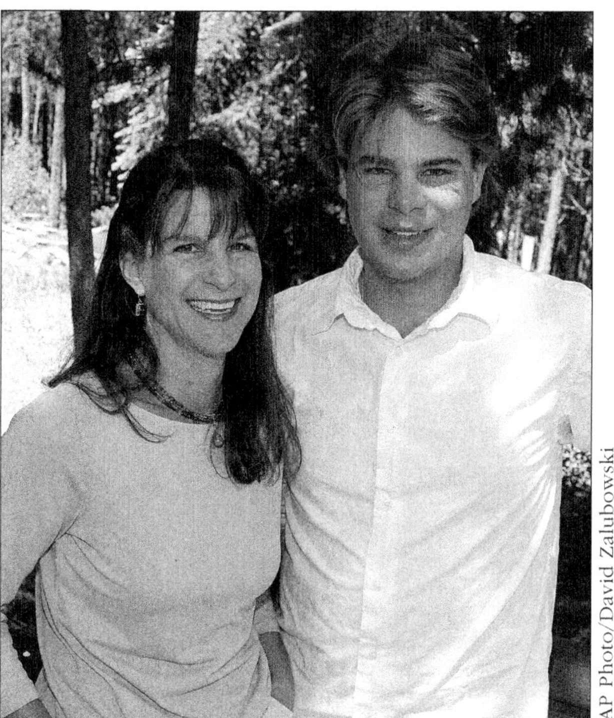

AP Photo/David Zalubowski

Wendy Kramer of Nederland, Colo., and her son Ryan — who was conceived through donor insemination — founded and run the Donor Sibling Registry to help donor-conceived children locate siblings and learn about their genetic lineage. Ryan has learned of six half-sisters to date. As of February, more than 6,200 siblings have been connected via the online registry, which was launched in 2000.

The cost to the health-care system of multiple births is enormous. "The cost of caring for the octuplets would probably cover more than a year of providing IVF for everyone in L.A. County who needed it," says David L. Keefe, professor of obstetrics and gynecology at the University of South Florida, in Tampa. "The likelihood that some of those kids will get cerebral palsy means they'll need a lifetime of care."

The high-profile Suleman case has spurred calls for government regulation of fertility medicine — sometimes called assisted reproductive technologies, or ART. (*See box, p. 464.*) Like U.S. medicine generally, ART is not regulated by the federal government and only lightly supervised by state agencies. Since 1978 — when the world's first IVF baby, Louise Brown, was born in England — more than 3 million ART babies have been born worldwide, and some experts and ethicists fear the field's rapid expansion leaves too much room for abuses. [3]

Others argue that lack of insurance coverage for IVF is the biggest problem with ART in the United States. Fertility treatments can cost more than $12,000 per cycle, pushing cash-strapped would-be parents to opt for the higher-risk, multiple-embryo implantation to increase their chances of a pregnancy.

By contrast, in most European countries — where IVF procedures are paid for through universal health-care systems — doctors generally implant only one fertilized embryo at a time. In Sweden and Finland, for instance, where the procedure is covered by insurance, doctors perform single-embryo implantations 70 percent and 60 percent of the time, respectively, compared to only 3.3 percent of the time in the United States. [4] (*See graph, p. 457.*)

In fact, some European governments prohibit multiple-embryo transfers for women under 36 and limit older women to no more than two embryos per cycle. As a result, "Triplets have virtually disappeared in Europe," a Danish doctor told European colleagues at a 2006 fertility conference. [5]

Self-regulation of ART in the United States clearly isn't working, said Marcy Darnovsky, associate executive director of the Oakland, Calif.-based Center for Genetics and Society, which advocates for responsible use of genetic technologies. According to the federal Centers for Disease Control and Prevention (CDC), to which ART clinics

Most States Don't Require Infertility Coverage

Only 12 states require all state-regulated health insurance plans to cover infertility diagnosis and treatment. Two states — California and Texas — require only that every insurer offer at least one plan with fertility coverage.

States Mandating Infertility Insurance Coverage

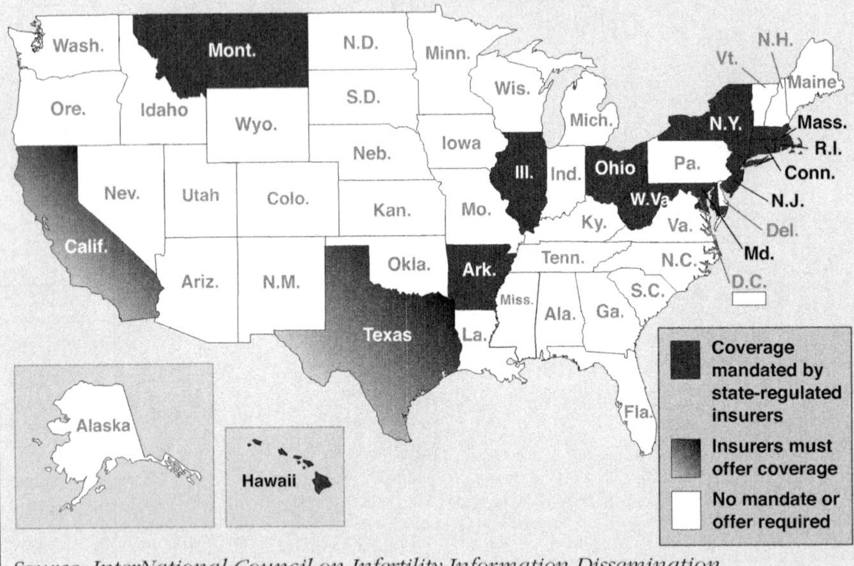

Source: InterNational Council on Infertility Information Dissemination

must report data, 80 percent of programs do not strictly follow American Society for Reproductive Medicine guidelines, making government regulation "long overdue," she said. [6]

"In reproductive matters, individuals are making decisions [that affect] not just themselves, but . . . others as well," which makes regulation appropriate, said Johns Hopkins University scholars Franco Furger and Francis Fukuyama. Reproductive medicine is headed toward giving prospective parents "a range of . . . techniques to make specific choices about a baby's health and sex and eventually about other attributes," said Furger, a research professor, and Fukuyama, a professor of international political economy, both at the Paul H. Nitze School of Advanced International Studies in Washington, D.C. "It would be misguided to take a wait-and-see attitude." [7]

Industrialized countries that pay for IVF through their universal health-care systems strictly regulate which services may be provided, says Susannah Baruch, director for law and policy at the Genetics & Public Policy Center, a think tank at John Hopkins funded by the Pew Charitable Trusts. The services typically include pre-implantation genetic diagnosis (PGD) — genetic testing of embryos. While PGD to detect serious genetic illnesses is conducted routinely, many countries strictly limit other PGD uses, such as selecting a child's gender, because they aren't considered in the public interest, she says.

However, in the United States — even though U.S. reproductive-medicine experts roundly criticize Kamrava's implantation of multiple embryos in the Suleman case — many ART experts also argue that government regulation of the industry is not necessarily a solution.

Suleman's case is much more of an outlier today than it would have been 15 years ago, when it wasn't unusual to have six embryos transferred, says Josephine Johnston, a research scholar at the Hastings Center for bioethics research in Garrison, N.Y. "I would have bet money that it was not IVF" that led to the octuplet birth, she says, but the use of ovary-stimulating drugs — a much cheaper, far less controllable method of assisted reproductive technology.

Multiple-embryo implantation is being phased out as ART technologies improve, Johnston says, and six-embryo implantation is "so far outside the guidelines it's amazing that a physician would do it."

Such hair-raising cases are virtually always outliers and shouldn't be used to hastily enact laws, some analysts say.

For example, ever since artificial insemination was introduced sperm banks have promised would-be parents a genetic lineage of intelligence, athleticism and good looks for babies born from donor sperm, says R. Alta Charo, a professor of law and bioethics at the University of Wisconsin Law School. But "it hasn't undermined Western culture as we know it," she says. "So why do we think that people are very likely to go through much more onerous PGD to choose traits?" Very few will try to use it to enhance their baby's intelligence or appearance, so there would be little point in prohibiting such behavior, she says.

A recent study by New York University's Langone Medical Center supports Charo's view somewhat. Of 999 patients who completed a survey on traits they thought warranted use of PGD screening, solid majorities named potential conditions such as mental retardation, blindness, deafness, heart disease and cancer. Only 10 percent said they might use PGD to choose a child with exceptional athletic ability and 12.6 percent, high intelligence. [8]

"People are after different things" in calling for ART regulation, making legislation difficult, Charo says. Some may want limits on the number of embryos implanted per cycle, but most are calling for rules to enforce "personal morality," such as whether gay couples should become parents or whether lower-income mothers should be allowed to have very large families, Charo says. "We must then ask why we would regulate these [reproductive] personal choices differently from other personal choices."

ART-related law would likely be based on the unusual cases that make headlines, "and bad cases make bad policy," she says.

Opposition to regulation might drop considerably if insurance covered IVF and other artificial reproduction procedures, but today only 12 states require such coverage. (*See map, p. 452.*)

For instance, limitations on multiple-embryo implantations might be acceptable if insurance covered several single-embryo implantations for all patients who have experienced six months of proven infertility, suggests Ronald M. Green, a professor of ethics and human values at Dartmouth College.

Because of the high cost of IVF treatments, the lack of insurance coverage has deprived "the vast majority of the middle class" in America, as well as the poor, from the modern ART "revolution," says Keefe at the University of South Florida. "Once you have the middle class covered, then I have no trouble saying, 'We're not going to pay' " for multiple-embryo implantation.

Furthermore, the procedure doesn't have to cost $12,000 per cycle, as evidenced by the lower amounts accepted by IVF clinics when insurance companies that are required to cover the procedure negotiate lower fees, he says. "It's a lot cheaper [for society] to pay for IVF at $3,000 or $4,000 per procedure and deliver only singletons," thus avoiding the harrowing medical problems and high costs associated with multiple births, he says.

Mandating coverage not only reduces the number of multiple births but also increases access for the middle class. "I practiced in Massachusetts and Rhode Island [which require coverage], where sheet-metal workers and

Majority of ART Pregnancies Result in a Live Birth

About 82 percent of the U.S. pregnancies resulting from assisted reproductive technology (ART) in 2006 resulted in live births. More than half were a single-child birth, and a quarter were multiple-infant births. Nearly three-quarters of U.S. ART procedures use fresh, non-donor sperm or eggs.

Outcomes of Pregnancies Resulting From ART Cycles Using Fresh, Non-donor Eggs or Embryos, 2006

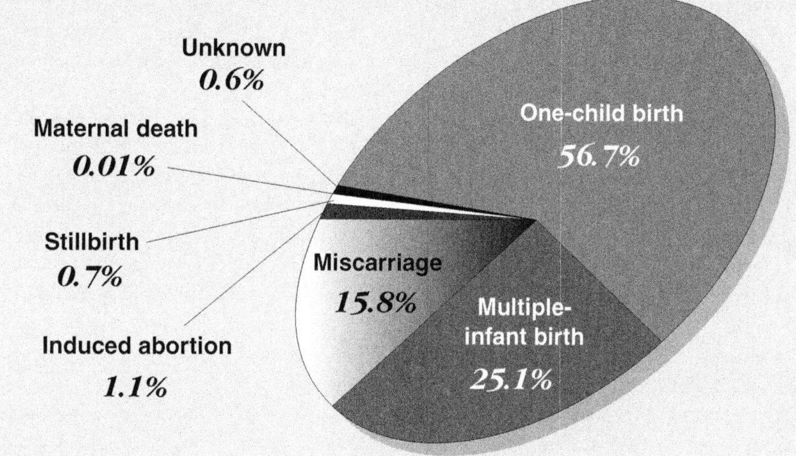

** Percentages do not total 100 due to rounding.*

Source: "Assisted Reproductive Technology Success Rates 2006," Centers for Disease Control and Prevention, 2008

heiresses from Newport" mingled at IVF clinics because insurance picked up the tab, Keefe says.

However, not all fertility doctors would opt into a fully insured system, says Dawn Gannon, director of professional outreach for RESOLVE, the National Infertility Association, which advocates that insurance companies treat infertility like any other medical condition. For example, when New Jersey mandated coverage, in 2001, "some clinics didn't take insurance at all, and some started taking it and then stopped," she says, because "they got less money per procedure."

If the United States enacts universal health-care coverage, advocates for the infertile hope ART will be covered as it is in other industrialized countries.

But universal coverage would still leave thorny issues unsettled, such as whether taxpayer subsidies should support ART for unmarried women or women over 40. For older women, the debate centers on whether it is appropriate for health insurance to subsidize an infertility problem that is the result of natural aging and not the result of a medical condition. Also, pregnancy is riskier for both the older mother and the child.

Earlier in IVF's history, many clinicians routinely refused ART to single women, older women, lesbians and, in some cases, poor people. A 1993 survey of Finnish ART clinics found that many doctors "preferred not to treat either lesbian or single women," arguing that they "wanted to protect children from having inappropriate parents, primarily 'bad mothers,' " according to Maili Malin, a medical sociologist at Finland's

As Technology Advances, Questions Emerge

Multiple births threaten poor families.

Ghazala Khamis and her husband, a farmworker, had three daughters, but they longed for a son. Last year, the 27-year-old Egyptian woman gave birth to healthy septuplets, four boys and three girls, by Caesarian section near the end of her eighth month of pregnancy. Before the septuplets, she had not conceived for five years. [1]

Khamis conceived the septuplets using one of the oldest fertility technologies, introduced in the 1950s and '60s — fertility drugs that stimulate women's ovaries to produce multiple eggs. While effective for many, the drugs — which are becoming cheap and widely available around the world — are also among the most dangerous and unpredictable treatments, often leading to multiple births, and as they spread into poor communities the consequences can be dire.

"I'm really scared," Khamis said, soon after her delivery. "We live in a mud hut with only two rooms. I don't know how we're going to afford 10 children." [2]

The positive side of the medications' increased availability is that poor people have the greatest risk of infertility and, until recently, had literally no access to help. "The less money you have, the more likely you are to have difficulty conceiving," wrote Liza Mundy, author of a 2007 book on fertility medicine, *Everything Conceivable.* "Much infertility has always been caused by infections that can damage reproductive passageways," and "the lower your tax bracket, the less likely you are to have received the fairly simple medical treatment that can stave off these consequences." [3]

But the spread of the hard-to-control drugs, coupled with many families' desire for sons, can create tragedies in poor communities, especially in the developing world. Khamis' delivery ultimately went well, but because Egypt doesn't have enough respirators for newborns, doctors held back from performing the Caesarian section until long after Western doctors would have removed the children. "We were simply blessed by God that no complication happened," Khamis' physician, Mahmoud Meleis, said. "If there had been a complication, Ghazala would have died." [4]

As older fertility technologies spread, newer ones are being created, sometimes solving problems but sometimes creating new ones.

A fledgling technique — freezing women's eggs, rather than embryos, for later use — could eventually help solve two problems with fertility treatments, says John Jain, head of an IVF clinic in Santa Monica, Calif., and an early U.S. adopter of egg freezing, which began in 2005 in Italy. First, freezing eggs can offset the fertility problems often caused by the upward creep in the age at which people start families. Second, freezing eggs causes fewer moral and religious qualms than freezing embryos,

"I have patients flying in because I will freeze eggs rather than embryos," thus allowing women to bank their own eggs against future infertility, whatever its cause, such as cancer treatment or aging, he says. "The pregnancy rate from frozen eggs is as good as from frozen embryos."

But others warn that egg freezing hasn't been fully tested. "The biggest misconception coming down the pike is freezing eggs,' " says David L, Rosenfeld, director of the Center for Human

National Institute of Public Health. A single woman's marital status and "wish to have a child" were both "considered indications of . . . questionable mental health." [9]

Whatever the outcome, the coverage debate will generate intense emotion. "So much of your life feels out of control when you want a child but find that you can't have one," says Jan Elman Stout, a clinical psychologist in Chicago. "This is often the very first challenge that people encounter in their lives that, no matter how hard they work at it, it may not work out for them."

As ethicists, lawmakers and physicians debate how best to provide access and oversight for reproductive medicine, here are some of the questions being asked:

Should fertility medicine be regulated more vigorously?

Should a mother of six with limited income be allowed to give birth to eight additional children through IVF? If a man donates sperm that results in hundreds of babies — technically making them all half brothers and sisters — should the offspring be given the identity of their biological father so they won't end up dating or marrying a half-sibling? Is a father whose child was the product of donated egg and sperm liable for child support if the couple divorces?

These are just a handful of the sticky ethical questions that have emerged from the brave, new world of sperm and egg donation. [10]

Of course, outlier cases like that of the California octuplets quickly spur vociferous calls for government limits on in vitro fertilization. And others say the well-being of patients demands at least some rules. Finally, since many ART-related questions wind up in court, judges say they need more legislative guidance than the current case-by-case approach being used to settle IVF cases.

"No matter what one thinks of artificial insemination, and — as now appears in the not-too-distant future, cloning and even gene splicing — courts are still going to be faced with the problem of determining legal parentage," declared a unanimous California Court of Appeals ruling in the 1998 case *Buzzanca v. Buzzanca.* "Courts can continue to make decisions on an ad hoc basis . . . or the legislature can act to improve a broader

Reproduction at the North Shore-Long Island Jewish Health System in Manhasset, N.Y. "It's experimental, and right now the public expectations are unreal." Currently it's unknown how long frozen eggs can be stored — whether they'll be like embryos and sperm, which can be stored long term without apparent harm, or more fragile. "The technology will improve, but expectations are running way ahead of that," he says.

Like all reproductive technology, egg freezing could still raise ethics issues. In April 2007, a Canadian woman triggered a bioethical debate when she froze some of her own eggs so that her 7-year-old daughter, who has a genetic disorder that causes infertility, could use them as an adult.

A daughter potentially giving birth to her mother's child is unusual enough so that "we have to look very carefully into what we're doing here," said Margaret Somerville, an ethicist at McGill University in Toronto.

But other ethicists aren't troubled a bit. "It's hard for me to see what difference it'd make to the child that one of her gametes came from her grandmother [rather] than her mother," said Wayne Summer, a University of Toronto philosophy professor. [5]

Meanwhile, a new sperm-donation technique is drastically changing fertility medicine. Intra-cytoplasmic sperm injection, or ICSI, allows even a single, weak sperm to fertilize an egg. ICSI is quickly displacing sperm donation, once widely used by heterosexual infertility patients but increasingly used only by single women and lesbian couples. ICSI now allows many men to become fathers who previously could not have conceived, and it's spread like wildfire in the past decade. In Europe in 2005 — the most recent year for which data has been analyzed — the technique was used in 63.3 percent of all assisted-reproduction cases, up from 34.7 percent in 1997, when European data collection began. [6]

Using ICSI and other techniques, "you're probably helping people have a child that Mother Nature wouldn't have allowed for," and that has both risks and benefits, says Angeline Beltsos, medical director of the Chicago-based Fertility Centers of Illinois.

Indeed, evidence is growing that sons conceived through ICSI inherit their father's infertility, raising questions about consequences generations down the road.

"We may have tens of thousands of boys born with infertility," said Tommaso Falcone, head of obstetrics and gynecology at the Cleveland Clinic. [7]

---

[1] For background, see Hadeel Al-Shalchi, "Egypt Septuplets Stir Debate on Fertility Drugs," The Associated Press, ABC News Web site, Aug. 26, 2008, http://abcnews.go.com/print?id=5661108.

[2] Quoted in *ibid.*

[3] Liza Mundy, *Everything Conceivable* (2007), p. xiv.

[4] Quoted in Al-Shalchi, *op. cit.*

[5] Quoted in "Assisted Human Reproduction: Regulating and Treating Conception Problems," CBC News Web site, Feb. 5, 2009, www.cbc.ca.

[6] "Fertility Treatments: Researcher Says that ICSI May Be Over-used in Some Countries," *Science Daily* Web site, July 9, 2008, www.sciencedaily.com.

[7] Quoted in JoNel Aleccia, "Pass It On: Sons of Infertile Men May Be Next," MSNBC.com, Sept. 27, 2008, www.msnbc.msn.com.

order which . . . would bring some predictability to those who seek to make use of artificial reproductive techniques," said the justices in a case involving a divorcing husband who claimed no financial responsibility for his daughter, conceived from donor egg and sperm and borne by a surrogate mother. [11]

Creating a federal-government registry of information on egg and sperm donors would give adults born from donated gametes (sperms or eggs) access to their genetic history in order to prevent half-siblings from marrying each other. It would also allow limits on the numbers of children created through one person's donations, said Naomi Cahn, a research professor at the George Washington University Law School. In England, no more than 10 children can be created from a single donor's sperm. [12]

The federal government should exercise more aggressively the authority it already has to oversee the safety and efficacy of some ART technologies, say some experts.

For instance, inserting one woman's egg into another woman's body is arguably a type of tissue transplant — a procedure over which the Food and Drug Administration (FDA) has jurisdiction but has been lax in regulating, says the University of Wisconsin's Charo. "That's an appropriate place to step in to ask whether we have assurance of safety for the stuff that's being developed," she says.

The FDA has a role in determining whether genetic tests are safe and whether they work or are medically useful, says Baruch of the Genetics & Public Policy Center. For instance, many labs manufacture genetic tests that they don't market to other companies — called "home-brew" tests — but the FDA "has chosen not to regulate them," she says. "We believe that they have the authority" and would like to see them do it.

Genetic testing of embryos — preimplantation genetic diagnosis or PGD, which requires permanent removal of one cell from an eight-cell embryo — is much more technically difficult than other forms of genetic testing but gets less government scrutiny, according to Baruch's organization. And, the center points out, even the general quality standards for laboratories under the federal Clinical Laboratory Improvement Amendments of 1988 are not being applied to PGD labs. [13]

Most ART Cycles Don't End in Deliveries

Approximately 100,000 assisted reproductive technology (ART) cycles were performed in 2006 using fresh, non-donor eggs or embryos. Of that amount, less than 35,000 resulted in pregnancies. Only about 28,000 actually resulted in live-birth deliveries.

Outcome of ART Cycles Using Fresh, Non-donor Eggs or Embryos, 2006

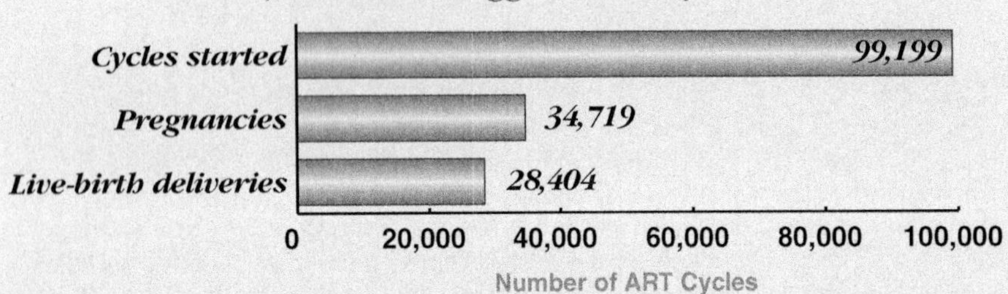

Source: "Assisted Reproductive Technology Success Rates 2006," Centers for Disease Control and Prevention, 2008

But aside from testing the safety and efficacy of medical products and drugs, the U.S. government does not, in general, regulate the practice of medicine, says Wisconsin's Charo. "That being the case, the issue of regulating fertility clinics actually becomes, 'Should they be regulated differently from the rest of medicine?' " she says. "It would be difficult to make that case."

"Muddling through" without regulation "is a respectable policy option, especially for a pragmatic people faced with irreconcilable moral quandaries" such as those often posed by ART, said John A. Robertson, a professor at the University of Texas College of Law in Austin. "This non-system 'system' has served well to date — even if not all the time and never perfectly — both in other contexts and for assisted reproduction." The current system can deal with even thorny issues, he adds, such as questions surrounding the "genetic screening of embryos . . . and the other edge technologies looming ahead." [14]

Furthermore, he pointed out, the President's Council on Bioethics appointed by George W. Bush examined the ART field for more than a year and found that the biggest problems were "on the margins, not at the core." The panel recommended only "tinker[ing] with ways to get more data" and making professional self-regulation more effective. [15]

National Infertility Association Executive Director Barbara L. Collura also advocates caution in regulating ART. While limiting the number of embryos implanted per cycle may seem like a no-brainer, she says, such a rule could be prohibitively difficult because of the wide variety of medical conditions that could occur. For example, she argues, while the American Society of Reproductive Medicine strongly recommends transferring only one — or at most two — embryos at a time, if a woman has already had three or four cycles of IVF and her embryo quality is poor, a doctor could easily justify implanting multiple embryos. "How do you put that into a law?" she asks.

And some fertility doctors argue that they're already more regulated than most other U.S. physicians. "FDA put in tons of rules a few years ago . . . [that] added hundreds of dollars to the cost," says John Jain, who heads a fertility clinic in Santa Monica, Calif. The guidelines, which mainly dealt with disease-testing of donated gametes, involved "viruses I've never seen in my life." He fears that other regulations "will add to the already exorbitant cost."

David L. Rosenfeld, director of the Center for Human Reproduction at the North Shore-Long Island Jewish Health System in Manhasset, N.Y., makes the same point. "We're already highly scrutinized," he says. Thanks to the CDC's fertility-clinic database, he adds, reproductive-medicine specialists are "the only physicians in the country whose numbers are published nationally."

Sanctions for outlier physicians already exist at state licensing boards such as the one scrutinizing Suleman's doctor, says Jain. "As a physician, how far do I need to be policed? If there are poor outcomes, a level of public scrutiny" emerges — as it has in the octuplets' case — which helps rein in doctors inclined to go too far, he says.

Finally, some doctors contend that having light government oversight allows U.S. medicine to advance rapidly.

"We are probably leaders in the field of reproductive medicine because we can advance without government interference," says Angeline Beltsos, medical director of the Chicago-based Fertility Centers of Illinois. "Creating guidelines is critical, but legislating is dangerous."

Should parents be allowed to choose their babies' characteristics, such as gender?

When pre-implantation genetic diagnosis is used in combination with in vitro fertilization, parents can select specific embryos for their characteristics, raising a variety of ethical questions. [16]

Today, PGD — which removes one cell from an eight-cell embryo — can generally test for only one trait. But soon "we're going to be able to look for many markers at once," opening the door to choosing various characteristics, explains Baruch of the Genetics & Public Policy Center. For instance, eventually hair and eye color will be on the list, "and that'll give people pause."

Many analysts see no problem with allowing parents to opt for PGD, since it seems unlikely that many would go through the rigors of IVF just for the chance to choose a child's gender or appearance.

"We've exercised the ability to choose characteristics for a long time, by deciding who we'll marry or by carefully choosing" a sperm donor for artificial insemination, yet history shows that few people put much effort into choosing traits that might produce a "superior" human, the University of Wisconsin's Charo says. "I'm the only person sent by Congress on taxpayer money to see" the so-called Nobel Prize-winner sperm bank, the Repository for Germinal Excellence, in Southern California, and "I found that nobody ever used that sperm."

Some bioethics experts say there's nothing necessarily wrong with choosing a baby's gender. "I'm the mother of four boys and . . . my sons are marvelous, but at the same time, I certainly would have liked to have had a girl," said University of Chicago professor of medicine Janet D. Rowley during a 2003 deliberation by the President's Council on Bioethics. "This is an area we should leave alone . . . unregulated." [17]

Sex selection to achieve what some call "gender balance" in a family is probably acceptable, says Robertson of the University of Texas. "I have a hard time finding sexism or bias" in a family with three daughters using PGD to have a son, he says.

Meanwhile, Robertson says selecting out genes for non-medical conditions or attributes like looks, personality and abilities probably won't be possible anytime soon. "Most conditions aren't controlled by a single gene," he explains, and scientists don't know which genes make the difference for potentially desirable traits like athleticism or intelligence. Even for single-gene traits, like "fast-twitch muscles" that help some athletes, "the idea of going through IVF when your child won't necessarily become a top athlete anyway seems outlandish," he says. "I think the fears of designer babies are overblown."

Single-Embryo Use Is Rare in U.S.

In countries where insurance pays for IVF procedures, doctors generally implant single embryos in women. By contrast, single-embryo implantation is rare in the United States, where the procedure is not usually covered by insurance, which forces women to have multiple implantations.

Percent of IVF Cycles Involving Single-Embryo Transfers

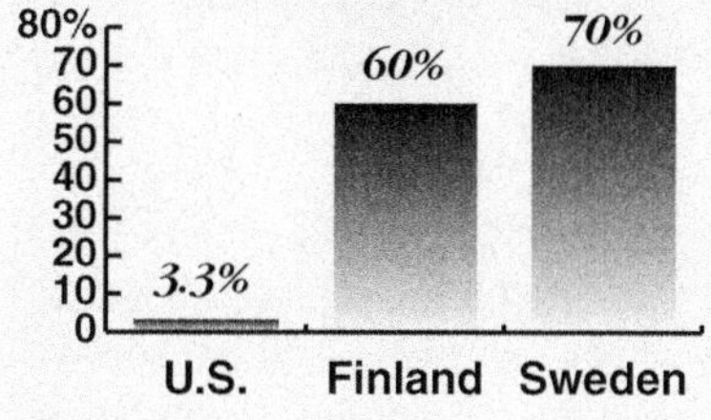

Country	Percent
U.S.	3.3%
Finland	60%
Sweden	70%

Source: BBC News, June 26, 2008, http://news.bbc.co.uk/2/hi/health/7475392.stm

Likewise, Paul Miller, a former commissioner of the Equal Employment Opportunity Commission, thinks fears are probably unfounded that allowing parents to select against characteristics like shortness or baldness would increase stigmatization of those traits. "There have been opportunities to terminate fetuses with Down's syndrome . . . for a generation," Miller said, "and yet I don't believe that individuals . . . with Down's syndrome are any more or less excluded or that . . . society has the sense that [such] a child . . . should have been prevented." [18]

But others say there's more interest among the public in choosing traits like gender than had been expected and that it's worrisome.

"Looking to the future, some observers view PGD, or any technology that allows parents to choose the characteristics of their children, as having the potential to fundamentally alter the way we view human reproduction and our offspring," noted researchers from the Genetics & Public Policy Center think tank. Rather than viewing "reproduction as a mysterious process that results in the miraculous gift of a child," children may become viewed as a commodity, created by a "series of meticulous, technology-driven" parental choices, said a center report. [19]

Potentially, wealthier people could increase their social advantage because they could afford to create babies with "genes selected to increase their chances of having good looks, musical talent . . . or whatever," thus worsening social inequalities, said the report. In addition, if trait selection becomes common, children born with genetic traits such as hereditary deafness or small stature could face increased social stigma, and parents could face pressure to use PGD to avoid having such children, center analysts speculated. [20]

While Baruch finds it difficult to believe anybody would go through IVF and PGD just to choose their child's gender, recent data indicate that there has been an unexpected uptick in interest in sex selection. "I have heard directly from IVF clinics who were surprised to have people come in primarily for sex selection," she says. Nevertheless, "we need to see better numbers before we call for regulation."

Researchers are finding evidence that some Asian immigrant families, for instance, are using ART to have sons. In some Asian countries, boys are so highly valued over girls that many families have selectively aborted or even murdered girl babies, leading to whole generations in which boys greatly outnumber girls. [21]

Separate research from scholars at Columbia University and the University of Texas concludes that some Asian families in the United States have used and are using whatever technology is available to produce sons, especially for second, third and subsequent children. In the 1990s, the chosen technique was most likely gender-selective abortion, but today more families appear to be using PGD as well. [22]

The researchers found that during the 1990s Chinese, Indian and Korean families' first children mirrored the gender balance in non-Asian families, but their subsequent children included significantly higher proportions of sons. Among Indian families in Santa Clara County, Calif., for example, University of Texas economist Jason Abrevaya found a 58-percent likelihood that a third child would be a son — significantly higher than the natural 51-percent chance of having a boy. [23]

In 2004, at least 70 percent of the parents using the Fertility Institute of Los Angeles wanted to choose their child's gender — far more than those who wanted the clinic's services to test for genetic diseases, reported Deborah L. Spar, a professor of business administration at Harvard Business School. [24] The clinic's medical director, Jeffrey Steinberg, generated some controversy in February when *The Wall Street Journal* reported that his clinic would now offer not only gender selection but selection for physical traits like eye and hair color, which he dubbed "cosmetic medicine." [25]

From some religious perspectives, PGD is immoral for any purpose, including ensuring a child will be free of a deadly genetic disease, wrote Marilyn E. Coors, associate professor of bioethics and genetics at the University of Colorado at Denver. In Catholic teaching, she wrote, PGD is "intrinsically immoral, because it involves the creation and destruction of human lives, replaces the conjugal act and involves third-party intervention in conception." [26]

Some ethicists warn that trait selection of any kind "treats the children . . . as 'products' as we try to mix the right characteristics," said Toby L. Schonfeld, assistant professor of medical ethics at the University of Nebraska Medical Center. "The increased pressure on these children to fulfill the goals of the parents . . . seems to minimize their autonomy and even exploit them." [27]

The proper use of PGD is for curing or averting disease, and "sex is not a disease," said PGD pioneer Mark Hughes, founder of the Genesis Genetics Institute in Detroit, Mich., explaining why he opposes gender selection. [28]

"I . . . fear . . . that clinics offering trait selection to satisfy the whims of parents will turn people against a procedure that can save lives," said Allen Goldberg, a marketing executive from Washington, D.C., whose 7-year-old son Henry died in 2002 of a rare genetic disease, Fanconi anemia. In the late 1990s, Goldberg and his wife tried unsuccessfully to use PGD to conceive a disease-free sibling who could donate umbilical-cord blood to Henry; other families have used the approach successfully.

However, some ethicists also condemn this use of PGD, arguing that the trait-selected newborn is being unfairly used as a tool to serve the medical needs of its sibling. [29]

Should doctors be able to refuse ART services to gay, older or single people?

The University of South Florida's Keefe says that a gay, male couple came into his clinic in Tampa and were at their wits' end. They had been to several assisted reproductive technology (ART) clinics seeking services, only to be turned away because center officials said they didn't want to be known as a clinic that welcomed gay families.

"These were taxpaying Americans who were very loving to each other, and they'd been bounced from one place to another," says Keefe, who helped the couple conceive a child using donor eggs and a surrogate.

Indeed, some doctors refuse to provide IVF to would-be parents because of their single, gay or elder status, usually citing religious or ethical reasons — or, in the case of older parents — concern about the long-term welfare of the child.

Some ethicists say clinics must first consider the welfare of the children in choosing whom to treat, and questions of religion and conscience figure strongly in such decisions.

In a 2007 report, the ethics committee of the American College of Obstetricians and Gynecologists described a California physician who refused to perform artificial insemination for a lesbian couple, "prompted by religious beliefs and disapproval of lesbians having children." In reproductive medicine, the report said, "health-care providers may find that providing indicated, even standard, care would present for them a personal moral problem — a conflict of conscience." The committee upheld doctors' right to refuse care on those grounds, but said doctors who refuse service must refer patients to other providers. [30]

Because the desire to raise children is not a medical need, physicians may ethically refuse to help people seeking IVF services, argued Julien S. Murphy, a professor of philosophy at the University of Southern Maine. In general, "it is assumed that physicians have a duty to treat 'medical conditions,' " she wrote, "but addressing the fulfillment of reproductive possibilities" opened up by new technology "is an optional matter." [31]

A 2005 survey of fertility doctors found that only 44 percent believed doctors do not have the right to decide who is fit to procreate, according to *Everything Conceivable* author Mundy. Nearly half the physicians surveyed said they'd refuse services to a gay couple, 40 percent said they'd refuse service to a couple on welfare who wanted to pay with Social Security disability checks and 20 percent said they would turn away a single woman. [32]

Continued on p. 461

Chronology

1980s-1990s

First U.S. in vitro fertilization (IVF) clinics open, with early success rates around 5 percent. Concerns grow about fate of frozen IVF embryos.

1981
Elizabeth Jordan Carr is first U.S. IVF baby, the 15th worldwide.

1982
The Sperm Bank of California opens in Berkeley to serve lesbians and single women; the next year it launches first U.S. program allowing donors to release their identities to offspring.

1984
Sweden is first nation to give grown offspring access to sperm donors' identities.

1985
Maryland requires all insurance plans to cover IVF.

1987
Massachusetts and Hawaii require all insurance plans to cover IVF. . . . Texas requires all insurers to offer a plan that covers IVF.

1989
Rhode Island requires all insurance plans to cover IVF. . . . Connecticut requires all insurers except HMOs to offer a plan covering IVF.

1991
Illinois requires all insurance plans to cover IVF.

1992
Congress requires all fertility clinics to report success rates annually.

1993
Richard Paulson, a University of Southern California fertility scientist, demonstrates that women in their 50s can become pregnant with donated eggs. . . . Canada's Royal Commission on New Reproductive Technologies says fertility doctors aren't following professional standards and that stronger laws are needed.

1995
Congress passes Dickey-Wicker amendment, banning government funding of research that may harm a human embryo. Subsequently, it is passed annually in spending bills for the Department of Health and Human Services.

1997
Californian Arceli Keh becomes a first-time mother at 63, after falsely telling IVF doctor Paulson she is in her 50s. . . . Denmark, widely considered a gay-friendly nation, limits government-provided artificial-insemination services to women in relationships with men, effectively shutting out lesbians and single women.

2000s

Fertility treatments become more widely available worldwide.

2001
American Society of Reproductive Medicine (ASRM) enrages some feminist groups with public-service announcements that list a woman's advancing age as among the top threats to fertility. . . . New Jersey requires all insurance plans to cover IVF.

2003
Norway revises its reproductive-medicine laws, ending anonymity for sperm donors but retaining a ban on egg donation.

2004
Canada bans sale of human eggs and sperm and sex selection of children. . . . ASRM recommends that parents inform IVF children they were born from donated eggs or sperm.

2005
Sperm donors in the United Kingdom must release identifying information to grown offspring. . . . Food and Drug Administration requires sperm banks to test for HIV and other communicable diseases.

2006
Canada establishes Assisted Human Reproduction Agency to regulate reproductive medicine.

2008
An impoverished 27-year-old Egyptian mother of three delivers septuplets after taking inexpensive fertility drugs now available worldwide, including in countries lacking health-care facilities to manage multiple births. . . . Colorado voters reject a referendum to amend the state constitution to consider a human embryo a legal "person."

2009
A 33-year-old California woman, Nadya Suleman, has octuplets after requesting that her doctor implant six frozen embryos created by IVF. . . . Reproductive tourism to Italy, one of the few European countries that don't regulate IVF, is up 75 percent since 2003. . . . England's reproductive-medicine regulatory agency says it will inform donor-conceived children at age 16 whether they're genetically related to a person they plan to be sexually intimate with. . . . Georgia legislature considers but doesn't enact law granting personhood to embryos. . . . California and Missouri legislatures consider legislation to regulate fertility clinics.

Searching the Web for Biological Parents

The era of anonymous egg and sperm donors may be ending.

The 15-year-old American boy had been conceived by his mother using an anonymous sperm donor. But the youth wanted to know the identity of his biological father, and in 2005 he made news and perhaps history by tracking down the donor online.

"This is the first time that I know of it being done," said Bryan Sykes, a geneticist at the University of Oxford in the United Kingdom. [1]

The case raises the question of whether the anonymity long promised to many egg and sperm donors is realistic in the 21st century.

Indeed, as happened over the past few decades with adoption, egg and sperm donation is gradually becoming an open process, analysts say.

"We're moving toward giving donors the opportunity to be contacted or identified," as more donation-organizations offer this option and online donor registries are established, says John A. Robertson, a professor at the University of Texas College of Law at Austin. "As a psychological matter, there's wide agreement that it's good to disclose, but you won't see anything in the United States as draconian as in England, where you can't be anonymous."

The American teenager sent his own DNA to an online genealogy Web site for testing and then was able to contact two men with closely matching DNA who were likely relatives. Using their surnames, plus information his mother had received about the donor's date and place of birth, he paid another online site for a list of everyone born in that place on that day. In less than two weeks, he had made contact with the donor. [2]

The incident reveals the "hunger for . . . connection and an understanding of this invisible part of themselves" that many donor offspring experience, according to Wendy Kramer, a Colorado mother who launched a voluntary Internet registry for donors, donor-conceived children and their families. [3]

"This boy did wonder why it was always assumed that the rights of a donor to remain anonymous trumped a child's right to know his genetic heritage" since he "had not entered into . . . anonymity agreements with anyone," wrote Kramer, who started the Donor Sibling Registry with her donor-conceived son Ryan about nine years ago. "Will every kid who swabs his cheek find his donor? Probably not. But we can expect this to happen with greater frequency as DNA data banks swell." [4]

The move away from anonymity and toward establishing a registry is spurred by more than young people's curiosity, says Jan Elman Stout, a clinical psychologist in Chicago. As the number of children born from donor sperm has increased, so has the likelihood that children from the same donor might unknowingly fall in love, have sexual relations or marry.

That possibility is particularly strong in smaller nations, which are acting to head off the problem. Beginning this October, for example, teens 16 and older in the United Kingdom who plan to become sexually intimate can contact the government's reproductive-medicine agency to find out whether they are genetically related to their partners. [5]

Statisticians say the United States is below the threshold where there's much chance sperm donors' children will meet and marry, "but I'm not sure the reporting of successful births is reliable enough" to be certain, says Stout. Some U.S. mental-health professionals are championing establishment of a centralized donor registry, but there's pushback both from patients and doctors, who worry that an end to anonymity will mean many fewer men will donate sperm, she says.

Laws in several countries ending donor anonymity are too new to draw firm conclusions.

When two Australian states abolished anonymity, donations fell off drastically. Western Australia, with a population of 1.4 million people, ended up with only 35 available sperm donors. Some Australian clinics offered all-expense-paid tours of their country — complete with free visits to dance clubs and other night spots — to Canadian college students, in return for sperm donations. [6]

But widespread concern that laws abolishing donor anonymity will cut the number of donors permanently may not be justified, according to Ken Daniels, a professor of social work at the University of Canterbury in Christchurch, New Zealand. For the most part, surveys showing that donors are super-leery of being identified have only polled people who had donated before disclosure laws had taken effect and could be expected to be biased against it, he said. [7]

Under new non-anonymity laws, a new and different group of potential donors — possibly older, married people with children — may come forward, inspired by their own parenthood to help others conceive, Daniels predicts. He recounts a conversation with a donor who said that, as a young man, he donated for the money, but "having his own children has made him aware of the child's perspective and the possible need for information." [8]

---

[1] Quoted in Alison Motluk, "Anonymous Sperm Donor Traced on Internet," *New Scientist online*, Nov. 5, 2005, www.newscientist.com.

[2] *Ibid.*

[3] Wendy Kramer, "DNA and the Exploding Myth of Donor Anonymity," Donor Sibling Registry Web site, www.donorsiblingregistry.com.

[4] *Ibid.*

[5] *The HFEA Register*, Human Fertilisation and Embryology Authority Web site, www.hfea.gov.uk/.

[6] Liza Mundy, *Everything Conceivable* (2007), p. 187.

[7] Ken Daniels, "Donor Gametes: Anonymous or Identified," *Best Practice & Research: Clinical Obstetrics and Gynecology*, February 2007, pp. 113-128.

[8] Quoted in *ibid.*, p. 119.

Continued from p. 458

Such ethical debates are not limited to the United States. Arguing for a ban on ART for single or lesbian women, a member of the Danish Parliament stated that such women have "completely, freely chosen to live" in a manner that "cannot naturally produce children," making providing ART to them "completely against nature, artificial and absurd." [33]

Many English fertility clinics will not serve single women, said Clare Murray, a psychologist at City University London. "Clinics treat lesbian couples at the drop of a hat, but still won't treat single women. They're the pariahs of the assisted-reproduction field." [34]

And University of Pennsylvania bioethicist Arthur L. Caplan argues that physicians have every right — and perhaps a moral duty — to refuse ART for people who are too old. He was commenting on the 2005 Caesarian-section birth of a daughter to 66-year-old Adriana Iliescu, an unmarried professor in Bucharest, Romania.

Such pregnancies are medically risky, Caplan noted. For instance, in Iliescu's IVF treatments, she initially had a miscarriage, then a stillbirth and, finally, a live child born prematurely from a "life-threatening emergency C-section." Furthermore, he pointed out, when the daughter enters high school, Iliescu will be 80, too old to raise a teenager to adulthood.

Caplan said he would refuse ART to single people over 65 or to a couple with one member who is 65 or older, making their total age higher than 130, and to any woman age 55 or older who could not pass "a rigorous physical examination." [35]

But other physicians say that — aside from screening out patients with severe mental disorders — deciding who may have children should not be up to the doctor. "How does that become my responsibility?" says Beltsos, of the Fertility Centers of Illinois. The case of octuplet-mother Suleman is "a tough one, but just because I might think it's inappropriate or irresponsible to have 14 kids, does that mean I can decide for someone else? Where does the line get drawn?"

As for worrying about the welfare of the child, the Hastings Center's Johnston says that IVF clinics deal with people who fervently want children. "This is not the population where the real child-welfare problem is," she says. "We take wanting a child as kind of placeholder for doing a pretty good job with the child," so she says she probably wouldn't support clinics adding child-welfare considerations to their protocols for accepting ART patients.

In August 2008, the California Supreme Court ruled that denying ART services to a lesbian constitutes unlawful discrimination under a law requiring businesses to guarantee all persons "full and equal accommodations." [36]

In *North Coast Women's Care Medical Group, Inc. v. Superior Court* the court ruled in favor of Guadalupe Benitez, a lesbian in a long-term relationship who sued the facility after two physicians refused to artificially inseminate her and referred her to another clinic. The doctors argued that their rights to religious liberty would be violated if they were required to provide ART to all comers. But the court said the state's civil rights law trumps the religious-liberty claim and requires the clinic to either offer ART to no one or have at least one physician on staff who will provide it to all clients. [37]

An American Society of Reproductive Medicine ethics committee declared in 2006 that, "as a matter of ethics, we believe the ethical duty to treat persons with equal respect requires that fertility programs treat single persons and gay and lesbian couples equally with married couples in determining which services to provide." [38] ■

Sixty Percent of ART Users Are Over 35

About 60 percent of women who turned to assisted reproductive technology (ART) in 2006 were over age 35. Women's fertility begins to drop off around age 24 and declines steeply after 35.

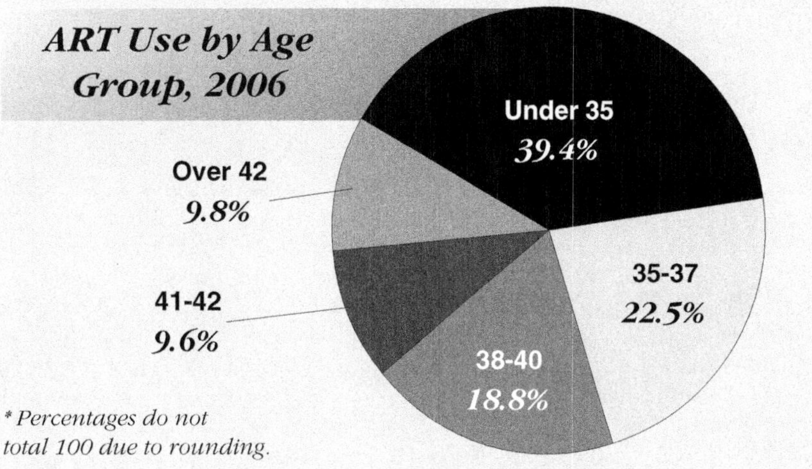

Source: "Assisted Reproductive Technology Success Rates 2006," Centers for Disease Control and Prevention, 2008

BACKGROUND

Stigma and Silence

Throughout history, many childless couples have struggled to have a child to call their own. [39]

Insurance Coverage Affects Fertility Decisions

More people use IVF when insurance covers the procedure.

With more and more patients turning to alternative means of reproduction over the past two decades, 14 states have enacted legislation offering at least some insurance coverage to help people have the families they long for.

Most of these states require all insurers under state regulation to include at least some infertility coverage in all insurance plans they sell, while two states, California and Texas, only require all insurers to "offer" everyone coverage — that is, insurers must offer at least one plan that covers infertility treatments.

While the laws may be similar, the actual coverage provided is anything but. States run the gamut from covering only screening tests to ascertain whether a couple is infertile to full coverage of multiple in vitro fertilization (IVF) treatments. Each state also limits who can access infertility treatment. For example, a state might limit the medical condition of infertility to apply only to a married couple who have tried unsuccessfully for a specified amount of time to conceive. In that state, an unmarried woman would not be eligible for any treatment coverage.

Insurance mandates definitely improve access. In Europe, for example, where IVF often is funded by government-financed health coverage, up to 4 percent of children are born following some kind of fertility procedure, compared to only about 1 percent in the United States. [1]

Increasing access by helping people pay for infertility treatments matters because "the less money you have, the more likely you are to have difficulty conceiving," wrote reporter Liza Mundy, author of the 2007 book *Everything Conceivable*. "Much infertility has always been caused by infections that can damage reproductive passageways," and "the lower your tax bracket, the less likely you are to have received the fairly simple medical treatment that can stave off these consequences." [2]

Insurance coverage — or the lack of it — "greatly impacts the decisions that doctors and patients make," says Angeline Beltsos, medical director of the Chicago-based Fertility Centers of Illinois. Illinois will pay for four IVF tries for a first baby for an infertile woman, regardless of her age.

In a state without an insurance mandate, a couple with a one-in-five chance of conceiving through IVF is highly likely to look at the average $12,000 price tag for one IVF cycle and simply give up, trying donor eggs, adoption or cheaper drug or surgical interventions instead, Beltsos says. "But here in our state you get a very different approach. Here, people say, 'OK, let's try IVF before we try donor eggs.' " Even some "younger couples who probably could get pregnant without IVF" opt for it because it costs them little.

And few Illinois patients try lower-tech drug or surgical procedures — which also may not work — Beltsos says. "They just go into IVF" instead, and "don't waste years and years with things that may not work very well, ultimately ending up in IVF only when they're so old" that simple, age-related fertility decline may doom IVF to failure, she says.

Once IVF treatment begins, patients in insured states again behave differently, Beltsos says. For example, "no insurance covers the $200 to $1,000 cost of freezing extra embryos," so people with IVF coverage are more likely to say "go ahead and destroy" the extras, she says. "But if you had paid for that cycle, they'd be begging to have the embryos frozen" since doing so "would significantly reduce the cost" of subsequent cycles, she says.

— Additional reporting by Vyomika Jairam

[1] Liza Mundy, *Everything Conceivable* (2007), pp. 3-4.
[2] *Ibid.*, p. xiv.

The biblical book of *Genesis* describes how Sarah, the infertile wife of Israelite patriarch Abraham, was so distraught over the couple's childlessness that she offered her maid Hagar as a surrogate mother with whom Abraham conceived a child, his son Ishmael. [40]

In England, King Henry VIII married wife after wife, primarily in order to satisfy his desire for a male heir. That 16th-century saga not only demonstrates how fierce the desire for children can be but also how the concept of fertility is intertwined with male virility. "The wives of Henry VIII knew all too well how women tend to be blamed for male-factor [fertility] issues," since several ended up divorced, with their marriages involuntarily annulled or even beheaded in Henry's quest for sons, observed *Everything Conceivable* author Mundy. [41]

Ironically, the "father of our country," U.S. President George Washington, was most likely infertile. But he blamed his wife Martha when he could not father children, "despite the rather glaring evidence of her fertility, provided by four children from a recent prior marriage," wrote Mundy. [42]

Bemoaning his childless state at age 54, Washington wrote that "if Mrs. Washington should survive me, there is a moral certainty of my dying without issue." Furthermore, he wrote, "should I be longest lived, the matter . . . is hardly less certain for . . . I shall never marry a girl; and it is not probable that I should have children by a woman of an age suitable to my own." [43]

Despite clear evidence of Washington's infertility, it is hardly ever mentioned in historical accounts of his life, said John K. Amory, associate professor of medicine at the University of Washington School of Medicine in Seattle.

The silence probably results from a "frequent erroneous assumption that infertility is mostly female in origin," Amory wrote, and fear that discussion of Washington's infertility "would diminish him in some way," even though infertility has nothing to do with one's other characteristics and occurs "without regard to [one's] historical stature." [44]

Stigma and silence may also help keep fertility treatment out of the mainstream of American medicine, some analysts say. Unlike most medical specialties, except plastic surgery, fertility medicine is largely provided on a cash-pay basis because it is not covered by insurance.

By definition, "infertility is an illness" — an "impairment of normal biological functioning that causes great distress," says Dartmouth's Green. "Nevertheless, we don't think of it that way because it affects only a few people. I teach an ART course to undergraduates, and they often don't get it, because at their age the big problem for most is keeping their fertility in check. But when you are ready to have a child, it becomes a grave, grave matter." The "mental suffering is as bad as that for cancer."

Nevertheless, it's been difficult to assemble a strong advocacy community around expanding IVF insurance coverage because "there's still a lot of public stigma," says Collura of the National Infertility Association. "We're where breast cancer was 25 years ago."

Breast-cancer and AIDS patients eventually "came out" and forced the public to confront those diseases, but igniting such a movement may be even harder for infertility, she says. "It's such a personal, private thing, so emotionally painful; and because people are private about it, we don't realize the extent of it."

But even with public recognition of how many people infertility affects, some experts doubt the U.S. health-care system — in which more than 45 million people lack coverage entirely — can afford to add more services, especially one as costly as IVF. [45]

ART "can be quite expensive," notes the National Conference on State Legislatures (NCSL). "On average each cycle of IVF costs $8,158 plus an average of $4,000 for medications — and debate exists about whether insurance plans should be required to cover them." Estimates of the monthly cost to mandate IVF coverage range from $.20 to $2.00 per insurance-plan member, according to the NCSL. [46]

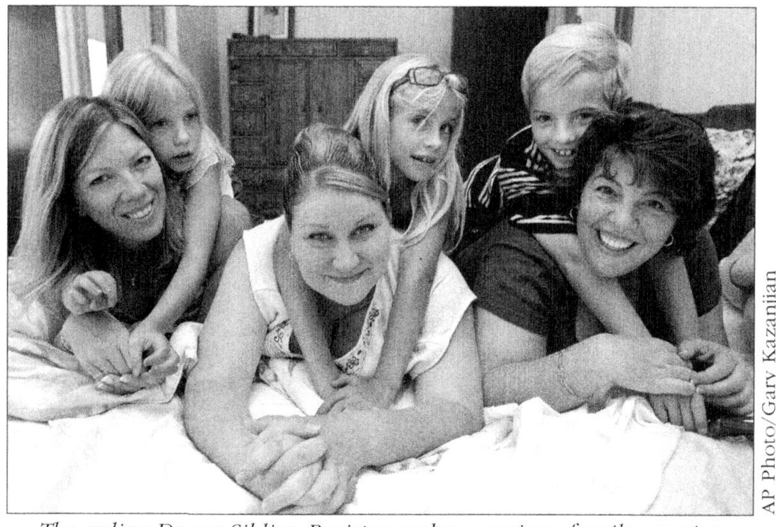

AP Photo/Gary Kazanjian

The online Donor Sibling Registry makes a unique family reunion possible in Fresno, Calif., for three mothers and their children. The children were all conceived after their mothers were artificially inseminated by sperm from the same donor and thus are half-siblings. From left: Dawn Warthen and Allyson, Michelle Jorgenson and Cheyenne, and Jenafer Elin and Joshua.

"Not having these treatments covered is unfortunate, but it is not unfair," because, "in fact, people don't have the [legal] right to any health care in this country except emergency care," said George J. Annas, professor of health law and bioethics at the Boston University School of Public Health. "To mandate [ART coverage], given the growing numbers of uninsured people, makes no legal, economic or health-care sense." [47]

Moreover, notes the NCSL, the use of ART over the years has raised overall health-care costs by contributing to an increase in multiple births, which have a higher rate of prematurity than single births. By 2004, for example, the percentage of babies considered to have low birth weight had risen to 8.1 percent, the highest level since the early 1970s, driven largely by ART-caused multiple births. [48]

Advocates of insurance coverage argue that it might eventually lower health-system costs, because there would be fewer high-risk multiple births if parents-to-be could opt for several single-embryo procedures rather than one multiple-embryo implantation. "The rate of triplets in insurance-mandate states is much lower," says Keefe, of the University of South Florida.

"In states where infertility treatments are not paid for, physicians run up expensive tabs for services that aren't needed, like surgery to reconnect scarred fallopian tubes," argues Green. Fertility doctors in those states may also spend too much time trying to diagnose the condition — because the diagnostics are often paid for by insurance — when it would have been cheaper just to try IVF immediately, he adds.

Since the 1980s, 14 states — Arkansas, California, Connecticut, Hawaii, Illinois, Maryland, Massachusetts, Montana, New Jersey, New York, Ohio, Rhode Island, Texas and West Virginia — have required insurers to either cover or offer at least one plan that covers some ART, although not necessarily IVF, according to the NCSL. (*See map, p. 452, and sidebar, p. 462.*)

Using Assisted Reproductive Technology

The ART birth cycle from beginning to end

Here are the steps toward pregnancy and live birth using assisted reproductive technology (ART) and fresh, non-donor eggs or embryos:

1. Cycle starts: *Woman starts taking medication to stimulate the ovaries to develop eggs or, if no drugs are given, the woman begins having her ovaries monitored for natural egg production.*

2. Egg retrieval: *If eggs are produced, a surgical procedure is used to collect them from the ovaries.*

3. Egg and sperm combine: *In vitro fertilization combines egg and sperm in the laboratory. If fertilization is successful, one or more of the resulting embryos are transferred, most often into the uterus through the cervix.*

4. Pregnancy: *If one or more embryos implant within the uterus, the cycle may progress to pregnancy.*

5. Birth: *The pregnancy may progress to the delivery of one or more live-born infants.*

Two of the states, California and New York, explicitly exclude IVF from the coverage mandate while covering other services such as diagnosis of infertility problems. [49] However, in 2002, New York authorized a demonstration program — still ongoing — to test the effects of IVF coverage by picking up a share of the costs for some patients, with the subsidy prorated by income. [50]

Fertility Industry

Physicians see advantages and disadvantages in fertility medicine's "cash-only" status.

"There are very few fields" in medicine as lucrative, says Jain of the Santa Monica Fertility Specialists.

As a result, when it comes to technical innovation, "I don't think there's a field that's evolved as rapidly as ours in the last 20 years," says Rosenfeld of New York's North Shore-Long Island Jewish Health System. With no public insurers and few private insurers involved, "we don't have any oversight — only our peers — so there's a lot more room for freelancing, for entrepreneurialism," Jain says.

Entrepreneurialism can lead to innovation but can also in many cases "be a euphemism for exploitation," Jain says. For example, "some will overrecommend IVF because it's so lucrative," rather than saving IVF as a last resort and taking patients through less-extreme procedures first, according to Jain.

The CDC keeps a database of fertility-clinic data as an oversight tool, in lieu of stronger policing, but when that information is combined with the highly competitive nature of the business, it can backfire, says Rosenfeld.

"How do people decide which clinic to choose?" he asks. They go online to the database, Rosenfeld says, and find that one clinic, for example, has a 46-percent success rate and another, 48 percent. But they don't realize that a clinic with a higher success rate might accept only patients with a higher probability of conceiving, so the data reporting process provides an incentive for physicians to "do things they might not otherwise do," such as rejecting patients with a low likelihood of conception or using the data as a marketing tool, without including caveats about what it actually means, he says.

The University of South Florida's Keefe headed an American Society of Reproductive Medicine committee on the CDC registry and "wanted to put a "Click to see [patient] inclusion criteria' " button on each clinic's statistics to help patients understand them better, he recalls. "But everybody said, 'That would be too confusing,' " so it didn't happen.

The profit motive extends to egg donation, according to author Mundy. In the early days of IVF, many donors were women who'd finished childbearing and wanted to help others, and "women helping women" was the byword of the then-nonprofit organizations that arranged for donation, she said. Today, most donors are young women in need of cash and, because some donors "are paid a lot" — based on physical and intellectual characteristics, such as an Ivy League diploma — private commercial agencies have gotten more aggressive in procuring eggs, she said. [51]

The profit motive in egg donation may be dangerous both to donors and potential offspring, Tucson, Ariz.-based physician Jennifer Schneider told a congressional briefing in November 2007. Schneider's college-age daughter Jessica donated eggs to supplement her income and, six years later, at age 29, died of colon cancer, a condition that her mother suspects could have been related to the donation process, in which women take fertility drugs to stimulate multiple egg production. [52]

Unfortunately, "I'm here to tell you that hardly anything is known" about an egg-donation-colon-cancer link — also present in several other cases of unusual colon cancers in young women — "because once a young woman walks out of an IVF clinic, she is of no interest to anyone," Schneider told lawmakers.

Continued on p. 466

At Issue:

Should egg and sperm donors be paid?

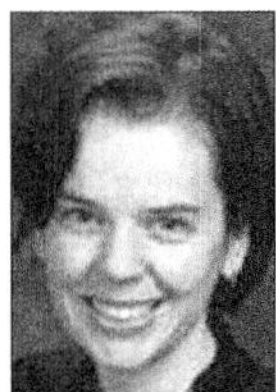

JOSEPHINE JOHNSTON
DIRECTOR OF RESEARCH OPERATIONS
THE HASTINGS CENTER

WRITTEN FOR *CQ RESEARCHER*, MAY 2009

Modest payments for gametes are fair, necessary for some kinds of fertility treatment and show respect for the autonomy and dignity of donors. Egg donors should receive more than sperm donors given the invasive and sometimes painful procedures they endure.

Sperm donation isn't as quick or pleasurable as one might assume, but it isn't terribly arduous either. Eggs are another story. Egg donors are medically assessed before beginning the daily routine of mixing and injecting themselves in the stomach or thigh with hormones to suppress and then dramatically increase egg production. They visit the fertility clinic regularly over the month-long process for blood tests and ultrasounds to monitor egg development. They then undergo minor surgery to remove the eggs, followed by a day of bed rest. The hormones and the surgery carry physical risks and often result in discomfort or pain. The drugs can cause emotions to fluctuate, and some anxiety often accompanies the process (how will her body respond to the drugs, what does an unsuccessful attempt imply about her own fertility?).

In the United States, sperm donors are usually paid (not much, but they can donate every five days). Egg donors receive far more, from $2,000 to tens of thousands of dollars. Technically, the money is for time and effort, not the gametes produced. Whether or not you buy that distinction, egg donation in particular can provide significant income.

I share the concern that $10,000 or $50,000 could easily persuade someone to undergo procedures without proper consideration of the risks. But the average egg donor receives just over $4,000 for the weeks she spends in and out of physician's offices, the daily self-administered injections and surgical retrieval of her eggs. Not to mention the discomfort, pain and apprehension. Would you do this for free? Few do.

While money for sperm rarely raises concern, many remain uneasy about paying egg donors. Is it because eggs, even if plentiful, are more difficult to remove and (perhaps) limited in number? If it's the risks, isn't doing it for free just as dangerous? Or does the unease represent an unexamined desire to control women's bodies, particularly their reproductive capacity, and a mistrust of their ability to make medical and reproductive decisions?

This society allows young women to make the same life-changing choices as any other adult. If few will donate their eggs for free, we should trust that they can make an ethical decision to do so for pay.

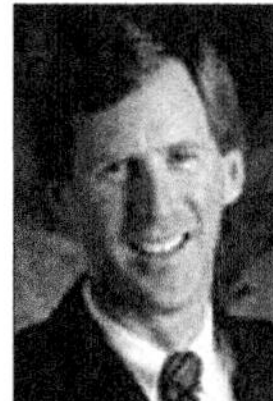

SCOTT B. RAE
PROFESSOR OF CHRISTIAN ETHICS
TALBOT SCHOOL OF THEOLOGY
BIOLA UNIVERSITY

WRITTEN FOR *CQ RESEARCHER*, MAY 2009

Paying sperm and egg donors should be discouraged. Egg selling involves often unrecognized health risks to the donor. The egg-harvesting process is highly invasive. Women run a short-term risk of ovarian hyperstimulation syndrome (OHSS). OHSS can cause potentially serious long-term thrombosis, liver and renal problems and respiratory distress — and in rare instances, death. Over time, donors risk future infertility and, potentially, development of cancers related to the synthetic hormones used to hyperstimulate the ovaries. Bear in mind, the egg donor is an otherwise healthy woman, not an infertile "patient" who chooses to assume these risks for the benefit of a baby.

Granted, sperm "donors" are not paid that much, and sperm "donation" does not entail risks to donors, but other concerns still apply.

Paying "donors" may undermine a child's right to know his or her biological parents. Most donors do not want to be identified, and in countries where the law requires identification, not surprisingly, the number of donors has diminished quickly. The Donor Sibling Registry has thousands of children still looking for their other biological parent. And, while they may not find their fathers, they often connect with many (10 or more) half-siblings, with uncertain consequences. One site (donorsibling.com) has traced over 100 children back to a single donor.

An apparent interest in eugenics has moved society toward "designer children," another issue potentially exacerbated by donor payments. One advertisement for an egg donor offered $75,000 if the donor was 5'10" or above, blond, blue-eyed, athletic and scored above 1400 on her SAT exams. In a culture that values diversity, producing designer children risks reinforcing damaging stereotypes.

Another concern comes with new types of families that are being intentionally preplanned. "Single mothers by choice" are increasingly common, yet a growing body of empirical evidence shows the importance of fathers to children's well-being. That is not to say that single-parent families that result from widowhood or divorce can't adequately raise children. But those situations are different from preplanned single-parent families.

Increasing the number of gamete donors by offering payment could also lead to a decrease in traditional adoptions or adoptions of existing embryos. I often suggest adoption of embryos to couples contemplating using donor eggs, because it provides the experience of pregnancy and birth but avoids using a "procreative pinch-hitter."

Continued from p. 464

Egg brokers "make enormous sums" of money and want to maximize the number of eggs they have, giving them "every reason to avoid follow-up of egg donors and studies of their possible long-term risks," she said. When she called Jessica's broker to warn that children born of her eggs should be tested, since the cancer may be genetic, Schneider was told that the records had already been destroyed, and offspring could not be tracked. [53]

Research Stinted

Fertility research has not been funded through the traditional routes, such as the National Institutes of Health (NIH), says fertility specialist Jain. Although the NIH funds most medical research in America, fertility medicine gets little NIH attention because the field operates largely without public and private insurance and because legislators have religion- and morality-based qualms about research using human embryos.

"IVF has had a 30-year life span," says Jain. "It came out of Ph.Ds who worked in zoos," conducting embryo research on animals. "But there's an absence of NIH funding for the basic science in human embryology. The field has had to sponsor its own studies."

After 30 years of IVF, there have been no multi-center studies — large-scale research coordinated at several clinical sites — the gold standard of medicine, says Dartmouth's Green. In the early 1990s, the National Institute on Child Health and Development (NICHD) tried to get research going, he says, after an advisory panel that he served on recommended increased federal funding.

But in 1995, Congress not only rejected NICHD's pitch but banned federal funding of any "research in which a human embryo or embryos are destroyed, discarded or knowingly subjected to risk of injury or death." Congress has included the ban as a part of annual appropriations legislation ever since then. [54]

While discussions of the ban usually focus on its effect on stem-cell research, it also significantly limits what scientists know about infertility and the early stages of human development. "We know very little about what is a good and what's a bad embryo," says Collura of the National Infertility Association. As a result, one of the top questions for any embryologist is which among a group of embryos are most likely to produce a full-term baby. "But if you have 10 different embryologists in a room, you'll get 10 different answers."

Knowing the answer would help reduce multiple births. "If you want singletons, it's important to know which embryos are the right ones to transfer," she says. ■

CURRENT SITUATION

Regulating IVF

In the wake of the octuplets' birth, a California legislator introduced a proposal that the state regulate fertility clinics, [55] and the Georgia legislature considered limiting the number of eggs that may be fertilized and embryos implanted during IVF. [56]

In the past year, a spate of state proposals have addressed fertility medicine, many by granting legal "personhood" to embryos, about 500,000 of which now sit frozen in fertility clinics around the country, their ultimate fate undecided since many of the families who created them are now finished with childbearing. [57] No bill has yet gained much traction, however.

The California bill, which would bring fertility clinics under the jurisdiction of the Medical Board of California and set accreditation standards, is one of a handful that would increase government oversight of fertility clinics. Missouri's House Bill 810, for instance, would require doctors to follow American Society of Reproductive Medicine (ASRM) guidelines on embryo implantation or face sanctions. [58]

"The people of this state don't need to be paying millions of dollars for some woman who has eight babies at once," said the bill's sponsor, Republican Missouri state Rep. Bob Schaaf. [59]

ASRM supports Schaaf's proposal. "We are very supportive of the bill," said Sean Tipton, ASRM director of public affairs, "because it defers to medical knowledge and experience and protects both women and unborn children." [60]

Legislative efforts to grant "personhood" to embryos — such as Colorado's proposed constitutional Amendment 48 defeated by voters last November — are heavily criticized by the reproductive-medicine community but win plaudits from right-to-life groups.

After fierce legislative wrangling and numerous language changes, Georgia's Senate-passed personhood bill was not brought to the House floor before the 2009 legislative session ended in March. The Georgia Right to Life group praised the bill for its attempt to limit the number of embryos created.

"The human embryo is one of us, fully human with great potential," and "we do not . . . need to sacrifice human life for money and economic development or the remote possibility of a medical cure for someone else," said Daniel Becker, the group's president. [61]

But ASRM's Tipton said the measure would hurt infertile people by presuming "that politicians know what is best . . . and not physicians." [62]

"Some of the people writing legislation don't understand ART," says Collura of the National Infertility Association. For example, some Georgia lawmakers backed language allowing doctors to fertilize only two eggs per

IVF cycle. That's unworkable, she says, because currently IVF is a process in which as many eggs as possible are fertilized in order to improve the chances that some embryos will be viable.

Those who would ban processes like embryo freezing don't realize how many people would be hurt, including cancer patients who can bear children after their ovaries are surgically removed only if their embryos are frozen before the treatment, she says.

Social Changes

Powerful social trends make it likely that usage of advanced assisted reproductive technology will increase.

The delay in childbearing until women are older, for instance, has increased the incidence of infertility. Human biology "is not built for a society where [women] first go to medical school" before bearing children, says Dartmouth's Green, so "we are seeing increasing infertility."

In addition, some large-scale recent studies have suggested — though not proven — that men's sperm counts have been declining for a half-century or so, mainly in industrialized countries. For example, a large 2000 study by Shanna Swan, professor of obstetrics, gynecology and environmental medicine at the University of Rochester's School of Medicine and Dentistry in New York state, suggested that sperm counts were dropping by about 1.5 percent a year in the United States and 3 percent annually in Europe and Australia. Rural areas seemed to have the lower counts, perhaps due to agricultural chemicals. [63]

Increasing the pressure on those hoping to start a family, the number of infants available for adoption in the United States has dropped steadily for decades. Before 1973, for example, nearly 20 percent of never-married, white, pregnant women relinquished the babies to adoption. By the mid-1990s, the percentage had plummeted to 1.7 percent — a "dramatic decline" that shows no signs of a turnaround, according to the Department of Health and Human Services. [64]

During the 1990s, international adoptions by Americans skyrocketed, partly compensating for the declining availability of U.S. infants, but recently some countries have clamped down on such adoptions out of fear of baby selling. [65]

Meanwhile, most people remain unaware of how quickly the average woman's fertility declines after age 30 and how many women and men have other medical issues that decrease fertility.

Celebrity births to women over age 40 and even over 50 — hyped in the media with no mention that virtually all resulted from IVF and, in many cases, donor eggs — contribute to a false public impression, said author Mundy. "A parade of high-profile women . . . have made 40-something motherhood seem almost natural," she wrote, citing actresses Jane Seymour, who had a baby at 44; Susan Sarandon, 46; Geena Davis, twins at 47; Holly Hunter, twins at 47; and the late playwright Wendy Wasserstein, who had a premature daughter at 48. [66]

"They're perpetuating a false impression" that fertility wanes less quickly than it does, says psychologist Stout. "They're also perpetuating a cultural notion that all of this is secret," thus helping maintain the social stigma that surrounds ART, she says. "The more we open up, the better." ■

OUTLOOK

Health-care Reform

Congress and the Obama administration plan to propose massive health-care reform. If the United States moves to a health-care system with guaranteed coverage for all, intense debate will surround the question of which services should be covered.

Coverage for a procedure can easily be nixed if enough people say, "I'm a taxpayer and I object to that," since everyone would be subsidizing the system, says Wisconsin's Charo. Although all other industrialized countries have universal health care, and most pay for a very broad range of ART services, including IVF, discussions in the United States would be difficult "because women's sexuality and childbirth resonate so strongly" with many religious groups here, she says.

Some countries, such as Australia, subsidize IVF partly to boost birthrates, a goal the government and much of the public support, says Washington-based health-care consultant Gleason, but even in such situations, payment for ART bumps up against the economic reality that there aren't enough dollars to go around.

Today "we use [services like IVF] only a tenth as much as France and Israel," for example, says Keefe of the University of South Florida. "There's a huge, unmet need."

Universal coverage would lead to more regulation, including holding clinics accountable for following medical guidelines, Keefe says. "You wouldn't give coverage for it just the way it's done now," he says.

Questions would be raised as to "whether you'd cover IVF generally and for what purposes you'd cover PGD," says Baruch at the Genetics & Public Policy Center. Another question, she says: Could people still pay privately for whatever additional services they want or would some procedures be banned altogether?

If universal coverage is provided, "we'll have to get used to drawing lines" regarding coverage, and not just for ART, says Dartmouth's Green. "In Great Britain, for example, nobody over age 65 gets dialysis," he says. When it comes to IVF, government might well say, "We won't pay after you've already had two children."

Whether universal coverage would help or hurt ART "would depend on how they restricted care," says Rosenfeld at the North Shore-Long Island Jewish Health System. "If they started restricting it like they do in Europe" — where some countries outlaw implantation of more than one or two embryos, for example — "it would be a problem."

Oregon and Massachusetts have both experimented with universal coverage — Oregon in the 1990s and Massachusetts currently — and ART fared differently in each of those states, Rosenfeld notes. In Massachusetts, a state law mandates IVF coverage, but when Oregon deliberated over which services to cut, given budget constraints, reproductive medicine "fell below the line and wasn't paid for," offering a sobering example of how universal coverage mandates can cut both ways, he says. ■

Notes

[1] "Medical Society Probes Octuplets' Conception," The Associated Press, MSNBC.com, Feb. 10, 2009, www.msnbc.msn.com/id/29123731.

[2] Liza Mundy, *Everything Conceivable* (2007), p. 217.

[3] For background, see "Three Million Babies Born Using Assisted Reproductive Technologies," *Medical News Today*, June 25, 2006, www.medicalnewstoday.com.

[4] See Marcy Darnovsky, *Biopolitical Times blog*, Center for Genetics and Society, Feb. 27, 2009, www.biopoliticaltimes.org/article.php?id=4550.

[5] See " 'One Egg' IVF Strategy Launched," BBC News, June 26, 2008, www.news.bbc.co.uk/2/hi/health/7475392.stm. Also see Mundy, *op. cit.*, p. 214.

[6] Marcy Darnovsky, "Voluntary Isn't Working," *Modern Healthcare*, April 13, 2009, www.modernhealthcare.com/apps/pbcs.dll/article?Date=20090413&Category=SUB&ArtNo=304139998&SectionCat=&Template=printpicart.

[7] Franco Furger and Francis Fukuyama, "A Proposal for Modernizing the Regulation of Human Biotechnologies," *Hastings Center Report*, July/August 2007, pp. 16-20.

[8] "Consumers Desire More Genetic Testing, But not Designer Babies," *ScienceDaily*, Jan. 26, 2009, www.sciencedaily.com/releases/2009/01/090126100642.htm.

[9] Maili Malin, "Good, Bad and Troublesome: Infertility Physicians' Perceptions of Women Patients," *European Journal of Women's Studies*, August 2003, pp. 301-319.

[10] For background, see Brian Hansen, "Cloning Debate," *CQ Researcher*, Oct. 22, 2004, pp. 877-900.

[11] *Buzzanca v. Buzzanca*, Cal. App. 4th 1410 (1998), quoted in Linda S. Maule and Karen Schmid, "Assisted Reproduction and the Courts: The Case of California," *Journal of Family Issues*, April 1, 2006, pp. 464-482.

[12] Naomi Cahn, Necessary Subjects: The Need for a Mandatory National Donor Gamete Registry, April 2008, *DePaul Journal of Healthcare Law*, http://papers.ssrn.com/sol3/papers.cfm?abstract_id=1120389.

[13] Audrey Huang and Susannah Baruch, "Oversight of PGD," issue brief, Genetics & Public Policy Center, July 2007, www.dnapolicy.org/policy.issue.php?action=detail&issuebrief_id=8.

[14] John A. Robertson, "The Virtues of Muddling Through," *Hastings Center Report*, July/August 2007, pp. 26-28.

[15] *Ibid.*

[16] For background, see David Masci, "Designer Humans," *CQ Researcher*, May 18, 2001, pp. 425-440.

[17] Transcript, discussion of staff working paper, "Ethical Aspects of Sex Control," President's Council on Bioethics, Jan. 16, 2003, http://bioethicsprint.bioethics.gov/transcripts/jan03/session4.html.

[18] Quoted in "Reproductive Genetic Testing: Issues and Options for Policymakers," Genetics & Public Policy Center, 2004.

[19] "Preimplantation Genetic Diagnosis: A Discussion of Challenges, Concerns, and Preliminary Policy Options Related to the Genetic Testing of Human Embryos," Genetics & Public Policy Center, January 2004, www.dnapolicy.org/pub.reports.php?action=detail&report_id=8.

[20] *Ibid.*, p. 7.

[21] For background, see Scott Baldauf, "India's 'Girl Deficit' Deepest Among Educated," *The Christian Science Monitor*, Jan. 13, 2006, www.csmonitor.com/2006/0113/p01s04-wosc.html, and "Female Deficit in Asia," conference proceedings, Committee for International Cooperation in National Research in Demography, December 2005, www.cicred.org/Eng/Seminars/Details/Seminars/FDA/FDdraftpapers.htm.

[22] Mike Swift, "It's a Boy! Asian Immigrants Use Medical Technology to Satisfy Age-old Desire: A Son," *San Jose* [California] *Mercury News*, Jan. 7, 2009.

[23] *Ibid.*

[24] Deborah L. Spar, *The Baby Business: How Money, Science, and Politics Drive the Commerce of Conception* (2006), p. 99.

[25] For background, see Gautam Naik, "A Baby, Please. Blond, Freckles — Hold the Colic," *The Wall Street Journal*, Feb. 12, 2009, p. A10.

[26] Marilyn E. Coors, "Genetic Enhancement: Custom Kids and Chimeras," United States Conference of Catholic Bishops, Secretariat for Pro-Life Activities, www.usccb.org/prolife/programs/rlp/coors05finaleng.pdf.

[27] Toby L. Schonfeld, "Smart Men, Beautiful Women: Social Values and Gamete Commodification," *Bulletin of Science, Technology and Society*, June 2003, p. 168.

[28] Quoted in Ronald M. Green, *Babies by Design* (2007), p. 45.

[29] Allen Goldberg, *Dear Henry blog*, March 8, 2009, http://henrystrongingoldberg.blogspot.com.

[30] "The Limits of Conscientious Refusal in Reproductive Medicine," American College of Obstetrics and Gynecology, Committee on Ethics, November 2007.

[31] Julien S. Murphy, "Should Lesbians Count as Infertile Couples? Antilesbian Discrimination in Assisted Reproduction," in Anne Donchin and Laura Martha Purdy, eds., *Embodying Bioethics* (1999), p. 107.

About the Author

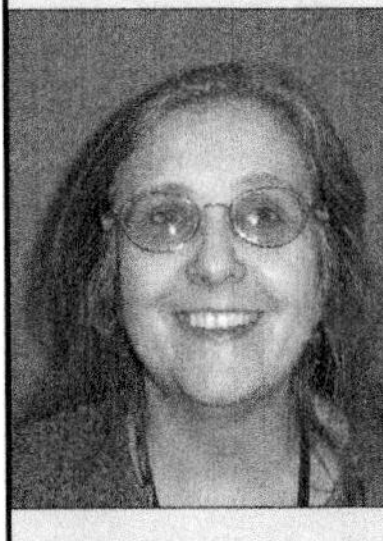

Staff writer **Marcia Clemmitt** is a veteran social-policy reporter who previously served as editor in chief of *Medicine & Health* and staff writer for *The Scientist*. She has also been a high-school math and physics teacher. She holds a liberal arts and sciences degree from St. John's College, Annapolis, and a master's degree in English from Georgetown University. Her recent reports include "Preventing Cancer" and "Public-Works Projects."

[32] Mundy, *op. cit.*, p. 202.
[33] Quoted in Ingrid Lüttichau, " 'We Are Family': The Regulation of 'Female-Only' Reproduction," *Social and Legal Studies*, March 2004, pp. 81-101.
[34] Quoted in Mundy, *op. cit.*, p. 160.
[35] Arthur L. Caplan, "How Old Is Too Old to Have a Baby?" *The American Journal of Bioethics*, Bioethics.net, Jan. 24, 2005, www.bioethics.net.
[36] For background, see Joanna Grossman, "The California Supreme Court Rules that Fertility Doctors Must Make Their Services Available to Lesbians, Despite Religious Objections," *FindLaw.com*, Sept. 2, 2008, http://writ.lp.findlaw.com.
[37] *Ibid.*
[38] "Access to Fertility Treatment by Gays, Lesbians, and Unmarried Persons," Ethics Committee of the American Society for Reproductive Medicine, Fertility and Sterility, November 2006, p. 1333.
[39] For background, see Susan C. Phillips, "Reproductive Ethics," *CQ Researcher*, April 8, 1994, pp. 289-312; see also Mundy, *op. cit.*
[40] *Genesis*, ch. 16.
[41] Mundy, *op. cit.*, p. 72.
[42] *Ibid.*
[43] Quoted in John K. Amory, "George Washington's Infertility: Why Was the Father of Our Country Never a Father," *Fertility and Sterility*, March 2004, pp. 495-499.
[44] *Ibid.*
[45] For background, see Marcia Clemmitt, "Rising Health Costs," *CQ Researcher*, April 7, 2006, pp. 289-312; Marcia Clemmitt, "Universal Coverage," *CQ Researcher*, March 30, 2007, pp. 265-288.
[46] "State Laws Related to Insurance Coverage for Infertility Treatment," National Conference of State Legislatures, www.ncsl.org/programs/health/50infert.htm.
[47] Quoted in Esther B. Fein, "Calling Infertility a Disease, Couples Battle With Insurers," *The New York Times*, Feb. 22, 1998, www.nytimes.com/specials/women/warchive/980222_2181.html.
[48] "State Laws Related to Insurance Coverage for Infertility Treatment," *op. cit.*
[49] *Ibid.*
[50] "NYS Infertility Demonstration Program," New York State Department of Health, www.health.state.ny.us/community/reproductive_health/infertility.
[51] Mundy, *op. cit.*, p. 59.
[52] Jennifer Schneider, "It's Time for an Egg-Donor Registry and Long-term Follow-up," Nov. 14, 2007, www.geneticsandsociety.org.
[53] *Ibid.*
[54] For background, see Adriel Bettelheim, "Embryo Research," *CQ Researcher*, Dec. 17, 1999, pp. 1065-1088; Marcia Clemmitt, "Stem Cell Research," *CQ Researcher*, Sept. 1, 2006, pp. 697-720.
[55] For background, Malcolm Maclachlan, " 'Octomom' Inspires Bill to Regulate Fertility Clinics," *Capitol Weekly*, March 5, 2009, www.capitolweekly.net/article.php?xid=xt1wfvpujdxifs.
[56] For background, see Betsy McKay, "In-Vitro Fertilization Limit Is Sought," *The Wall Street Journal online*, March 3, 2009, http://online.wsj.com/article/SB123603828823714509.html.
[57] For background, see Liza Mundy, "Souls on Ice: America's Embryo Glut and the Wasted Promise of Stem-Cell Research," *Mother Jones*, July/August 2006, p. 39, www.motherjones.com/politics/2006/07/souls-ice-americas-embryo-glut-and-wasted-promise-stem-cell-research.
[58] For background, see Michael Bushnell, "Missouri House Bill Seeks Limits on Embryo Implants," *Columbia Missourian*, March 5, 2009, www.columbiamissourian.com.
[59] *Ibid.*
[60] *Ibid.*
[61] "Georgia Takes Action: SB 169 to Protect Human Embryos," press release, Georgia Right to Life, Christian NewsWire, March 9, 2009, www.christiannewswire.com/index.php?module=releases&task=view&releaseID=9682.
[62] Quoted in Bushnell, *op. cit.*
[63] Mundy, *Everything Conceivable*, *op. cit.*, p. 69.
[64] "Voluntary Relinquishment for Adoption," Child Welfare Information Gateway, 2005, www.childwelfare.gov/pubs/s_place.cfm.
[65] "International Adoption Facts," Adoption Institute, www.adoptioninstitute.org/FactOverview/international.html.
[66] Mundy, *Everything Conceivable*, *op. cit.*, p. 54.

FOR MORE INFORMATION

American Society of Reproductive Medicine, 1209 Montgomery Highway, Birmingham, AL 35216-2809; (205) 978-5000; www.asrm.org/. Publishes information on infertility medicine and legal and legislative developments related to assisted reproduction.

The Center for Bioethics and Human Dignity, Trinity International University, 2065 Half Day Road, Deerfield, IL 60015; (847) 317-8180; www.cbhd.org. Explores Christian viewpoints on assisted reproduction and other bioethics issues.

Center for Genetics and Society, 436 14th St., Suite 700, Oakland, CA 94612; (510) 625-0819; www.geneticsandsociety.org. Promotes responsible oversight of genetic technologies.

Centers for Disease Control and Prevention, Assisted Reproductive Technology, 1600 Clifton Rd., Atlanta, GA 30333; (404) 639-3311; www.cdc.gov/ART. Federal agency that provides information and data on assisted reproduction, including success rates for U.S. clinics.

Donor Sibling Registry, P.O. Box 1571, Nederland, CO 80466; www.donorsiblingregistry.com. Provides information on donor-gamete issues and a forum for donor-conceived children to locate genetic relatives.

Genetics & Public Policy Center, 1717 Massachusetts Ave., N.W., Suite 530, Washington, DC 20036; (202) 663-5971; www.dnapolicy.org. Research center connected to Johns Hopkins University that analyzes and proposes public policy on genetic technologies.

The Hastings Center, 21 Malcolm Gordon Rd., Garrison, NY 10524; (845) 424-4040; www.thehastingscenter.org. Researches and provides information on bioethics issues from various ethical perspectives.

Human Fertilisation and Embryology Authority, 21 Bloomsbury St., London, UK, WC1B 3HF; 020 7291 8200; www.hfea.gov.uk. The United Kingdom's oversight agency for assisted reproduction; sets standards of practice and provides information on assisted reproduction.

RESOLVE: The National Infertility Association, 1760 Old Meadow Rd., Suite 500, McLean, VA 22102; (703) 556-7172; www.resolve.org. Advocates for improved access to infertility services and provides support for patients.

Bibliography

Selected Sources

Books

Green, Ronald M., *Babies by Design*, Yale University Press, 2007.

A Dartmouth University ethicist lays out probable scenarios for the choices genetic technology will soon lay before parents and argues that such "directed human evolution" can operate for humanity's good.

Knowles, Lori P., and Gregory E. Kaebnick, eds., *Reprogenetics: Law, Policy, and Ethics*, The Johns Hopkins University Press, 2007.

Bioethicists from Canada's University of Alberta (Knowles) and the Hastings Center in New York assemble essays discussing international regulatory schemes for assisted reproductive technology (ART) and related issues.

Mundy, Liza, *Everything Conceivable: How the Science of Assisted Reproduction Is Changing Men, Women, and the World*, Anchor, 2008.

A science writer reports on the rapidly changing landscape of assisted reproduction, based on interviews with parents, gamete donors, doctors and scientists.

Spar, Debora L., *The Baby Business: How Money, Science, and Politics Drive the Commerce of Conception*, Harvard Business School Press, 2006.

A professor of business at Harvard describes the commercial workings of reproductive medicine and adoption in the United States, including gamete donation and fertility clinics, and discusses possibilities for regulating the field.

Articles

Al-Shalchi, Hadeel, "Egypt Septuplets Stir Debate on Fertility Drugs," The Associated Press, Aug. 26, 2008, www.msnbc.msn.com/id/26408452.

Cheap, unpredictable fertility drugs pose dilemmas in developing countries.

Hopkins, Jim, "Egg-Donor Business Booms on Campuses," *USA Today*, March 15, 2006, p. A1.

College women are the most sought-after donors in the growing market for human eggs.

Naik, Gautam, "A Baby, Please. Blond, Freckles — Hold the Colic," *The Wall Street Journal*, Feb. 12, 2009, p. A10.

Preimplantation genetic diagnosis (PGD) — the technique of testing three-day-old in vitro fertilization (IVF) embryos for genetic characteristics — is increasingly used for choosing children's traits, not just to screen for serious genetic diseases, as in the past.

Roan, Shari, "On the Cusp of Life, and of Law," *Los Angeles Times*, Oct. 6, 2008.

Some 500,000 embryos are preserved in freezers in the U.S., some destined for further IVF cycles but many belonging to mothers who've finished with childbearing and now struggle to decide whether to discard the leftover embryos.

Reports and Studies

"2006 Assisted Reproductive Technology Success Rates," *National Summary and Fertility Clinic Reports*, Centers for Disease Control and Prevention/American Society for Reproductive Medicine, November 2008, www.cdc.gov/ART/ART2006.

The report analyzes practices and outcomes in U.S. fertility medicine in 2006, based on mandatory reporting by fertility clinics nationwide.

***The Hastings Center Report, July-August 2007*, Hastings Center, July 2007, Vol. 37, No. 4, www.thehastingscenter.org/Publications/HCR/Default.aspx?id=752.**

Scholars discuss the potential for regulating ART from various legal and ethical perspectives.

"Old Lessons for a New World; Applying Adoption Research and Experience to Assisted Reproductive Technology," Evan B. Donaldson Adoption Institute, February 2009, www.adoptioninstitute.org.

A nonprofit advocacy group for improved adoption practices argues that reproductive medicine would benefit from adopting state regulation and establishing a national database of adoptees' records.

"Reproductive Genetic Testing: Issues and Options for Policymakers," Genetics & Public Policy Center, 2004, www.dnapolicy.org/images/reportpdfs/ReproGenTestIssuesOptions.pdf.

A nonprofit think tank lays out the pros and cons for policy questions, such as, Should governments ban or establish strict rules for reproductive genetic testing, and Should doctors increase the amount of genetic counseling they provide to prospective parents?

"Reproductive Genetic Testing: What America Thinks," Genetics & Public Policy Center, 2004, www.dnapolicy.org/images/reportpdfs/ReproGenTestAmericaThinks.pdf.

Americans are divided over the morality of genetic testing of embryos, but many agree that it's probably acceptable to use the technology to avoid giving birth to a child with a life-threatening childhood illness or to try to conceive a child who could donate tissue to a sick sibling.

The Next Step:

Additional Articles from Current Periodicals

Insurance

Davidson, Terri, "State's Infertility Mandate Is Friendly Toward Family Values," *Telegram & Gazette* (Massachusetts), June 28, 2007, p. A19.
Massachusetts became the first state to provide mandated fertility insurance coverage in 1987.

Graham, Judith E., "Couples' Fertility Care Threatened," *Chicago Tribune*, Jan. 30, 2009, p. A27.
A contract dispute between a chain of fertility centers in Illinois and the state's largest HMO threatens to disrupt the medical care of hundreds of couples trying to become pregnant.

Henry, Ray, "R.I. Governor Blocks Bill Requiring Infertility Treatment Coverage for the Unmarried," The Associated Press, July 20, 2007.
Rhode Island Gov. Don Carcieri has vetoed a bill requiring health insurers to cover infertility treatments for unmarried couples.

Yee, Chen May, "Miracles for Sale," *Star Tribune* (Minnesota), Oct. 22, 2007, p. 1A.
Infertile couples are finding their insurance coverage is the primary factor in making it possible to have a child.

Refusal

Moran, Greg, "High Court Hearing Pits Religious vs. Equal Rights," *San Diego Union-Tribune*, May 29, 2008, p. B1.
A California lesbian is suing doctors at a fertility clinic for refusing to perform a fertility procedure.

Tarkan, Laurie, "Lowering the Odds of Multiple Births," *The New York Times*, Feb. 19, 2008, p. F1.
Many fertility centers are trying to reduce multiple births by limiting the number of embryo transfers per patient.

Turner, Allan, "Time Running Out in Fight for Embryos," *Houston Chronicle*, April 10, 2008, p. B1.
A Houston woman is trying to persuade the Supreme Court to give her control of three embryos doctors refused to inseminate after her husband changed his mind.

Registries

Campbell, Colleen Carroll, "Children's Rights Often Overlooked in Today's Brave New World," *St. Louis Post-Dispatch*, April 16, 2009, p. A15.
Assisted reproductive technologies can make donor-conceived children's natural longing to understand their origins particularly confusing and painful.

Goldberg, Carey, "The Search for DGM 2598," *The Boston Globe*, Nov. 23, 2008, p. A1.
More children of anonymous donors want to know who fathered them, but sperm banks say donor supplies would drop dramatically if anonymity is prohibited.

Montgomery, Rick, "Through the Web, Kids of Sperm-Donor Dads Connect With Siblings," *The Kansas City Star*, March 22, 2009, p. A1.
Thousands of individuals conceived from sperm or egg donations have found relatives through the Donor Sibling Registry.

Regulation

Barlow, Rich, "In Baby Business, What Are the Rules?" *The Boston Globe*, March 15, 2008, p. B2.
Proponents of fertility regulation say fertility clinics should disclose the health risks of any procedure as well as the relevant success rates.

LaFee, Scott, "Octuplet Case Sparks Calls for Fertility-Industry Curbs," *San Diego Union-Tribune*, Feb. 12, 2009, p. A1.
Fertility doctors generally oppose government regulation, arguing that the industry has been good at policing itself.

Yoshino, Kimi, "Fertility Industry Oversight Is Urged," *Los Angeles Times*, March 5, 2009, p. A8.
The Center for Genetics and Society wants Congress to examine the largely unregulated $3 billion fertility industry.

Zarembo, Alan, "Does In-Vitro Need Rules?" *Orlando Sentinel*, Feb. 16, 2009, p. A2.
Fertility treatment is a private matter between doctors and patients that is insulated from outside influences and free from government regulation.

CITING *CQ* RESEARCHER

Sample formats for citing these reports in a bibliography include the ones listed below. Preferred styles and formats vary, so please check with your instructor or professor.

MLA STYLE

Jost, Kenneth. "Rethinking the Death Penalty." CQ Researcher 16 Nov. 2001: 945-68.

APA STYLE

Jost, K. (2001, November 16). Rethinking the death penalty. *CQ Researcher, 11*, 945-968.

CHICAGO STYLE

Jost, Kenneth. "Rethinking the Death Penalty." *CQ Researcher*, November 16, 2001, 945-968.

CHAPTER

7

Abortion Debates

By Kenneth Jost

Excerpted from the CQ Researcher. Kenneth Jost. (September 10, 2010). "Abortion Debates." *CQ Researcher*, 725-748.

Abortion Debates

BY KENNETH JOST

THE ISSUES

Mike Flood is a lawyer and a radio station owner, not a doctor or scientist. But after listening to medical experts on both sides of the issue, Flood is convinced that a fetus is capable of feeling pain by the 20th week of pregnancy. And as speaker of the Nebraska Senate, Flood relied on that conclusion in sponsoring and guiding to enactment a new state law that imposes an outright ban on abortions at the 20th week.

Opponents say the law, set to go into effect on Oct. 15, is wrong both medically and legally. They say medical evidence does not show that a fetus experiences pain until later in a pregnancy. And they claim the law is unconstitutional because it directly contradicts Supreme Court precedents that allow states to ban abortions only after a fetus is viable — generally considered to be no sooner than the 22nd week of pregnancy.

KEEP ABORTION LEGAL
KEEP ABORTION LEGAL
NOW
Getty Images/Mark Wilson

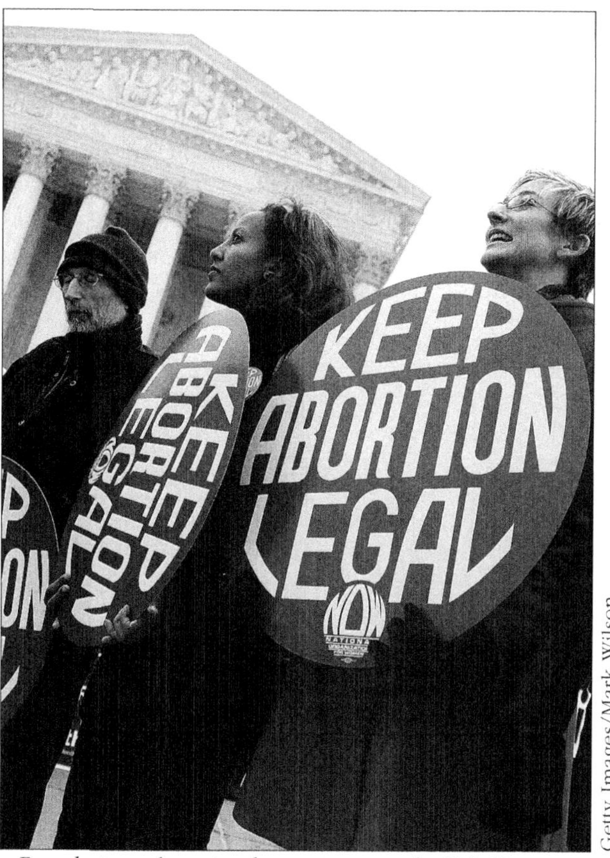

Pro-choice advocates demonstrate at the U.S. Supreme Court on Jan. 22 to commemorate the 37th anniversary of the court's landmark Roe v. Wade *decision legalizing abortion. Today anti-abortion groups say new state restrictions on abortion reflect a gradual shift in public opinion in favor of so-called "pro-life" views. Abortion-rights advocates disagree about the state of public opinion but acknowledge they face a difficult political climate.*

Flood, now in his sixth year in the nonpartisan, unicameral legislature and fourth year as speaker, acknowledges the difference of medical opinion on the subject. But he says that the Supreme Court's most recent abortion-related decision opens the ways for states to restrict abortions even if medical issues are disputed.

"I think the state of Nebraska has a substantial interest in protecting the life of a fetus that can feel pain by the 20th week of pregnancy," Flood says in a telephone interview from his home in Norfolk, in northeastern Nebraska. He acknowledges the new law is "a departure" but notes that the Supreme Court in 2007 upheld a federal ban on certain late-term abortions called by opponents "partial birth abortion" despite disagreement among experts about the medical need for the procedure.

For their part, abortion-rights advocates view Nebraska's Pain-Capable Unborn Child Protection Act as a direct challenge to the Supreme Court's landmark 1973 *Roe v. Wade* decision. "We believe it is unconstitutional, that it is in defiance of *Roe v. Wade* by banning abortion pre-viability without regard to the woman's health or welfare," says Jill June, president of Planned Parenthood of the Heartland, which covers Iowa and Nebraska. "That clearly to us is a frontal attack on *Roe v. Wade*." [1]

The new law is one of several ambitious anti-abortion measures enacted in the states during the past legislative season. Another Nebraska statute requires additional screening procedures before an abortion, including informing the woman of any resulting "complications" from an abortion identified in any peer-reviewed journal on the subject. In Oklahoma, a new law requires a physician to display an ultrasound image of a fetus for the patient before performing an abortion, although the woman is permitted to turn away from the display if she chooses. A somewhat comparable Louisiana law requires a physician to give a copy of an ultrasound to the woman before an abortion.

All three of those measures have been blocked from going into effect by federal judges in suits filed by three abortion-rights groups: Planned Parenthood and the American Civil Liberties Union (ACLU) in Nebraska and the New York-based Center for Reproductive Rights (CRR) in Oklahoma and Louisiana. So far, those groups have not decided whether to challenge Nebraska's fetal-pain measure. But Nancy Northrup, president of CRR, called the law "clearly unconstitutional" in a letter in April unsuccessfully urging Republican Nebraska Gov. David Heineman to veto the bill.

The new variations on abortion regulations came as legislatures in several states were considering proposals to limit coverage of abortion in the

U.S. Abortions Have Been Declining

Both the total number of abortions and the nation's abortion rate have been declining for the past two decades. In 2005, the year with the most recent data available, 1.2 million abortions were performed, down from 1.58 million in 1985 (top graph). The abortion rate has dropped from a high of 29.3 abortions per 1,000 women in 1981 to 19.4 in 2005. From 1973, when the Supreme Court's Roe v. Wade *decision legalized abortion, to 2005, more than 45 million legal abortions were performed.*

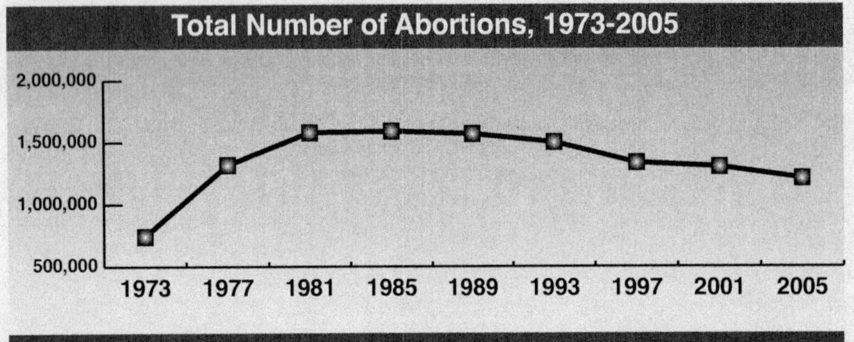

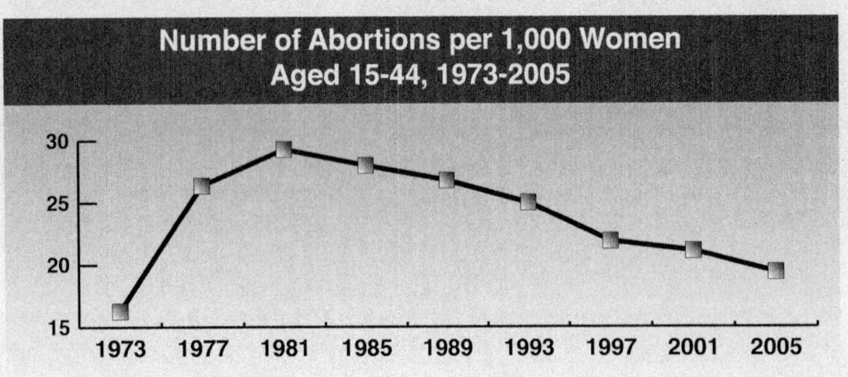

Source: "Facts on Induced Abortion in the United States," Guttmacher Institute, May 2010

insurance exchange plans to be established under the new federal health-care law pushed by President Obama over the past two years. Most private health insurance plans provide abortion coverage, but anti-abortion groups want to bar any federal subsidies or support for abortion coverage under the insurance plans to be established under the new federal law. [2]

The legislative battles demonstrate that abortion remains a contentious issue — and an intensely emotional one — now nearly four full decades after the Supreme Court established a qualified right to abortion in *Roe v. Wade.* Almost immediately, Congress and state legislatures began passing laws to regulate abortions.

Since the 1970s, Congress and about two-thirds of the states have passed laws barring the use of taxpayer funds to pay for abortions for poor women except in cases of rape, incest or danger to the woman's life. And state legislatures continue to devise increasingly intricate laws regulating abortion procedure, often — as in the case of Nebraska's screening law — with the stated purpose of reducing abortion "whenever possible." [3]

Anti-abortion groups say the legislated restrictions reflect a gradual shift in public opinion in favor of what has come to be called "pro-life" views. "Recent polling shows that more Americans characterize themselves as pro-life than pro-choice," says Mary Harned, staff counsel with Americans United for Life (AUL). She says that "a strong majority" of Americans oppose government funding for elective abortions and that even abortion-rights supporters "accept" such restrictions as bans on late-term abortions and informed-consent laws, which require patients to be told of potential risks from a procedure.

Abortion-rights advocates disagree about the state of public opinion but acknowledge they face a difficult political climate. "The vast majority of Americans remain pro-choice," says Donna Crane, policy director for NARAL Pro-Choice America, formerly the National Abortion Rights Action League. But she concedes that states have been "extremely active" in passing "hundreds of laws" over the past two decades since the Supreme Court reaffirmed *Roe v. Wade* in somewhat modified form in 1992. "Women's access to medical care has definitely suffered as a result," Crane says.

Public opinion is, in fact, nearly as ambivalent as the opposing groups' different descriptions suggest, but support for abortion does appear to be declining, according to two recent public opinion surveys. As anti-abortion groups note, a Gallup survey in May 2009 found for the first time in 15 years of polling that more Americans describe themselves as pro-life than pro-choice (51 percent to 42 percent). Somewhat similarly, a *Washington Post*-ABC News poll in August 2009 found that only a bare plurality — 47 percent to 45 percent — believe that abortion should be legal instead of illegal in all or most cases; only once before in the past 15 years had support for legal abortions dropped below a majority. [4] (*See graphs, p. 729.*)

More Americans Are Now Pro-Life

Since 1995, the ratio of pro-life versus pro-choice Americans has flip-flopped. More than half of all Americans now consider themselves pro-life, an 18-point increase from the mid-1990s. During the same period, the percentage of pro-choice Americans dropped below 50 percent.

Would you consider yourself to be pro-choice or pro-life?

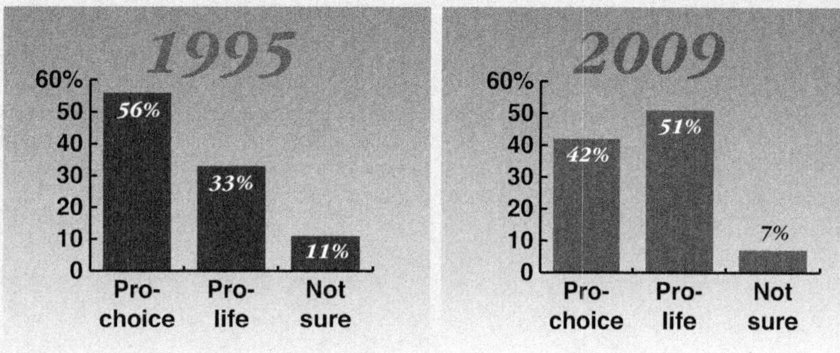

Source: Lydia Saad, "More Americans 'Pro-Life' Than 'Pro-Choice' for First Time," Gallup, May 2009

Meanwhile, the abortion rate in the United States has been declining steadily since 1980 after a sharp rise in the years immediately after *Roe v. Wade*, according to the Guttmacher Institute, a research center that supports abortion rights. The absolute number also appears to be falling: from 1.3 million abortions in 2000 to 1.2 million in 2005, the most recent year available. The center's data show that women in their 20s account for more than half of the abortions, with teenagers another 18 percent. The vast majority of abortions — 88 percent — occur within the first trimester of pregnancy (by 12 weeks); only 1.5 percent of the total are after the 20th week of pregnancy. [5] (*See graph, p. 732.*)

Anti-abortion advocates say restrictive laws are helping drive down the abortion rate. Abortion-rights advocates say many women face significant barriers in access to abortion services. They cite the cost — an average of about $413 for the procedure in a clinic — and the declining number of doctors performing abortions. Guttmacher says the number of abortion providers declined slightly from 1,815 in 2000 to 1,787 in 2005 and that 87 percent of all U.S. counties lack any abortion provider at all. [6]

Abortion became a pivotal issue in the congressional health care endgame as President Obama pushed for passage of legislation aimed primarily at ensuring coverage for the estimated 46 million Americans without health insurance. Anti-abortion Democrats in the House won passage of an amendment in November 2009 prohibiting any coverage for abortion in the federally subsidized health plans; in the Senate, anti-abortion Democrat Ben Nelson of Nebraska also insisted on an anti-abortion provision, though less restrictive, as his price to support the measure.

With Nelson's provision in the final bill, Obama secured the anti-abortion Democrats' votes in the House only after promising to issue an executive order to tighten the ban on any federal funding for abortion under the law. Anti-abortion forces remain dissatisfied even as abortion-rights advocates harshly criticize the restrictions. Meanwhile, states are also considering measures to limit abortion coverage in the insurance exchanges that the federal law calls to be created by 2014 in order to increase access for individuals and small businesses to affordable coverage.

At the same time, court challenges continue to newly enacted abortion restrictions even as anti-abortion forces look to ballot measures in the fall and a new legislative season in 2011 as opportunities for additional initiatives. Abortion-rights advocates say they expect more battles and are mobilizing both politically and legally to counter them.

As those battles continue, here are some of the major questions being debated:

Will federal health care reforms result in taxpayer funding of abortion?

President Obama made it a major media event on March 23 when he signed into law the landmark health-care bill after a hard-fought political battle that extended over more than a year. But the next day, the White House allowed no live coverage when Obama signed an executive order guaranteeing that the new law prohibits federally funded abortions.

The executive order fulfilled Obama's promise to anti-abortion House Democrats, persuading them to vote for the bill. The two-page order reiterates the prohibition that the White House says is already in the law against any funding of abortion services under the law, including tax credits and cost-sharing reduction payments, except in cases of rape or incest or danger to the life of the woman. The order directs the secretary of the Department of Health and Human Services (HHS) to propose regulations for state health commissioners to use to accomplish that goal within 180 days — that is, by the end of September. [7]

White House press secretary Robert Gibbs said the order "maintains the status quo" limiting federal funding of abortions. Anti-abortion groups dismissed the executive order. A "transparent political fig leaf," said Douglas Johnson, national legislative director of the National Right to Life Committee. Abortion rights groups, on the other hand, said they were disappointed with Obama's action. "Women will be worse off under health care reform," said Vicki Saporta, president of the National Abortion Federation (NAF), which represents abortion providers. [8]

Five months later, opposing groups continue to disagree about the practical effect of the executive order, as well as the underlying policy. The administration claims that any subsidy for abortion coverage under the federal law will be prevented by a "two-check" requirement, as dictated by the Nelson amendment. Anyone covered under a federally subsidized health plan will have to make one payment for principal coverage and a separate payment for abortion coverage.

Abortion rights advocates call the requirement onerous and unnecessary. "This creates a really significant disincentive," says Vania Leveille, an ACLU legislative counsel. "Women across the country can find themselves in an insurance market that offers them no option for abortion coverage."

"Abortion services and abortion care are a fundamental part of women's health care needs," says Laura MacCleary, government relations director for the Center for Reproductive Rights. "Insurance coverage should absolutely be available to women when they need those services."

From the other perspective, anti-abortion groups say the two-check requirement does not prevent government funding from leaking into abortion coverage in insurance plans. "If you are paying a premium on an insurance plan and that plan covers abortion, your premiums could be used to pay for abortion," says Harned at Americans United for Life.

Abortion opponents also continue to complain that Congress adopted the less-restrictive Nelson amendment instead of the provision backed by anti-abortion House Democrats that would have prohibited abortion coverage in subsidized health plans altogether.

"Congress went directly against what most Americans want," says Wendy Wright, president of Concerned Women for America, a conservative women's group. "Even people who are not pro-life don't want their tax dollars subsidizing abortions. The health care bill subsidizing abortion garners opposition from both pro-life and those who don't necessarily identify themselves as pro-life."

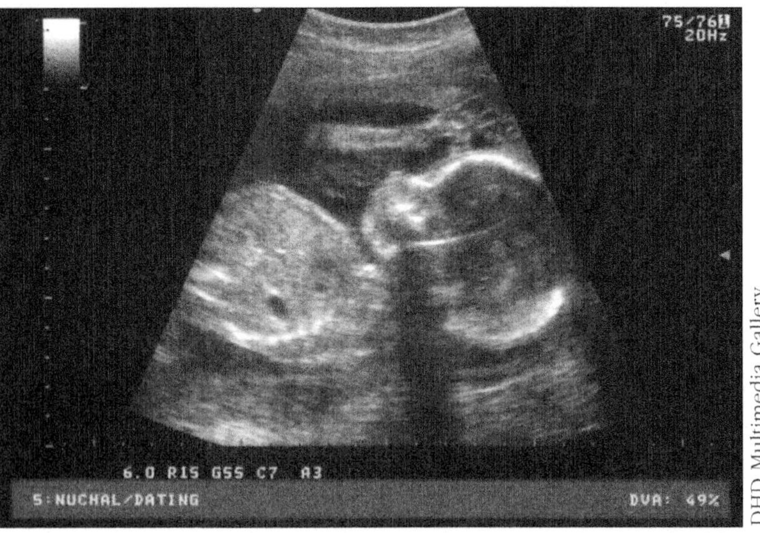

DHD Multimedia Gallery

Ultrasound images, or sonograms, are used to monitor the growth of the fetus and the mother's condition during pregnancy. Although ultrasound is a pain-free, low-cost and non-invasive process, two medical groups recommend restraint in using ultrasound. And the Food and Drug Administration recommends strongly against taking "keepsake" videos of the fetus.

Both sides are waiting for the rules that HHS will be proposing by the end of September for insurance companies to follow in segregating payments for abortion coverage. MacCleary says she hopes the rules will make the requirement "more reasonable in practice." For her part, Harned says even if the rules for segregating payments are "airtight," anti-abortion groups still oppose any abortion coverage by insurance plans under the law.

Meanwhile, the Obama administration moved to bar abortion coverage through the temporary "high-risk pools" to be established under the federal law to help ensure coverage for people with pre-existing medical conditions until 2014, when the law's major provisions are to take effect. The $5 billion program is completely federally funded, but states can assume responsibility for its administration. It may cover up to 400,000 people when implemented.

As enacted, the law did not bar abortion coverage in the high-risk pools. Anti-abortion groups objected strongly after the administration approved some state plans with abortion coverage. The administration moved to squelch the controversy with rules issued by HHS on July 29 barring any abortion coverage under the plans.

Abortion rights groups deplored the decision. "The Obama administration has put up an unnecessary barrier to comprehensive health care to the women who need it most by singling out abortion in these high-risk pools," said Laura Murphy, the ACLU's Washington legislative director.

Continued on p. 732

Cautious Use of Ultrasound Recommended

Negative side effects can't be ruled out, scientists warn.

Long before their baby is born, expecting parents come back from the doctor's office with a picture fit to be framed: a sonogram image of the fetus taken by an ultrasound procedure.

A sonogram is not only a memento but also a valuable diagnostic tool, periodically performed during the nine months of a pregnancy to monitor the baby's growth. In addition, states increasingly are passing legislation requiring a woman who wants an abortion to have ultrasound and to be given the chance to view the image of the fetus.

Although ultrasound is a pain-free, low-cost and noninvasive imaging process that does not involve radiation, the American Institute of Ultrasound in Medicine, the American College of Radiology and the American College of Obstetricians and Gynecologists recommend restraint. In a joint guideline, the groups say "this diagnostic procedure should be performed only when there is a valid medical indication, and the lowest possible ultrasonic exposure setting should be used to gain the necessary diagnostic information." [1]

During an ultrasound procedure, a handheld device called a transducer uses sound waves with an extremely high frequency (over 20,000 vibrations per second) to check the development of the fetus in the womb. Because ultrasound does not work correctly through air, the ultrasound technician puts a clear gel on the woman's abdominal region and places the transducer on the target area. The sound waves reflect from bones, tissues and organs, carrying signals back to a computer, creating ultrasound pictures. [2]

Ultrasound is used throughout the pregnancy to monitor the condition of the woman and the fetus. It is performed during the first trimester to confirm the pregnancy and then to determine a heart rate, set a likely birth date, check to see if there is more than one fetus, measure the baby's head and gauge the chances of a miscarriage or determine if there are any issues with the cervix, uterus or placenta. Ultrasound also can reveal the development of an ectopic pregnancy, in which the fertilized ovum develops outside the uterus.

During ultrasound procedures in the second and third trimesters, doctors not only can monitor the baby's health, positioning and growth but also can see if it has birth defects or placenta previa, in which the placenta is implanted in the lower part of the uterus, causing bleeding. Detecting problems early allows doctors and patients to plan for the most favorable outcome possible. [3]

While ultrasound of a fetus produces no known negative side effects, researchers say they cannot be completely ruled out. In a paper published in August, three scientists from the U.S. Food and Drug Administration (FDA) warn that "ultrasound energy delivered to the fetus cannot be regarded as completely innocuous." [4] They point to studies that show ultrasound can produce vibration and a rise in tissue temperature.

Other researchers caution that current ultrasound technology "has significantly higher output potential than older machines used in most clinical studies" and that the safety profile for modern machines is unknown. [5] Some advocacy groups have even speculated that the increased use of fetal ultrasound has contributed to the rise in autism, although a journal article published a year ago found no such correlation. [6]

Proud prospective parents who might be tempted to purchase a "keepsake ultrasound video" from a private company should also think twice. One such company says "it's a great way to preserve the memory of this special time shared with your child for years to come" and encourages parents to come "as often as you wish." [7]

But the FDA strongly recommends against videos. "In some cases, the ultrasound machine may be used for as long as an hour to get a video of the fetus," says the FDA. "We are concerned about this misuse of diagnostic ultrasound equipment." [8] A little more than a year ago, Connecticut banned keepsake ultrasounds. [9]

— Barbara Mantel and Caroline Young

---

[1] "AIUM Practice Guideline for the Performance of Obstetric Ultrasound Examinations," *Journal of Ultrasound Medicine*, American Institute of Ultrasound in Medicine, 2010: 29: 157-166, www.jultrasoundmed.org/cgi/content/full/29/1/157.

[2] Mary Bellis, "The History of Ultrasound," About.com:Inventors, July 2010, http://inventors.about.com/library/inventors/blultrasound.htm.

[3] "Pregnancy Ultrasounds," Genesis-Ultrasound.com, July 22, 2010, www.genesis-ultrasound.com/Pregnancy-ultrasounds.html.

[4] R. A. Phillips, *et al.*, "Safety and U.S. Regulatory considerations in the nonclinical use of medical ultrasound devices," *Ultrasound in Medicine and Biology*, 2010 Aug; 36(8): 1224-28, www.ncbi.nlm.nih.gov/pubmed/20447750.

[5] L. E. Houston, *et al.*, "The safety of obstetrical ultrasound: a review," Prenatal Diagnosis, 2009 Dec; 29(13):1204-12, www.ncbi.nlm.nih.gov/pubmed/19899071.

[6] Judith K. Grether, *et al.*, "Antenatal Ultrasound and Risk of Autism Spectrum Disorders," *Journal of Autism and Developmental Disorders*, published online Sept. 1, 2009, www.ehib.org/papers/Antenatal_Ultrasound_Risk_ASD.pdf.

[7] "Welcome to Med Life Imaging," Med Life Imaging, http://medlifeimaging.com/?tid=g31b&gclid=CKfmmJPa8KMCFZJ95QodrCBt3w.

[8] "Fetal Keepsake Videos," Food and Drug Administration, www.fda.gov/MedicalDevices/Safety/AlertsandNotices/PatientAlerts/ucm064756.htm.

[9] "Conn. governor signs keepsake ultrasound ban," The Associated Press State & Local Wire, June 24, 2009.

Continued from p. 730

But anti-abortion groups remained dissatisfied. In a press release, the National Right to Life Committee said the episode showed that "there is no language in the new health care law, and no language in Obama's politically contrived March 24 executive order, which effectively prevents federal subsidies for abortion on demand." [9]

Should states limit insurance coverage for abortions?

Gov. Haley Barbour was exultant as he signed a law making Mississippi the third state to prohibit general coverage for abortions in the new health care exchanges to be established for individuals and small businesses as part of President Obama's health insurance reform.

"Mississippi continues to be the safest place to be an unborn child in America today," the Republican chief executive said on May 24 as he signed the state's Federal Abortion-Mandate Opt-Out Act. "This bill ensures that taxpayers' money will not fund abortions if the health insurance exchanges are implemented under the federal health care law." [10]

Two other states, Arizona and Tennessee, had enacted similar "opt-out" laws earlier in the legislative season; two more, Louisiana and Missouri, followed suit later. Mississippi and two of the others permitted abortion coverage under limited exceptions, but Louisiana's and Tennessee's barred abortion coverage without exception.

Insurance coverage for abortion had not been a high-profile issue until Congress began considering Obama's call for federal health care reform. The vast majority of employer-provided health insurance plans — more than 80 percent — included coverage for surgical or medical abortions, according to a study by Guttmacher Institute researchers. Five states, however, prohibited private insurance coverage for abortion: Idaho, Kentucky, Missouri, North Dakota and Oklahoma. And 12 prohibited abortion coverage for state employees. [11]

Most U.S. Abortions Occur in First Trimester

Nearly 90 percent of abortions in the United States occur in the first 12 weeks of pregnancy — or first trimester — with most of those taking place at nine weeks or less. Fewer than 2 percent occur after 20 weeks, the point where anti-abortion proponents say the fetus can feel pain.

When Women Have Abortions, 2006

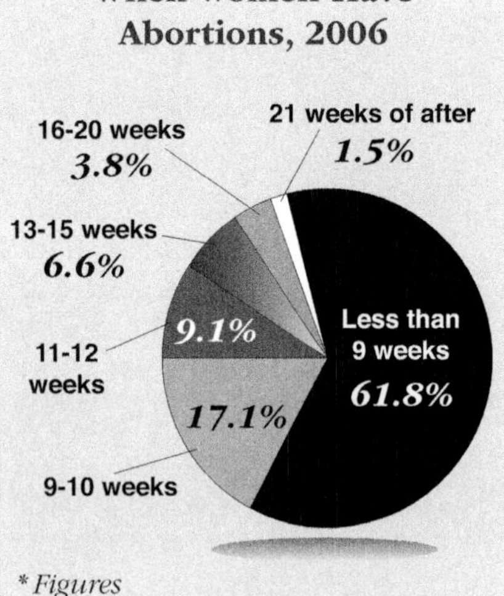

** Figures do not total 100 due to rounding.*

Source: "Facts on Induced Abortion In the United States," Guttmacher Institute, May 2010

By proposing a limited federalization of private health insurance, Obama made abortion coverage a national instead of a state issue. The Nelson amendment added in the Senate specifically authorizes states to "prohibit abortion coverage in qualified health plans offered through an exchange."

"The debate around health care reform clearly has politicized the idea of private insurance coverage of abortion," says Adam Sonfeld, a senior policy associate at Guttmacher and lead author of the insurance coverage study. "It has put this issue in the political sphere in a way we haven't seen in many years. And there is no reason to think the genie in the bottle is going back anytime soon."

Anti-abortion groups say the moves to bar abortion coverage by the health insurance exchanges called for in the new law simply reflect the broad public opposition to any use of public funds to pay for abortions. "The American people do not want their tax dollars to go for abortions," says Mary Spaulding Balch, director of the National Right to Life Committee's Department of State Legislation.

"The abortion movement claims that it's a woman's choice," says Wright of Concerned Women for America, "and now they are demanding that other people pay for her choice."

Abortion rights advocates counter that the laws will have the effect of reducing women's access to abortion coverage in private health insurance. "Abortions can be very expensive," says Jordan Goldberg, state advocacy counsel with the Center for Reproductive Rights. "Right now, most women do have coverage for this. So these insurance bans are going to change the status quo."

"Abortion coverage should be part of any basic insurance plan," says NARAL's Crane. "These laws are all about taking away a basic procedure."

Besides the five states that enacted opt-out laws, legislatures in Oklahoma and Florida approved similar provisions, but the measures were vetoed. Oklahoma's Democratic governor, Brad Henry, vetoed the bill in his state because an exception allowing coverage in event of rape or incest would have applied only if the offense had been reported to law enforcement within 48 hours. In Florida, Charlie Crist, the state's Republican-turned-Independent chief executive, vetoed a bill that included an opt-out provision as well as a new requirement requiring women to view an ultrasound image of the fetus before an abortion.

Balch notes that several other states considered opt-out provisions, but the bills were introduced too late in legislative sessions to advance. She expects more states to pass such laws in the 2011 legislative season. NARAL's Crane similarly expects the issue to continue to roil next year. "The Nelson restriction has certainly shown a spotlight on this issue," she says. "States that have anti-choice legislatures are certain to take up that opportunity."

Should states pass additional laws regulating abortion procedures?

Campaigning as a Republican for the U.S. Senate early in 2010, Florida's Gov. Crist promised to support "pro-life legislative efforts." In June, however, Crist disappointed his former supporters among social conservatives by vetoing a bill to require a woman to view an ultrasound of her fetus before having an abortion.

The bill "places an inappropriate burden on women seeking to terminate pregnancy," said Crist, who had dropped his GOP affiliation in late April to run as an independent in the face of eroding support among Republicans. The veto also killed a separate provision to bar abortion coverage in the insurance exchanges to be created under the federal health care reform, but Crist did not address that section in his veto message. [12]

Crist's veto was a disappointment for anti-abortion groups in a legislative season when they enjoyed successes in several other states. In all, 15 states passed new abortion-related laws in 2010, according to the Guttmacher Institute. Ultrasound laws were enacted in five states, bringing the number of states with such laws to 20.

Two other states added other counseling or waiting-period provisions. Provisions added in two states required abortion clinics to post notices that a woman cannot be coerced to have an abortion. Three states provided funding for alternatives for abortion services. And one state, Montana, required that a woman be told that a fetus feels pain during an abortion and that an abortion ends the life of "a separate, unique, living human being."

Anti-abortion groups say the laws are all aimed at making sure that women are fully informed before deciding to have an abortion. "The woman deserves adequate informed consent, and that includes literature and the fact that this is a human being, not a blob," says Joseph Cook, a Detroit physician and vice president of the American Association of Pro-Life Obstetricians and Gynecologists. "You can be polite and say 'terminate pregnancy,' but women should really be told what is actually happening: the unborn child is being killed."

Abortion rights supporters say the laws are both intrusive and ineffective. "We shouldn't take away or restrict a woman's decision-making ability and allow politicians to make decisions for her," says the ACLU's Leveille. "These laws represent political interference in a woman's most personal, private medical decisions."

"We hear regularly from our members that these laws do not deflect women from going ahead with their decision of having an abortion," says Saporta with the National Abortion Federation. "They are ineffective in doing their stated goal of making it more difficult to access abortion care. They are ill-advised, and they don't work."

Cook and Saporta disagree in particular on the issue of fetal pain. Cook supports laws that require a physician to tell a woman that a fetus does experience pain.

"There are some mindless comments out there that the baby doesn't feel anything in the first 20-29 weeks," Cook says. "In actual scientific terms, when there's a baby at six to 18 weeks, they can experience pain. If we poke a needle in there, they jump."

"There is no scientific evidence to support that a fetus feels pain prior to the third trimester," Saporta replies. "So those laws are based on faulty science."

The ultrasound laws vary significantly. Ten states merely require a doctor to offer the patient the opportunity to view the image if an ultrasound is performed as part of the preparation for the abortion. But six require an ultrasound to be performed — two only after the first trimester and four at any point during the pregnancy. The doctor in those states is required to offer the opportunity to view the image.

Oklahoma's newly enacted law goes furthest by requiring the doctor to display and describe the image. A state court judge, ruling in a case brought by attorneys with the Center for Reproductive Rights, has temporarily blocked the law from going into effect pending a further hearing scheduled for Jan. 21, 2011.

Goldberg, the center's state legislative counsel, calls the ultrasound laws "particularly demeaning" to women. "Women seeking abortions have carefully considered their options and life circumstances," she says, "and these requirements serve only as an attempt to shame them and make them feel guilty about their decisions."

Harned with Americans United for Life disagrees. "Laws like fetal pain and ultrasound requirement actually inform women what abortion is and the effects it has on women," she says. Women, she adds, "often have abortions without being fully informed about the choice they are making." ■

BACKGROUND

An Ambivalent History

Over the course of two centuries, abortion went from a legal, unregulated procedure in the United States to a criminal but rarely prosecuted offense and then to a constitutional right subject to regulation up to an uncertain point. For nearly half a century, the issue has been a divisive issue on the national legal and political agenda even as public opinion has remained in a state of fairly constant ambivalence supporting a right of abortion — up to an uncertain point. [13]

Abortion had been a legal and somewhat common procedure in ancient Greece and Rome, in early modern Europe and England, and in colonial America. In 19th-century America, advertisements for "abortifacents" were common even if the substances' use for that purpose was purportedly disapproved of. Beginning with Connecticut in 1821, however, states in the 19th century passed laws criminalizing abortion. The medical establishment first pushed the laws to protect women from botched abortions; later, Protestant and Catholic groups added moral condemnation of abortion to the reasons for the laws.

By the mid-20th century, laws against abortion had been on the books for so long as to be largely beyond public debate, especially at a time when contraception itself was illegal in some jurisdictions. The laws did not eliminate abortion, however. Instead, women used back channels of communication to find doctors or unlicensed practitioners willing to perform the procedure, either in the United States or abroad. The dangers of in-the-shadows medicine, especially for low-income women with limited access to qualified physicians, helped give rise by the 1960s to an abortion reform movement led by many religious leaders, which gained strength with the advance of the broader rise in feminist consciousness.

By the first years of the 1970s, the abortion reform movement had won passage in a few states of model laws generally legalizing the procedure when deemed necessary for the woman's life or health. The legislative reform movement was cut short, however, by the Supreme Court's landmark ruling in *Roe v. Wade* establishing a qualified constitutional right to abortion. Whether or not abortion reform would have advanced with less contentiousness without the Supreme Court's decision — that debate can never be settled — the ruling lastingly reversed the political dynamics of the issue. Since *Roe*, opponents of abortion have been forced to lobby for legislated restrictions on the procedure, while abortion rights supporters had federal courts as a backstop for any restrictions that were enacted. [14]

In an early and vitally important pair of decisions, the Supreme Court upheld state and federal laws limiting government funding of abortions for poor women. In 1977, the Court upheld on a 6-3 vote a Connecticut law barring Medicaid funding of abortion unless a doctor certified the procedure was medically necessary for the woman's physical or mental health. Three years later, the Court upheld on a 5-4 vote a federal provision — known as the Hyde Amendment after its principal House sponsor, Rep. Henry Hyde, R-Ill. — that barred federal Medicaid funding unless an abortion was necessary to protect a woman's life or the pregnancy resulted from rape or incest. The federal law has remained on the books, and about two-thirds of the states have the same restrictions on use of their own Medicaid funds. [15]

Through the 1970s and '80s, the justices charted a more difficult-to-follow course on other regulations in a series of closely divided decisions. The court struck down laws requiring spousal or parental consent but upheld parental-notification requirements as long as a minor, under some circumstances, could go to court for permission for the abortion without notifying parents, known as a judicial bypass procedure. The court struck down so-called "informed-consent provisions," mandatory 24-hour waiting periods and provisions requiring abortions be performed in hospitals, not clinics.

Throughout the period, anti-abortion groups attacked *Roe* as constitutionally unsound and hoped for a decision to overrule it. Under two Republican presidents — Ronald Reagan and George H. W. Bush — the government urged the court to scrap *Roe*. In 1989, four justices — one short of a majority — called for overturning what Chief Justice William H. Rehnquist termed *Roe*'s "rigid framework."

Three years later, anti-abortion groups hoped that a Pennsylvania case would give a court with a fortified conservative majority the vehicle for finally jettisoning *Roe*. Instead, however, the court reaffirmed what Justices Sandra Day O'Connor, Anthony M. Kennedy and David H. Souter called in a jointly authored opinion *Roe*'s "essential framework." Even so, the decision in *Planned Parenthood v. Casey* upheld restrictions previously struck down, including an informed-consent provision and a 24-hour waiting period.

Policy Swings

Abortion politics swung back and forth in the 1990s and the first decade of the new century depending on the political party that controlled the White House. Abortion rights advocates made gains under a Democratic president, Bill Clinton, while anti-abortion forces gained the upper hand under the Republican president, George W. Bush, who had a GOP-controlled Congress for most of his eight years in office. Bush's role in naming two Supreme Court justices was pivotal in the court's upholding a federal ban on so-called partial birth abortions after having earlier struck down a comparable state law. Meanwhile, anti-abortion groups

Continued on p. 736

Chronology

Before 1970

Abortion is illegal in most states; reform movement forms, advances in 1950s, '60s.

1970s-1990s

Supreme Court establishes constitutional right to abortion; decision ignites political battles; court upholds some restrictions, strikes down others.

1973
Supreme Court's landmark *Roe v. Wade* decision establishes qualified right to abortion; 7-2 ruling guarantees right to abortion in first trimester of pregnancy, permits regulation of procedure in second trimester and allows a ban in final trimester as long as exceptions are permitted for woman's life or health.

1977, 1980
Supreme Court rules that states, federal government can deny Medicaid funding for abortion for poor women.

1980s
Supreme Court upholds some abortion regulations, strikes down others; four justices vote to overrule *Roe v. Wade* in 1989, one vote short of majority. . . . Abortion rates begin to decline after all-time high in 1985.

1992
Three-justice plurality provide pivotal votes for reaffirming *Roe v. Wade* while permitting state regulations as long as they do not impose "undue burden" on woman's right to abortion.

1996, 1997
President Bill Clinton vetoes bills passed by Congress to ban "partial-birth abortions."

2000-Present

Abortion rate continues to decline in United States; Bush appointments to Supreme Court shift balance on abortion; Obama's health-care plan is entangled in abortion politics.

2000
Supreme Court strikes down Nebraska law banning late-term or "partial-birth" abortions; Justice Sandra Day O'Connor says modified law might be upheld.

2003
Congress passes and President George W. Bush signs federal ban on "partial-birth" abortions.

2005
President Bush chooses two past critics of *Roe v. Wade* for Supreme Court vacancies: John G. Roberts Jr. as chief justice and Samuel A. Alito Jr. as associate justice, succeeding O'Connor.

2006
South Dakota voters repeal abortion ban passed by legislature; two years later, voters similarly reject effort to enact law through voter initiative.

2007
Roberts and Alito provide pivotal votes in Supreme Court decision to uphold federal ban on partial-birth abortions; majority opinion says medical dispute on procedure eliminates need for health exception in law.

2008
Democrat Barack Obama elected president; took pro-choice positions in campaign; Democrats gain House, Senate seats, but both chambers are closely divided between pro-choice and pro-life blocs.

2009
Obama takes modest pro-choice steps in first months in office; makes health-care overhaul major domestic priority. . . . States continue to enact anti-abortion measures; ambitious Arizona, Oklahoma laws blocked by federal courts in fall. . . . Abortion emerges as major sticking point on Obama's health-care overhaul; House votes 240-194 to bar abortion coverage in any publicly subsidized health insurance; Senate leaders accept less stringent restriction to gain 60th vote needed for passage.

2010
House passes Senate's health-care bill without changes after anti-abortion lawmakers are promised an executive order to tighten anti-abortion provisions (March 23); Obama issues executive order next day. . . . Several states consider, some enact bills to opt out of health-care plan, bar abortion coverage in planned insurance exchanges; five states, including Oklahoma and Louisiana, also pass laws to require women to have access to sonograms before abortion. . . . Guttmacher Institute data show abortion rate in the United States is at lowest level since 1975. . . . Nebraska legislature approves precedent-testing law to ban abortion after 20th week of pregnancy because fetus is capable of feeling pain by that point; abortion rights groups say bill is unconstitutional, weigh possible challenge before law takes effect on Oct. 15. . . . Midterm elections on Nov. 2 could shift balance on abortion issues in Congress.

Anti-Abortion Groups Cite Fetal Pain

New Nebraska law says fetuses feel pain at 20th week.

Abortion proponents and opponents as well as medical professionals strongly disagree about when a fetus feels pain.

Lawmakers in Nebraska have already enacted tougher abortion restrictions based on the belief that a fetus can feel pain as early as the 20th week of gestation. The state's Pain Capable Unborn Child Protection Act prohibits performing abortions after 20 weeks except for the most extreme conditions — such as if giving birth were to threaten the mother's life — and requires that women before having abortions be screened for mental health or other problems. The law goes into effect on Oct. 15.

"Nebraska does have an interest in protecting unborn lives when it can be established that the baby feels pain," said Speaker of the House Mike Flood. [1]

Anti-abortion groups say the law is grounded in credible scientific research conducted since the Supreme Court's landmark *Roe v. Wade* decision legalized abortion, with certain restrictions, in 1973.

"It is time our laws caught up with our science — all human beings are persons and deserve equal rights," says Johanna Dasteel, senior congressional liaison for the American Life League, a grassroots Catholic pro-life organization in Virginia. "And it is the purpose of our laws to recognize and protect these rights for the weakest and most vulnerable among us — especially those in the womb."

Nebraska's new law is likely to end up in the Supreme Court because it challenges one of the principal tenets of *Roe v. Wade*: that abortion is legal until the "viability" of the fetus, or its ability to live outside the womb, generally held to begin at 22 to 24 weeks. Nebraska is likely to ask the high court to take into account research conducted since *Roe*, and push the legal threshold back further.

When *Roe* was decided, it was widely believed that the nervous systems of even newborns were too immature to feel pain, and doctors didn't use anesthesia during surgical operations on newborns. Twenty-five years ago, however, Kanwaljeet Anand of Oxford University noticed that babies coming to his neonatal intensive care unit after surgery were exhibiting massive stress responses, indicating they had experienced pain. His research into the phenomenon shifted medical opinion, and today's most premature newborns are given anesthesia during surgery. [2]

"It is as early as 20 weeks, and there is data that shows 16 weeks and even earlier, many of these infants feel pain and have negative outcomes from it," Jean Wright, chair of pediatrics at the Mercer School of Medicine in Georgia, told the House Judiciary Committee. [3]

"We're speaking to more and more professionals who are looking at the latest research, the latest from the medical community and the shift we're seeing is an acknowledgment of the preborn child as another patient," says Dasteel. "More medical professionals are seeing the inherent injustice of a procedure that would deprive a human being, their patient, of a fundamental human right — the right to life."

The research, however, is far from conclusive. In June, the Royal College of Obstetricians and Gynaecologists in London reported there is no evidence showing fetuses feel pain in the womb prior to 24 weeks, suggesting no need to scale back abortion limits in the United States.

"Although we may speculate that these [pain-sensitive] regions [of the brain] will also be functionally active from 24 weeks, similar to primary sensory cortex, there is no evidence for this at the moment," the report suggests. [4]

"That report comes up with the conclusion that the fetus doesn't feel pain, suggesting that the justification for the Nebraska law isn't correct," says Tracy Weitz, director of the Advancing New Standards in Reproductive Health program at the University of California, San Francisco. "We continue to misuse science to justify new regulations on abortion and whittle down the Supreme Court decision in *Roe v. Wade*, instead of focusing on the larger ethical issue of whether or not a woman can terminate her pregnancy."

— Darrell Dela Rosa

[1] Dan Harris, *et al.*, "Nebraska Passes Controversial Abortion Ban," ABC News, April 13, 2010, abcnews.go.com/WN/Supreme_Court/nebraska-passes-controversial-abortion-ban/story?id=10361705.

[2] Marc A. Thiessen, "Bringing Humanity Back to the Abortion Debate," *The Washington Post*, April 19, 2010, www.washingtonpost.com/wp-dyn/content/article/2010/04/19/AR2010041902082.html.

[3] "Pain of the Unborn," House Judiciary Committee, Nov. 1, 2005, ftp.resource.org/gpo.gov/hearings/109h/24284.pdf.

[4] "Fetal Awareness: Review of Research and Recommendations for Practice," Royal College of Obstetricians and Gynaecologists, March 2010, www.rcog.org.uk/files/rcog-corp/RCOGFetalAwarenessWPR0610.pdf.

Continued from p. 734

won enactment of new restrictions at the state level and claimed the laws were helping to reduce the overall number of abortions.

Clinton's election in 1992 put an abortion-rights supporter in the White House for the first time in 12 years, along with a Democratic-controlled Congress. Within days of taking office in 1993, Clinton rescinded some anti-abortion policies, including a Reagan-era ban on abortion counseling at federally funded clinics that the Supreme Court had upheld in 1991. The next year, Congress passed and Clinton signed into law the Freedom of Access to Clinic Entrances Act, aimed at thwarting anti-abortion groups' blockades of women's health clinics. In his first two years in office, Clinton also strengthened the abortion-rights majority on the Supreme Court with the appointment of two pro-choice justices, Ruth Bader Ginsburg and Stephen G. Breyer.

Bush's election in 2000, along with the GOP's continued control of Congress since the 1994 midterm election, resulted in some anti-abortion regulatory and legislative initiatives. Bush in 2001 restored a Reagan-era directive — the so-called Mexico City policy — that bars foreign recipients of State Department-administered family-planning grants from performing abortions or counseling women about abortions. Bush did not, however, attempt to reimpose the ban on abortion counseling at federally funded clinics within the United States. The administration also pleased anti-abortion groups with a regulation defining a fetus as a "child" eligible for government-subsidized health care. Most significantly, Bush in his second term appointed two members of the Supreme Court — Chief Justice John G. Roberts Jr. and Justice Samuel A. Alito Jr. — who both had criticized *Roe v. Wade* while serving in the Justice Department during the Reagan administration.

The Supreme Court became the focal point of perhaps the most emotional issue of the two decades: the effort to ban an infrequent, late-term procedure that anti-abortion groups labeled "partial birth abortions." The procedure — in medical terms, an "intact dilation and extraction" or D&E — entails the partial delivery of the fetus from the uterus before being aborted. Through the 1990s, anti-abortion forces won passage of laws banning the procedure in around 30 states; Congress approved a comparable ban, but Clinton vetoed the measure. In 2000, however, the Supreme Court ruled one of the laws, Nebraska's, unconstitutional in a 5-4 decision. The majority faulted the definition of the procedure as too broad and the failure to include an exception to permit the procedure if necessary to protect the woman's health. In a concurring opinion, O'Connor said a narrower law might pass constitutional muster.

With Bush in the White House, the GOP-controlled Congress passed a federal ban modified somewhat to accommodate the Supreme Court decision but again with no exception for a woman's health. The constitutional challenge to the law reached the court in 2007 after Alito had succeeded O'Connor. With Alito casting the decisive vote, the court upheld the federal law in a 5-4 ruling. For the majority, Kennedy said the ban did not extend to more common D&E procedures. He went on to conclude that no health exception was needed because of the debate over whether the specific procedure was ever medically necessary. For the dissenters, Ginsburg said the ruling contradicted a basic premise of *Roe v. Wade* — requiring a health exception in any legislation banning late-term abortions. [16]

As Bush prepared to leave office in 2008, anti-abortion groups were touting their successes outside Washington in passing restrictive legislation in the states. Americans United for Life claimed success in "a systematic and strategic effort" in the states to enact laws that provided immediate "incremental gains" while "laying the groundwork for much larger gains in the future." From the opposite perspective, NARAL Pro-Choice America criticized what it called the "relentless attacks on a woman's right to choose in legislatures throughout the country." [17]

Anti-abortion advocates failed, however, in their most ambitious attempt: an effort in South Dakota to write into law an outright ban on abortions that would directly challenge *Roe v. Wade*. The measure won approval from the South Dakota legislature in 2006 only to be repealed in a referendum in November. Two years later, anti-abortion forces proposed a similar measure by initiative, but it went down to defeat at the polls in November 2008.

Health Care Battle

Barack Obama won the presidency in November 2008 after a campaign that put health care reform at the top of his domestic-policy agenda. Abortion financing and funding proved to be a major hurdle for the administration in the protracted health care fight in Congress. Obama secured final passage of legislation in March 2010 only after promising anti-abortion Democrats to issue an executive order aimed at ensuring no federal funding or insurance subsidies for abortions. Anti-abortion groups remained dissatisfied even as abortion rights advocates denounced the restrictions. Meanwhile, states continued to enact new abortion restrictions, including several that acted to bar coverage for abortion in the insurance exchanges to be established under the federal legislation by 2014.

Abortion was not a major issue in the 2008 presidential campaign, but Obama and his Republican opponent, John McCain, took diametrically opposite positions on the topic. Obama supported *Roe v. Wade*, while McCain called for overruling the decision; McCain supported the partial-birth abortion ban, while Obama opposed banning the procedure without a health exception. [18] Along with Obama's election, Democrats increased the majorities they had gained in the House and Senate in 2006. But NARAL depicted both chambers as somewhat evenly balanced between pro- and anti-choice members with "mixed choice" lawmakers holding the balance of power in each. The 2008 elections left a comparable balance of power in the states, NARAL said. Out of 100 legislative chambers, 33 were rated as having pro-choice majorities, 44 with anti-choice majorities and 23 as "mixed choice." [19]

Once in office, Obama pleased abortion rights advocates by rescinding the Mexico City policy restricting aid to family-planning organizations overseas. The administration proposed but has not yet adopted a regulation to ease the late Bush administration directive allowing health care workers to refuse to provide abortion counseling or referrals on religious grounds. In Congress, abortion rights advocates similarly put pro-choice initiatives on a back burner in deference to the significant number of anti-abortion lawmakers in Democratic ranks. The Democratic leadership left unchanged the Hyde Amendment's restrictions on abortion funding — enacted annually as an appropriations rider. And sponsors decided not to press for action on a bill, the Freedom of Choice Act, aimed at codifying in federal law the right to abortion established in *Roe v. Wade*. [20]

Congressional leaders' efforts to skirt the abortion issue fell victim to the need to satisfy anti-abortion Democrats whose votes were needed to get a health care overhaul through both the House and the Senate. In the House, Democrat Bart Stupak of Michigan, chairman of the Congressional Pro-Life Caucus, proposed an amendment to bar any coverage for abortion in the publicly subsidized health insurance plans to be created. Stupak's amendment was approved on Nov. 7, 2009, by a vote of 240-194, with 64 Democrats voting for it. In the Senate, Nebraska Democrat Ben Nelson agreed to provide the needed 60th vote for that chamber's health care bill only after a less restrictive provision was added that merely requires abortion coverage in federally subsidized insurance plans to be paid for through separate, non-subsidized premiums. [21]

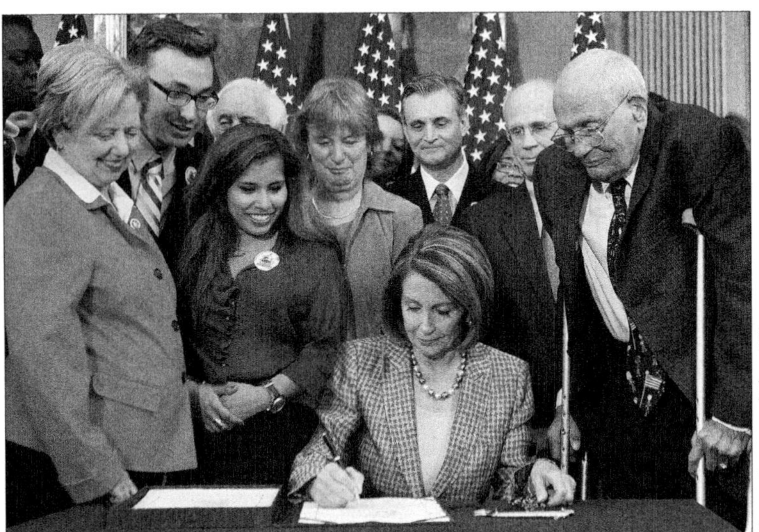

Getty Images/Alex Wong

Speaker of the House Nancy Pelosi, D-Calif., signs the revised Health Care and Education Reconciliation Act, flanked by other House members. To pass the bill, Pelosi negotiated a compromise with Rep. Bart Stupak, D-Mich., who had proposed an amendment to bar any insurance coverage for abortion in the publicly subsidized health insurance plans to be created by the legislation.

When the Senate bill was brought to the House floor, Stupak wanted to insist on his more restrictive provision. But any amendment to the Senate bill threatened to delay or even derail final passage. House Speaker Nancy Pelosi, D-Calif., worked hard to peel off some of Stupak's supporters, eventually forcing Stupak to settle for a compromise. The Nelson amendment would stay in the final bill, but Obama would issue an executive order to specify no federal funding for abortions. With that agreement, the House passed the health care bill on March 21 by the barest of margins: 219-212. And Obama issued the executive order three days later, on March 24, just one day after signing the bill itself. [22]

In the states, meanwhile, anti-abortion forces continued to win enactment of new restrictions that abortion-rights advocates challenged in court, with some success. In 2009, NARAL counted enactment of 29 anti-choice measures, bringing the total since 1995 to 610. (In its compilation, Americans United for Life counted 60 pro-life measures in 2009.) Two of the most ambitious of the laws, however, were blocked from going into effect by state court judges.

In Arizona, Maricopa County Superior Court Judge Donald Daughton in Phoenix issued a preliminary injunction in September 2009 blocking several provisions of an anti-abortion law, including specifications that a physician personally inform a patient of risks of complications from the procedure. Daughton said lawyers for Planned Parenthood had demonstrated a "substantial likelihood" of prevailing on the merits and that women faced the possibility of "irreparable injury" if the law were to go into effect. The ruling is on appeal. [23]

In Oklahoma, Oklahoma County District Judge Dan Owens ruled on Feb. 19 that an omnibus measure passed in 2009 violated the state constitution's "single-subject" rule for legislation. Among the law's several provisions was a requirement to report a patient's age, education and marital status to the state's health department. Another provision prohibited an abortion requested based on sex selection of the fetus. The state did not appeal the decision, but Oklahoma legislators in 2010 split the law into separate bills and passed most of them again. [24] ■

CURRENT SITUATION

Court Battles

Abortion rights groups are still mulling whether to challenge Nebraska's new "fetal pain" law banning abortions after the 20th week of pregnancy, even as they are winning court rulings blocking other new anti-abortion measures from going into effect.

Planned Parenthood and the Center for Reproductive Rights both call the new law unconstitutional because it bans abortions outright before the accepted standard for determining when a fetus can survive outside the womb. But with the law set to take effect on Oct. 15, both organizations were still saying in early September that no decision has been made on whether to file a federal court challenge to the law.

The wait-and-see posture persists even as Planned Parenthood's Nebraska chapter is celebrating a final court ruling striking down the state's other newly enacted anti-abortion measure, which had sought to impose elaborate screening requirements for women before an abortion. The state's attorney general, Jon Bruning, had set the stage for the court victory by announcing on Aug. 15 that the state would not contest a federal judge's decision a month earlier to issue a preliminary injunction against the law.

Bruning said the state was likely to lose the case and end up paying legal fees for Planned Parenthood's lawyers. "We will not squander the state's resources on a case that has very little probability of winning," Bruning's spokeswoman, Shannon Kingery, said. [25]

The law — sometimes identified by its bill number, LB 594 — had expanded a previous requirement for "voluntary and informed" consent before an abortion by requiring a health care worker to evaluate whether a woman was being pressured or coerced to agree to the procedure. In addition, the physician would have been required to inform the woman of any abortion-related "complications" or "risk factors" identified in any peer-reviewed publication and to certify that the patient faced only a "negligible" risk of suffering such a complication.

In her 35-page ruling on July 14 granting a preliminary injunction against the law, U.S. District Judge Laurie Smith Camp said the bill created "substantial, likely insurmountable, obstacles in the path of women seeking abortions in Nebraska." She also concluded the law was unconstitutionally vague. Camp made the injunction permanent on Aug. 24 after Bruning's office and Planned Parenthood's lawyers agreed on the terms. [26]

Flood, sponsor of the fetal pain law, says he approves of Bruning's move. "If the legislature wants to redesign LB 594, I think that's a better approach than spending taxpayer dollars in fighting a case in court that won't be successful," Flood says. "I think he made a good decision."

Flood says he had expected a challenge to his fetal-pain bill but is now uncertain because of the noncommittal stance by abortion rights groups. The likely plaintiff in a suit, LeRoy Carhart, an abortion provider in the Omaha suburb of Bellevue and plaintiff in previous cases challenging partial-birth abortion laws, is making no comment but referring media calls to the Center for Reproductive Rights, which represented him in the previous cases. As of early September, Dionne Scott, the center's spokeswoman, says no decision has been made about challenging the law.

In Washington, National Right to Life Committee state director Balch says anti-abortion groups are wary of contesting the law. "I think this is a debate that they do not want to have," says Balch. "They don't want the American people discussing whether an unborn child at 20 weeks in the womb is capable of feeling pain."

"We welcome debate on this or any other restriction on a woman's fundamental rights," replies Janet Crepps, deputy director of the center's U.S. legal program, "but we do not discuss legal strategy in public."

Lawyers from the center are representing abortion providers in Oklahoma and Louisiana in challenging those states' newly enacted ultrasound laws. The Oklahoma law would require a physician to display and describe an ultrasound for a patient before an abortion, although the woman could avert her eyes from the image. The Louisiana law included a provision requiring a physician to give a copy of an ultrasound to a woman along with separate provisions that the woman be offered a description of the image.

The Oklahoma law is now on hold following a July 19 preliminary injunction issued by Oklahoma County District Court Judge Norma Gurich. The injunction will remain in effect at least until the next scheduled hearing on Jan. 21. [27]

In Louisiana, U.S. District Judge Ralph Tyson in New Orleans issued a preliminary injunction against the mandatory provision of the ultrasound law on Aug. 11 after the state's attorneys agreed not to enforce it. The other parts of the law went into effect on Aug, 15. The center is continuing to challenge a separate law that denies abortion providers the liability protections afforded physicians under the state's medical malpractice law. [28]

Washington Fights

Abortion politics flares up regularly in the nation's capital, with pro-life and pro-choice groups clashing most recently over the Food and

Four in 10 Unintended Pregnancies Are Aborted

Nearly half of pregnancies among American women are unintended, and four in 10 of these are terminated by abortion.

Twenty-two percent of all pregnancies end in abortion.

Forty percent of unintended pregnancies are terminated by abortion.

Each year 2 percent of women ages 15-44 have an abortion.

Women in their 20s account for 57% of all abortions.

Teenagers account for 18% of abortions.

Women who have never married and are not cohabiting account for 45% of abortions.

Three-fourths of women who have an abortion say they cannot afford a child; or that a baby would interfere with work, school or caring for other dependents.

Forty-two percent of women obtaining abortions have incomes below the poverty level.

Source: "Facts on Induced Abortion In the United States," Guttmacher Institute, May 2010

Drug Administration's decision to approve a new "emergency contraceptive" for use in the United States.

Abortion rights groups hailed the FDA's decision on Aug. 13 to approve the prescription drug being marketed under the name Ella, which has been shown to prevent pregnancy if taken as long as five days after unprotected sexual intercourse. But anti-abortion groups sharply criticized the decision, claiming that the drug is unsafe for women and that its use amounts to an abortion. [29]

The regulatory decision is one of many issues where anti-abortion groups have lined up against the Obama administration in the past two years. Anti-abortion groups were among the most vocal opponents of President Obama's Supreme Court nominee, Elena Kagan, who won Senate confirmation in a mostly party-line vote on Aug. 5. They fought against congressional passage of Obama's health care reform law and are now calling for its repeal. And they strongly oppose the administration's liberalized rules on use of human embryos in stem cell research, which a federal judge struck down on Aug. 23.

Abortion rights groups have generally lined up in support of Obama administration policies, but they have voiced deep disappointment with the administration's concession to anti-abortion lawmakers on provisions in the health care overhaul. "Do we agree with every single action by the administration? No," says NARAL policy director Crane. "Do we expect to keep the pressure on even our friends? Yes. That's our job."

Ella becomes the second emergency contraceptive approved by the FDA following the agency's approval of Plan B in 1999. Plan B originally required a prescription, but the Bush administration in 2006 approved its sale to women 17 years of age or older without a prescription. It prevents pregnancy if used within three days after sex.

The new drug, manufactured by the French company HRA Pharma, will require a prescription for any users. It will be sold in the United States by Watson Pharmaceuticals beginning sometime in October; the company has not announced the price to be charged.

Both drugs operate by interfering with the hormone progesterone, which is crucial for pregnancy. The abortifacent RU-486, which the FDA approved for use by prescription in the United States in 2000, similarly represses progesterone. It is effective within the first two months of pregnancy. These so-called medical abortions accounted for about 13 percent of all abortions in the United States in 2005, according to the Guttmacher Institute. [30]

The FDA's approval of Ella followed the recommendation by an independent advisory panel in mid-July. Abortion rights groups hailed both actions as giving women an additional option for preventing an unplanned pregnancy. "Emergency-contraception options like ella are a safe, effective back-up method when something goes wrong, such as if a condom breaks, or in tragic situations when a woman is sexually assaulted," said Keenan, president of NARAL Pro-Choice America.

Anti-abortion groups denounced the FDA's action. Charmaine Yoest, a physician and president of Americans United for Life, called the FDA's action "irresponsible" because the agency had not required sufficient studies of the drug's use on women's health.

Anti-abortion groups argue that emergency contraceptives in fact are equivalent to abortifacents. "Women deserve to be fully informed that Ella may interfere with and kill a developing embryo and does not only prevent conception," AUL says.

Continued on p. 742

At Issue:

Can the fetus feel pain before the 24th week of pregnancy?

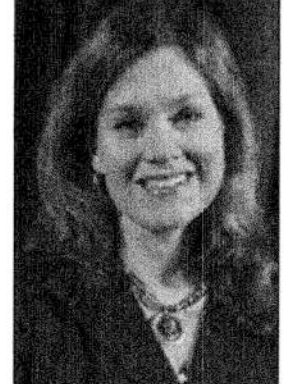

JEANNE MONAHAN
DIRECTOR, CENTER FOR HUMAN DIGNITY, FAMILY RESEARCH COUNCIL

WRITTEN FOR *CQ RESEARCHER*, SEPT. 5, 2010

The abortion industry is clamoring to draw attention to a report released earlier this summer by the UK's Royal College of Obstetricians and Gynaecologists (RCOG), in which a false and alarming conclusion was made, "that a fetus cannot feel pain before 24 weeks because the connections in the fetal brain are not fully formed." Note that the claim that fetuses cannot feel pain prior to 24 weeks of development very much hinges on how one defines "feeling pain." RCOG claimed that in order for a human being to have the sensation of pain, a person's cortex must be fully developed.

On the contrary, a wealth of scientific research suggests otherwise. For example, a number of studies show that early second-trimester babies respond to invasive procedures performed at 18-20 weeks with an elevated heart rate and secretion of stress hormones. Bjorn Merker, a Swedish neuroscientist who has done extensive research on children born without fully developed cortexes, has suggested that the cortex may not be necessary for the perception of pain. He wrote: "The tacit consensus concerning the cerebral cortex as the organ of consciousness may have been reached prematurely, and may be seriously in error."

Some scientists would even offer that children as young as 20-30 weeks of development can feel pain more severely than full-term or newborn babies. It is during this stage in the mother's womb that a fetus has the highest number of pain receptors per square inch. Fibers that help moderate pain do not begin to develop until 32-34 weeks. In the words of fetal pain expert Kanwaljeet Anand of Oxford University, "the human fetus possesses the ability to experience pain from 20 weeks of gestation, if not earlier and the pain perceived by a fetus is possibly more intense than that perceived by term newborns or children."

The truth is that abortion proponents are uncomfortable with the concept of fetal pain. They continually try to debunk the wealth of scientific research upon which it stands, not because the evidence is lacking, but because an understanding of fetal pain destroys their strategy of portraying an unborn baby as a lifeless blob of tissue.

The concept of fetal pain exposes the stark reality that abortion takes the life of a developing person; a person who will live, breathe, have emotions and, yes, feel pain (long before 24 weeks of development).

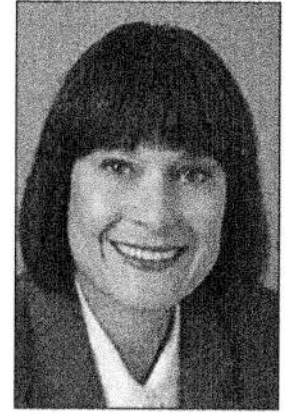

VICKI SAPORTA
PRESIDENT, NATIONAL ABORTION FEDERATION

WRITTEN FOR *CQ RESEARCHER*, SEPT. 5, 2010

Although abortion opponents often use arguments about fetal pain to advance an anti-choice political agenda, the body of scientific evidence clearly demonstrates that a fetus is incapable of feeling pain prior to the 24th week of gestation, and possibly throughout pregnancy.

As the professional association of abortion providers in North America, the National Abortion Federation (NAF) is committed to ensuring that women seeking reproductive health care receive the highest quality care, which includes accurate and complete information integral to their health care decisions. As such, we believe this information must be based on scientific evidence.

Earlier this year, the Royal College of Obstetricians and Gynaecologists (RCOG) published a report commissioned by the British government entitled "Fetal Awareness: Review of Research and Recommendations for Practice," which reviewed the latest evidence and found that "the fetus cannot experience pain in any sense" prior to 24 weeks gestation.

As the RCOG report explains in a chapter addressed to women and parents, "to be aware of something or have pain, the body has to have developed special sensory structures and a joined-up nerve system between the brain and the rest of the body to communicate such a feeling. Although the framework for the nervous system in the growing fetus occurs early, it actually develops very slowly. Current research shows that the sensory structures are not developed or specialised enough to experience pain in a fetus less than 24 weeks."

The RCOG report also states that "after 24 weeks, it is difficult to say that the fetus experiences pain because this, like all other experiences, develops postnatally along with memory and other learned behaviours. In addition, increasing evidence suggests that the fetus never enters a state of wakefulness inside the womb. The placenta produces chemicals that suppress nervous system activity and awareness."

Those who argue that a fetus can feel pain at 20 weeks do so contrary to credible scientific evidence and without support from leading international experts. Their goals are to dissuade women from choosing abortion and to pass legislation that restricts women's access to abortion care.

Women deserve the facts, not inflammatory, unsubstantiated rhetoric. Responsible medicine requires that patients and doctors make treatment decisions together, based on medically accurate, unbiased information.

Continued from p. 740

Abortion rights groups vigorously disagree. "Emergency contraception prevents a pregnancy," says NARAL's Keenan. "It does not cause abortion." [31]

Anti-abortion groups are also the leading critics of the administration's decision in March 2009 to allow use of stem cells harvested from discarded embryos for use in federally funded research. They are praising a federal judge's ruling on Aug. 23 to strike down guidelines issued by the National Institutes of Health (NIH) as violating a 1996 law intended to prevent the destruction of embryos. [32]

The law, first passed by Congress in 1996 and renewed annually since, prohibits NIH from funding research in which embryos "are destroyed, discarded, or knowingly subjected to risk of injury or death." The Bush administration eased the restriction somewhat in 2001 by permitting research using previously created lines of stem cells. In March 2009, Obama directed NIH to ease the restrictions further by permitting use of stem cells obtained after embryonic destruction — most commonly, embryos discarded during in vitro fertilization.

In his 15-page ruling, Chief U.S. District Judge Royce Lamberth in Washington, D.C., said the policy violated Congress' "unambiguous intent" to prohibit any use of federal funds on research with cells from destroyed embryos. The ruling came in a suit filed on behalf of two scientists by the Alliance Defense Fund, a conservative public-interest law firm that has been involved in anti-abortion litigation.

Yoest said the ruling "reconfirms what we already knew, that administration policy is in violation of the law." Abortion rights groups have not been vocal on the issue. But NIH officials and research groups warned the decision could effectively shut down stem cell research and its potential for treating currently untreatable diseases and conditions. The Justice Department says it will appeal. ■

OUTLOOK

'Fatigue Factor'?

Archbishop George Lucas spent a recent Saturday afternoon leading 200 of Omaha's faithful in prayer at a construction site in a shopping center along one of the city's major arteries. Their mission: prevent Planned Parenthood of the Heartland from completing its construction of the city's third abortion clinic.

"Women and their unborn children deserve better than to suffer the violence of abortion," Lucas said in a pastoral statement issued a few days before the July 31 vigil. "Please pray," the prelate concluded, "for a greater respect for all human life, from conception to natural death."

Planned Parenthood says it is proceeding with plans for the fall opening of the clinic, which will offer women cancer screenings, annual exams, birth control and adoption referrals as well as abortion services. "Abortion has been a legal medical service in the United States for well over 30 years," says June, the group's president. "And it is important that women have access to safe and legal abortions because when they do not, they suffer and die from illegal and unsafe abortions." [33]

The episode points to the continuing divide between abortion rights and anti-abortion activists, but it also suggests the limited effectiveness of tactics on both sides. The women's clinic is apparently destined for completion, with hearts and minds on both sides seemingly unchanged.

In much the same way, the abortion wars appear now to be at a kind of stalemate, with only marginal gains by one side or the other in legislative arenas, in courtrooms or in the court of public opinion. And some evidence suggests that the public at large is weary of the fight and either in support of or reconciled to the ambivalent status quo in which abortion is a legal right that can be regulated more or less closely depending on the prevailing political climate.

In their analysis of polling data, the Pew centers on religion and public opinion note that fewer Americans all across the ideological spectrum today list abortion as a critical issue than their counterparts did in 2006. Overall, about 13 percent of respondents to an ABC News/*Washington Post* survey listed abortion as a critical issue in August 2009 compared to 28 percent in March 2006. The decline is especially sharp among liberal Democrats — from 34 percent in 2006 to 8 percent in 2009 — but smaller drops were also found among conservative and moderate Republicans, independents and moderate Democrats. [34]

Whatever lack of engagement in the public at large, activists on both sides are mobilizing and digging in for more fights, especially in the states. "The states are doing well," says Balch with the National Right to Life Committee. "They're very active in passing protective legislation." NARAL communications director Ted Miller says "anti-choice attacks" are likely to continue at their current level — and could increase "depending on what happens in the 2010 elections."

In Washington, too, the midterm congressional elections in November could reshape abortion politics somewhat. The widely expected Republican gains in the House could strengthen anti-abortion sentiment in the lower chamber. Likely GOP gains in the Senate could also make the upper chamber somewhat friendlier to anti-abortion initiatives.

Still, with an abortion rights supporter in the White House, freestanding anti-abortion initiatives face a possible presidential veto. And, as the FDA's emergency contraceptive decision indicates, the administration can execute some pro-choice policies without any need for congressional approval.

The Supreme Court, which might have to rule on the constitutionality of Nebraska's fetal-pain bill, remains precariously divided on abortion-related issues. Kagan is widely expected to join three other liberal justices in supporting abortion rights, but she replaces a strong pro-choice justice, John Paul Stevens.

Among conservatives, Antonin Scalia and Clarence Thomas remain willing to overrule *Roe*, while Roberts' and Alito's votes on the partial-birth abortion ban show their willingness at least to narrow existing precedents. That leaves the balance of power with Kennedy, who has voted to uphold virtually all abortion regulations before the court even in the pivotal 1992 decision where he joined in reaffirming *Roe*'s "essential holding."

Over time, however, the political and legal battles are likely to become less significant, according to Jean Reith Schroedel, a professor at Claremont Graduate University in Pomona, Calif., who cites "a certain fatigue factor."

"People are tired," Schroedel says. "For some people, it's been decades that they have been hearing about abortion from both sides that the sky is falling, the sky is falling — and the sky hasn't fallen on either side." ■

About the Author

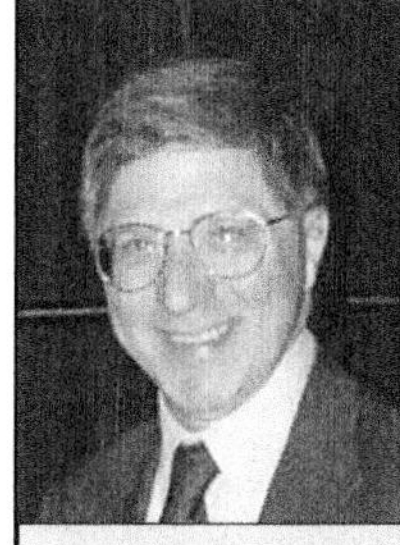

Associate Editor **Kenneth Jost** graduated from Harvard College and Georgetown University Law Center. He is the author of the *Supreme Court Yearbook* and editor of *The Supreme Court from A to Z* (both *CQ Press*). He was a member of the *CQ Researcher* team that won the American Bar Association's 2002 Silver Gavel Award. His previous reports include "Abortion Showdowns" (with Kathy Koch). He is also author of the blog *Jost on Justice* (http://jostonjustice.blogspot.com).

Notes

[1] The text of the Nebraska law and its legislative history can be found on the Nebraska legislature's Website: www.nebraskalegislature.gov/bills/view_bill.php?DocumentID=10024. For coverage, see Nate Jenkins, "Neb. governor signs landmark abortion bills," The Associated Press, April 14, 2010; JoAnne Young, "Governor signs first-of-kind abortion laws," *Lincoln Journal Star*, April 14, 2010, p. A1. The Supreme Court cases are *Gonzales v. Carhart*, 550 U.S. 124 (2007); *Roe v. Wade*, 410 U.S. 113 (1973).

[2] For an overview of the issues, see FactCheck.org, "The Abortion Issue," April 1, 2010, www.factcheck.org/2010/04/the-abortion-issue/. For background on the health-care law, see Marcia Clemmitt, "Health-Care Reform," *CQ Researcher*, June 11, 2010, pp. 505-528.

[3] For background, see these *CQ Researcher* reports: Kenneth Jost and Kathy Koch, "Abortion Showdowns," Sept. 22, 2006, pp. 769-792; Kenneth Jost, "Abortion Debates," March 21, 2003, pp. 249-272; Sarah Glazer, "Roe v. Wade at 25," Nov. 28, 1997, pp. 1033-1056.

[4] Lydia Saad, "More Americans 'Pro-Life' Than 'Pro-Choice' for First Time," Gallup Poll, May 15, 2009, www.gallup.com/poll/118399/more-americans-pro-life-than-pro-choice-first-time.aspx; *Post*-ABC poll cited in "Support for Abortion Slips," from 2009 "Annual Religion and Public Life Survey," Pew Forum on Religion and Public Life/Pew Research Center on the People and the Press, Oct. 1, 2009, http://pewforum.org/uploadedfiles/Topics/Issues/Abortion/abortion09.pdf.

[5] "Facts on Induced Abortion in the United States," Guttmacher Institute, May 2010, www.guttmacher.org/pubs/fb_induced_abortion.pdf.

[6] *Ibid*.

[7] "Executive Order: Ensuring Enforcement and Implementation of Abortion Restrictions in the Patient Protection and Affordable Care Act," March 24, 2010, www.whitehouse.gov/the-press-office/executive-order-patient-protection-and-affordable-care-acts-consistency-with-longst. Peter Nicholas and James Oliphant, "Little cheer about deal on abortion;" *Los Angeles Times*, March 25, 2010, p. A9.

[8] Johnson quoted in Mimi Hall, "Both sides of abortion issue dismiss presidential order," *USA Today*, March 25, 2010, p. 10A; Saporta quoted in Rob Stein, "Order on abortion care angers core backers," *The Washington Post*, March 25, 2010, p. A8.

[9] See Julian Pecquet, "Abortion coverage restricted in high-risk insurance pools," Healthwatch: THE HILL's health care blog, July 29, 2010, http://thehill.com/blogs/healthwatch/health-reform-implementation/111615-obama-administration-restricts-abortion-coverage-in-high-risk-pools.

[10] Quoted in Steven Ertelt, "Mississippi Governor Haley Barbour Signs Health Care Abortion Funding Opt Out," LifeNews.com, May 24, 2010, www.lifenews.com/state5119.html. For earlier coverage, see Elizabeth Crisp, "Abortion measure sent to governor," *The Clarion-Ledger* (Jackson, Miss.), April 29, 2010, p. B1.

[11] See Adam Sonfeld, *et al.*, "U.S. Insurance Coverage of Contraceptives and the Impact of Contraceptive Coverage Mandates, 2002," *Perspectives on Sexual and Reproductive Health*, Vol. 36, No. 2 (March/April 2004), p. 75, www.guttmacher.org/pubs/psrh/full/3607204.pdf.

[12] John Frank and Lee Logan, "Crist Vetoes Abortion Bill," *St. Petersburg Times*, June 12, 2010, p. 1A; a different version appeared the same day in *The Miami Herald*. *Times* reporter Frank and *Herald* reporter Logan work together in the *Herald/Times* joint Tallahassee bureau.

[13] Background drawn in part from N.E.H. Hull and Peter Charles Hoffer, Roe v. Wade: *The Abortion Rights Controversy in American History* (2000).

[14] For a compact summary of Supreme Court abortion decisions through 2000, see Kenneth Jost, "Abortion," in Clare Cushman (ed.), *Supreme Court Decisions and Women's Rights* (2001), pp. 188-206.

[15] The Supreme Court decisions are *Maher v. Roe*, 432 U.S. 464 (1977) and *Harris v. McRae*, 448 U.S. 297 (1980). For current state laws, see National Conference of State Legislatures, "Abortion Laws," www.ncsl.org/default.aspx?tabid=14401.

[16] The decision is *Gonzales v. Carhart*, 550 U.S. 124 (2007). For a full account, see Kenneth Jost, *Supreme Court Yearbook 2006-2007* (2007).

[17] See Americans United for Life, *Defending Life 2009: Proven Strategies for a Pro-Life America* (2009), pp. 45-46; NARAL Pro-Choice America, *Who Decides? The Status of Women's Reproductive Rights in the United States* (January 2009), pp 4-5.

[18] Katherine Seelye, *et al.*, "On the Issues: Social Issues," Election 2008: *The New York Times*, http://elections.nytimes.com/2008/president/issues/abortion.html.

[19] See *Who Decides? op. cit.*, pp. 6-7. NARAL included the District of Columbia Council in its state listing and noted that Nebraska has a unicameral legislature.

[20] James Oliphant, "Abortion laws on Democrats' back burner," *Los Angeles Times*, Feb. 10, 2009, p. A14. NARAL's listing of major federal abortion-related provisions was not changed from 2009 to 2010.

[21] See Drew Armstrong, "2009 Legislative Summary: Health Care Overhaul," *CQ Weekly*, Jan. 4, 2010; Alex Wayne, "2009 Key House Votes: Abortion Funding," *ibid.*

[22] See Clea Benson, "A New Kind of Abortion Politics," *CQ Weekly*, March 29, 2010.

[23] Casey Newton, "New abortion laws halted," *The Arizona Republic*, Sept. 30, 2009, front section, p. 1.

[24] Nolan Clay and Michael McNutt, "Judge overturns abortion statute," *The Oklahoman* (Oklahoma City), Feb. 20, 2010, 1A.

[25] Quoted in Timberly Ross, "Future of Nebraska's other abortion law murky," The Associated Press, Aug. 18, 2010. Some other background taken from account.

[26] The case is *Planned Parenthood v. Heineman*, U.S. District Court-Nebraska, 4:10-cv-03122-LSC-FG3. For coverage, see Josh Funk, "Judge blocks Neb. abortion screening law," The Associated Press, July 14, 2010.

[27] The case is *NOVA Health Systems v. Edmondson*. For coverage see Nolan Clay, "State abortion law on hold," *The Oklahoman* (Oklahoma City), July 20, 2010, p. 9A.

[28] The case is *Hope Medical Group for Women v. Caldwell*. The temporary restraining order is available on the center's Website: http://reproductiverights.org/sites/crr.civicactions.net/files/documents/Order%20granting%20TRO_8.11.10.pdf. For coverage see Ed Anderson, "Abortion laws take effect Sunday," *The Times-Picayune* (New Orleans), Aug. 15, 2010, p. A2.

[29] For coverage, see Rob Stein, "5-day-after contraceptive wins FDA approval," *The Washington Post*, Aug. 14, 2010, p. A1; Gardiner Harris, "U.S. approves a 2d after-sex contraceptive," *The New York Times*, Aug. 13, 2010, p. A1. For background see Marcia Clemmitt, "Birth-Control Debate," *CQ Researcher*, June 24, 2005, pp. 565-588.

[30] Guttmacher Institute, "Facts on Induced Abortion," *op. cit.*

[31] For opposing positions see AUL's Website: www.aul.org/2010/08/yoest-on-approval-of-ella-drug-by-the-fda/; and NARAL's: www.prochoiceamerica.org/media/press-releases/2010/statement-on-fda-approval-of.html.

[32] The decision is *Sherley v. Sebelius*, Civ. No. 1:09-cv-1575 (RCL) (Aug. 23, 2010), https://ecf.dcd.uscourts.gov/cgi-bin/show_public_doc?2009cv1575-44. For coverage see Gardiner Harris, "Judge calls halt to stem cell aid backed by Obama," *The New York Times*, Aug. 24, 2010, p. A1; Rob Stein and Spencer Hsu, "Judge blocks stem cell rules," *The Washington Post*, Aug. 24, 2010, p. A1. For background see Marcia Clemmitt, "Stem Cell Research," *CQ Researcher*, Sept. 1, 2006, pp. 697-720.

[33] See Zack Colman, "Abortion opponents hold vigil," *Omaha World-Herald*, July 31, 2010.

[34] Pew Forum on Religion and Public Life/Pew Research Center for the People and the Press, *op. cit.*, p. 2.

FOR MORE INFORMATION

American Association of Pro-Life Obstetricians and Gynecologists, 339 River Ave., Holland, MI 49423; (616) 546-2639; www.aaplog.org. Special interest group promoting the dignity of human life in all stages of development.

American College of Obstetricians and Gynecologists, P.O. Box 96920, Washington, DC 20090; (202) 638-5577; www.acog.org. Nonprofit organization of women's health-care physicians advocating for the highest standards of practice.

American Life League, P.O. Box 1350, Stafford, VA 22555; (540) 659-4171; www.all.org. Grassroots Catholic pro-life organization opposing all forms of abortion.

Americans United for Life, 655 15th St., N.W., Suite 410, Washington, DC 20005; (202) 289-1478; www.aul.org. Public-interest policy organization seeking legal protection for the unborn.

Center for Reproductive Rights, 120 Wall St., 14th Floor, New York, NY 10005; (917) 637-3600; www.reproductiverights.org. Global legal organization dedicated to advancing women's reproductive health, self-determination and dignity as basic human rights.

Guttmacher Institute, 125 Maiden Lane, 7th Floor, New York, NY 10038; (212) 248-1111; www.guttmacher.org. Working to advance sexual and reproductive health through social science research, policy analysis and public education.

NARAL Pro-Choice America, 1156 15th St., N.W., Suite 700, Washington, DC 20005; (202) 973-3000; www.prochoiceamerica.org. Engages in political action to oppose restrictions on abortion.

National Abortion Federation, 1660 L St., N.W., Suite 450, Washington, DC 20036; (202) 667-5881; www.prochoice.org. Private association of abortion providers advocating for private medical decisions by women.

National Conference of State Legislatures, 444 N. Capitol St., N.W., Suite 515, Washington, DC 20001; (202) 624-5400; www.ncsl.org. Provides research and technical assistance for policymakers to exchange ideas on the most pressing state issues.

National Right to Life Committee, 512 10th St., N.W., Washington, DC 20004; (202) 626-8800; www.nrlc.org. Largest pro-life organization in the United States working through legislation and education to advocate against abortion.

Bibliography

Selected Sources

Books

Ehrlich, J. Shoshanna, *Who Decides? The Abortion Rights of Teens*, Praeger, 2006.
An associate professor at the University of Massachusetts-Boston's College of Public and Community Service provides an overview of Supreme Court decisions regarding abortion rights of teenagers along with the experiences of 26 young women in Massachusetts who went to court to obtain authorization for an abortion instead of seeking their parents' consent. Includes notes, four-page list of resources.

Greenhouse, Linda, and Reva B. Siegel (eds.), *Before Roe v. Wade: Voices That Shaped Abortion Debate Before the Supreme Court's Ruling*, Kaplan, 2010.
The book includes source documents dating from the 1960s and continuing up to and including selected briefs from the landmark abortion rights case *Roe v. Wade* and Supreme Court Justice Harry A. Blackmun's bench announcement of the 1973 decision. Greenhouse covered the Supreme Court for *The New York Times* for nearly 30 years until her retirement; she now teaches at Yale Law School. Siegel is a professor of constitutional law at Yale.

Hull, N.E.H., and Peter Charles Hoffer, *Roe v. Wade: The Abortion Rights Controversy in American History*, University Press of Kansas, 2001.
The book provides a lucid and balanced history of the abortion-rights issue from colonial times through 2000. Includes five-page chronology, 11-page bibliographical history. Hull and Hoffer, husband and wife, are professors, respectively, at Rutgers Law School and the University of Georgia. Along with their son, William James Hoffer, they are co-editors of *The Abortion Rights Controversy in America: A Legal Reader* (University of North Carolina Press, 2004), a compilation of primary sources from the criminalization of abortion in the 19th century through Supreme Court decisions from *Roe v. Wade* through *Stenberg v. Carhart* (*Carhart I*).

Palmer, Louis J., Jr., and Xueyan Z. Palmer, *Encyclopedia of Abortion in the United States* (2d ed.), McFarland & Co., 2009.
The 600-page encyclopedia comprehensively covers a full range of abortion-related topics, including entries on all Supreme Court decisions through 2007, on advocacy groups on both sides of the issue and on legislation in individual states. Includes a three-page bibliography. Louis Palmer is an attorney for the West Virginia Supreme Court of Appeals and author of other encyclopedias on legal issues; his wife Xueyan Palmer is also an attorney.

Rose, Melody, *Safe, Legal, and Unavailable? Abortion Politics in the United States*, CQ Press, 2007.
An associate professor of political science at Portland State University in Oregon provides an up-to-date overview of the abortion controversy with a major focus on restrictions to abortion access at the state and federal levels.

Articles

Bazelon, Emily, "The New Abortion Providers," *The New York Times Magazine*, July 18, 2010, pp. 30 et seq.
Physicians and medical students are seeking to strengthen women's access to abortions by encouraging obstetricians and gynecologists to make the procedure part of their normal practice, performed in their offices instead of referring patients to stand-alone clinics.

Ruggles, Rick, "When can fetus feel pain?," *The* (Omaha) *World-Herald*, Feb. 14, 2010, www.omaha.com/article/20100214/NEWS01/702149910.
The article by one of the newspaper's health and medicine writers provides a thorough and balanced account of the medical evidence and political debate over fetal pain; it appeared as Nebraska legislators were beginning consideration of the bill eventually enacted to ban abortions after the 20th week of pregnancy on the premise that a fetus can feel pain by that point of development.

Reports and Studies

"Defending Life 2010: Proven Strategies for a Pro-Life America," Americans United for Life, 2010.
The advocacy group's 832-page report includes an overview of state laws along with individual state rankings as well as the texts of model legislation. Information available at www.aul.org/defending-life/.

"Who Decides? The Status of Women's Reproductive Rights in the United States," NARAL Pro-Choice America, January 2010.
The advocacy group's 19th annual report, 90 pages long, surveys state and federal laws affecting women's reproductive health and individually grades states on reproductive rights. The publication is updated daily online (www.ProChoiceAmerica.org/whodecides).

"Support for Abortion Slips," Pew Forum on Religion and Public Life/Pew Research Center on the People and the Press, from 2009 Annual Religion and Public Life Survey, Oct. 1, 2009, http://pewforum.org/uploadedfiles/Topics/Issues/Abortion/abortion09.pdf.
The 35-page analysis of public opinion data on abortion by the two Pew centers finds slightly less support for abortions even though a plurality say abortion should be legal in most cases and a majority oppose making abortions more difficult. At the same time, the number of Americans who view abortion as a critical issue has declined.

The Next Step:

Additional Articles from Current Periodicals

Fetal Pain

"Committee Supports Fetal Pain Information Bill," The Associated Press, Feb. 24, 2009.
A Utah Senate committee has advanced a bill that would require doctors to inform women considering an abortion that the fetus might feel pain during the procedure.

Blow, Charles M., "Abortion's New Battle Lines," *The New York Times*, May 1, 2010, p. A19.
Several states have rushed to restrict access to abortion, such as through scientific research on fetal pain and through health-insurance limitations.

Borgmann, Caitlin, "Backdoor Attack On Abortion," *Los Angeles Times*, April 25, 2010, p. A29.
Nebraska's attempt to block abortions on the grounds of fetal pain is not rooted in the most objective scientific principles.

Jenkins, Nate, "Nebraska Governor Signs Landmark Abortion Measures," *The Boston Globe*, April 14, 2010, p. A2.
Nebraska Republican Gov. Dave Heineman has signed a bill banning abortions after 20 weeks on the assertion that fetuses feel pain at that point.

Insurance

Childress, Gregory, "BOG Responds to Abortion Concerns," *Herald-Sun* (North Carolina), Aug. 13, 2010, p. A1.
Anti-abortion forces are protesting a new insurance program for University of North Carolina students because it covers abortions.

Eaton, Sabrina, "Boehner Statement on Abortion Wrong," *Plain Dealer* (Ohio), Aug. 2, 2010, p. B1.
Republicans such as Rep. John Boehner wrongly claim that high-risk insurance pools will provide a backdoor way for the federal government to fund abortions.

Hall, Mimi, "Abortion Issue Snarls Health Bill," *USA Today*, Nov. 12, 2009, p. 5A.
A ban on abortion coverage in health-care legislation is being interpreted differently by both sides of the abortion debate.

Hoey, Mike, "Sen. McCaskill Jeopardizing Health Care Reform," *St. Louis Post-Dispatch*, Dec. 17, 2009, p. A18.
Senators who want to include federally funded abortions in health-care legislation are denying coverage to millions of Americans who have no insurance at all.

Jacobson, Louis, "Maddow Says Stupak Amendment Bars Those With Subsidies From Getting Abortion Coverage," *St. Petersburg Times*, Nov. 16, 2009.
An amendment to the House health-care bill limiting abortion coverage continues to inspire political passions.

Koranda, Jeannine, "Bill Would Make Abortion Coverage Extra," *Wichita* (Kansas) *Eagle*, Feb. 12, 2010, p. A1.
Abortion opponents in Kansas want the state to bar private insurance companies from automatically covering elective abortions.

Levine, Phillip B., "False Alarm On Abortion," *The New York Times*, Nov. 25, 2009, p. A31.
Insurers could decide to drop all abortion coverage in order to ensure eligibility to participate in exchanges that allow Americans to purchase public insurance.

Ratnayake, Hiran, "Abortion Foes Seek to Limit Help With Premiums," *News Journal* (Delaware), Dec. 10, 2009.
Fifty-five percent of Americans say abortion should not be included as a guaranteed medical benefit under any government health-care plan.

Roberts, Jerry, "Health Care Win, Pro-Choice Loss," *Santa Barbara* (California) *Independent*, Nov. 12, 2009, p. 17.
Women's access to reproductive care has been greatly sacrificed by the addition of an anti-abortion amendment.

Seelye, Katharine Q., "Another Standoff May Be Looming On Abortion Issue," *The New York Times*, Nov. 15, 2009, p. A26.
The abortion issue has members of Congress contemplating whether to resist legislative efforts limiting access to insurance for abortions.

Personhood

Abcarian, Robin, "The (Legal) Concept of a 'Person,' " *Los Angeles Times*, Sept. 28, 2009, p. A1.
Many abortion foes are reviving efforts to write their definition of a "person" into state constitutions.

Adams, John S., "Pro-Life Group Holds 'Personhood' Event," *Great Falls* (Montana) *Tribune*, Oct. 16, 2009, p. 1M.
Supporters of a Montana constitutional ballot initiative that would redefine "personhood" are organizing a rallying conference.

Bauer, Laura, "New Anti-Abortion Tactic: Redefine 'Personhood,' " *St. Paul* (Minnesota) *Pioneer Press*, April 10, 2010.
Anti-abortion activists are trying to stretch the legal definition of a "person" in their state constitutions.

Draper, Electa, "Personhood Group Unveils Strategy," ***The Denver Post*, July 27, 2010, p. B3.**
A 2008 ballot proposal in Colorado — rejected by nearly three-fourths of voters — sought to define "personhood" as beginning with a fertilized human egg.

Vogel, Ed, "Initiative Part of U.S. Drive," ***Las Vegas Review-Journal*, Oct. 24, 2009, p. 1B.**
A "personhood" amendment petition drive seeks to come up with a legal argument that can overturn *Roe v. Wade*.

Whittenberger, Gary J., and Richard Hull, "Zygote Fanatics Push Personhood Amendment," ***Tallahassee* (Florida) *Democrat*, Nov. 28, 2009.**
The proper stage in fetal development during which "personhood" should be defined is when the mind begins to operate.

Procedural Laws

Klepper, David, "Lawmakers Again Try to Tighten Late-Term Abortion Laws in Kansas," ***Kansas City Star*, March 31, 2010, p. A12.**
Kansas lawmakers are proposing a bill that would require physicians who sign off on late-term abortions to report the diagnosis used in justifying the procedure.

Krajacic, Zach, "Serious About Reducing Abortion? Make Women See an Ultrasound of the Procedure," ***The Christian Science Monitor*, Jan. 7, 2010.**
A law requiring abortion-seeking women to watch an ultrasound video of the procedure could save lives and enhance "choice."

Leininger, Kevin, "Proposal Would Regulate Abortion Doctors," ***News-Sentinel* (Indiana), Dec. 18, 2009.**
An Indiana county commissioner is introducing a bill regulating certain medical procedures — including abortions — performed outside hospitals.

Lorentzen, Leslie, "Parents Legally Responsible for Teen's Care Should Have Say On Abortion," ***Anchorage* (Alaska) *Daily News*, May 15, 2009, p. A13.**
In Alaska, a parent must give consent for all medicine and medical care for their child except for procedures related to abortion.

Maze, Rick, "Measure Would Lift Abortion Ban At Military Hospitals," ***Air Force Times*, June 7, 2010, p. 13.**
A Senate committee has approved legislation that would permit abortions in U.S. military hospitals so long as patients pay for the procedure.

Olkon, Sara, "Teen Abortion Law to Begin Tuesday," ***Chicago Tribune*, Nov. 2, 2009, p. A8.**
A new notification act requires Illinois parents of girls 17 or younger to be told if their daughters are having abortions.

Reckdahl, Katy, "Group of Abortion Clinics Challenges New Louisiana Laws," ***Times-Picayune* (Louisiana), Aug. 8, 2010, p. A4.**
A group of abortion clinics has filed a federal lawsuit challenging two Louisiana laws that require ultrasounds for women getting abortions and block medical malpractice insurance for doctors who perform the procedure.

Rodriguez, Salvador, "Lawsuits Filed to Block New Arizona Abortion Law," ***Arizona Republic*, Sept. 15, 2009.**
Lawsuits have been filed at the state and federal levels against a new Arizona law that would require women to make two trips to a physician's office prior to obtaining an abortion.

Steitzer, Stephenie, "Senate Panel OKs Abortion Ultrasound Bill," ***Courier-Journal* (Kentucky), Jan. 15, 2010.**
A Kentucky Senate panel has approved a measure requiring doctors to show ultrasound images of fetuses to women preparing to have an abortion.

Walker, Julian, "S.C. Abortion-Clinic Law Could Foreshadow Changes in Va.," ***Virginian-Pilot*, Aug. 29, 2010, p. A1.**
A federal court has upheld a South Carolina law requiring abortion clinics to meet hospital-like standards.

White, Josh, "Federal Court Upholds Midterm Abortion Ban," ***Virginian-Pilot*, June 25, 2009, p. A1.**
A federal appeals court has ruled constitutional a Virginia law that bans "partial-birth abortion."

Zeman, Jill, "Arkansas House Votes to Ban Late-Term Abortion," The Associated Press, Feb. 13, 2009.
The Arkansas House has voted to ban a late-term abortion procedure that opponents call "partial-birth abortion."

Citing *CQ Researcher*

Sample formats for citing these reports in a bibliography include the ones listed below. Preferred styles and formats vary, so please check with your instructor or professor.

MLA STYLE

Jost, Kenneth. "Rethinking the Death Penalty." CQ Researcher 16 Nov. 2001: 945-68.

APA STYLE

Jost, K. (2001, November 16). Rethinking the death penalty. *CQ Researcher, 11*, 945-968.

CHICAGO STYLE

Jost, Kenneth. "Rethinking the Death Penalty." *CQ Researcher*, November 16, 2001, 945-968.

CHAPTER

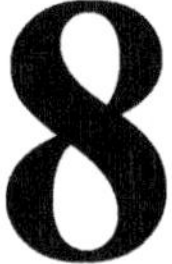

Breast Cancer

By Barbara Mantel

Excerpted from the CQ Researcher. Barbara Mantel. (April 2, 2010). "Breast Cancer." *CQ Researcher*, 289-312.

Breast Cancer

By Barbara Mantel

The Issues

Nearly everyone knows somebody with breast cancer. Kathy Kivelson Hecht of West Windsor, N.J., knows two women with the disease — her sisters.

Her mother died of cancer in 1989, but doctors could not identify the originating site. A year later, her 37-year-old middle sister was diagnosed with breast cancer and opted for a lumpectomy.

"We'd had a very traumatic year," says Kivelson Hecht, who was at her sibling's bedside after the surgery, along with their older sister. "I was just 35, and when the surgeon walked into my sister's room, she insisted he speak to us about our chances of breast cancer."

"He strongly recommended that we go home and talk with our own gynecologists," she recalls. She did and has had annual mammograms ever since.

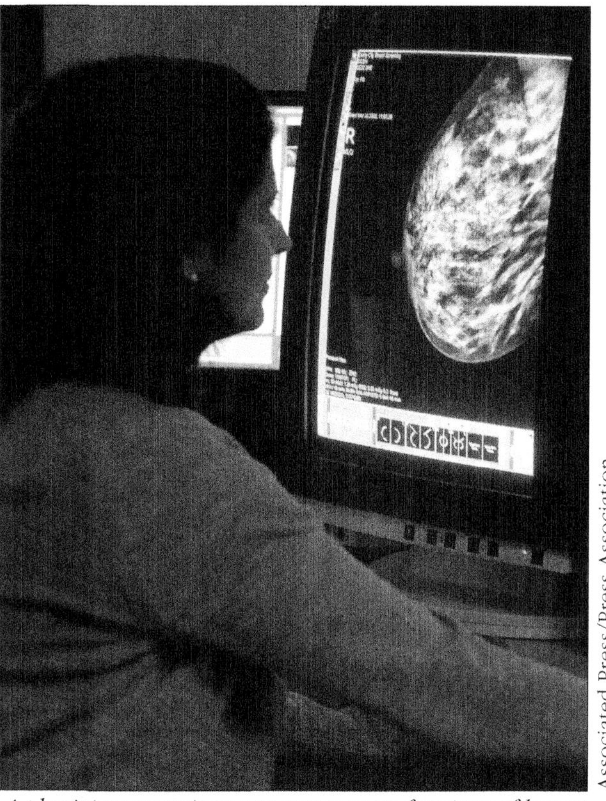

Associated Press/Press Association

A physician examines a mammogram for signs of breast cancer, the most frequently diagnosed cancer in women, next to skin cancer, and the second-leading cause of cancer death in women. In a controversial move last November, an independent panel of doctors and scientists reversed its own mammogram advice from seven years ago and recommended against routine mammography for most women in their 40s.

But seven years later, the middle sister's cancer spread to her other breast, requiring a mastectomy, and her oldest sister also eventually got breast cancer.

Not a year goes by, says Kivelson Hecht, that she doesn't say to herself: " 'OK, it's going to be there.' But so far I've been lucky."

Changes in DNA can cause normal breast cells to become cancerous. About 2 percent of adult women in the United States inherit mutations that are associated with a high risk of the disease — Kivelson Hecht tested negative — but most DNA changes that can lead to cancer are not inherited and occur in a woman's breast cells during her lifetime. [1] (A small number of men also get breast cancer.)

Researchers do not know exactly what causes those mutations or the alterations in surrounding tissue that might allow cancer cells to spread, but there are known risk factors, including dense breasts, early menstruation and late menopause, alcohol use, obesity and use of menopausal hormone therapy. (*See box, p. 302.*)

Breast cancer is the most frequently diagnosed cancer in women, next to skin cancer. (*See glossary and a list of common types of breast cancer, pp. 294-295.*) That's despite a 2.2 percent drop in the incidence rate each year from 1999 through 2005 — the most recent figures available — after increasing for more than two decades. The decline in the incidence rate may reflect the sharp reduction in the use of hormone-replacement therapy for menopausal women following a well-publicized report in 2002 that tied hormone replacement to increased risk of heart disease and breast cancer. [2] The drop in breast cancer cases may also reflect a small decline in detection, as the percentage of women 40 and older who opted for mammography declined from 70.1 percent in 2000 to 66.4 percent in 2005. [3]

Breast cancer is also the second-leading cause of cancer death in women; only lung cancer kills more. Yet death rates from breast cancer have steadily decreased since 1990, the result of advances in both earlier detection and improved treatment. [4] For instance, drugs have been developed that help prevent breast cancer in women at high risk, and therapies that disrupt hormones are now prescribed for breast cancers with hormone receptors. Antibodies have also been developed to target cancer cells with too much of the protein Her2/neu. Finally, genetic testing of tumor tissue is helping oncologists determine which patients will most benefit from chemotherapy.

Amidst these advances in treatment, however, one thing seems to never change: the long-running debate about the efficacy of mammography screening for women in their 40s.

Last November, an independent panel of doctors and scientists recommended against routine screening mammography for most women in this age bracket, a reversal from its recommendation of seven years earlier. In both announcements, however, the United States Preventive Services Task

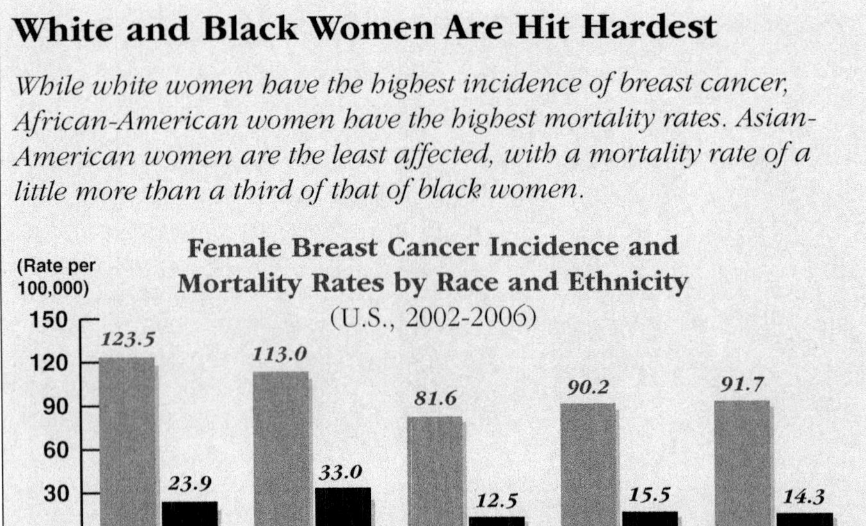

Force (USPSTF) emphasized that each woman should weigh the benefits and harms of screening mammography and make her own decision. [5]

This is not the first time that scientists have changed course on breast screening. In 1987, the National Cancer Institute (NCI) recommended that healthy women, beginning at age 40, should get mammograms every one to two years. In 1993, it dropped that recommendation, only to adopt it again in 1997. With each switch, confusion and debate followed. This time was no different.

A media storm erupted almost immediately. Celebrities lined up to denounce the task force's new guidelines, including singer/actress Olivia Newton-John, diagnosed at 43, who said, "We are not data, we are human beings." [6] The American Cancer Society and the American Congress of Obstetricians and Gynecologists issued statements continuing to recommend screening for women in their 40s, as did the American College of Radiology, which issued a press release titled "USPSTF mammography recommendations will result in countless unnecessary breast cancer deaths each year." [7]

Even Secretary of Health and Human Services (HHS) Kathleen Sebelius, to whom the task force reports, distanced herself and the Obama administration from the panel. "They do not set federal policy, and they don't determine what services are covered by the federal government," Sebelius said in a statement. "Indeed, I would be very surprised if any private insurance company changed its mammography coverage decisions as a result of this action." [8]

Gail Wilensky, a former official in George W. Bush's HHS, called Sebelius's statement "appalling and outrageous and a very good reminder of how hard it is going to be to move to evidence-based medicine whenever it goes against a sacred cow." [9]

Meanwhile, several leading women's health groups endorsed the task force's recommendation, including the National Breast Cancer Coalition, Breast Cancer Action and the National Women's Health Network, all of which had been saying for years that the benefits of mammograms for younger women have been oversold and do not outweigh the potential harms, such as false positives and unnecessary biopsies.

The timing of the USPSTF announcement further complicated the public reaction. A hyper-emotional and increasingly heated debate was raging over Democrats' proposed health-care reform legislation, and Republicans had claimed the plan would amount to the rationing of health care based on cost. In early December, when a subcommittee of the House Energy and Commerce Committee asked task force members to come and explain their mammography recommendations, Chairman Henry A. Waxman, D-Calif., felt compelled to defend the USPSTF's motives.

"While that judgment may be contentious, I have no doubt it was driven by science and by the interpretation of science — and not by cost or insurance coverage or the ongoing health reform debate," Waxman said. [10]

Advocates for African-American women raised particular concerns. "These recommendations completely ignore the impact of well-known breast cancer disparities affecting us," said Eleanor Hinton-Hoytt, president and CEO of Washington-based Black Women's Health Imperative. [11] African-American women are more often diagnosed with breast cancer at a later stage than whites and also are more likely to die of the disease.

African-American women — for unknown reasons — account for a disproportionate number of "triple negative" breast cancer, a particularly aggressive form of the disease. But lack of medical coverage, barriers to early detection and screening and unequal access to treatment may also contribute to black women's higher mortality rate, according to the NCI. [12]

For instance, a recent study showed that black women are less likely than white women to receive radiation therapy after a lumpectomy, the standard of care for early stage breast cancer. The authors did not know if fewer black women are receiving radiation "simply because it is not offered to them, because they decline the treatment or perhaps because they are unable to complete a whole course of treatment due to other health problems." [13] More studies are needed, they said.

Here are some of the questions that breast cancer sufferers, physicians, researchers, advocacy groups and politicians are debating:

Most Victims Are Women Over 45

An estimated 40,000 women died from breast cancer in 2009, and more than 192,000 invasive cases were diagnosed.

Estimated New Female Breast Cancer Cases and Deaths by Age Group, 2009

Age	In situ cases	Invasive cases	Deaths
Younger than 45	6,460	18,640	2,820
45 and older	55,820	173,730	37,350
Younger than 55	24,450	62,520	8,890
55 and older	37,830	129,850	31,280
Younger than 65	40,940	120,540	17,200
65 and older	21,340	71,830	22,970
All ages	62,280	192,370	40,170

Source: "Breast Cancer Facts and Figures 2009-2010," American Cancer Society

Is mammography oversold?

Early detection is the key to saving the lives of cancer victims. That's been the message from much of the medical community for decades. But research is calling that notion into question.

Physicians are debating the usefulness of prostate cancer screening for middle-aged men, and new guidelines for cervical cancer screening now say women should start having PAP smears at age 21; the medical community had previously recommended young women start screening three years after beginning to have intercourse, even if a teenager. [14] But perhaps most contentious of all was last November's recommendation by the influential United States Preventive Services Task Force (USPSTF) that most women under 50 should no longer have routine breast cancer screening and that women between 50 and 74 should no longer have mammograms every year but rather every other year. The new recommendation does not apply to the small number of women who are at high risk for the disease.

The task force's guidelines are intended to reduce potential harms from screening, like overtreatment of noninvasive cancer and the anxiety and unnecessary biopsies that result from false positives.

But the uproar that erupted immediately following their release caught the task force and its supporters by surprise.

"I'm not sure why it created such a firestorm," says Fran Visco, president of the National Breast Cancer Coalition. "I was taken aback." Her group supports the task force's findings and, like several other women's health organizations, has been vocal for years about the limitations of screening mammography for younger women.

Opposition to the task force's change of course ranged from measured to outraged. "This is one screening test I recommend unequivocally . . . to any woman 40 and over, be she a patient, a stranger or a family member," said Otis Brawley, the American Cancer Society's chief medical officer, who also acknowledged that reasonable experts can disagree. [15] The American Congress of Obstetricians and Gynecologists said it "maintains its current advice" that women in their 40s continue mammography screening [16] while the American Society of Breast Surgeons "strongly opposed" the new guidelines. [17] And the American College of Radiology said flatly if the guidelines became policy, "countless American women may die needlessly from breast cancer each year." [18]

Perhaps the angriest challenges came from individual women, like Gena Knutson, a 13-year breast cancer survivor diagnosed at age 35, who wrote a letter to the editor of her local newspaper: "With my history, you can imagine my shock regarding the federal recommendation that mammograms before age 50 are not medically necessary. This recommendation puts lives at risk." [19]

Task force members believe their true message got obscured in the media storm. "If you really look at what the task force was saying in 2002 [the last time it issued guidelines], it's not a lot different from what they were saying in 2009," says Russell Harris, a professor of medicine at the University of North Carolina in Chapel Hill and a former task force member.

In 2002, the task force had recommended that women get screened every one to two years beginning at age 40, but it went on to say that the

A Breast Cancer Glossary

Here are key breast cancer terms and a list of the most common types of breast cancer. Many other types of less common breast cancer are not listed here. Sometimes a breast tumor can be a mix of these types or a mixture of invasive and in situ cancer.

Understanding Key Terms

Adenocarcinoma — A type of cancer that starts in gland tissue (tissue that makes and secretes a substance). The ducts and lobules of the breast are gland tissues because they make breast milk, so cancers starting in these areas are often called adenocarcinomas.

Breast lumps — Most breast lumps are benign (not cancerous). Benign breast tumors are abnormal growths, but they do not spread outside of the breast and are not life threatening. But some benign lumps can increase the risk of getting breast cancer. Most lumps are caused by fluid-filled sacs known as cysts, which can cause breast swelling and pain. They often happen just before a woman's period is about to start. The breasts may feel lumpy, and sometimes there is a clear or slightly cloudy nipple discharge.

Carcinoma — A cancer that begins in the lining layer of organs such as the breast. Nearly all breast cancers are carcinomas (either ductal carcinomas or lobular carcinomas).

Carcinoma in situ — The early stage of cancer, when it is still only in the layer of cells where it began. In breast cancer, in situ means that the cancer cells are only in the ducts or lobules and have not spread into deeper tissues in the breast or to other organs. Sometimes called non-invasive or pre-invasive breast cancers.

Duct — Small tubes in the breast that carry milk to the nipple.

Invasive (infiltrating) carcinoma — A cancer that has already grown beyond the layer of cells where it started. Most breast cancers are invasive carcinomas — either invasive ductal carcinoma or invasive lobular carcinoma.

Lobule — Glands that make breast milk.

Sarcoma — Sarcomas are cancers that start from connective tissues such as muscle tissue, fat tissue or blood vessels. Sarcomas of the breast are rare.

precise age at which the benefits (a reduced death rate) justify the potential harms (false positive results and unnecessary biopsies) is a "subjective judgment" and that clinicians should tell women that the balance improves with age. In other words, women should make up their own minds.

"But very few people read or took to heart that message," says Harris, "and because of that, organizations and physicians assumed the task force said screen everybody over 40, and that's not really what they said."

So in 2009, after reviewing the data again, the task force decided to change "the tone" of its recommendation, according to Harris, saying it could no longer recommend screening for women in their 40s but continuing to stress that the judgment was subjective and up to each individual and her doctor.

Some of the panel's critics said task force members underestimated the potential benefit of screening mammography. The panel ignored information from more recent population-based studies, says Carol Lee, a radiologist at Memorial Sloan Kettering Cancer Center in New York City and the chair of the American College of Radiology's Commission on Breast Imaging. "Where the older, randomized trials showed a 15 percent reduction in mortality with screening for women in their 40s, the newer population trials show a 30 to 40 percent reduction in mortality."

Randomized controlled clinical trials enroll patients and then randomly assign them to various treatments, following up for years to determine the results. Population studies compare different parts of a country with different mammography rates, and if there is a change in mortality in one area versus another, they attribute it to screening.

Harris says that the new population studies were taken into account but that they are "methodologically weak." For instance, there could be many other differences between the two groups aside from screening that could account for variations in mortality.

Lee and other critics of the task force also say it overstated the potential harms from screening mammography. It's true that 1,900 women in their 40s need to be screened for 10 years in order to prevent one cancer death, and more than 1,000 false positive results will be generated in the process, leading to some unnecessary biopsies. [20] But Lee points to studies showing that the anxiety from receiving a false positive is short-lived. "And biopsy these days is much less invasive than it used to be," says Lee. "A needle biopsy can take as little as 15 minutes."

But Vasco says biopsies create scar tissue, which can mask problems that would show up in a mammography later, "when women are supposed to have routine screening in their 50s."

Besides false positives, the task force said that the increasing use of mammography has also resulted in the diagnosis and treatment of cancers that would never have become invasive and of slow-growing cancers that would not have shortened a woman's life.

And while the magnitude of overdiagnosis is unknown, Harris says, it is not trivial, as task force critics claim. "It is not zero, and it may be as much as 20 to 25 percent of all the breast cancers diagnosed," he says. [21]

To date, the new guidelines do not seem to have had an impact on insurance coverage, but it has opened up a divide between doctors and patients, if a recent survey in the *Annals of Internal Medicine* is any indication. Most doctors who responded said they would no longer offer routine screening to women in their 40s, while most women who responded said they would not give up their annual mammogram. [22]

"What this whole debate underscores is the urgent need to come up with better screening tools," says Eric Winer, director of the breast oncology center at the Dana-Farber Cancer Institute in Boston. If oncologists better understood who is most at risk, he says, then mammograms and MRIs [magnetic resonance imaging] could be devoted to those women. "When you do that, the false positives go down, and the true positives go up."

Major Types of Breast Cancer

Ductal carcinoma in situ (DCIS) — The most common type of non-invasive breast cancer, where the cancer is only in the ducts and has not spread into the breast tissue. Nearly all women with cancer at this stage can be cured. Often the best way to find DCIS early is with a mammogram. If there are areas of dead or dying cancer cells (called tumor necrosis) within the biopsy sample (when tissue is taken out to be looked at in the lab), the tumor is likely to grow and spread quickly (become more aggressive).

Lobular carcinoma in situ (LCIS) — Begins in the milk-making glands (lobules) but does not go through the wall of the lobules. It is not a true cancer, but having LCIS increases a woman's risk of getting cancer later, so it's important that women with LCIS should have regular mammograms and doctor visits.

Invasive (or infiltrating) ductal carcinoma (IDC) — The most common breast cancer, it starts in a duct, breaks through the duct wall and invades the tissue of the breast. From there it may spread (metastasize) to other parts of the body. IDC accounts for about eight out of 10 invasive breast cancers.

Invasive (infiltrating) lobular carcinoma (ILC) — Starts in the milk glands (lobules) and can spread (metastasize) to other parts of the body. About one out of 10 invasive breast cancers are ILCs.

Inflammatory breast cancer (IBC) — An uncommon type of invasive breast cancer that accounts for about 1 percent to 3 percent of all breast cancers. Usually there is no single lump or tumor. Instead, IBC makes the skin of the breast look red and feel warm. It also makes the skin look thick and pitted, something like an orange peel. The breast may get bigger, hard, tender or itchy. In its early stages, IBC is often mistaken for infection. Because there is no defined lump, it may not show up on a mammogram, which may make it even harder to catch it early. It usually has a higher chance of spreading and a worse outlook than invasive ductal or lobular cancer.

Source: American Cancer Society, Sept. 29, 2009

Should "stage zero" cancer be watched and not treated?

The increase in mammography screening since the late 1970s has led to a surge in diagnoses for ductal carcinoma in situ (DCIS), a kind of breast cancer rarely seen before 1980 but that now accounts for about 25 percent of all breast cancers diagnosed. [23]

Individual DCIS cells look just like invasive cancer under a pathologist's microscope, but unlike invasive cancer they are confined to the inside of the milk ducts. Some doctors call DCIS "zero stage" breast cancer, and the survival rate is high: Ten years after diagnosis, 96 to 98 percent of women are alive. [24]

However, the disease is typically treated much like early-stage invasive breast cancer — with a lumpectomy and radiation or even a mastectomy and often hormone treatment. And that bothers many clinicians and researchers.

Many DCIS patients do not need treatment since a significant number of cases will never progress to invasive cancer. Analysis of autopsy results and studies of DCIS that were missed at biopsy "suggest that the lifetime risk of progression must be considerably less than 50 percent." [25] That means thousands of women each year are actually harmed by treatment, suffering disfiguring surgery and the side effects of radiation and hormone treatment for no reason, most oncologists agree. The problem is that physicians have no sure way of distinguishing between the DCIS cases that will remain dormant and those that will spread.

With so much uncertainty, DCIS patients tend to overestimate their risk of invasive breast cancer, one study showed, and suffer unnecessary anxiety as a result. "You think you're going to die," said 40-year-old Barbara Laufer, a woman from Burbank, Calif., who was diagnosed with DCIS three years ago and had two lumpectomies and radiation and is taking the hormone treatment tamoxifen. [26]

Some physicians have proposed changing the name and removing the word "carcinoma" to reduce that anxiety. "Cancer usually implies invasion, and DCIS is specifically not invasive," says Carmen Allegra, chair of a National Institutes of Health panel on DCIS and chief of hematology and oncology at the University of Florida's Shands Cancer Center. "To call it cancer is probably an overstatement."

"You could rename it, for instance, in ductal intra-epithelial neoplasia," says Stephen Bauer, president of the College of American Pathologists and director of laboratories at Mercy San Juan Medical Center, near Sacramento, Calif. "It's been done with cervical cancer." Cervical intraepithelial neoplasia is the label now used instead of carcinoma in situ.

But the biggest harm is not anxiety but overtreatment, and a few physicians propose scaling back therapy.

"I've come to a very different approach to talking to patients with DCIS," says Shelley Hwang, a breast surgeon at the University of California, San Francisco, "and it's more of an evaluation of tradeoffs. So I present as one option active surveillance." That includes a mammogram every six months, possibly alternating with an MRI, and no surgery and no radiation. "But the patient has to know that the possibility of having invasive cancer will increase," explains Hwang, "although with surveillance the likelihood is that they would have a curable cancer. Hwang acknowledges that she is "definitely on the fringe" when it comes to her approach to DCIS treatment.

"It would be hard to not at least intervene surgically," says Allegra.

Pat Whitworth, a breast surgeon in Nashville, Tenn., and former chairman of the board at the American Society of Breast Surgeons, says he would consider active surveillance only rarely, with the following hypothetical patient: "She's physiologically elderly and frail. She's not going to tolerate a haircut well let alone a surgical procedure, and the biopsy appears to have removed the problem, and it was low-grade DCIS." But most of his patients would still opt for a little more surgery, Whitworth says.

Hwang says 90 percent of her patients also opt for some surgery. But Mary Jane Lapinski did not. The 55-year-old, single woman from Northern Virginia was diagnosed with DCIS seven years ago. Because she had DCIS in two locations, her surgeon recommended a mastectomy. "It was mind-boggling," she says. "I'm thinking, 'How can you tell me that I need a mastectomy for a noninvasive cancer when women with invasive cancer are getting lumpectomies?' It truly did not make any sense to me at all."

Lapinski went on the Internet, where all she read pointed to mastectomy, and she was about to schedule her surgery when she came across an article about a study conducted by Hwang. In the study, DCIS patients whose cancer cells have estrogen receptors were given the hormone treatment tamoxifen for three months before submitting to surgery.

Lapinski flew to San Francisco, signed up, and after three months and a discussion with Hwang about the pros and cons, opted to not have surgery and to leave the study. She remains on tamoxifen and returns to San Francisco every six months for an MRI. "Over the years, the whole area in my breast that was affected has shrunk significantly," says Lapinski.

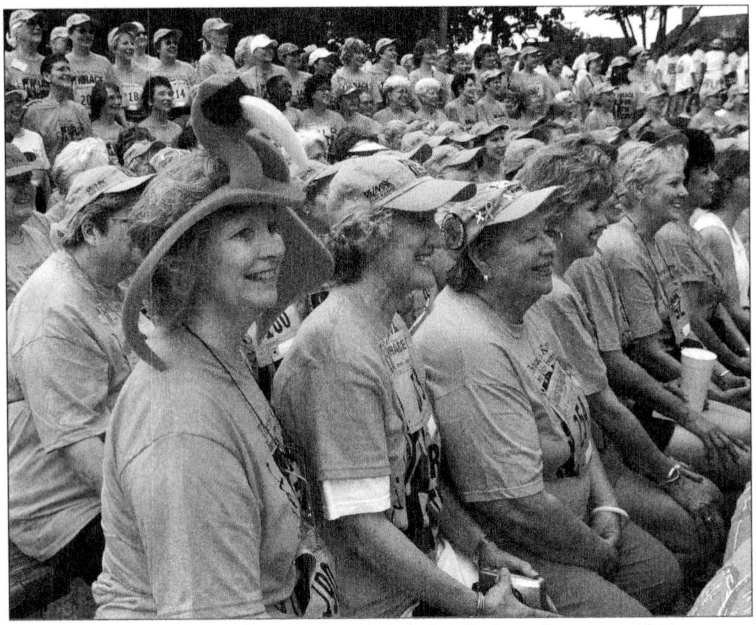

Hwang published the results of the study last year, reporting that cancer cells under the microscope look shriveled, and tissue markers that show how fast cells are dividing indicated that the growth rate had slowed down. [27] "It doesn't happen to the same extent in all patients, but it does happen to some patients big time," says Hwang. Those patients may benefit from longer-term hormonal therapy instead of surgery and instead of just pure active surveillance, she says. Hwang is also planning a study of six months of hormonal treatment before surgery.

AP Photo/Tyler Morning Telegraph/D.J. Peters

Cancer survivors sit for a portrait in pink before the annual Komen Race for the Cure in Tyler, Texas. Susan B. Komen for the Cure is a leading national grassroots advocacy organization that raises money for breast cancer research.

What would it take for other breast surgeons to consider discussing active surveillance with their DCIS patients? Whitworth says he would need to see a published study of post-menopausal women randomized to either standard treatment or active surveillance and followed afterward for five to 10 years. If data on recurrence and mortality "were fairly comparable, then I think we would see some shifting in treatment," he says.

Do chemicals in the environment cause breast cancer?

There is no single cause of breast cancer. Yet understanding the etiology of this complex disease is essential to understanding how to prevent it. While 5 to 10 percent of breast cancer cases are thought to be hereditary, the majority of women who develop the disease will never know why.

Scientists have identified certain risk factors, like early menstruation and late menopause, alcohol consumption and obesity, but "most of these risk factors account for very small increases or decreases in a woman's chances of developing breast cancer," according to the National Breast Cancer Coalition. [28]

Environmental chemicals may play a role, say some researchers, by damaging DNA, by mimicking hormones that signal tumor cells to grow or by altering mammary gland development early in life. They say the size of the dose may not be what matters most but how early in life and for how long the exposure occurs and to whom; some women may be more susceptible than others. "Breast cancer rates increased enormously over the decades since World War II at the same time that we have had increasing exposure to a wide variety of chemicals and radiation in the environment," says Janet Gray, director of the program in science, technology and society at Vassar College in Poughkeepsie, N.Y., who wrote an extensive review of the research on breast cancer and the environment for the Breast Cancer Fund, an advocacy group in San Francisco, Calif.

But correlation does not prove a link. For that, scientists turn to animal and human studies. One team of researchers reviewed hundreds of animal studies and found that 216 chemicals have been shown to cause mammary gland tumors, mostly through DNA mutations. There could be many others, since only a small fraction of the more than 80,000 chemicals used in the United States today have been tested in animals for carcinogenic potential. [29]

"The laboratory evidence is very strong that there are environmental chemicals that affect biological processes linked to breast cancer," says Julia G. Brody, who participated in the review of chemicals and is the executive director of the Silent Spring Institute in Newton, Mass., which researches the environment and women's health. The chemicals include benzene, found in gasoline; polycyclic aromatic hydrocarbons, found in vehicle exhaust, air pollution, tobacco smoke and charred foods; methylene chloride, a common solvent in paint strippers and glues; and some pharmaceuticals, like furosemide, a diuretic, and griseofulvin, an anti-fungal. [30]

Most of the 216 chemicals also caused tumors in multiple organs, not just mammary tissue, and in multiple species of animals. "These characteristics are generally believed to indicate likely carcinogenicity in humans," Brody's team reported. [31]

A growing number of animal studies also implicate endocrine-disrupting compounds (EDCs) — found in certain plastics, pesticides, flame retardants and personal care products — which mimic or block hormones. "There are literally hundreds of studies demonstrating that low doses of endocrine disruptors in early development have profound effects on mammary tissue, breast development and incidence of breast cancer, especially in a variety of rodent models," says Gray. [32]

But extrapolating from animal studies to the human experience is tricky. "We're on very thin ice inferring from animal models that there's a high probability that a chemical is a carcinogen in humans," says David Hunter, a professor of epidemiology at Harvard University in Cambridge, Mass. "There is a relatively low correlation between exposures that cause cancer in animals and those exposures causing cancer in humans," says Hunter. "And if there is a relationship, it's a different type of cancer in the human compared to the animal."

The gold standard would be human studies, but there haven't been many, and most that have been done have not found a link. Perhaps that's because human studies have mostly measured levels of a single chemical in adult women, while the critical period of exposure might be puberty, or early childhood, or even in utero. In addition, it might be exposure to a mix of chemicals that is important.

But it is extremely difficult to study early exposure to multiple chemicals. Most people don't know what chemicals they are exposed to now, let alone decades ago. And when interviewing women with breast cancer, "How do you know the diagnosis itself isn't influencing their recall of events?" asks James Lacey, a cancer epidemiologist at City of Hope, a comprehensive cancer center in Duarte, Calif. "People want to put a narrative to their experiences," he says. Researchers also may not be able to find an unexposed control group, since many chemicals are pervasive. And finally, chemicals may increase breast cancer risk only for women with certain genetic mutations.

Instead, some researchers have combed through state environmental data and medical records looking for reliable information. One group found blood samples taken from young women at the time they gave birth, measured their levels of the pesticide DDT, and then followed the women for two decades. Early exposure to DDT was associated with a fivefold increase in risk of developing breast cancer before age 50. [33] DDT, though banned in 1972, continues to linger in the environment.

"That is an important study, and it provides the kind of evidence that is very difficult to get," says Brody.

Four human studies show higher breast cancer risk from exposure to polychlorinated bipheyls (PCBs) in women with a gene mutation that affects how they metabolize these now banned chemicals that were once used in electrical equipment, but still linger.

But Hunter cautions that no single epidemiological study is definitive. "We only accept something as likely to be causal if the majority of studies point in the same direction," he says. Brody also calls the number of human studies sparse and says there are "huge knowledge gaps."

Experts say more chemicals must be tested — both in the lab and in animals and in forward-looking human studies — not dependent on memory. For instance, the federal National Children's Study will examine the effects of environmental influences on the health and development of 100,000 children in the United States, following them from before birth until age 21. [34]

"However, that doesn't help us right now," says Gray. That's why she and Brody both advocate relying on the animal data to propel action in the short term. "I don't think most families want to take unnecessary risks with their daughters," says Brody. A progressive policy, she says, would acknowledge that we know enough now to start reducing those exposures.

For Michael Thun, emeritus vice president of epidemiology and surveillance at the American Cancer Society, it's not so clear. "The precautionary principle says that if you have some evidence you should take action — you don't need conclusive evidence — but the question that remains unresolved is where do you draw the line?" says Thun.

Brody says the U.S. should look to Europe and Canada for a model of how to implement the precautionary principle. These countries have developed systematic programs for assessing the health consequences of synthetic chemicals — both old and new — as a prerequisite for use. [35] ■

BACKGROUND

Radical Surgery

In the late 19th century, the American surgeon William Stewart Halsted offered "an alternative, a choice, a possibility for breast cancer patients in a surgical world bereft of hope," writes James S. Olson in his book *Bathsheba's Breast: Women, Cancer & History.* [36] At the time, women, terrified of a breast cancer diagnosis, typically delayed consulting a doctor, who would then not see the cancer until it was large and often inoperable. When they did operate, tumors often returned, and most women died a brutal and painful death.

Halsted believed that cancer slowly spread through the body's lymphatic system, and he embraced the technique of removing lymph nodes during cancer surgery. But he also knew that cancer was a cellular disease, and he worried that "a careless surgeon who cut into the tumor with the scalpel, lifted the breast away with his hands, then . . . scooped out lymph nodes with his fingers probably scattered tumor cells all over." [37] Using the hands this way was advised in textbooks and was common practice at the time.

Instead, in the early 1890s Halsted called for removing the breast, lymph nodes and chest muscles in a single procedure, "cutting widely around the tumor, removing all the tissue in one piece." [38]

Over the next two decades, Halsted, his students and colleagues performed tens of thousands of these radical mastectomies, and Halsted began to collect a database on the 210 surgeries he himself had performed. Of the 60 women whose cancer had not spread to the lymph nodes, more than 85 percent were alive three years later. Of the 110 women whose cancer had spread to the lymph nodes, just 31 percent survived for three years. And for the 40 women with cancer in more remote lymph nodes, only 10 percent survived that long.

Olson writes that Halsted's conclusion was clear: "Women who received a radical mastectomy before the tumor spread to regional lymph nodes had excellent odds. Women who delayed treatment were doomed." [39] Halsted's results laid the foundation for a massive campaign 70 years later for early detection through mammography.

Mastectomy to Lumpectomy

But radical mastectomy was disfiguring and at times led to persistent pain and arm swelling known as lymphedema. As surgeons gained an appreciation of its side effects and learned more about the biology of cancer, the procedure attracted critics.

Among the most vocal was English physician Geoffrey Keynes, who questioned Halsted's basic assumption — that breast cancer "spread slowly through the lymph nodes, hypothesizing that the disease in fact entered

Continued on p. 300

Chronology

1800s Surgical techniques are refined; radiation is introduced.

1882
American William Stewart Halsted develops the radical mastectomy.

1896
Chicago physician Emil Grubbe treats breast cancer patients with X-rays. . . . Scotsman Thomas Beatson reports that removing ovaries results in improvement of breast cancer patients, laying foundation for modern hormone therapy.

1930s-1970s

Advances are made in breast cancer treatment and diagnosis.

1939
Congress establishes National Cancer Institute (NCI).

1969
Mammography machines introduced.

1975-76
Studies demonstrate that adjuvant chemotherapy — treatment after surgery — prolongs survival for breast cancer patients.

1978
Tamoxifen is approved as adjuvant therapy to prevent cancer recurrence.

1980s-1990s

Scientists begin to understand the genetics of breast cancer; mammography debate begins.

1980-83
Studies show combining treatments, like chemotherapy and radiation, helps certain breast cancers, changing the standard of care.

1987
NCI and the American Cancer Society (ACS) recommend that beginning at age 40, women should begin screening every one-to-two years.

1990
National Institutes of Health (NIH) says lumpectomy plus radiation is as effective as mastectomy.

1992
Study finds no evidence that low-fat or high-fiber diets protect against breast cancer. . . . Taxol, derived from yew tree bark, is approved to treat breast cancer after other drugs have failed.

1993
NCI drops its recommendation that women in their 40s get mammograms, saying no clear scientific evidence exists that regular screening reduces risk of dying; ACS continues to recommend screening for women in their 40s.

1997
Mutations to the BRCA1 and BRCA2 tumor-suppressing genes are linked to high lifetime chance of developing breast cancer. . . . After reviewing updated screening studies, NCI reverses course and recommends mammograms for women in their 40s every one-to-two years.

1998
Daily tamoxifen treatment is shown to reduce the incidence of invasive breast cancer by 45 percent and noninvasive breast cancer by 50 percent in high-risk women. . . . Food and Drug Administration (FDA) approves an antibody for women with certain types of metastatic breast cancer.

2000-Present

Genetic tests of breast tumors are developed while mammography debate continues.

2002
Hormone replacement therapy for postmenopausal women is shown to increase the risk of breast cancer and increase the odds of heart attack, stroke and blood clots.

2002
U.S. Preventive Services Task Force (USPSTF) recommends routine mammography for women in their 40s every one-to-two years, emphasizing that each woman must weigh potential benefits and harms.

2002-2004
Test for gene activity in breast tumor tissue is shown to predict recurrence likelihood and benefit of chemotherapy.

2005
Herceptin is shown to cut risk of tumors returning in women with early stage HER2-positive breast cancer by 50 percent; approved for this use in 2006.

2007
Studies describe common variations in DNA sequences associated with small increased breast cancer risk.

November 2009
After reviewing studies about false positives and overtreatment of non-invasive breast cancer, USPSTF no longer recommends routine mammography for women in their 40s. The task force also says that women between 50 and 74 should have mammograms every other year rather than every year and recommends against breast cancer self-exams because harms, like false positives, outweigh the benefits.

Few High-Risk Women Get Genetic Testing

Tests can spot mutations in genes that suppress breast cancer tumors.

Karen Kramer, a 45-year-old mother of three in Maryland, spent most of her adult life worried about breast cancer. "For me, it was not if I get it but when I get it," she says. Three generations of women on her father's side have had the disease, and her mother's sister as well.

Fifteen months ago, a mammography technician told Kramer that she had dense breasts, making detection more difficult. Already nervous about her family history, Kramer asked for advice, and the technician recommended a genetic counselor. Kramer went the same day and soon chose to be tested for harmful mutations in two tumor-suppresor genes, BRCA1 and BRCA2.

About 60 percent of women who have inherited BRCA mutations will develop breast cancer, compared to 12 percent of women in the general population. And 15 to 40 percent will develop ovarian cancer, compared to less than 2 percent of most women. [1]

But the dreaded mutations are rare. "If you are looking at non-Hispanic whites in the U.S., 1 in 800 carries a mutation," says oncologist Marc Robson, clinic director of the Clinical Genetics Service at Memorial Sloan-Kettering Cancer Center in New York. But for women of Ashkenazi Jewish descent, like Kramer, the chance is much higher: 1 in 40.

Three weeks after testing, Kramer sat in an oncologist's office with the counselor as they opened the results. "When they said it was positive, the oncologist handed me tissues," recounted Kramer. "And I said, 'You know what, I don't need tissues.' Honestly, I have not cried about it. I'm actually grateful because now I have choices."

The American Society of Clinical Oncology (ASCO) recommends testing for BRCA1 and BRCA2 mutations only if an individual has "a personal or family history suggestive of genetic cancer susceptibility." [2] But most high-risk women do not get tested. Kramer almost didn't. "I had told every gynecologist throughout the years what my family history was," says Kramer, "and nobody seemed to worry about it."

According to a recent study, about half of the women identified as high risk in a national survey knew about genetic testing, about 10 percent had discussed it with a health professional and less than 2 percent had been tested. [3]

A woman who tests positive has several options: She can take a medication like tamoxifen, which can reduce the risk of developing breast cancer; have more frequent cancer screenings and clinical exams; or have preventive surgery.

Kramer decided to have surgery to remove her ovaries, fallopian tubes, uterus and both breasts. "I did not want to live on pins and needles," she says. Her sister, who also tested positive, chose hysterectomy, no mastectomy and frequent breast screening.

Continued from p. 298

the bloodstream and spread throughout the body early in its course," writes Barron Lerner, in *The Breast Cancer Wars*. [40] If this were true, then removing lymph nodes would not reduce mortality.

Other critics suggested that the mortality of breast cancer patients depended less on early detection and surgery than on the innate aggressiveness of the cancer itself. One New York surgeon wrote that "cures depend . . . on a mystical something that pathologists are now exploring and which is spoken of as the biology of the tumor."

By the late 1920s, a few of these critics had begun to argue that radiation, "either by itself or accompanied by surgical removal of the tumor or breast alone, was as or more effective than radical mastectomy." Studies began to show survival rates comparable to radical mastectomy. [41]

Yet radical mastectomy remained the standard of care for decades. In fact following World War II and the development of potent antibiotics that prevented postoperative infections, a few surgeons went "superradical." University of Minnesota surgeon Owen H. Wangensteen believed that breast cancers that had reached the lymph nodes required even more aggressive surgery, which entailed "the splitting of a patient's clavicle, ribs and sternum (breast bone) in pursuit of cancer cells," writes Lerner. [42]

Meanwhile, more voices were challenging the notion of early treatment and curability, including biometricians who studied the statistical record. These new studies claimed, like the few lone voices 20 years earlier, that the biology of each breast cancer determined a woman's chances of survival. For instance, a Canadian biometrician, Neil McKinnon, published studies showing that breast cancer mortality in Ontario, England, Wales, Denmark and five U.S. states had remained stable from 1909 to 1947, despite surgery and greater public awareness of the benefits of early intervention, thanks to publicity by cancer societies. [43]

By the late 1950s, many researchers began to argue that the only way to compare the efficacy of different breast cancer therapies was to conduct randomized controlled clinical trials, which many surgeons interpreted as a direct assault on their authority and expertise. Roald Grant, a surgeon with the American Cancer Society, compared physicians who relied on such

Testing for BRCA1 and BRCA2 mutations clearly can lead to intervention, but experts say some new types of DNA analysis being offered to consumers have no clear clinical utility.

Researchers have found minor variations in DNA — called SNPS (single nucleotide polymorphisms) — that are associated with breast cancer. Unlike BRCA mutations, SNPs are fairly common, but the increased risk associated with each SNP is low — the equivalent, say, of postponing childbearing from age 30 to 35.

Robson doesn't favor testing for SNPs, because "it is not at all clear that SNPs indicate any change in intervention." And ASCO recommends that SNP testing be given only through clinical trials. [4] Moreover, a government advisory panel has called for the creation of a public registry of genetic tests so their validity can be studied. [5]

In the meantime, dozens of companies now offer genomic testing to individuals, who swab their cheeks or spit into a test tube and mail it in with a check.

For instance, Navigenics, a genetics-testing firm in Foster City, Calif., tests for markers associated with 28 health conditions, including seven different SNPs associated with breast cancer. Consumers can order their genomic profile directly or through a physician.

"Many of the physicians we work with use this to help refine screening recommendations for their patients," says Elissa Levin, Navigenics' director of genomic services. But ASCO says there are no scientific studies, at least so far, that validate this use of the tests.

Nevertheless, genomic screening may have some personal utility. Positive results, Levin says, may help motivate some women to make lifestyle changes that could lower their risk of cancer. But critics say it could make others anxious and confused.

To avoid that, Navigenics offers its customers genetic counseling by phone, and Levin says most of its clients use the service. But not all companies offer genetic counseling. In fact, neither do all physicians.

— Barbara Mantel

[1] "BRCA1 and BRCA2: Cancer Risk and Genetic Testing," National Cancer Institute fact sheet, May 2009, p. 2.

[2] Marc E. Robson, *et al.*, "American Society of Clinical Oncology Policy Statement Update: Genetic and Genomic Testing for Cancer Susceptibility," *Journal of Clinical Oncology*, Jan. 11, 2010, p. 3, http://jco.ascopubs.org/cgi/doi/10.1200/JCO.2009.27.0660.

[3] Douglas E. Levy, *et al.*, "Guidelines for Genetic Risk Assessment of Hereditary Breast and Ovarian Cancer: Early Disagreements and Low Utilization," abstract, *Journal of General Internal Medicine*, July 2009.

[4] Robson, *et al.*, *op. cit.*

[5] "U.S. System of Oversight of Genetic Testing: A Response to the Charge of the Secretary of Health and Human Services," Department of Health and Human Services, April 2008, p. 8.

trials and statistics to Nazi physicians who experimented on humans during World War II. [44]

Yet in 1966, in a series of papers following several clinical trials, University of Pittsburgh surgeon and pathologist Bernard Fisher "turned upside down the prevailing logic of malignancy and metastasis." He argued that from the very beginning of a breast tumor's life, cancer cells slough off into the lymphatic system and the blood stream. "Cells without a future succumbed to the immune system, but others . . . waited to take root somewhere else in the body." Olson writes that the papers had enormous impact, removing the rationale for emergency surgery — to catch the cancer quickly before it can spread — and giving women time to explore their options. [45]

Fisher's research also set the stage for the expanded use of chemotherapy — chemical agents that destroy cancer cells throughout the body. He argued that the only hope for cancer was for surgeons to reduce the tumor so any remaining cancer cells could be destroyed by the patient's immune system and anticancer drugs.

Ten years later, Fisher was responsible for delivering the obituary on radical mastectomy. He tracked nearly 2,000 women in Canada and the United States for six years, who either had had a radical mastectomy or a simple mastectomy (removal of the breast that leaves the lymph nodes and chest muscles intact) followed by radiation. The survival rates were virtually the same. [46]

In 1990, the National Institutes of Health announced that lumpectomy (removing the tumor but leaving most of the breast intact) plus radiation is as effective as simple mastectomy. But the ensuing debate about lumpectomy did not completely subside until 2002, when Fisher and colleagues published the results of a randomized trial showing that women with relatively small breast cancers treated with lumpectomy plus radiation were as likely to be alive and disease-free 20 years later as women treated with mastectomy. [47]

Non-surgical Breakthroughs

Despite advances in surgery and chemotherapy, mortality rates for breast cancer barely budged from 1950-1990 — remaining at about 28 deaths per 100,000 people. [48] Since

Risk Factors for Breast Cancer

Several factors affect women's likelihood to get breast cancer, including age and family history. Several other risk factors are preventable, such as a woman's recent use of birth control pills.

Risk Factors That Aren't Preventable:

Gender: Women are 100 times more likely than men to get breast cancer.

Age: About two-thirds of women with invasive breast cancer are at least 55.

Genetics: About 5 to 10 percent of breast cancers may be linked to mutations in certain genes.

Family history: A woman with a mother, sister or daughter with breast cancer is twice as likely to get it.

Personal history: A woman with breast cancer is more likely to get a new cancer in her other breast or elsewhere in the same breast.

Race: White women are most likely to get breast cancer. African-American women are most likely to die from it. Asian, Hispanic and Native American women are less likely to get breast cancer.

Breast tissue density: Women with denser breast tissue have more gland tissue and less fatty tissue and are at a higher risk for breast cancer.

Menstrual periods: Women who began having periods before age 12 or who began menopause after age 55 have been exposed to more estrogen and progesterone.

Earlier breast radiation: Women treated for another cancer with radiation to the chest have a greatly increased risk of getting breast cancer.

Risk Factors That May Be Preventable:

Not having children or having them later in life: Women who haven't had children or had their first child after age 30 are more likely to get breast cancer.

Recent use of birth control pills: Women using birth control pills are at a higher risk for breast cancer, but that risk subsides once they stop taking them.

Using post-menopausal hormone therapy: Some doctors prescribe estrogen and progesterone to relieve menopause symptoms, which may make women more likely to get breast cancer and die from it.

Not breast-feeding: Because breast-feeding lowers a woman's total number of menstrual periods, it slightly lowers her risk of breast cancer.

Alcohol: Women who have between two and five drinks per day are one-and-a-half times more likely to get breast cancer than women who don't drink alcohol.

Being overweight: Women who are overweight or obese have a greater risk of breast cancer, especially after beginning menopause or if they became overweight or obese during adulthood.

Lack of exercise: A study found that only an hour-and-a-quarter to two-and-a-half hours of brisk walking weekly reduced risk of breast cancer by 18 percent.

Source: "What Causes Breast Cancer?" American Cancer Society

then, however, the death rate has declined steadily, thanks to earlier detection, improved treatment and a better understanding of the genetics of breast cancer.

In 1990, while teaching at the University of California, Berkeley, geneticist Mary-Claire King determined that 5-10 percent of breast cancer cases resulted from an inherited mutant gene on the long arm of chromosome 17, later identified as BRCA1, a tumor suppressor gene. The mutations allow tumor cells to grow.

King — who had spent 15 years studying Jewish women of Ashkenazi decent, who have a high incidence of breast cancer — later discovered a second, similar gene called BRCA2. Since her breakthroughs, scientists have developed drugs that help prevent breast cancer in women of high risk. [49]

But not all women with the mutations go on to develop breast cancer. Since a woman inherits two copies of the gene, one from each parent, perhaps the normal copy must also mutate during a patient's lifetime for cancer to grow. Some researchers have speculated that environmental toxins may cause that mutation.

As scientists made strides in understanding the biology of breast cancer, they began to develop therapies geared to the particular characteristics of tumor tissue. For instance, drugs like tamoxifen are given to patients who have early-stage breast cancer with estrogen receptors on the cells' surfaces. The drugs block the receptors, preventing estrogen from binding to the cell and causing the cancer to grow. Taking tamoxifen after surgery for five years cuts the chances of recurrence by about half, but the drug has side effects and may increase a woman's chance of developing endometrial cancer and blood clots. [50]

Continued on p. 304

Do Social Isolation and Stress Lead to Breast Cancer?

Experiments with mice and rats suggest a possible link.

Suzanne Conzen is an associate professor of hematology/oncology at the University of Chicago's Pritzker School of Medicine. She and behavioral biologist Martha McClintock are studying the link between stress, social isolation and breast cancer in mice and rats. They also have teamed up with sociologists to study socially isolated African-American women on Chicago's South Side who are newly diagnosed with breast cancer. Here are highlights from CQR contributing writer Barbara Mantel's recent interview with Conzen.

CQR: What happens to female mice and rats when they are isolated, compared to rats living in groups?

SC: For reasons that are not completely understood, this strain of rats has been known in older age to develop breast cancer. We have found that these rats develop tumors much earlier, and the tumors end up being larger when the rats are socially isolated.

CQR: Why?

SC: Martha noticed that these isolated rats were much more jumpy and vigilant than those in groups and wondered if they have differences in their stress response brought on by their social isolation. She found the levels of the stress hormone corticosterone [cortisol in humans] were much higher and lasted much longer in reaction to a superimposed, unexpected stress in the isolated rats.

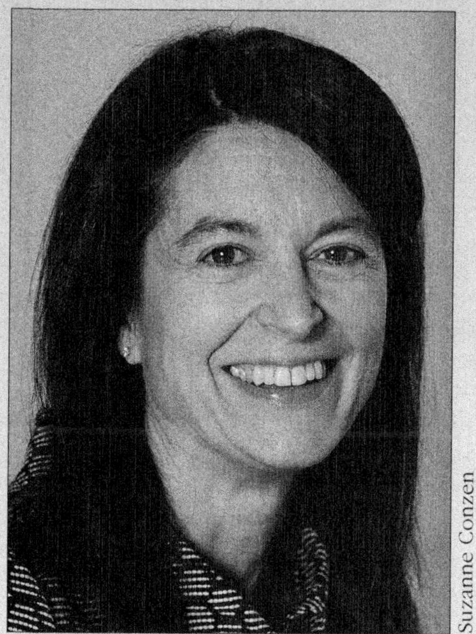
Suzanne Conzen

Suzanne Conzen.

CQR: What do you mean by superimposed unexpected stress?

SC: This was [physical] restraint; it is supposed to mimic a burrow collapsing.

CQR: So you did the same experiment with mice that are designed to get cancer, known as transgenic mice?

SC: Yes, we separated the female mice at weaning into isolation or group housing. And indeed these socially isolated transgenic mice develop earlier and larger tumors.

CQR: Did you also measure the stress hormones?

SC: Yes, and we found a very similar response to a superimposed stressor. Their corticosterone levels increased significantly more rapidly and to a higher degree than the group-housed mice. This is interesting because this is a genetically inbred strain of mice that are used for cancer biology experiments, and the only difference had been their housing.

CQ: How would stress hormone affect the development of breast cancer?

SC: One possibility is that chronic social isolation is causing an increase in the circulating stress hormones, and this may be related to changes in the gene expression that we see in the mouse mammary gland. This hormone, corticosterone, is actually known to turn genes on and off.

CQR: Do you know which genes?

SC: What surprised us is that we thought the genes that would be regulated in association with this stress would be primarily cell survival genes, genes that affect whether a cell lives or dies. What we found, in fact, was that they were genes more closely associated with the metabolism of sugars and fats.

CQR: So how did the increase in stress make these tumors grow faster and larger?

SC: That's what we don't know. All we know is that it has changed the gene expression in the mammary gland so that there is more efficient production of fatty acids, which are absolutely critical for cancer cells to grow.

CQR: Does this research in the lab have much to say about women, stress and breast cancer?

SC: I think it is not directly translatable at this point, except to say it raises the possibility that the social environment is a player in changing the physiology that is relevant to cancer development. In that way, it is paradigm shifting.

CQR: You've teamed up with sociologists, in particular Sarah Gehlert of Washington University in St. Louis, to study African-American women newly diagnosed with breast cancer who live on the South Side of Chicago. Why?

SC: My interest was instigated by my patients, many of whom are from the South Side of Chicago, who were convinced that stress played a role in their cancer.

CQR: Gehlert's team is interviewing the women, analyzing crime statistics and neighborhood conditions, measuring their stress hormone and studying tumor biopsies. How does it all work?

SC: Sarah measures the women's cortisol levels to see if their history of stress — for instance, divorce, murders in the family — associate with abnormal cortisol secretion. What we'd like to do is get a sense of what happens to these patients. How does the cortisol correlate with the kinds of breast cancers that they get?

Continued from p. 302

The antibody trastuzumab is given to breast cancer patients with too much HER2 protein in the cancer cell membrane, which causes cells to reproduce uncontrollably. The drug binds to the protein, effectively deactivating it. Studies have shown that the drug in combination with chemotherapy improves survival, but patients have often developed resistance. Heart problems can also result.

The holy grail of treatment is personalized medicine, and the introduction in 2004 of a new genetic test called Oncotype DX is a start down that path for breast cancer patients. The test measures the expression of 21 genes in breast tumor tissue and generates a prediction of recurrence. Clinicians have begun to use the test to determine who best benefits from chemotherapy after surgery in hopes of avoiding unnecessary toxic treatment. ■

CURRENT SITUATION

Task Force Authority

The historic health care legislation signed into law by President Obama on March 23 includes a controversial — but little discussed — provision that expands the authority of the U.S. Preventive Services Task Force. Created in 1984, the independent panel of private-sector experts evaluates the scientific evidence for the effectiveness of preventive services, like mammography. Until March 23, its recommendations were considered authoritative, but primarily advisory.

Now USPSTF guidelines will have the weight of law. Under health care reform, all insurance plans eventually will have to cover at little or no cost to patients all preventive services that the task force rates as "A" or "B," indicating that science shows the service provides a net benefit that is moderate to substantial.

Late last year, when this provision was inserted into both the Senate and the House versions of health care reform, opposition was vigorous.

Critics quickly warned that the task force would ration care. "We're starting down a path, in my opinion, of socialization of medicine in this country," said Rep. Joe L. Barton, R-Texas, at a congressional hearing. "We don't want rationing of health care in America. We don't want to intervene between the doctor-patient relationship." [51]

Task force supporters disputed that charge. "Nothing could be further from the truth," said Rep. Waxman. The legislation simply established a minimum coverage, and insurers would be free to cover services given a lower rating, said Waxman. [52] In fact, the exact wording of the legislation is quite clear:

"Nothing in this subsection shall be construed to prohibit a plan or issuer from providing coverage for services in addition to those recommended by United States Preventive Services Task Force or to deny coverage for services that are not recommended by such Task Force." [53]

But critics worried the task force's ratings would serve as a benchmark, tempting insurers to withdraw coverage of lower-rated services, like mammograms for women in their 40s, which got a C rating last November.

So in early December, the Senate sprang into action and carved out an exception for mammography, delivering a significant blow to the credibility of the USPSTF. Because the Senate bill was eventually passed by the House and signed by the President into law, this exception now stands.

"As I reviewed the bill, I felt we could do more to enhance and improve women's healthcare," said Sen. Barbara Mikulski, D-Md., at the time. [54]

Mikulski and Olympia Snow, R-Maine, sponsored, and the Senate passed, an amendment requiring insurers to cover, without any costs to patients, preventive care and screenings for women approved by a federal agency, the Health Resources and Services Administration.

But an amendment offered by Sen. David Vitter, R-La., and passed by the Senate specifically set aside the USPSTF's November guidelines for the purposes of insurance coverage. "The current recommendations of the United States Preventive Services Task Force regarding breast cancer screening, mammography, and prevention shall be considered the most current other than those issued in or around November 2009." [55] In other words, the task force's B rating from 2002 is the one that counts. So insurers will have to cover screening mammography for women in their 40s.

Task Force Accountability

Besides expanding the authority of the USPSTF, the original House version of the health care reform measure had tried to make the panel's proceedings more transparent and its members more diverse.

The measure would have expanded the task force from 16 to 30 members, including specialists in women's health and geriatrics, for instance. Its meetings would have been made more public, and it would have had to consult a "stakeholder's board" made up of representatives from the public, advocacy groups and the insurance industry. [56]

"People who follow the USPSTF have long recognized some of the problems

Continued on p. 306

At Issue:

*Should the courts overturn patents for genes linked to elevated breast cancer risk?**

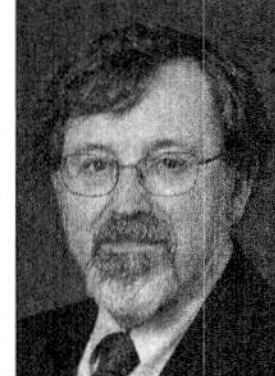

JEFFREY A. KANT
DIRECTOR, DIVISION OF MOLECULAR DIAGNOSTICS, UNIVERSITY OF PITTSBURGH MEDICAL CENTER; MEMBER, COLLEGE OF AMERICAN PATHOLOGISTS MOLECULAR PATHOLOGY WORKGROUP

WRITTEN FOR *CQ RESEARCHER*, APRIL 2010

Lawyers from the American Civil Liberties Union (ACLU) have laid out legal arguments challenging patents issued to Myriad Genetics for the genes known as BRCA1 and BRCA2. Mutations of the two genes provide a significant hereditary predisposition for breast and ovarian cancer. The case could set a landmark precedent. The College of American Pathologists is among 19 plaintiffs, representing thousands of medical researchers, physicians and patients who oppose the issuance of patents on human genes.

The College believes patents on genes, genetic variants and genotype-phenotype correlations — when enforced to restrict diagnostic genetic testing — violate longstanding prohibitions against patenting natural phenomena and laws of nature. The College's opposition to gene patents is rooted in principle and practice. Genes including their range of DNA sequence variants are naturally occurring products of nature, hence issuing a patent on an isolated gene — including mutations of that gene — violates legal principles restricting patents on products or laws of nature. As the law is currently written, patenting human genes limits patient access to medical care, jeopardizes the ability to practice medicine in the best interest of patients and raises the cost of care.

A patent holder may authorize a single lab to test a patented gene or require such high licensing fees that a wider range of laboratories are prevented from providing diagnostic services, second opinions or developing improved tests. As medical specialists in the diagnosis of disease, pathologists have an abiding interest in ensuring that gene patents do not restrict the ability of physicians to provide quality diagnostic services to the patients they serve. Multiple surveys have indicated that gene patents limit laboratory offerings as well as a patient's access to testing for specific genes and disorders.

Recently, the Department of Health and Human Services Secretary's Advisory Committee on Genetics, Health and Society voted to recommend exemptions from certain patents, which would allow medical researchers to study more genes and develop more diagnostic tests based on already patented human genes without the threat of a patent-infringement lawsuit. Recognition by this prestigious advisory group underscores the importance of addressing gene patents for the future of medical research, genetic testing and personalized health care.

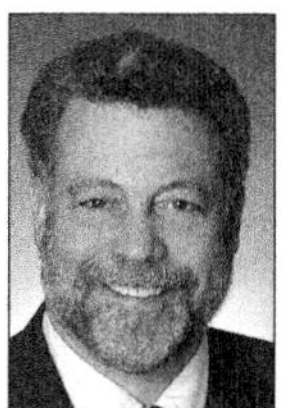

KEVIN E. NOONAN
PATENT ATTORNEY AND MOLECULAR BIOLOGIST, CHICAGO, ILL.

WRITTEN FOR *CQ RESEARCHER*, APRIL 2010

Patents for any invention do two things: protect from copiers (thereby promoting commercialization) and facilitate disclosure. U.S. patent law fulfills both these goals. Patent rights are granted for only 20 years from the application's filing date; after a patent expires, the invention is freely available to all — forever — and cannot be repatented or its availability otherwise restricted. Also, a patent applicant must provide a complete description of how to make and use the invention, ensuring that it is fully disclosed.

Isolated DNA is patentable for several reasons that contradict some of the misinformation spread by those opposed to the practice. First, patented DNA must be isolated from a cell, so that no one owns "your" DNA. Second, patented DNA is changed from its chemical form in the body, and this chemical conversion is more extensive than the types of purification of naturally occurring compounds, such as antibiotics and anti-cancer drugs, which are clearly patentable. Third, the genetic information contained in a patented gene is unpatentable and can be freely used. Fourth, gene patents do not prevent basic research on genes: The research database PubMed contains more than 7,000 research papers on the BRCA1 and BRCA2 genes, most of them published after the patents on these genes were granted. Finally, without patent protection, university researchers would be performing uncompensated research and development for corporations that would be able to use their inventions freely, since university scientists publish their work.

Most diseases are not like BRCA-linked breast or ovarian cancer; more than one gene is affected during the development of the disease. Imagine a world where isolated DNA was not patentable. Researchers could survey tissue samples to identify genes and alterations involved in common diseases like diabetes and cancer. Bio-informatics methods using "gene chips" containing 10,000 genes could then be used to provide a diagnosis without identifying the specific genes or mutations involved. The complexity of such systems would make them very hard to reverse-engineer, so developers could keep them a trade secret. The public would not benefit from the expiration of a patent or the disclosures that accompany patenting.

Critics of gene patenting do not take these disadvantages of banning such patenting into account. In addition, the reliance on emotional — and in some cases dishonest — appeals should raise serious questions about the motivations and cogency of these arguments.

---

* *Editor's note: On March 29, 2010, U.S. District Judge Robert W. Sweet struck down patents on two genes linked to breast and ovarian cancer, BRCA1 and BRCA2. Myriad Genetics, the patent holder, said it would appeal the decision.*

Continued from p. 304

with it," says Dick Woodruff, senior director of federal relations for the American Cancer Society's Cancer Action Network, which opposed the task force's revised mammography guidelines. "They operate several levels down in the bureaucracy, the meetings are closed and the membership is small," he adds.

Transparency and public trust are worthy goals, says former task force member Harris, "and I think there are good ways and bad ways to do it." It would help to allow for public comments on proposed task force guidelines before the panel takes its final votes, he said. But making every meeting public, he says, "would turn the proceedings into a circus."

Expanding the size of the task force could make meetings unwieldy, and the membership is already diverse, he says. "There are physicians, health economists, nursing specialists, pediatric people and ob-gyn," Harris says, and all of them have been trained in biostatistics. They know how to summarize, examine, and critically appraise the thousands of published studies of preventive services for which the task force issues guidelines, he says.

"We need to make sure the task force's evaluations remain free from advocacy, politics and economics," said Ned Calonge, the task force's chairman. [57]

Although the House provisions did not make it into the final health care reform legislation, supporters hope they will eventually become law. "Congress is legislating all the time," says Woodruff. "Hopefully, there will be opportunities in the future to improve upon the bill."

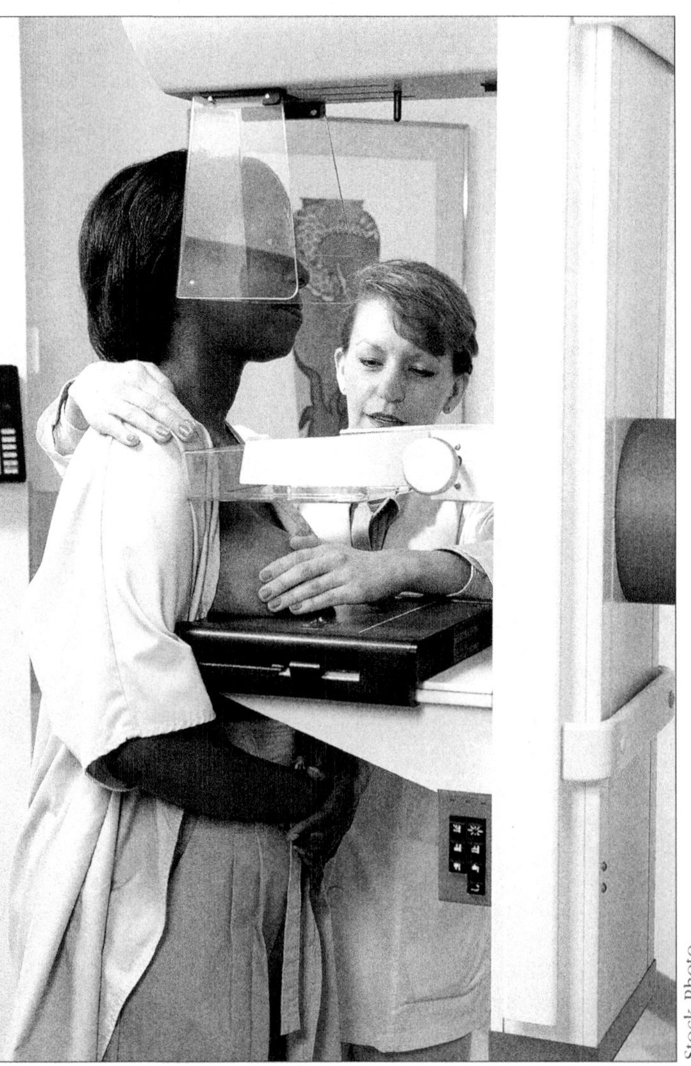

Stock Photo

Debate over the efficacy of regular mammography screening for women in their 40s has been going on for decades, and shows no sign of ending. Last November, an independent scientific panel recommended against routine screening for most women in this age bracket, reversing its recommendation of seven years earlier. In 1987, the National Cancer Institute recommended that healthy women, beginning at age 40, should get mammograms every one to two years. In 1993, it dropped that recommendation, only to adopt it again in 1997.

Breast Cancer Education

The health care reform law contains the Breast Cancer Education and Awareness Learning Young Act, or EARLY Act. Its controversial original version, introduced a year ago, directed the federal government to conduct a public education campaign to teach young women how to detect and prevent breast cancer, by encouraging breast exams, genetic counseling and lifestyle changes.

But critics worried that such a campaign would do more harm than good by raising unnecessary alarm among younger women, especially those in their 20s and 30s for whom breast cancer is a rare disease. Breast self exams might lead to false alarms and to unneeded mammograms and biopsies. And making lifestyle changes to reduce risk, these critics say, is not always feasible.

Two professors of medicine at the Dartmouth Institute for Health Policy and Clinical Practice pointed out that the most common risk factor for breast cancer is delaying childbirth, and the risk begins to rise if a woman has not had her first full-term pregnancy by age 20. In addition, some evidence indicates that young women with increased body mass have a lower risk of breast cancer. "It is hard to believe that the EARLY Act's sponsors would want to launch a public health campaign encouraging teens to become pregnant or gain weight," the professors wrote in a newspaper opinion piece. [58]

Susan Love, a breast cancer surgeon in Santa Monica, Calif., and president of the Dr. Susan Love Research Foundation, argued against passage of the EARLY Act. Young women may be led to overestimate their risk of dying from the disease, she said, and "once you have made women more 'aware' of their potential risk, you will have nothing to tell them to do," she wrote in a letter to the bill's sponsors. [59]

The American Cancer Society and its Cancer Action Network also opposed the EARLY Act, and the organization proposed revisions, which were eventually adopted.

"The key to the rewrite," says Woodruff, "was to give the secretary [of Health and Human Services] much broader authority to look at the evidence and the science and figure out how best to communicate to young women about breast health in general." Gone were specific recommendations for dietary changes, genetic counseling and breast self-exam.

But is the bill so watered down as to be unnecessary? "Our job is to look at the legislation and help to develop a bill that makes the most sense under the circumstances," says Woodruff. ■

OUTLOOK

Personalized Treatment

More than half of American women diagnosed with breast cancer each year have estrogen receptor positive cancer that has not spread to the lymph nodes. The standard treatment is surgery, plus radiation and hormonal therapy, which cures about 80 to 85 percent of patients. Yet most women with this diagnosis are also advised to receive often toxic chemotherapy to prevent the cancer's return. [60]

"The vast majority of people that we are treating with chemotherapy are not benefiting from the treatment" because they don't need it, says Joseph Sparano, MD, the director of the Breast Evaluation Center at the Montefiore-Einstein Cancer Center in the Bronx. Doctors are still refining the tools that would identify the minority of patients at risk of recurrence.

One of those tools is Oncotype DX, which marks a breakthrough in personalized medicine for breast cancer patients. It is a test that measures the activity of 21 genes in tumor tissue and allows doctors to customize treatment. The test generates a score ranging from 0 to 100; the higher the score, the greater the chance a woman has of a recurrence without chemotherapy. According to the National Cancer Institute, Oncotype DX is more accurate at estimating recurrence risk than standard measures, like tumor size. [61]

Since Oncotype DX came on the market in 2004, physicians have ordered it for more than 100,000 patients, and the American Society of Clinical Oncology has recently endorsed it. [62] In one study published this year, oncologists changed treatment recommendations for 31.5 percent of patients based on the Oncotype DX recurrence score, with the most common change from chemotherapy plus hormonal therapy to hormonal therapy alone. [63]

But the test's benefit is unclear for the majority of women receiving it, those whose scores fall in the 11 to 25 range. For women with scores below or above, Sparano says the treatment direction after surgery is clear: hormonal therapy alone for those with low scores and hormonal therapy plus chemotherapy when the score is high. But, he says, "We don't have really definitive information that a woman with a score in the mid-range really benefits from chemotherapy."

Sparano is recruiting patients into a nationwide study called TAILORx, designed to determine the benefit of chemotherapy to those women. Women with low or high scores will receive the accepted treatment for their scores, but women with a recurrence score of 11 to 25 will be randomly assigned to receive hormonal therapy, with or without chemotherapy. A total of 11,000 women are expected to be enrolled by mid-2011. The women will be studied for 10 years.

Personalized medicine is also being tested for women with high risk, fast growing breast cancers. In March, a public-private partnership led by the Foundation for the National Institutes of Health launched a national trial that would administer promising new drugs to women based on genetic markers in their tumors. The drugs would be given, along with chemotherapy, prior to surgery to help shrink tumors. [64]

"Personalized treatment of cancer is the future," says Dr. Edith Perez, director of the Mayo Clinic's Breast Program in Jacksonville, Fla., who is also recruiting patients for the TAILORx study. Perez runs the clinic's Breast Cancer Translational Genomics Program, whose purpose, she says, "is to eventually be able to do a complete genomic profiling of tissue from a woman's tumor, look for abnormalities and then customize treatment." ■

Notes

[1] "Can Breast Cancer Be Prevented?" American Cancer Society, September 2009, p. 1, www.cancer.org.

[2] For background, see David Masci, "Women's Health," *CQ Researcher*, Nov. 7, 2003, pp. 941-964.

[3] "Cancer Facts & Figures 2009," American Cancer Society, p. 9, www.cancer.org.

[4] *Ibid.*

[5] "Screening for Breast Cancer," United States Preventive Services Task Force, Agency for Healthcare Research and Quality, Department of Health & Human Services, November 2009, updated December 2009, www.ahrq.gov/clinic/USpstf/uspsbrca.htm#summary.
[6] "Hollywood Breast Cancer Survivors Speak Out Against New Mammogram Guidelines," "Access Hollywood," Nov. 18, 2009, www.accesshollywood.com.
[7] "USPSTF Mammography Recommendations Will Result in Countless Unnecessary Breast Cancer Deaths Each Year," American College of Radiology, Nov. 16, 2009, www.medicalnewstoday.com/articles/171247.php.
[8] "Secretary Sebelius Statement on New Breast Cancer Recommendations," Dept. of Health and Human Services, news release, Nov. 18, 2009, www.hhs.gov/news/press/2009pres/11/20091118a.html.
[9] Alice Park and Kate Pickert, "The Mammogram Melee," *Time*, Dec. 7, 2009, p. 40.
[10] "Opening Statement of Rep. Henry A. Waxman," Hearing on Breast Cancer Screening Recommendations, Subcommittee on Health, Dec. 2, 2009, http://energycommerce.house.gov./Press_111/20091202/waxman_opening.pdf.
[11] "New Mammography Guidelines, A Death Sentence for Black Women," Nov. 19, 2009, http://breakingoursilence.com.
[12] "Cancer Health Disparities," National Cancer Institute, March 11, 2008, www.cancer.gov/cancertopics/factsheet/cancer-health-disparities/disparities.
[13] "M.D. Anderson Study Finds Racial Disparities Exist in Radiation Therapy Rates for Early Stage Breast Cancer," news release, MD Anderson Cancer Center, Dec. 14, 2009, www.mdanderson.org/newsroom.
[14] Sandra Young, "New cervical cancer screening guidelines released," CNN, Nov. 20, 2009, www.cnn.com/2009/HEALTH/11/20/cervical.cancer.guidelines/.
[15] "American Cancer Society Responds to Changes to USPSTF Mammography Guidelines," American Cancer Society, Nov. 16, 2009, www.cancer.org.
[16] "ACOG Statement on Revised US Preventive Services Task Force Recommendations on Breast Cancer Screening," American Congress of Obstetricians and Gynecologists, Nov. 16, 2009, www.acog.org.
[17] "Society Responds to USPSTF Changes in Mammography Guidelines," American Society of Breast Surgeons, www.breastsurgeons.org.
[18] "USPSTF Mammography Recommendations Will Result in Countless Unnecessary Breast Cancer Deaths Each Year," *op. cit.*
[19] "New mammography guidelines a disservice," letter to the editor, *The San Diego Union-Tribune*, Dec. 27, 2009, p. B7.
[20] Robert Aronowitz, "Addicted to Mammograms," *The New York Times*, op-ed., Nov. 20, 2009.
[21] "Screening for Breast Cancer, Recommendation Statement," Agency for Healthcare Research and Quality, U.S. Department of Health & Human Services, December 2009, p. 2.
[22] Roni Caryn Rabin, "Doctor-Patient Divide on Mammograms," *The New York Times*, Feb. 16, 2010, p. D7.
[23] Beth A. Virnig, *et al.*, "Diagnosis and Management of Ductal Carcinoma in Situ (DCIS)," Agency for Healthcare Research and Quality, U.S. Department of Health and Human Services, September 2009, p. 1.
[24] Liz Szabo, " 'New' type of breast cancer stops women in their tracks; Mystery condition called DCIS sparks treatment debate," *USA Today*, Oct. 12, 2009, p. 5D.
[25] H. Gilbert Welch, *et al.*, "The Sea of Uncertainty Surrounding Ductal Carcinoma in Situ: The Price of Screening Mammography," *Journal of the National Cancer Institute*, Feb. 20, 2008, p. 228.
[26] Szabo, *op. cit.*
[27] Y. Y. Chen, *et al.*, "Pathologic and biologic response to preoperative endocrine therapy in patients with ER-positive ductal carcinoma in situ," *BMC Cancer*, Aug. 18, 2009.
[28] "Environmental Risk Factors for Breast Cancer," National Breast Cancer Coalition, September 2006, p. 2, www.stopbreastcancer.org.
[29] Ruthann A. Rudel, *et al.*, "Chemicals Causing Mammary Gland Tumors in Animals Signal New Directions for Epidemiology, Chemical Testing, and Risk Assessment for Breast Cancer Prevention," *Environmental Factors in Breast Cancer*, supplement to *Cancer*, June 15, 2007, pp. 2635-2636.
[30] Julia Green Brody and Ruthann A. Rudel, "Environmental Pollutants and Breast Cancer: The Evidence from Animal and Human Studies," *Breast Diseases: A Year Book Quarterly*, Vol. 19, No. 1, 2008, p. 17.
[31] Rudel, *et al.*, *op. cit.*
[32] Julia G. Brody, "Everyday Exposures and Breast Cancer," *Reviews on Environmental Health*, Vol. 25, No. 1, 2010, p. 3.
[33] Janet Gray, ed., "State of the Evidence: The Connection Between Breast Cancer and the Environment," Breast Cancer Fund, 2008, p. 9.
[34] "What is the National Children's Study?" www.nationalchildrensstudy.gov/Pages/default.aspx.
[35] Brody, *op. cit.*, p. 4.
[36] James S. Olson, *Bathsheba's Breast: Women, Cancer & History* (2002), p. 61.
[37] *Ibid.*
[38] *Ibid.*
[39] *Ibid.*, pp. 62-63.
[40] Barron H. Lerner, *The Breast Cancer Wars* (2001), p. 33.
[41] *Ibid.*, pp. 33-35.
[42] *Ibid.*, p. 69.
[43] *Ibid.*, p. 101.
[44] *Ibid.*, p. 115.
[45] Olson, *op. cit.*, p. 129.
[46] Bernard Fisher, "United States trials of conservative surgery," *World Journal of Surgery*, Vol. 1, No. 3, May 1977, www.springerlink.com/content/j1313t7453876666/.
[47] B. Fisher, *et al.*, "Twenty-year follow-up of a randomized trial comparing total mastec-

About the Author

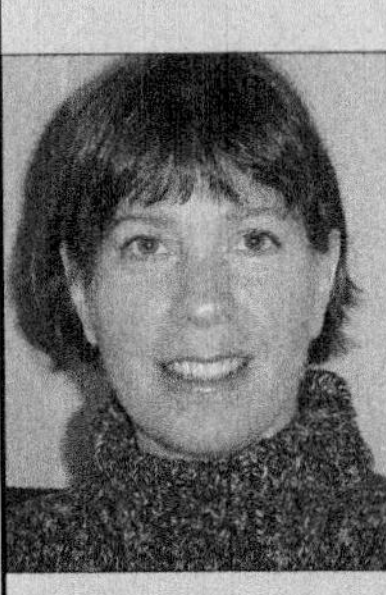

Barbara Mantel is a freelance writer in New York City whose work has appeared in *The New York Times*, the *Journal of Child and Adolescent Psychopharmacology* and *Mamm Magazine*. She is a former correspondent and senior producer for National Public Radio and has won several journalism awards, including the National Press Club's Best Consumer Journalism Award and the Front Page Award from the Newswomen's Club of New York for her April 18, 2008, *CQ Researcher* report "Public Defenders." She holds a B.A. in history and economics from the University of Virginia and an M.A. in economics from Northwestern University.

tomy, lumpectomy, and lumpectomy plus irradiation for the treatment of invasive breast cancer," *New England Journal of Medicine*, Oct. 17, 2002.

[48] Aronowitz, *op. cit.*

[49] "Gene BRCA1," The Chemical Heritage Foundation, 2001, www.chemheritage.org/EducationalServices/pharm/chemo/readings/brca1.htm.

[50] "Hormone Therapy," American Cancer Society, Sept. 18, 2009, www.cancer.org.

[51] Rob Stein, "In wake of mammography guidelines, U.S. health task force faces new scrutiny," *The Washington Post*, Dec. 20, 2009, p. A3.

[52] *Ibid.*

[53] Patient Protection and Affordable Care Act, Sec. 2713, http://thomas.loc.gov/cgi-bin/query/F?c111:7:./temp/~c111kVSix:e51492.

[54] Emily P. Walker, "Senate Affirms Screening Mammography for 40-Year-Olds," *MedPage Today*, Dec. 3, 2009.

[55] "Patient Protection and Affordable Care Act," Sec. 2713, *op. cit.*

[56] Stein, *op. cit.*

[57] *Ibid.*

[58] Steven Woloshin and Lisa M. Schwartz, "The EARLY Act is not what the doctor ordered," *Los Angeles Times*, July 31, 2009, http://articles.latimes.com/2009/jul/31/opinion/oe-woloshin31.

[59] Natasha Singer, "In Push for Cancer Screening, Limited Benefits," *The New York Times*, July 17, 2009, p. A1.

[60] "New Genetic Test for Personalized Treatment of Breast Cancer," Montefiore Medical Center, www.montefiore.org/whoweare/stories/Sparano/.

[61] "Personalized Treatment Trial for Breast Cancer Launched," National Cancer Institute, www.cancer.gov/newscenter/pressreleases/TAILORxRelease.

[62] Susan Jenks, "Gene tests avert chemotherapy," *Florida Today*, June 2, 2009, p. 1D.

[63] Shelly S. Lo, *et al.*, "Prospective Multicenter Study of the Impact of the 21-Gene Recurrence Score Assay on Medical Oncologist and Patient Adjuvant Breast Cancer Treatment Selection," *Journal of Clinical Oncology*, abstract, Jan. 11, 2009, jco.ascopubs.org/cgi/content/abstract/JCO.2008.20.2119v1.

[64] "The Biomarkers Consortium Launches I-Spy 2 Breast Cancer Clinical Trial," Foundation for the National Institutes of Health, March 17, 2010, www.biomarkersconsortium.org/images/stories/docs/ispypress031710.pdf.

FOR MORE INFORMATION

Agency for Healthcare Research and Quality, 540 Gaither Road, Suite 2000, Rockville, MD 20850; (301) 427-1364; www.ahrq.gov. A Department of Health and Human Services agency that uses research to improve health care practice and policy.

American Cancer Society, 250 Williams St., N.W., Atlanta, GA 30303; (404) 320-3333; www.cancer.org. A nationwide, community-based health organization that sponsors cancer research, educates the public and advocates for policies and laws.

Breast Cancer Action, 55 New Montgomery St., San Francisco, CA 94105; (415) 243-9301; http://bcaction.org. Advocates for policy changes in treatment, environmental exposures and health care inequities.

Breast Cancer Fund, 1388 Sutter St., Suite 400, San Francisco, CA 94109; (415) 346-8223; www.breastcancerfund.org. Advocates for elimination of environmental and other preventable causes of breast cancer.

Centers for Disease Control and Prevention, Division of Cancer Prevention and Control, 4770 Buford Hwy, N.E., MS K-64, Atlanta, GA 30341; (800) 232-4636; www.cdc.gov/cancer/breast. Federal agency that collects information about cancer, including who gets it, at what stage it is diagnosed and how it is treated.

Dr. Susan Love Research Foundation, 811 Wilshire Blvd., Suite 500, Santa Monica, CA 90403; (310) 828-0060; www.dslrf.org. Works to eradicate breast cancer and improve the quality of women's health through research, education and advocacy.

National Breast Cancer Coalition, 1101 17th St., N.W., Suite 1300, Washington, DC 20036; (202) 296-7477; www.stopbreastcancer.org. Lobbies national, state and local governments for increased funding for cancer research and improved health care access for women.

National Breast Cancer Foundation, 2600 Network Blvd., Suite 300, Frisco, TX 75034; (469) 252-0075; www.nationalbreastcancer.org. Funds free mammograms for women in need.

National Cancer Institute, 6116 Executive Blvd., Bethesda, MD 20892; (301) 496-6641; www.cancer.gov. The principal federal agency for cancer research and training.

National Women's Health Network, 1413 K St., N.W., 4th floor, Washington, DC 20005; (202) 682-2640; http://nwhn.org. Promotes a critical analysis of health issues in order to affect policy and support consumer decision-making.

RxList, c/o WebMD, 111 8th Ave, 7th Floor, New York, NY 10011; (212) 624-3700; www.rxlist.com. An online medical resource providing detailed and current pharmaceutical information on brand and generic drugs.

Silent Spring Institute, 29 Crafts St., Newton, MA 02458; (617) 332-4288; www.silentspring.org. Investigates research into the links between the environment and women's health, with particular emphasis on breast cancer.

Susan G. Komen for the Cure, 5005 LBJ Freeway, Suite 250, Dallas, TX 75244; (877) 465-6636; www.komen.org. A worldwide grassroots network of breast cancer survivors and activists that raises money for research through its Race for the Cure.

Bibliography

Selected Sources

Books

Lerner, Barron H., *The Breast Cancer Wars: Hope, Fear, and the Pursuit of a Cure in Twentieth-Century America*, Oxford University Press, 2001.

A Columbia University professor of medicine examines the medical and cultural history of the battle against breast cancer in the United States.

Olson, James S., *Bathsheba's Breast: Women, Cancer & History*, The Johns Hopkins University Press, 2002.

A history professor at Sam Houston State University in Huntsville, Texas, describes the history of breast cancer through the stories of historical figures like Abigail Adams and Betty Ford.

Articles

Park, Alice, and Kate Pickert, "The Mammogram Melee," *Time*, Dec. 7, 2009.

The furor over the new breast cancer screening guidelines from the U.S. Preventive Services Task Force could be a sign of things to come.

Rabin, Roni Caryn, "Doctor-Patient Divide on Mammograms," *The New York Times*, Feb. 16, 2010.

Many doctors are inclined to accept the new breast cancer screening guidelines, while many patients reject them.

Stein, Rob, "In wake of mammography guidelines, U.S. health task force faces new scrutiny," *The Washington Post*, Dec. 20, 2009.

Members of the U.S. Preventive Services Task Force testify before Congress about breast cancer screening and the task force's expanded role under health care reform.

Szabo, Liz, " 'New' type of breast cancer stops women in their tracks," *USA Today*, Oct. 12, 2009.

Doctors are treating ductal carcinoma in situ (DCIS) aggressively even though not all cases will develop into invasive breast cancer.

Welch, H. Gilbert, Steven Woloshin and Lisa M. Schwartz, "The Sea of Uncertainty Surrounding Ductal Carcinoma in Situ —The Price of Screening Mammography," *Journal of the National Cancer Institute*, Feb. 20, 2008.

A journal editorial argues it may be time to consider reserving biopsy for lesions that can be palpated.

Reports and Studies

"Screening for Breast Cancer: Recommendation Statement," U.S. Preventive Services Task Force, November 2009, updated December 2009, www.ahrq.gov/clinic/uspstf09/breastcancer/brcanrs.htm.

The task force no longer recommends routine screening for most women in their 40s and recommends screening for women 50-74 only every other year.

Allegra, Carmen J., "National Institutes of Health State-of-the-Science Conference Statement: Diagnosis and Management of Ductal Carcinoma In Situ Sept. 22-24, 2009," *Journal of the National Cancer Institute*, Vol. 102, Issue 3, Feb. 6, 2010.

The statement assesses the current data on diagnosis and management of DCIS.

Brody, Julia Green, *et al.*, "Environmental Pollutants and Breast Cancer: Epidemiologic Studies," *Cancer*, May 14, 2007, www3.interscience.wiley.com/cgi-bin/fulltext/114261513/PDFSTART.

The authors review the limited research on links between environmental pollutants and breast cancer risk in humans.

Gray, Janet, ed., "State of the Evidence: The Connection Between Breast Cancer and the Environment," Breast Cancer Fund, 2008, www.breastcancerfund.org/media/publications/state-of-the-evidence.

The author summarizes hundreds of studies examining links between breast cancer and chemicals and radiation in the environment.

Robson, Mark E., *et al.*, "American Society of Clinical Oncology Policy Statement Update: Genetic and Genomic Testing for Cancer Susceptibility," *Journal of Clinical Oncology*, Jan. 11, 2010, http://jco.ascopubs.org/cgi/doi/10.1200/JCO.2009.27.0660.

The professional group revises its testing recommendations for genetic mutations associated with breast cancer risk and raises concerns about genetic tests marketed directly to consumers.

Rudel, Ruthann A., *et al.*, "Chemicals Causing Mammary Gland Tumors in Animals Signal New Directions for Epidemiology, Chemicals Testing, and Risk Assessment for Breast Cancer Prevention," *Environmental Factors in Breast Cancer*, Supplement to *Cancer*, May 14, 2007.

The authors identify 216 chemicals associated with increases in mammary gland tumors in animals.

Virnig, Beth A., "Diagnosis and Management of Ductal Carcinoma In Situ (DCIS)," Agency for Healthcare Research and Quality, AHRQ Publication No. 09-E018, September 2009, www.ahrq.gov/clinic/tp/dcistp.htm.

The authors review the literature on the incidence and treatment of DCIS and recommend further avenues for research.

The Next Step:

Additional Articles from Current Periodicals

Early Detection

Begley, Sharon, "The Myth of Early Detection," *Newsweek*, April 6, 2009, p. 44.
Many breast cancer survivors say early detection saved their lives, but early detection does not necessarily produce clear and unquestionable benefits.

Frellick, Marcia, "Breast Cancer Research Advancing," *Chicago Tribune*, Oct. 4, 2009, p. A24.
Mammograms are still vital to fighting breast cancer, but new tools for detection are more promising than ever.

Tatum, Cheryl, "New HMC MRI Aids Breast Cancer Detection," *The Tennessean*, March 30, 2009.
A Tennessee hospital has installed new MRI technology that can detect previously undetectable breast cancers.

Health Care Proposals

Park, Alice, and Kate Pickert, "The Mammogram Melee," *Time*, Dec. 7, 2009, p. 40.
New breast cancer recommendations from the U.S. Preventive Services Task Force may be difficult for Americans to accept.

Pear, Robert, and David M. Herszenhorn, "Senate Backs Preventive Health Care for Women," *The New York Times*, Dec. 4, 2009, p. A21.
The Senate has voted to require health insurance companies to provide free mammograms for women while rejecting a Republican challenge to Medicare savings that would finance most of the bill.

Yamamura, Kevin, "Health Policy Very Personal for Fiorina," *Sacramento Bee*, Nov. 26, 2009, p. A1.
U.S. Senate candidate Carly Fiorina, R-Calif., is a breast cancer survivor and opposes any health policy recommending that women get fewer mammograms.

Mammography

Brawley, Otis W., "Cancer Society: Let's Stick With Mammograms," *News Journal* (Delaware), Nov. 23, 2009.
Many women would not be candidates for breast-conserving therapy without mammograms, according to the American Cancer Society.

Brinker, Nancy, "Debating Mammograms," *Newsweek*, Dec. 21, 2009, p. 20.
Mammograms are not perfect, but they are still the best breast cancer screening tool widely available.

Rabin, Roni Caryn, "Benefits of Mammogram Under Debate in Britain," *The New York Times*, March 31, 2009, p. D5.
Mammograms diagnose breast cancer in many women that is so slow-growing that it would never threaten their lives.

Smith, Stephen, "Breast Screening Advice Upended," *The Boston Globe*, Nov. 17, 2009, p. 30.
The U.S. Preventive Services Task Force has concluded that mammograms save the lives of very few women ages 40 to 49.

Voskuil, Scott, "Digital Mammography Offers Many Advantages," *Herald Times Reporter* (Wisconsin), Oct. 19, 2009, p. 1B.
Digital mammography offers several advantages over regular mammography largely because images can be manipulated after they are recorded.

Risk Factors

Charles-Harris, Hakan, "Black Women More Likely to Die From Breast Cancer," *Miami Times*, April 1, 2009, p. 15B.
Breast cancer is the leading cancer among white and black women, but black women are more likely to die from the disease.

Fahrner, Mari Anne, "Medications Decrease Risk of Breast Cancer, Studies Find," *St. Louis Post-Dispatch*, Aug. 27, 2009, p. B2.
Several prevention trials provide evidence that women with above average risks for breast cancer can decrease the risks with medication.

Simmons, Shannon, "Diet, Exercise May Help Prevent Breast Cancer," *Statesman Journal* (Oregon), Oct. 8, 2009, p. 1.
A healthy diet and regular exercise can help reduce a woman's weight, which in turn reduces her risk for breast cancer.

CITING *CQ RESEARCHER*

Sample formats for citing these reports in a bibliography include the ones listed below. Preferred styles and formats vary, so please check with your instructor or professor.

MLA STYLE

Jost, Kenneth. "Rethinking the Death Penalty." CQ Researcher 16 Nov. 2001: 945-68.

APA STYLE

Jost, K. (2001, November 16). Rethinking the death penalty. *CQ Researcher, 11*, 945-968.

CHICAGO STYLE

Jost, Kenneth. "Rethinking the Death Penalty." *CQ Researcher*, November 16, 2001, 945-968.

CHAPTER

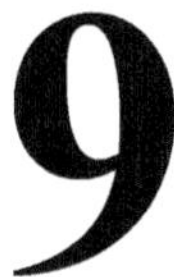

Preventing Cancer

By Marcia Clemmitt

Excerpted from the CQ Researcher. Marcia Clemmitt. (January 16, 2009). "Preventing Cancer." *CQ Researcher*, 25-48.

Preventing Cancer

BY MARCIA CLEMMITT

THE ISSUES

When Sen. Edward M. Kennedy, D-Mass., was diagnosed with brain cancer in May 2008, it wasn't the first time a Kennedy had confronted the deadly disease. Two of Kennedy's three children have been diagnosed with cancer.

An above-the-knee leg amputation followed by then-experimental chemotherapy cured his 12-year-old son Edward of bone cancer in 1973. In 2002, Kennedy's daughter, Kara, then 42, was diagnosed with lung cancer, which was also halted by surgery. In 1988, Kennedy's other son, Rep. Patrick Kennedy, D-R.I., then 20, was diagnosed with a benign spinal tumor, which was surgically removed. [1]

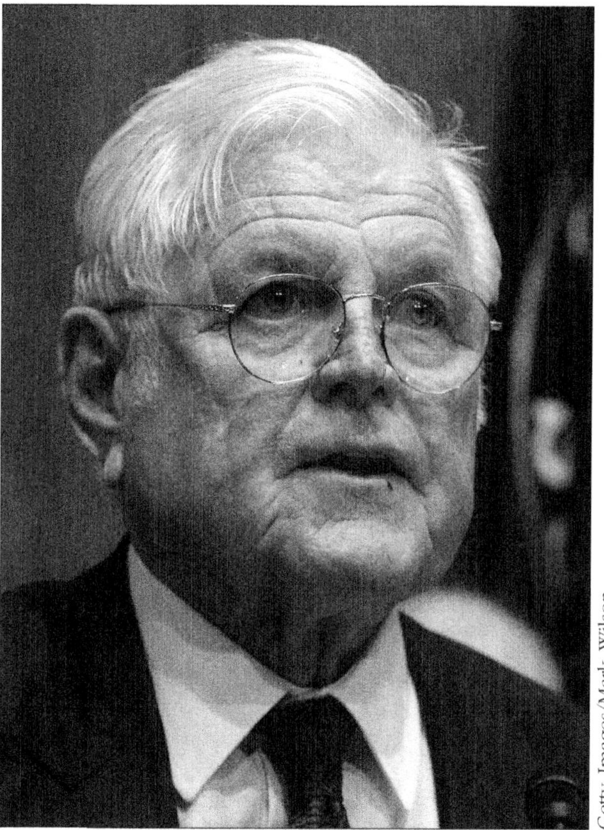

Getty Images/Mark Wilson

Sen. Edward M. Kennedy, D-Mass., is back in the Senate after having a cancerous brain tumor surgically removed last summer. Both Kennedy and President-elect Barack Obama plan to push for more aggressive action on cancer research this year. But many experts say the most effective strategy would be to focus more on detection and prevention.

In each case, Sen. Kennedy was an aggressive advocate, seeking out a range of medical opinions before choosing a course, and observers have no doubt that he's taking the same approach with his own cancer. "This family has had cancer laid in front of it, and each time they have beaten it," said David J. Sugarbaker, chief of thoracic surgery at Boston's Brigham and Women's Hospital, who operated on Kara Kennedy. "They have an insatiable appetite for information and answers." [2]

Sen. Kennedy's tumor was surgically removed last summer, but brain cancer is harder to beat than many other cancers, partly because it's more difficult to remove the entire tumor.

Now back in the Senate, Kennedy hopes to shepherd to passage a comprehensive cancer bill — conceived of before his diagnosis — to improve the process of turning lab science into effective drugs to treat cancer. With President-elect Barack Obama, whose mother died of ovarian and uterine cancer, also hoping to overhaul the federal cancer program's clinical initiatives, 2009 could be a banner year for cancer patient advocates. However, many experts say effective cancer treatments are, and will remain, elusive and that the most effective strategy in the future would be to focus more on detection and prevention.

Cancer drugs are "particularly likely to fail in development compared to other therapies," according to an expert panel at a September 2008 conference at the Brookings Institution think tank in Washington. "One estimate shows that 60 percent of cancer-drug development programs fail in the late clinical phase." [3]

Eventually, scientists are likely to uncover key cell molecules that can be targeted with drugs that will keep some cancers in check, but gene science is in its infancy, says Kenneth W. Kinzler, a professor of oncology at the Johns Hopkins School of Medicine. Thus, he says, "from a practical point of view, prevention, early diagnosis and behavioral modification" — to squelch cancer-causing habits like smoking — "are really important."

Furthermore, individuals' cancers mutate in such a way that they eventually become resistant to even drugs that were initially effective, says Kinzler, whose lab has produced the first genetic profiles of colon, breast, pancreatic and brain tumors. Thus, no single drug treatment is likely to outrun cancer over the long haul.

In short, cancer remains such a formidable force that prevention is a far more potent anti-cancer strategy than previously imagined, said Kinzler's colleague Bert Vogelstein, co-director of Hopkins' Kimmel Cancer Center. "It's accurate to say that 99 percent of applied cancer research now goes toward developing new therapeutics," Vogelstein said, but "it is . . . apparent from [gene] studies like ours that it is going to be even more difficult . . . than previously expected to derive real cures from such therapies. The proportion of effort and funding devoted to other ways of managing cancer, such as prevention and early detection, should be greatly increased." [4]

Pancreatic Cancer Is Most Lethal Form

Only 5 percent of Americans with pancreatic cancer survive for five years, compared with 15 percent of lung cancer victims and 89 percent of those with breast cancer. Lung and colorectal cancer cause the most deaths each year in the United States.

Most Common Forms of Cancer in the U.S.
(Listed in order of lethality)

Type of Cancer	5-Year Survival Rate	No. of Deaths	Risk Factors
Pancreatic Cancer	5%	34,300	Smoking, chewing tobacco and being heavily exposed to chemicals, dyes and pesticides increase risk. Mainly strikes people over age 55.
Lung Cancer	15%	161,840	Most deaths are related to tobacco smoke. Lung cancer is also the largest cause of cancer deaths worldwide.
Stomach Cancer	24%	10,900	Though rare in the U.S., it's the second-biggest cancer killer worldwide, with 900,000 deaths. Infection with *Helicobacter pylori,* a common bacterium also associated with ulcers, may be a major cause, but most who carry it don't get the disease. Smoking doubles risk.
Brain/Nervous-System Tumors	29%	Over 13,000	Even "benign" brain tumors can fatally damage the brain. Risk factors largely unknown.
Multiple Myeloma	34%	10,700	African-Americans are twice as likely as whites to get the immune system disease.
Ovarian Cancer	45%	Over 15,500 women	Family history, obesity, childlessness, use of estrogen as hormone replacement therapy and use of talcum powder in the genital area are risk factors.
Leukemia	50%	21,700	Exposure to high levels of radiation and to certain chemicals, such as benzene and some chemotherapy drugs, increase risk.
Colorectal Cancer	64%	50,000	Nine of 10 cases occur in people over age 50. Mortality higher among long-term smokers than nonsmokers.
Non-Hodgkin's Lymphoma	79%	Over 19,000	Can occur at any age. Risk factors largely unknown.
Breast Cancer	89%	40,500 women	Five to 10 percent of breast cancers are inherited. Having more than two alcoholic drinks daily, being overweight and having extra fat at the waist increase risk.
Prostate Cancer	99%	28,600	Two out of three cancers occur in men over age 65. Eating large amounts of red meat or high-fat dairy products increases risk.

Source: National Cancer Institute

Cancer prevention can make a huge difference, experts insist. For example, ending smoking "could cut the cancer burden by 30 percent," says Gerald N. Wogan, a professor emeritus of chemistry at the Massachusetts Institute of Technology.

In fact, U.S. smoking rates have been declining for about two decades, but the rate of decline has slowed recently. In 2007, the percentage of people over 18 who smoke dropped below 20 percent — to 19.8 percent, amounting to about 43 million smokers — for the first time since at least the 1960s. But the percentage of high school students who smoked remained constant, at 20 percent, between 2003 to 2007. [5]

But prevention continues to receive fewer funds and less attention than treatment, say many experts. Prevention-related findings routinely are ignored for years after evidence emerges, says Samuel Epstein, professor emeritus of environmental and occupational medicine at the University of Illinois School of Public Health.

For example, the National Cancer Institute (NCI) waited until 2002 to declare that hormone-replacement therapy raised women's cancer risks, although at least a decade's worth of earlier studies strongly suggested the connection, he says. And as early as 1994, research strongly linked talcum powder use to lethal ovarian cancer, especially in black women, but the Food and Drug Administration (FDA) "ignored it," he says. "Today the evidence of the connection is overwhelming," but in the United States, "the idea is, if you get cancer, it's your own fault" for smoking or eating fatty foods, and manufactured products aren't to blame.

Meanwhile, recent drug-development research has swallowed up billions of dollars and years of scientists' time while producing relatively few results, says Guy B. Faguet, author of the 2008 book *The War on Cancer* and a professor emeritus of medicine at the Medical College of Georgia. The World

Health Organization lists 17 cancer drugs that really make a difference, "and they were all developed before 1970," he says.

In addition, science has "fads and fashions, mostly driven by technology," says Wogan. And thanks to new, lightning-fast gene-sequencing technology, "genetics is everything" is the fashion today, while research on prevention-related questions — such as how cancer-promoting substances or processes (carcinogens) interact with cells to cause cancer — is being "left by the wayside."

Tobacco has been the subject of the highest-profile debate over carcinogens. But some environmental-health experts say cancerous changes in our cells result from a lifetime of mostly low-level exposure to a variety of substances, including many industrial chemicals, and that U.S. law takes this too lightly.

"A growing body of evidence from both human and animal models indicates that exposure of fetuses, young children and adolescents to radiation and environmental chemicals puts them at considerably higher risk for later-life breast cancer diagnosis," according to the Breast Cancer Fund. Furthermore, the rising incidence of breast cancer after World War II "paralleled the proliferation of synthetic chemicals," says the group. [6]

Many other countries take a more cautious approach to potential carcinogens, says Richard Clapp, a professor of environmental health at the Boston University School of Public Health. The World Health Organization's International Agency for Research on Cancer (IARC) issues a consensus listing of more than 100 substances that cause cancer in humans. "A third of the substances are industrial in origin," and many European governments limit the use of all items on the list, "since we now understand that long-term low-dose exposure" — generally construed as harmless by U.S. regulatory agencies — can actually have a cumulative carcinogenic effect, he says.

Cancer Survival Rates Steadily Increasing

The five-year survival rates for many types of cancer have increased from three decades ago. Breast cancer had one of the largest increases: jumping 14.8 points, from 74.4 percent to 89.2 percent.

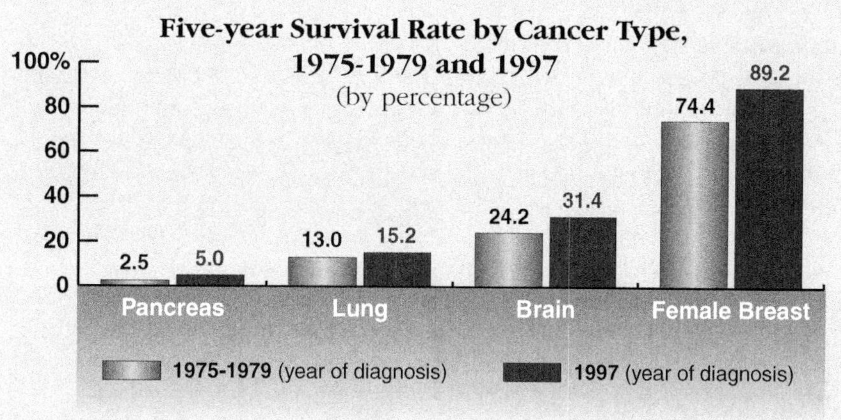

Source: Surveillance, Epidemiology and End Results Program, National Cancer Institute

"In the workplace, we have [Occupational Safety and Health Administration] lists of carcinogens, but we aren't enforcing them," Clapp says. The new science of "green chemistry" — which seeks to develop less toxic compounds and processes — can develop non-carcinogenic substitutes for toxic chemicals, he says. "It's not like life will fall apart if we don't use trichloroethylene to clean oily parts."

But others argue that lifestyle causes — like cigarette smoking — remain the real cancer threat and that most of the to-do over potential industrial carcinogens is misplaced.

"Some environmental pollutants, like pesticides, have been shown to induce cancer in laboratory animals at high doses, but they pose little risk to most people because of very low concentrations in air, land or water," said the American Institute for Cancer Research (AICR). And while "some workers come into regular contact with known carcinogens, such as asbestos, nickel, cadmium, uranium, radon, vinyl chloride, and benzene . . . it is important to remember that the vast majority of Americans are not exposed" to these risks. [7]

Besides preventive efforts, finding cancers early, when they can be cut out surgically or killed by drugs and radiation more easily than later-stage cancers, is crucial for future progress, many scientists say. Like prevention, however, screening has been less of a focus than treatment.

It's now known that every cancer contains a multitude of mutated genes, which means the war on cancer will be "more of a guerrilla war" than previously thought, said Kinzler. "The best long-term strategy may be early detection of tumors, when the number of guerrilla warriors is still small and more easily handled." [8]

At present, Americans don't do a very good job of detecting cancers early, says University of Chicago professor of medicine Richard L. Schilsky, chairman of the country's oldest National Cancer Institute-sponsored clinical-trials group, the Cancer and Leukemia Group. For example, only about half of the Americans who should be screened for colon cancer are screened, even though early detection is known to decrease mortality for colon cancer, says Schilsky, president of the American Society of Clinical Oncology (ASCO).

But others warn that much screening is imperfect and carries its own risks. Mammography screening "finds too many cancers," for example, said H. Gilbert Welch, a professor of medicine at Dartmouth Medical School in New Hampshire. "Because doctors don't know which cancers will be harmful, we treat all of them," unnecessarily exposing some women to disfiguring surgery and chemotherapy side effects. [9]

As lawmakers, physicians and patient groups mull the future of cancer control, here are some of the questions being asked:

Are we screening enough people for cancer?

Many experts insist that screening more patients for cancer would save lives and money. But there's reason to believe that some widespread screening is picking up conditions that aren't dangerous.

Early detection is vital for two reasons: Surgery can cure some early-stage cancers, unlike drug treatment and radiation, which only delay cancer's progress. Moreover, in later stages cancers have accumulated genetic mutations that increase their ability to evade both drug treatments and the body's own defenses, says Johns Hopkins' Kinzler.

Although current screening methods cannot catch all or most cancers, screening is still "a conceptually viable" way to control cancer, because improved screening methods likely will emerge from the human genome database, according to Faguet at the Medical College of Georgia. [10]

Responsibility falls on primary-care doctors to screen for cancer and all other diseases, but sparse communication among medical specialties makes that difficult, says the University of Chicago's Schilsky. "It's not as easy as you'd like" to get up-to-date screening recommendations, since there is no one-stop shop that covers cancer and all the other diseases primary-care physicians should screen for, he says.

Nationwide screening for colon cancer beginning at age 55 would save at least two dollars for every dollar it costs, according to Scott Tenner, an associate professor of medicine at the State University of New York's Health Sciences Center in Brooklyn. But lack of insurance coverage and other barriers keep many people from being screened until they enter Medicare at age 65, when cancers that could have been surgically cured have advanced to become lethal and expensive to treat, he said. [11]

But Medicare patients aren't getting recommended screenings either, according to the federal Agency for Healthcare Research and Quality. For example, from 1998-2004, only 25 percent received colorectal cancer screenings, the agency said. [12]

And screening tests are desperately needed for other big killers, some of which are considerably more deadly and rarer — such as pancreatic cancer — than cancers that we have screening tests for, says A. William Blackstock, Jr., an associate professor of radiation oncology at the Wake Forest University School of Medicine. "If you catch a disease late, there's not much you can ever do about it," and lack of screening methods mean lethal diseases like pancreatic cancer are virtually always caught late, he says.

Nevertheless, the rate of cancer screening has increased enormously over the past few decades. For example, mortality from cervical cancer declined long ago in the United States, largely because of widespread screening with Pap tests, which began in the 1950s, says John Bailar, a former chief of the NCI's demography section.

But some physicians warn that aggressive screening is not a panacea, because screening methods can't fully distinguish between deadly and benign tumors. For every 1,000 women who have regular mammography screening over a 10-year period, one woman will live longer because a cancer was detected at a treatable state, but five others will receive unnecessary cancer treatment, according to an analysis of international data. [13]

"Whether this is too high a price to pay is open to debate," but women and policy makers should consider it as they make decisions, the authors wrote. [14]

Prostate-cancer screening based on finding PSA — prostate specific antigen — in men's blood has a similar statistical picture, according to Thomas A. Stamey, a professor emeritus of urology at the Stanford University School of Medicine. "It's immoral for surgeons not to tell patients that we [men] all get prostate cancer as we age," said Stamey, who, at age 76, said he hadn't been screened for several years. "Do we really want to screen 100,000 men to save 226 from dying of prostate cancer?" he asked. "It's about the same chance of my not driving home safely tonight." [15]

"The media have taken it on ourselves to promote everybody getting screened for everything," believing that's the right public-health message, says medical journalist Shannon Brownlee, author of *Overtreated: Why Too Much Medicine Is Making Us Sicker and Poorer.* In international comparisons, U.S. survival rates for some cancers — such as a 99 percent five-year survival rate for prostate cancer — "make us look like geniuses," says Brownlee. But "if you're treating a lot of things that didn't need to be treated [in the first place], of course people are going to survive."

And screening doesn't always lengthen lives. In a 2007 study of computed tomography (CT) scanning of current and former smokers, researchers from New York's Memorial Sloan-Kettering Cancer Center found nearly three times as many lung cancers as predicted but also found that the early detection and treatment "did not lead to a corresponding decrease in advanced lung cancers or a reduction in deaths." [16]

In fact, too much screening for all kinds of ills actually is raising our cancer risk, says Brownlee. Increasingly, physicians order CT scans for many medical complaints and even to pick up hidden ills in healthy people. Within the next few years, "Americans will be getting 100 million scans a year, and each is one hell of a dose of radiation" — at least 100 times a chest X-ray, says Brownlee. "It's very clear that we are causing cancer."

Are too few resources devoted to cancer prevention?

Critics say prevention has long been downplayed by the cancer establishment, even though organizations like the American Cancer Society and the NCI insist they are just as serious about preventing cancer as they are in treating it, citing efforts to stamp out cigarette smoking as an example of prevention programs.

"We very firmly believe in prevention," says Christy Schmidt, senior director for policy of the society's Cancer Action Network.

In fact, interest in cancer prevention research appears to be increasing as health-care costs continue to rise, said a 2007 report from the President's Cancer Panel, a group of experts that monitors the cancer landscape. For example, larger employers and some state and local governments are devising and implementing "wellness programs," including such cancer-prevention activities as smoking cessation and exercise classes. [17]

Moreover, 21st-century research that highlights cancer's complexities has intensified the focus on prevention — including environmental factors — say some cancer researchers. [18] In the past, "everybody was convinced cancer was genetic and assumed it came from what you were born with," says H. Kim Lyerly, director of Duke University's Comprehensive Cancer Center. Scientists assumed that identical twins, for instance, would be susceptible to cancer in exactly the same way, he says. "Then it turned out that it was only a 10-15 percent chance," he says.

Thus, the environment — ranging from chemicals in the air and water to differing hormone levels in the body — accounts for the other 85-90 percent of cancer risk, Lyerly says. And since many environmental factors are avoidable, this new knowledge has led scientists to focus heavily on prevention, he says.

"We already have enough data to be able to say that a third of cancers could be prevented with healthy eating, weight management and exercise and another third with stopping tobacco use," says AICR nutrition education consultant Karen Collins.

Yet, prevention efforts can take a long time to pay off. Recent improved cancer mortality and incidence numbers are the fruit of prevention efforts long in the pipeline, physicians point out. For example, smoking-cessation efforts launched in the 1970s have finally paid off with fewer cancer cases in 2008, according to the latest numbers, says Blackstock at Wake Forest. But many analysts say that if significant new strides are to be made, prevention efforts must be greatly enhanced.

Bailar, the former head of the NCI's demography section, says an unbiased review of new cancer mortality statistics reveals a pattern: The improvement in cancer death rates is more related to prevention and early detection than to cancer treatment, even though research funding has traditionally run about four to one the other way.

Prevention and detection have long been "the poor stepsisters" of cancer medicine, says Bailar. When he started out in cancer research in the mid-1950s, he says, "the interest was moving to treatment, and it's been there ever since."

Prevention research funding "is still quite limited" compared with support for research on detection and treatment, the President's Cancer Panel said in 2007. Especially lacking is research on how to help people change unhealthy behaviors and how policy changes — such as city planning —

Smoking Is the Biggest Cause of Cancer

Scientists agree that smoking is the single, biggest cause of cancer. In addition to lung cancer, smoking significantly increases the risk for pancreas, stomach, kidney and bladder cancer.

Smoking. . . .

Causes more than a quarter of cancer deaths in developed countries.
Will kill around half of current smokers if they continue to smoke, including up to 40 percent of them in middle age.
Causes 9 in 10 cases of lung cancer.
Causes two out of three cases of bladder cancer in men and one in three in women.
Doubles the risk of kidney cancer.
Is the only preventable cause of pancreatic cancer.
Causes about one in five cases of stomach cancer.

Source: Cancer Research UK

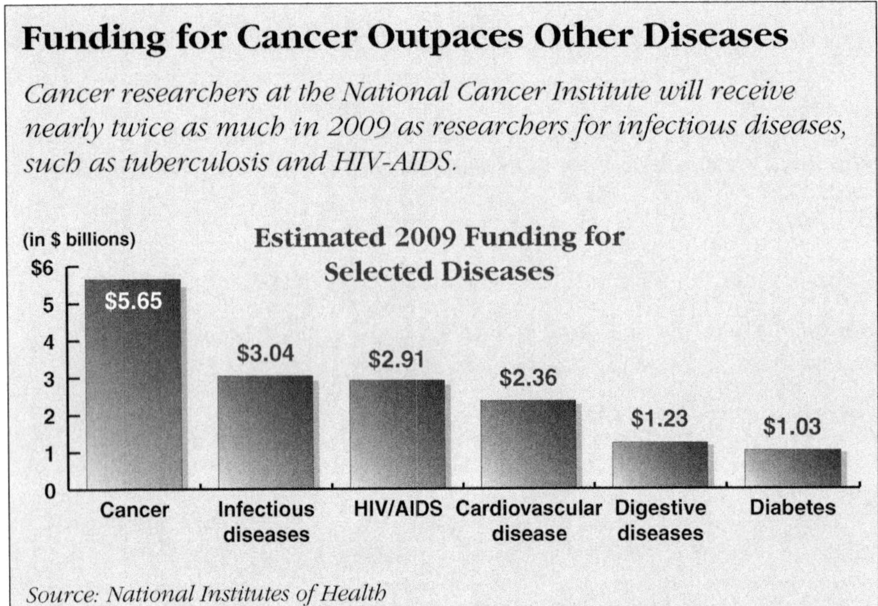

could get people to exercise more, the group said. [19]

In addition, many millions of Americans — especially low-paid and part-time workers, the uninsured and minorities — continue to lack access to wellness services like smoking-cessation programs, said the panel. [20]

And as for exposure to workplace carcinogens, the federal Occupational Safety and Health Administration (OSHA) specifies what substances are carcinogenic and at what levels and can legally limit workers' exposure, "but we haven't been using those tools," says Boston University's Clapp.

Anti-tobacco efforts also could go much further, says Ross Brownson, co-director of the Prevention Research Center at the Saint Louis University School of Public Health. States such as California and Massachusetts have seen smoking rates plummet in response to strong anti-smoking programs, he says. "But we haven't had a national strategy."

In the late 1990s, when the tobacco industry settled two landmark lawsuits brought by the states, the $246 billion settlement was intended to fund model anti-smoking initiatives nationwide, he says. "But the money ultimately didn't go where it was supposed to go," funding roads and other priorities instead, Brownson says. [21]

The AICR would like to see industries finance more research on cancer risk. For example, "the meat industry has a lot at stake" in knowing exactly what it is about red meat that causes its consumption to increase the consumer's risk of developing cancer, says Collins. For instance, it may be the form of iron, called heme iron, that reddens the meat, she says. And do less-studied meats, such as bison, pose the same risks as beef? she asks. "This is an area where we've thought that private organizations might step forward and recommend cooking meats in a certain way" to cut carcinogens, she says.

Chemoprevention, a more controversial form of prevention, may forestall development of cancer in high-risk people. Some chemoprevention drugs have been discovered — such as tamoxifen and raloxifene for women at high risk for breast cancer — but "are not widely used," says the University of Chicago's Schilsky. More research is needed to profile the highest-risk people, he says, since "it's probably not cost effective" to use the drugs for a broad population because they must be taken for many years.

But critics say chemoprevention is oversold. Breast cancer takes 12 to 15 years to develop, and research establishing chemoprevention as a successful therapy lasted no more than five years, making it unclear whether the drugs actually prevent breast cancer "or merely delay its onset," said Maryann Napoli, associate director of the New York City-based Center for Medical Consumers, which disseminates evaluations of medical treatments.

Trials involving women believed to be at high risk for breast cancer showed that 1.7 percent developed breast cancer during the five-year trial of the chemoprevention drug if they took a drug while 3.4 percent of those who didn't take the drug developed cancer. With such low numbers of supposedly high-risk women developing cancer even without the preventive therapy, more research is needed to determine who is at high risk, particularly since the drugs can raise the risk of uterine cancer, blood clots and strokes, said Napoli. [22]

Have we paid too little attention to carcinogens in the environment?

Exposure to carcinogens likely contributes to many if not all cancers. Carcinogens range from those outside the body — such as chemicals or radiation — to those inside, such as hormones or physical changes that occur when organs suffer inflammation.

But debate has long raged over how heavily to focus on possible triggers such as industrial chemicals, largely because tracing environmental causes is an uncertain business, leaving regulators to make decisions based on inconclusive data.

"There are a lot of people who have a vested interest in not looking at the environment issue" because chemical use by industries permeates modern life, says Alice Shabecoff, co-author with her husband, former *New York Times* environment reporter Philip Shabecoff, of *Poisoned Profits: The Toxic Assault on Our Children*.

"It is not a coincidence that the decrease in carcinogen-control regulations, studies and government publications corresponds to the rapid shrinkage of the United States' industrial workforce and . . . trade unions" because industry advocacy, not science, has convinced the government to back off, said Jeanne Mager Stellman, professor of environmental and occupational health sciences at the State University of New York's Downstate Medical Center in Brooklyn. [23]

But fears that regulating carcinogenic substances will drive companies out of business are overblown, Shabecoff says. "When toxics are found, why can't you just make a different kind of product?" she asks. For every product with toxic ingredients, "we found another comparable product that doesn't have them," proving that it can be done, she says.

For example, while many deodorants have been found to contain potentially toxic chemicals called phthalates, a few commercial products, such as Dove Powder Anti-Perspirant Deodorant and Lady Speed Stick Soft Anti-Perspirant, do not, according to the University of Illinois' Epstein. [24]

Currently, many U.S. companies are reformulating products to meet tough, new European Union standards for chemical toxicity (*see p. 39*).

In the United States, when concerns are raised that a product or process contributes to cancer, many industries routinely respond by funding research to raise doubts about the finding, says David Michaels, a research professor of environmental and occupational health at The George Washington University School of Public Health. "How ridiculous can it get? There is widespread agreement in the scientific community that broad-spectrum ultraviolet radiation, whether from sunlight or from tanning lamps, causes skin cancer," he wrote. "Yet trade associations representing the indoor tanning industry have attempted to derail the 'cancer-causing' designation by questioning the scientific evidence." [25]

Industry-sponsored research is "strongly associated with pro-industry conclusions," according to Michaels. For example, in studies of lung-cancer risk for workers exposed to beryllium — a lightweight metal often combined with other metals to strengthen them — "three government-funded analyses find an elevated risk while the one industry-funded analysis . . . does not." [26]

Moreover, recent research has shown that cancer-causing agents combine their effects in unknown ways, says Boston University's Clapp, undercutting the argument that the carcinogenic effect of one chemical can be ignored because its individual cancer-causing effect appears small. For example, someone exposed to tobacco smoke or asbestos may have a 10-times greater risk of developing cancer than someone exposed to neither, he says, but someone exposed to both has a 55-times greater risk. Thus, even agents that don't increase cancer risk significantly on their own may interact with other exposures to greatly increase risk and should be considered carcinogenic, Clapp says.

Industry advocates say if a chemical is found to cause cancer only in large doses, it shouldn't be banned if most people are exposed only to small amounts at a time. But that argument doesn't hold water, said French virologist Luc Montagnier, winner of the 2008 Nobel Prize for medicine, since over time people develop an "accumulation of these doses — they all add up. A little dose of radiation here, and exposure to some chemical there, a little bit of something in your food and so on. . . . All of this adds up to create an oxidant field, and it's the totality of this field which does all the damage and may bring about a cancer." [27]

Testing chemicals for their carcinogenic effects lags woefully behind industrial developments, according to James Huff, associate director for chemical carcinogenesis at the National Institute of Environmental Health Sciences. The U.S. National Toxicology Program (NTP), established in 1978, has tested about 600 chemicals — 0.6 percent of chemicals on the market — for carcinogenesis and found nearly half to have some carcinogenic properties, he wrote. Likewise, the International Agency for Research on Cancer has tested about 950 chemicals and found about 100 to be carcinogenic and more than 300 probably or possibly carcinogenic. [28]

"The number of chemicals that have not yet been tested is staggering," and thousands enter the marketplace every year, Huff said. "We live in a chemical soup," he pointed out, while the NTP initiates, at most, only about five new bioassays per year. "We must test more chemicals for carcinogenicity than are currently being evaluated." [29]

But others aren't convinced that industry-related carcinogens are something to worry about. Bailar, the former chief of the NCI's demography section, is skeptical about apparent increases in childhood cancers, which some advocates blame on industrial products. He cites a "cautionary tale" from Japan, where concern rose in the 1980s about apparent increases in neuroblastoma in infants. But a government program that apparently found and treated "a lot of cancers" ended up having "no detectable effect on mortality rates," raising serious questions about whether the cancer epidemic actually existed in the first place, he says.

The NCI says it already pays adequate attention to the issue. The National Institutes of Health (NIH) will spend $705 million on breast-cancer research in fiscal 2008, including nearly $100 million on the role of the environment in breast-cancer development, according to the testimony of

Deborah Winn, associate director of NCI's epidemiology and genetics research program, before the House Energy and Commerce Health Subcommittee last May. [30]

Industries deny that they deliberately try to raise doubts about whether their substances cause cancer. Cleveland-based beryllium manufacturer Brush Wellman denies it's ever sought to downplay the health risks associated with its product. The company "first put warning labels on its products and sent letters to all of its customers warning them of . . . potential health hazards . . . in 1949" and continues to evaluate the potential exposure risks, wrote Marc Kolanz, a certified industrial hygienist employed by the company. [31]

Others say lifestyle-related behaviors, such as smoking and lack of exercise, are so significant that any potential carcinogenic effects of environmental chemicals are trivial by comparison. "Chemicals in our food and the environment do not have a significant impact on overall cancer risk in the United States," said Elizabeth M. Whelan, president of the American Council on Science and Health, a nonprofit science-information group that has frequently taken pro-industry stances. "Most cancers are related to lifestyle factors." [32]

The American Institute for Cancer Research, which studies the effect of diet and lifestyle on cancer, agrees that Americans greatly overestimate the health threats of industrial factors such as pesticides and electric power lines. "Scientists do have a good idea about which factors increase cancer risk," says the institute. "Yet they aren't the factors many people associate with cancer."

For example, an AICR survey found that 71 percent of Americans believed pesticide residues are a factor in cancer incidence, even though "there is no proven link between pesticide residues on produce and cancer occurrence." [33] ■

BACKGROUND

'War on Cancer'

Hope that science could defeat cancer surged in the 1960s, when the United States vowed to put humans on the moon by decade's end.

Leading the campaign ever since her husband Albert died of colon cancer in 1952 was New York philanthropist Mary Lasker. Her coalition of cancer activists persistently urged federal officials to launch an all-out government effort to find a cure. Lasker was able to finance her medical advocacy using the fortune her husband had amassed in advertising. Considered the father of modern advertising, Lasker, ironically, was the brains behind the Lucky Strike cigarette ad campaign "Reach for a Lucky instead of a sweet" — possibly the first ad to specifically target women to buy cigarettes, a major carcinogen. [34]

Mrs. Lasker's persistent advocacy efforts culminated in December 1969 — five months after U.S. astronaut Neil Armstrong became the first human to walk on the moon — when her Citizens Committee for the Conquest of Cancer ran a full-page *New York Times* ad imploring President Richard M. Nixon with the boldface headline: "Mr. Nixon: You Can Cure Cancer."

At the time, little was known about cancer's cellular and genetic bases. But faith in what science could accomplish was running high, and the ad boasted, "America can do this." It continued: "Dr. Sidney Farber, past president of the American Cancer Society, believes: 'We are so close to a cure for cancer. We lack only the will and the kind of money and comprehensive planning that went into putting a man on the moon.' "Why don't we try to conquer cancer by America's 200th birthday?" [35]

The advocates got their way. Just two years later, on Dec. 23, 1971, Nixon signed the National Cancer Act, saying it could be "the most significant action taken during this administration." Nixon and the U.S. Congress declared a "war on cancer," and ever since then heroic rhetoric has all but promised a pharmaceutical cure for cancer was just around the corner.

But while federal funding for cancer research has consistently outstripped spending on other diseases — $5.65 billion for cancer research at the NIH in 2009, for example, compared to $2.9 billion for HIV/AIDS and $2.4 billion for cardiovascular disease — cancer mortality statistics have barely budged. [36]

Losing the War

Declaring "recent advances in the knowledge of this dread disease" offered great opportunity, the National Cancer Act authorized large funding increases for the NCI. Patient advocates recommended breaking the institute out of NIH entirely — to free researchers from what some considered a stifling bureaucracy. While lawmakers rejected that radical notion, they gave the NCI's director unprecedented authority to submit annual budget requests directly to the president, rather than to the NIH.

Advocates and lawmakers who had backed the legislation were thrilled. But most of the scientists in the audience at the bill-signing ceremony "did not smile," said one observer. "The hoopla . . . implied the conquest of cancer in the near future because a couple of hundred million dollars a year more were to be channeled into cancer research. Those of us who knew the 'state of the art' had cause to worry." [37]

The worriers had it right, but they were drowned out by the misplaced enthusiasm and "self delusion," says the Medical College of Georgia's Faguet.

Continued on p. 36

Chronology

1930s-1960s

Research intensifies on using drugs to treat cancer along with radiation and surgery; chemotherapy helps reduce mortality from so-called liquid cancers like leukemia.

1937
Congress establishes National Cancer Institute (NCI) as an independent agency to research the causes and treatment of cancer.

1938
Science publishes an article showing non-smokers live a decade longer than smokers.

1939
Hormones are found to spur the growth of certain cancers.

1943
The "Pap" test is introduced for screening for cervical cancer, leading to an eventual 75 percent drop in U.S. deaths from cervical cancer.

1944
NCI is incorporated into the National Institutes of Health.

1946
A cousin of the chemical-warfare agent mustard gas becomes the first effective chemotherapy.

1948
As smoking continues to rise in popularity, lung cancer is found to have increased five times faster than other cancers.

1959
NCI environmental cancer chief Wilhelm Hueper submits a 20-page chronicle of political efforts to quash his research.

1964
Surgeon general releases first report linking lung cancer and smoking.

1970s-1990s

Scientists find cancer is caused by gene mutations, some inherited but most due to interactions between human cells and their environment.

1971
President Richard M. Nixon declares a "war on cancer." . . . National Cancer Act of 1971 gives NCI $1.6 billion over three years. . . . Cigarette ads on the radio are banned.

1979
American Medical Association states for the first time that cigarette smoking harms the lungs but stops short of saying it causes cancer.

1980
National Toxicology Program publishes list of 25 chemicals that cause cancer or gene mutations.

1992
Environmental Protection Agency declares secondhand tobacco smoke a Class A carcinogen — the most dangerous type.

1994
The BRCA1 and BRCA2 "breast cancer" genes are identified.

1998
Clinton administration allows Medicare to pay for some experimental cancer treatments. . . . States get windfall after settling a lawsuit against tobacco companies, but little of the money funds smoking-cessation programs.

2000s

Researchers seek new drugs that only target cancerous cell molecules, eschewing chemotherapy's cell-killing approach. Individual patients' cancers differ far more than expected.

2001
Food and Drug Administration approves Novartis' Gleevec, one of the first drugs to target a cellular molecule — an enzyme that runs amok in chronic myeloid leukemia — rather than simply killing cancer cells.

2002
NCI Director Andrew von Eschenbach is accused of politicizing the institute after he deletes from an online fact sheet a statement that abortion does not increase the risk of breast cancer.

2003
The human genome is deciphered.

2004
A 50-year British study finds long-time smokers die 10 years earlier than non-smokers, but quitting at age 50 halves the extra risk.

2006
NIH launches project to map the DNA of all cancers.

2008
Researchers discover the gene profile of glioblastoma, the deadliest brain cancer. . . . African-Americans continue to fall behind whites in cancer mortality rates, due to poorer screening and treatment. . . . Long-term incense use is found to raise the risk of respiratory-tract cancers. . . . President-elect Barack Obama promises to increase the number of patients in clinical trials. . . . Vitamin D deficiency is found to contribute to many cancers.

How Treatment Hype Hurts Cancer Care

When hope trumps science, it can be painful and costly.

Exaggerated hopes for new cancer treatment can sometimes prove painful and costly to patients. Take the use of bone-marrow transplants, coupled with high-dose chemotherapy, for advanced breast cancer. Beginning in the late 1980s, some oncologists began prescribing the controversial treatment, which had worked with some other cancers, even though only one small study seemed to show an effect with breast cancer, while other evidence suggested the treatments might make patients sicker. But with few other therapies available, hope soon displaced caution. [1]

The expensive, painful treatment quickly became the rage among oncologists, the media, litigators and lawmakers, all of whom pushed insurers to cover the procedure as women's last, best hope. "Hope trumped science" and "politics trumped policy," wrote George C. Halvorson, CEO of Kaiser Permanente, the big managed care organization, and George J. Isham, medical director of HealthPartners, an HMO based in Bloomington, Minn. "[G]ood-hearted lawmakers" and courts around the country required insurers to cover the procedure, they explained, despite warnings that clinical trials were needed to determine its effectiveness. [2]

As often happens, media coverage fueled enthusiasm, according to health writer Shannon Brownlee, a senior fellow at the nonpartisan New America Foundation think tank. "I looked at 1,000 stories," she says, and 90 percent portrayed the transplants as "women's last chance," framing the treatment as a Homeric epic with villains — the cancer and, eventually, insurance companies who refused to pay — a physician hero and a patient, suffering victim.

Entrepreneurship also played a role. Physicians and others set up local clinics to perform the therapy, further pressuring insurers to pay, says Richard A. Rettig, a co-author of the 2007 book *False Hope: Bone Marrow Transplantation for Breast Cancer.*

It was not the first time financial incentives trumped clinical judgment, said Guy B. Faguet, a professor emeritus of medicine at the Medical College of Georgia. For example, he said, when doctors own radiation facilities, radiotherapy use jumps 53 percent, charges rise 42 percent and consultation time between doctors and patients drops 18 percent, compared to the national average. [3]

Ironically, when clinical trials were launched to test the bone-marrow transplant idea, the existence of the trials themselves signaled clinicians that the treatment was worthwhile, says Rettig, encouraging even more doctors to offer it. And the rush to treat made it harder to recruit trial subjects: Women who knew they could get the treatment outside of the trials were reluctant to participate because they feared they might be placed in the no-treatment "control" section of the experiments, Rettig says.

By the mid-1990s the transplant frenzy led at least eight states to legally require insurers to cover the procedure. [4] In 1993, a California jury ordered the insurer HealthNet to pay cancer patient Nelene Fox $89 million for refusing coverage of the treatment. But in 1999, a large, definitive clinical trial found that the transplant/chemo combination treatment did not improve survival rates for breast cancer. And many women had suffered serious side effects, including heart failure, bone-marrow disease and even death.

Continued from p. 34

The cancer-research money pipeline opened up by the law has produced theory after theory that proponents hoped would quickly lead to highly effective treatments, if not cures. But none of these hypotheses led to significantly "more efficacious cancer management, and today the outcome of most cancer patients remains grim." [38]

For example, over the 30 years from 1973 to the early 1990s, the overall median survival rate for advanced lung cancer — the nation's biggest cancer killer — only edged up from 6.9 months to 7.3 months and the three-year survival rate after diagnosis rose from 2 percent to only 4 percent, said Faguet. "Since that time, no breakthroughs occurred," he said. "The No. 1 cancer killer in the U.S. remains essentially unaffected" after more than 50 years of clinical drug trials and 35 years of the cancer war. [39]

Moreover, says Faguet, the media collude with scientists to oversell the idea that there's been progress. "Ninety-nine percent of the treatment ideas scientists try fall through, but the media don't want to report stories that say, 'You remember that big discovery we told you about five years ago? Well, in practice it doesn't work,' " he says.

The belief that effective cancer treatments are just around the corner has helped foster the notion that it's OK to stint on prevention, says Bailar, the former NCI demography chief.

"When I came out of medical school in 1955, a friend advised, 'Don't go to NCI. The problems they deal with are just about solved,' " Bailar recalls. In the intervening half-century, however, heart disease mortality has been "dropping like a rock" while cancer mortality has decreased only marginally. "Even where we have drugs that work, they don't work as well as you'd expect."

"A number of years ago, there was a great excitement over Gleevec" (chemical name, imatinib) — one of the first of the new breed of drugs that target specific molecules that help cancer cells proliferate rather than simply killing dividing cells, he says. But while Gleevec has been successful with some cancers, such as a form of

By then at least 42,000 women had received the treatment, not including those in the clinical trials, at a total cost — at $80,000 per patient — of more than $3 billion.

Despite the costly bone-marrow transplant debacle, some cancer researchers and oncologists are optimistic that 21st-century cancer science — including understanding of genetic changes and molecular mechanisms — has advanced to the point where optimistic predictions about successful cancer treatments are no longer hype but reality. Food and Drug Administration chief Andrew von Eschenbach, who served as director of the National Cancer Institute (NCI) for four years, said in 2005 the institute had "committed itself [to] eliminate the suffering and death" caused by cancer by 2015. [5]

But other analysts caution that such grand visions can be more of a danger than a help in cancer medicine. "Some people with visions are hallucinating," says Paul Goldberg, editor of *The Cancer Letter*, a medical newsletter. When it comes to cancer science, "sometimes the worst thing you can have is somebody with a vision."

In fact, points out Goldberg's wife Kirsten — publisher of the newsletter — von Eschenbach's "grandiose vision" actually crippled the NCI by shifting the focus to "far-out things like nanotechnology" while shortchanging approaches that might have borne more fruit.

"A visit to the annual [American Society of Clinical Oncology] meeting will convince one how desperate we are for any sign, no matter how minor, that a treatment might work," said Joseph V. Simone, a professor emeritus of pediatrics and medicine at the University of Utah, referring to how oncologists grasp at even the slimmest hint that a new treatment might work. "We share our patients' desperation, but we do them no favor by adopting unproven therapies as the standard of care." [6]

Rettig favors a new partnership between the NCI, patient-advocacy groups and insurers that would issue formal public statements about which experimental treatments need clinical-trial evaluation. Insurers would then fund the clinical trials, promising to cover whatever procedures are proved safe and effective. Such a move, Rettig says, would protect insurers from the kinds of lawsuits they faced over bone-marrow transplants.

[1] For background, see Michelle M. Mello and Troyen A. Brennan, "The Controversy Over High-Dose Chemotherapy With Autologous Bone Marrow Transplant for Breast Cancer," *Health Affairs*, September/October 2001, pp. 101-117.

[2] George C. Halvorson and George J. Isham, *Epidemic of Care; A Call for Safer, Better, and More Accountable Health Care* (2003), p. 58.

[3] Guy B. Faguet, *The War on Cancer: An Anatomy of Hope, A Blueprint for Failure* (2008), p. 122.

[4] Kristianna Pettibone, Lisa Lineberger and Regina el Arculli, "State Legislative Mandates for Insurance Coverage of Breast Cancer Treatment Services," paper presented at the annual research meeting of the Academy for Health Services Research and Policy, June 23, 2002, www.scld-nci.net/presentations/breastcancer020623.pdf.

[5] Andrew von Eschenbach, "Eliminating the Suffering and Death Due to Cancer by 2015," *Medical Progress Bulletin*, Manhattan Institute, September 2005, www.manhattan-institute.org/pdf/mpb_01.pdf.

[6] Joseph V. Simone, "A Cautionary Tale," "Simone's OncOpinion" column, *Oncology Times*, July 10, 2007, p. 11.

leukemia and some stomach tumors, it hasn't turned out to be as broadly applicable as many observers initially expected, he says.

Furthermore, cancer is now understood to be not one but hundreds, perhaps thousands, of different diseases. "You'd need 150 Gleevecs just for breast cancer," says Paul Goldberg, editor of the Washington, D.C.-based *Cancer Letter*. "And there aren't going to be a hundred Gleevecs."

"That's the story of cancer," says Bailar. "We've spent 50 years with the best scientific talent working hard to find cures, and we're still floundering around. At a certain point, don't you need to say there's probably nothing magic out there waiting to be discovered?"

Environmental Consciousness

Even among cancer researchers who favor prevention, sparring has persisted for decades over whether environmental factors unique to the industrial age — such as radiation and synthetic chemicals — have received enough attention as potential causes.

Some of the earliest cancer research targeted environmental exposures. In the 18th century, Italian physician Bernardino Ramazzini noted the low incidence of cervical cancer and the relatively high incidence of breast cancer among nuns. The observation eventually led to the discovery that a sexually transmitted virus — human papillomavirus — caused most cervical cancer and that breast cancer was related to levels of a woman's own hormones. [40] In the same century, British physician Percival Potts described a cancer that afflicted London's chimney sweeps after soot collected under their scrotums, while his countryman, John Hill, linked tobacco smoking to cancer.

But while research on cancer treatments stirs up outsized hype and hopes — including researchers' dreams of fortune and fame — prevention studies have long been dogged by industry and government concerns that important substances or activities would be deemed carcinogenic.

Continued on p. 39

New Findings Raise New Questions

Genetics and therapeutic vaccines reveal new complexities.

New findings in genetics and the inner workings of cells may hold promise for major advances in cancer therapy, but the new findings also point to previously unimagined complexities in one of humanity's most feared diseases.

"We are the first generation who has read our genetic code, and it's been known for only four years," says Kenneth W. Kinzler, a professor of oncology at the Johns Hopkins University School of Medicine who researches the genetic basis of cancer. That means "we now have the road map of the enemy," he says. "So though we've been waging the war on cancer since 1972, this is a unique time" for cancer science, Kinzler says.

Not all the hot science is genetic, though.

For example, some scientists are pursuing so-called therapeutic vaccines — aimed at boosting a patient's immune system to fight cancer — based on a long-proposed but still highly controversial theory that cancers arise in our bodies repeatedly but are mostly rejected before they grow. The theory is bolstered by the fact that people with AIDS and other immunosuppressive conditions develop more cancers.

To date, however, "no therapeutic vaccines have been approved by the Food and Drug Administration," says Jeffrey Schlom, head of the National Cancer Institute (NCI) immunotherapeutics group.

Nevertheless, therapeutic vaccines are working in at least some patients, Schlom says.

Vaccinations against infectious diseases like the flu inject minute amounts of disease proteins into the body, triggering an immune system response to destroy the invaders. Some scientists think the same thing could be done with cancer. Earlier experiments, however, in which highly concentrated tumor proteins were injected into a cancer patient did not work, says Schlom. But more recent studies have found that if the immune system is revved up by injecting, for instance, a touch of smallpox virus (which a previously inoculated patient's body will already recognize) along with the tumor protein, the immune system *does* act against the cancer, Schlom says.

"It's the difference between just jumping and jumping on a trampoline" — keeping the immune system highly active to enhance its natural anti-tumor activity, he says.

Therapeutic vaccines will not work with advanced tumors or fast-moving cancers because the immune system's anti-tumor response is too subdued, even when enhanced, Schlom says. "But we can pick out those patients who have more indolent disease, and they'll benefit more from vaccines than from chemotherapy" and also avoid chemotherapy's painful side effects, he says. Recent vaccine trials in prostate cancer, for example, show increased survival for patients who get the vaccine, he says.

In the realm of cancer genetics, scientists discovered about a decade ago that women who inherited certain mutated forms of two genes — dubbed BRCA1 and BRCA2 — had greatly increased risk of developing breast or ovarian cancer.

Today, thousands of women undergo genetic screening to find out whether they have inherited mutated genes. Some women learn that they have mutations known to be harmful — and can then decide whether to take drugs or have surgery to ward off potential cancers. But many find themselves in a more perplexing category. They have mutations — sometimes ones that haven't even been seen before — but no one knows whether the gene variants they carry raise cancer risks or not.

"It's a matter of life or death," but the information gained through genetic screening often doesn't bring a doctor nearer to knowing whether the patient has increased cancer risk, says Shyam Sharan, head of the NCI's Genetics of Cancer Susceptibility Section.

That's where Sharan's mouse genetics laboratory comes in handy.

"In humans you look at the tumor and see hundreds of thousands of changes" in the DNA, but "you don't know what was the initial thing" in the chain of cancer causation, says Sharan. But thanks to advances in gene technology, biologists can place a mutated human gene into mice and see the result. In the mouse, "you can change things one at a time" and see what happens. Does the particular gene mutation "affect the normal development? Does it help the mouse survive a little longer?"

But cancer is not just a disease of genes but a disease of genes that have mutated through their interactions with the environment, says Gerald N. Wogan, a professor emeritus of chemistry at the Massachusetts Institute of Technology. Even identical twins — with identical gene profiles — don't develop the same cancers in most cases, for example.

For that reason, genetic studies "still will only leave us a catalog of what the changes are" in a cell that's turned cancerous but won't enlighten us on how and why those changes happen, says Wogan.

That's the realm of cancer-prevention research, at least in part, and it's changing, says Karen Collins, a nutrition education consultant to the American Institute for Cancer Research, which funds research on links between cancer and diet, physical activity and weight management.

For example, "There's a gene we all have, the tumor-suppression gene, and dietary changes can turn it on or off," says Collins. "That's leading prevention scientists to ask a startling question: What if the way you eat could change your genes? Ten years ago, that would have been so wild a thought that the question never would have been asked, but today it's a hot area."

Continued from p. 37

William Hueper, director of the NCI's environmental section from 1948 to 1964, was an early proponent of studying environmental links to cancer but was ultimately barred from pursuing some such studies because of concern his work would compromise advances in nuclear energy. [41]

Hueper launched a study of European uranium miners, who suffered high rates of lung cancer, but he was prevented from presenting his results about the uranium-cancer link to a medical-society meeting in 1952 after the federal Atomic Energy Commission objected. The NCI subsequently prevented him from conducting any further investigations into "the causation of cancer in man related to environmental exposure to carcinogenic chemical, physical, and parasitic agents," said Robert N. Proctor, a professor of the history of science at Stanford University. [42]

Many battles over government regulation of potential environmental carcinogens — which could cost industry or society significant amounts of money and inconvenience — turn on the question of what constitutes adequate scientific evidence to act.

"A 'known-to-be-a-human-carcinogen' determination should only be made if there is sufficient evidence of carcinogenicity from epidemiological studies that indicates a causal relationship between exposure to the . . . substance . . . and human cancer," said the American Chemistry Council, an industry group. "Mechanistic or other scientific information should not be used to bolster insufficient epidemiological evidence." [43]

Many environmental scientists disagree. Human epidemiological studies that definitively show a cause-effect link between environmental exposures and cancer are extremely difficult to carry out, they argue, so other types of evidence, such as animal studies, should also be considered.

In every case where epidemiological studies have followed up on rodent studies, the epidemiological research "has confirmed the mouse results," says the University of Illinois' Epstein. "I'm unaware of any mouse study in which there's contrary epidemiological data," he says. Furthermore, for reasons of funding and practicality, most rodent studies include relatively small numbers of animals. As a result, they are not very "sensitive" — they pick up only cancerous effects that are very large, affecting a large proportion of the population, Epstein says.

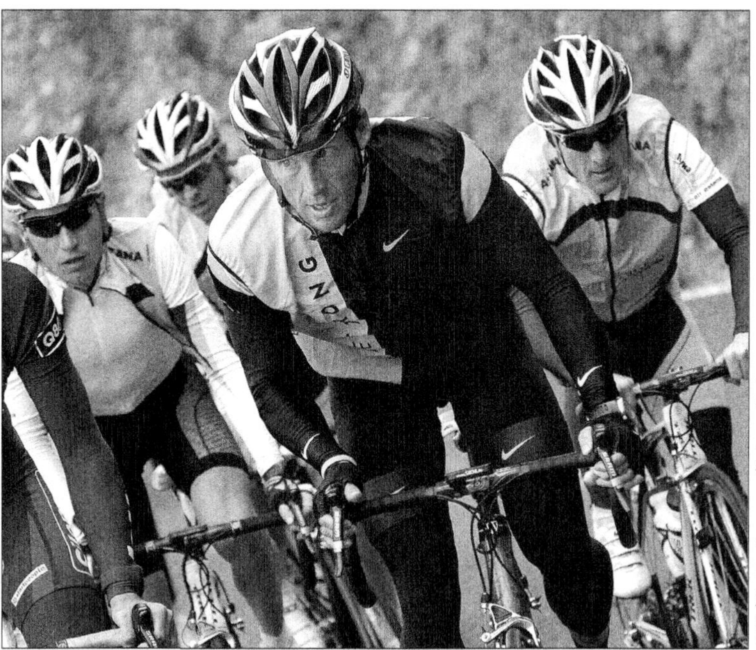
AFP/Getty Images/Jaime Reina

Tour de France champion American Lance Armstrong is dramatic proof that cancer is no longer a death sentence for everyone. He was diagnosed in 1996 with testicular cancer that had spread to his lungs, abdomen and brain. After surgery and chemotherapy, he was declared cancer-free and returned to racing.

Industries' influence on epidemiological research to protect their financial interests has hurt the public, argues Devra Davis, director of the University of Pittsburgh Cancer Institute's Center for Environmental Oncology. In 1988, for example, Davis said Sir Richard Doll, a celebrated epidemiologist from Britain's Oxford University, showed that the industrial chemical vinyl chloride caused only fatal angiosarcoma of the liver, not several other cancers, as the World Health Organization's International Agency for Research on Cancer had believed.

"As a result of this analysis by an eminent authority, workers who developed the more common tumors of the brain, liver and lung after exposures to vinyl chloride . . . were not able to get compensation for them," Davis said. But 12 years later it was revealed that Doll may not have been "a disinterested expert," as he had claimed, but since 1979 had been paid $1,500 a day as a consultant to the giant chemical manufacturer Monsanto. [44]

Many European environmental regulators, unlike those in the United States, hew to the "precautionary principle" — that it's better to act against a potential cause of serious public or environmental harm rather than wait for scientific certainty. That's the principle behind the European Union's 2006 REACH (Registration, Evaluation, Authorization and Restriction of Chemicals) initiative, which requires manufacturers and importers to report to a central database detailed information about industrial substances used in their products and

Getting Drugs from the Lab to the Bedside

Rare forms of cancer face unique obstacles.

With a slew of technical and scientific issues confronting biomedical researchers, analysts say the focus of federal cancer programs should shift to clinical research in an effort to move effective treatments quickly from the laboratory to the bedside.

Both Congress and President-elect Barack Obama say they'll propose legislation this year to bolster clinical research — studies that explore whether a proposed treatment is safe and effective in human patients — a move most analysts say should be a top priority.

But other obstacles remain. For instance, clinical studies are especially difficult to arrange for rarer cancers, leading some patient-advocacy groups to create clinical-trial infrastructures of their own. For instance, the Multiple Myeloma Research Foundation was started in 1998 by Kathy Giusti, then an executive for the drug company G. D. Searle, who had just been diagnosed with multiple myeloma, a relatively rare cancer of the immune system. When Giusti, of New Canaan, Conn., learned no drugs for her condition were in the development pipeline, she used her knowledge of the drug industry to change that.

The foundation raises funds to support laboratories worldwide conducting multiple myeloma research and has established a consortium of 14 research institutions pursuing research cooperatively — a rarity in the biomedical research world, where competition for academic prestige and lucrative patents keeps most research proprietary.

The foundation's streamlined administrative setup — bolstered by a joint tissue bank and signed agreements by participants to operate transparently — has sped up early-stage clinical trials on priority therapies, says Anne Quinn Young, the foundation's program director for communication, education and outreach.

The foundation provides "an incredible brain trust" for mutual assistance and avoids duplication of effort, which is a special boon to smaller biotech companies, where therapies often originate but "who need whatever help they can get" to further the work, says Young. "We went from no therapies to four approvals by the Food and Drug Administration [FDA] in four years," and last year alone "we opened seven trials."

Once a drug appears to be effective, getting it developed also proves tricky. Normally, cancer drugs are approved to treat one cancer and then are used "off label" in quasi experimentation by physicians to treat other cancers, says Paul Goldberg, editor of *The Cancer Letter* newsletter. "But you can't do that any more because drugs cost too darn much" — $10,000 a month or more for some recently approved treatments. As a result, public and private insurers now demand specific FDA approval for a drug for any kind of cancer, he says.

Moreover, today's experimental treatments don't kill cancer cells as with older chemotherapy drugs but are designed to impede cells' ability to proliferate by targeting particular molecules or processes.

Thus, cancer researchers and the FDA are looking for quicker ways to show that a drug works rather than waiting to see whether patients who take it survive longer. But so far that quest has led mostly to confusion, according to an expert panel at a September conference at the Brookings Institution think tank in Washington, D.C.

"Measures of disease progression, health-related quality of life, patient-reported symptoms and biomarkers" — such as a protein in the blood that indicates a cancer has progressed to a certain stage — "have been proposed and tested in clinical studies, but consensus has not been reached on the role of these endpoints in determining the overall benefit of a therapy," the group said. [1]

Measuring whether a drug lengthens a patient's "time to progression" — the amount of time between when a patient enters a study and when his or her disease progresses to a more advanced stage — has become popular for measuring drug effectiveness. But, in fact, nobody understands how to gauge time to progression accurately and without bias, Goldberg says.

Two recent drug approvals — of the kidney-cancer drug sorafenib (brand-name Nexavar) and the breast-cancer drug bevacizumab (brand-name Avastin) — were based solely on evidence of lengthened time to progression, with no statistical evidence the drugs helped patients survive longer. That underscores the critical need to agree on how the endpoint is defined and interpreted, said the Brookings panel. [2]

Further complicating matters, scientists now know that cancer is many diseases and that cancers vary from one patient to another. So drug therapy will need to become a "personalized" treatment in which drugs are prescribed only for patients whose cancers match certain criteria. That would require the FDA to figure out how to approve both a drug and a test to determine whether the drug suits the patient.

So far, "Nobody understands how to do that," Goldberg says.

[1] Raymond DuBois, *et al.*, "Issue Brief," Conference on Clinical Cancer Research, September 2008.
[2] *Ibid.*

to progressively phase out those the European Chemicals Agency deems too dangerous.

Some cancer experts say Europe's "precautionary" model has merit. Ronald B. Herberman, director of the University of Pittsburgh's Cancer Institute, cautioned university staff to use speakerphones or wireless headsets instead of cell phones and to limit children's cell phone use to emergencies. While researchers haven't found a clear link between cell phone use and cancer, "at the heart of my concern is that we

Continued on p. 42

At Issue:

Should phthalates and bisphenol in plastics be restricted?

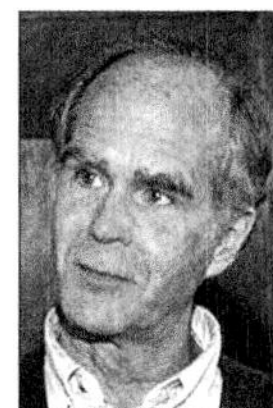

TED SCHETTLER
SCIENCE DIRECTOR, SCIENCE AND ENVIRONMENTAL HEALTH NETWORK

FROM TESTIMONY BEFORE HOUSE SUBCOMMITTEE ON COMMERCE, TRADE AND CONSUMER PROTECTION, JUNE 10, 2008

yes

The chemicals being discussed today are in the bodies of virtually every American. They are in fetuses, infants and children. Phthalates are produced in large amounts and used in many consumer products, including construction materials, insect repellants, paints, cosmetics, personal-care products, air fresheners and others. In general, phthalates are not tightly bound in these products, and people are exposed when they use them or from general environmental contamination.

People are not exposed to single phthalates but rather to mixtures of these chemicals. It is essential to consider these exposures collectively when drawing conclusions about the risks associated with exposures to any particular phthalate. . . .

Studies from the Centers for Disease Control and Prevention show that exposure to bisphenol A is widespread in the general population. Ninety-three percent of people in the representative study population had detectable levels of bisphenol A in their urine. Fetuses and infants have markedly reduced capacity to transform the active form of bisphenol A into the inactive form excreted in the urine and so are at particular risk.

Health effects . . . include neurobehavioral changes, impacts on reproductive-system development and function, abnormal numbers of chromosomes in dividing cells, predisposition to cancer and insulin resistance as it is seen in diabetes.

Animal testing shows that low-level bisphenol A exposures during fetal development or infancy modify the development of the prostate gland and breast, permanently altering their tissue architecture in ways that predispose them to later disease, including cancer. In some cases, these changes are themselves precancerous. These abnormalities occur in animal studies at levels of exposure similar to those to which people in the general public are now exposed.

I urge you to think about this from a public health perspective and ask what amount or strength of evidence we should require before taking action to reduce or eliminate exposures to these chemicals, particularly in vulnerable populations. That is a public policy decision, which should be informed by good science, and also by values and common sense. Do we wait for irrefutable proof of harm in people before taking action?

The limits of epidemiological research will always make it difficult to tease out some cause-and-effect relationships, even when they exist. It is particularly difficult when the entire population is already exposed to chemicals of concern. But policy makers need to decide when evidence is sufficient to act, even in the face of scientific uncertainty.

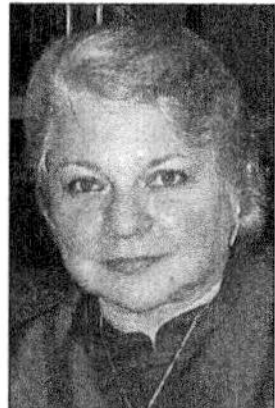

MARIAN K. STANLEY
SENIOR DIRECTOR, AMERICAN CHEMISTRY COUNCIL

FROM TESTIMONY BEFORE HOUSE SUBCOMMITTEE ON COMMERCE, TRADE AND CONSUMER PROTECTION, JUNE 10, 2008.

no

Phthalates are primarily used to make vinyl soft and flexible. Flexible vinyl products are used in our cars, home and workplaces. Both the U.S. National Toxicology Program and the European Union have performed risk assessments on phthalates and have generally found no significant risk to children from exposure.

The U.S. Centers for Disease Control and Prevention (CDC) has also tested thousands of Americans for evidence of exposure to phthalates. The CDC data show that average human exposure is far below levels set by the U.S. Environmental Protection Agency as protective of human health and that exposure levels are actually declining.

It is unfortunate that some media reports referred to a handful of studies that attempt to link phthalate exposure to adverse health effects. Many of the studies are biased in their design, test only a small sample size or have uncontrollable variables. Other studies ignore or exaggerate real-world human exposure. Some studies are based on findings in rodents at extremely high exposure levels. Similar studies in primates do not show these same effects.

In today's world, zero exposure to anything is impossible, and with today's advances in analytical techniques, incredibly tiny amounts can be measured. These levels do not necessarily constitute a health risk.

Bisphenol A (BPA) is a chemical building block used primarily to make polycarbonate plastic — a lightweight, highly shatter-resistant plastic with optical clarity comparable to glass — and epoxy resins. Both are used in a wide array of products, many of which improve health and safety. . . .

The Food and Drug Administration regulates the use of bisphenol A in food-contact materials, such as baby bottles, water bottles and coatings on food cans. . . . The agency said in July 2007 that "FDA is unaware of any specific study in which humans exposed to BPA through any food containers experienced miscarriages, birth defects or cancer. Human exposure levels to BPA from its use in food-contact materials is in fact many orders of magnitude lower than the levels of BPA that showed no adverse effects in animal studies.

From a toxicological perspective, BPA and phthalates are among the most well-defined chemicals on Earth. They have been the subject of hundreds of studies in lab animals and numerous government-sponsored assessments. Accordingly, based on the science and the use patterns for these compounds, no restriction on their uses is warranted at this time.

How to Lower Your Risk of Cancer

- ***Don't smoke, or, if you do smoke, quit.*** Smoking is linked to at least 15 different types of cancer and accounts for at least 30 percent of all cancer deaths. People who quit, even after decades as smokers, almost immediately begin reducing their risk.
- ***Limit your sun exposure.*** Sun damage throughout your lifetime can eventually cause cancer, as can tanning beds and sunlamps. And while generous use of sunscreen — at least a whole handful in each application — limits exposure to so-called UVB rays, it doesn't block all of them and frequently offers little or no protection against UVA rays, which also are dangerous. Avoid the midday sun, stay in the shade when you can and wear lightweight clothing and hats with brims to cut your exposure.
- ***Keep your weight down and eat a wide variety of plant-based foods, including whole grains, beans and at least five servings of fruits and vegetables daily.*** Variety is important because many "micronutrients" found in different foods play cancer-fighting roles in the body.
- ***Be physically active.*** Children and adolescents should aim for 60 minutes daily of moderately vigorous exercise, at least five days a week, and adults should aim for at least 30 to 45 minutes. Anything that makes you breathe harder, such as brisk walking or stair climbing, counts. Exercise can be spaced throughout the day.
- ***Drink alcohol only in moderation.*** Men who consume more than two drinks per day on average and women who consume more than one drink per day have a higher risk of developing several forms of cancer.

Source: American Cancer Society

Continued from p. 40

shouldn't wait for a definite study . . . but err on the side of being safe rather than sorry later," he said. [45]

In fact, in the early 2000s congressional Democrats, including Sen. Frank Lautenberg, D-N.J., drafted legislation "to overhaul U.S. regulations to resemble" the EU's then-proposed REACH reforms, said the University of Illinois' Epstein. [46]

But REACH is not a good model for the United States to follow and is opposed by both private industries and the Bush administration, said Joseph G. Acker, president of the Synthetic Organic Chemical Manufacturers Association. "Despite interest from far left-wing corners of Congress, which have a great interest in adopting a REACH-type system here in the U.S., REACH is losing steam as the new model." [47]

In recent meetings with government officials from several Asian-Pacific nations, "we described for them major trade challenges that U.S.-based chemical companies now have because of REACH," said Acker, and "it became clear . . . that these governments see more disadvantages to adopting REACH than advantages." [48] ■

CURRENT SITUATION

Action In Congress

Both Congress' Democratic majority and President-elect Obama plan to address cancer research and treatment with legislation.

This year "will be one of the most active legislative years in a long time," says Dick Woodruff, chief lobbyist for the American Cancer Society's Cancer Action Network.

Sens. Edward M. Kennedy, D-Mass., and Kay Bailey Hutchison, R-Texas, are developing a comprehensive bill, expected to be introduced early this year, to increase research funding, spur research on early detection and provide better access to screening and treatment for uninsured people.

"We need an entirely new model" to coordinate a "fragmented and piecemeal system of addressing cancer" by linking research, prevention and treatment into a "continuum of comprehensive cancer care," said Kennedy, then-chairman of the Health, Education, Labor and Pensions Committee, at a hearing in May, less than two weeks before he was diagnosed with a malignant brain tumor. [49]

The cancer-advocacy community also wants the FDA to regulate tobacco, says Woodruff. The House passed such a bill in July 2008, but the legislation languished in the Senate, so lawmakers will start again in the new year.

Woodruff expects the bill to become law this time. The legislation has at least 60 Senate cosponsors and will probably garner votes from 10 more senators, he says. "We will work with the Senate leadership so Republicans can offer the amendments they want on the floor, but there's only one senator who's said he wants to filibuster" the bill, and "that's not enough" to stop passage, Woodruff says.

Under the legislation, the FDA could require testing tobacco products to stop companies from making false health and safety claims, Woodruff says. By the time this is done, the health-warning label "will take up half the package," he predicts.

Also on the prevention front, Sens. Christopher J. Dodd, D-Conn., and Jack Reed, D-R.I., have introduced legislation to require the FDA to require labels warning that sunscreen products currently protect only against the sun's UVB rays, which cause sunburn and increase the risk of skin cancer, but not against UVA rays, which also cause skin cancer. [50]

Since Democrats took over control of Congress in 2007, committees also have been mulling tighter regulation of several potentially carcinogenic chemicals, such as bisphenol A, used in plastics manufacture. (*See "At Issue," p. 41.*)

Obama's Plan

President-elect Obama's cancer plan would double federal research funding over five years, increase the numbers of patients in clinical trials, eliminate Medicare and Medicaid patient copays for screening, expand funding for smoking cessation and provide guidance for patients navigating the treatment system. [51]

"Obama's goal to put 10 percent of patients in clinical trials is terrific," says *Cancer Letter* Editor Goldberg.

NCI funding for clinical research has "taken a big hit" in recent years as the agency has struggled to prop up basic-research initiatives amid slowed congressional funding, says his wife, *Cancer Letter* Publisher Kirsten Boyd Goldberg. Furthermore, even between 1998 and 2003, when Congress doubled NIH funding, money for NCI's cooperative groups — researchers, cancer centers and community doctors around the United States who do clinical research — only went up by 50 percent, she says.

"Physicians out there are subsidizing" NCI's clinical research — receiving $2,000 to support a patient's clinical-trial participation when a drug company would offer $6,000 or $8,000 — "and though the doctors do it because they truly believe in it, that can't go on forever," publisher Goldberg says.

It's important that the groups get support to continue their work because their research asks different questions than drug-company-sponsored researchers, who aim solely at getting a drug approved, says Paul Goldberg. By contrast, cooperative groups may even come out with conclusions like "Hey, don't use that drug," he says. "The more you squeeze the groups, the more you may lose" such valuable insights into what actually constitutes the best cancer care, he says.

Not everyone is so pleased with Obama's plan. The president-elect "is putting all the emphasis on oncology — there seems to be no emphasis on prevention in the plan at all," the University of Illinois' Epstein says.

There's also room to wonder whether the government can come up with cash for cancer in the midst of an economic meltdown.

"Money is the elephant in the room, the main stumbling block for all these things," says David Bernstein, senior science policy analyst for the American Association for Cancer Research. Nevertheless, "we're still optimistic about money because research is an economic stimulus," he says. ■

OUTLOOK

Prevention Ahead?

Shifting cancer science toward prevention won't be easy, but a growing worldwide cancer burden makes prevention efforts vital.

"We probably could get rid of 90 percent of lung cancer by ending smoking, but we don't know how to accomplish that, so we need research on how to help people quit who want to quit," as well as much more prevention research, says Bailar, the former head of the NCI's demography section.

Even so, "it's going to be a long, slow process to get that research program reoriented" because a prevention focus is a "totally different world" from a treatment focus, says Bailar. "You can't just turn a treatment person into a detection, screening and prevention researcher. It's sometimes hard even to persuade them that there's another path to be investigated."

The war on cancer launched a multibillion-dollar, multifaceted enterprise that is now set in its ways, and the scientists, physicians and companies involved have no incentive to change, according to *War on Cancer* author Faguet at the Medical College of Georgia.

"The information pipeline, generated by clinical researchers and supported by their sponsors and publishers, fosters standards of care that are reinforced by financial incentives and the extraordinary capacity of physicians for self-delusion and by unrealistic expectations of consumers, nurtured by the media," Faguet wrote. [52]

As developing countries make headway against some infectious diseases, and heart disease in industrialized countries recedes as a killer, cancer is taking a larger toll.

However, even though the approximately 4 million annual cancer deaths in low- and middle-income countries outnumber the 3 million annual deaths from AIDS, cancer remains low on those nations' health-care priority lists, according to a 2007 National Academy of Sciences report. Furthermore, in low-income countries, most people with cancer have no access to potentially curative treatments, and in middle-income countries treatment is "generally limited," said the report. [53]

Those facts strengthen the case for prevention, and some very successful approaches for addressing cancer in developing countries have been proposed, says MIT's Wogan. For example, the combined effects of hepatitis B infection and exposure to aflatoxins — fungi that contaminate stored crops — cause many developing-world cancers, "and an obvious approach is vaccination" against hepatitis B, he says.

Indoor air pollution from unventilated cooking fires also is "a huge problem globally," he says. "Just putting a chimney on the stove" constitutes effective prevention.

Implementing preventive measures "will only continue to grow more important as cancer rapidly overtakes heart disease as the No. 1 killer," Wogan says. ■

Notes

[1] For background, see Sally Jacobs, "Kennedy, His Children, and Cancer," *The Boston Globe*, May 25, 2008.

[2] Quoted in *ibid*.

[3] Richard Schilsky, Jeffrey Abrams, Janet Woodcock, Gwen Fyfe and Robert Irwin, "Issue Brief," Conference on Clinical Cancer Research, September 2008.

[4] Quoted in John Russell, "Cancer Studies Suggest Pathways Are Best Targets," *Bio-IT World*, Sept. 25, 2008, www.bio-itworld.com,

[5] Bill Hendrick, "Smoking Rate Is Declining in the U.S.," *WebMD*, Nov. 13, 2008, www.webmd.com/smoking-cessation/news/20081113/smoking-rate-is-declining-in-us.

[6] Janet Gray, ed., *State of the Evidence: The Connection Between Breast Cancer and the Environment*, Breast Cancer Fund (2008), p. 15.

[7] *Ibid*.

[8] "Comprehensive Genetic Blueprints Revealed for Lethal Pancreatic, Brain Cancers," press release, Johns Hopkins Medical Institutions, Sept. 4, 2008, www.hopkinskimmelcancercenter.org.

[9] H. Gilbert Welch, "Seek, and You'll Find," *Minneapolis Star Tribune*, Nov. 6, 2008, www.startribune.com.

[10] Guy B. Faguet, *The War on Cancer: Anatomy of Failure, A Blueprint for the Future* (2008), p. 156.

[11] "Colon Cancer Screening Before Medicare Age Could Save Millions in Federal Health Care Dollars," *Science Daily*, Oct. 6, 2008, www.sciencedaily.com.

[12] Quoted in "Recent Studies Confirm Significant Underuse of Colorectal Cancer Screening," *Science Daily*, Jan. 3, 2008, www.sciencedaily.com.

[13] Quoted in Maryann Napoli, "Mammography Screening — Both Good and Bad News," Center for Medical Consumers Web site, September 2005, www.medicalconsumers.org. The analysis is by Karsten Juhl Jorgensen and Peter C. Gotzsche of the Danish branch of the Cochrane Collaboration, an international nonprofit group that publishes evidence-based information on health-care procedures based on systematic review of the research.

[14] Quoted in *ibid*.

[15] Quoted in Maryann Napoli, "Early Promoters of PSA Screening for Prostate Cancer Do a Turnabout," Center for Medical Consumers Web site, February 2005, www.Medicalconsumers.org.

[16] 'Study Shows No Benefit for CT Screening for Lung Cancer," press release, Memorial Sloan-Kettering Cancer Center, March 6, 2007, www.mskcc.org; Peter B. Bach, *et al.*, "Computed Tomography Screening and Lung Cancer Outcomes," *Journal of the American Medical Association*, March 7, 2007, pp. 953-961.

[17] "Promoting Healthy Lifestyles: Policy, Program, and Personal Recommendations for Reducing Cancer Risk, 2006-2007 Annual Report," President's Cancer Panel, National Cancer Institute, August 2007, http://deainfo.nci.nih.gov/advisory/pcp/pcp07rpt/pcp07rpt.pdf, p. i.

[18] For background, see Nellie Bristol, "HPV Vaccine," *CQ Researcher*, May 11, 2007, pp. 409-432.

[19] "Promoting Healthy Lifestyles," *op. cit.*

[20] *Ibid.*, p. ii.

[21] For background, see Kenneth Jost, "Closing in on Tobacco," *CQ Researcher*, Nov. 12, 1999, pp. 977-1000.

[22] Maryann Napoli, "Drugs to Reduce Breast Cancer Risk: Is It Worth It?" Center for Medical Consumers Web site, May 2006, www.medicalconsumers.org.

[23] Jeanne Mager Stellman, "Delusions, Illusions and Ongoing Neglect of Hazard Recognition, Regulation and Control of Industrial Carcinogens," Presentation to the President's Cancer Panel, Sept. 16, 2008, www.firstscience.com/home/news/breaking-news-all-topics/immediate-action-needed-to-prevent-industrial-manslaughter-says-expert_52622.html.

[24] Samuel S. Epstein and Randall Fitzgerald, *Toxic Beauty* (forthcoming, 2009), p. 142.

[25] David Michaels, "Manufactured Uncertainty: Protecting Public Health in the Age of Contested Science and Product Defense," *Annals of the New York Academy of Sciences*, September 2006, pp. 149-162.

[26] *Ibid.*, p. 156.

[27] Quoted in Richard Clapp, *Industrial Carcinogens: A Need for Action*, The Collaborative

About the Author

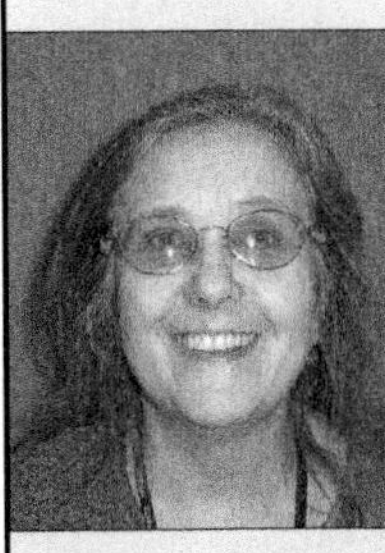

Staff writer **Marcia Clemmitt** is a veteran social-policy reporter who previously served as editor in chief of *Medicine & Health* and staff writer for *The Scientist*. She has also been a high-school math and physics teacher. She holds a liberal arts and sciences degree from St. John's College, Annapolis, and a master's degree in English from Georgetown University. Her recent reports include "Mortgage Crisis," "Climate Change," "Health Care Costs" and "Preventing Memory Loss."

on Health and the Environment Web site, Sept. 16, 2008, www.healthandenvironment.org/?module=uploads&func=download&fileId=558.

[28] James Huff, "More Toxin Tests Needed," letter to the editor, *Science*, Feb. 8, 2008, p. 725.

[29] *Ibid.*

[30] Deborah Winn, testimony before House Energy and Commerce Health Subcommittee, May 21, 2008.

[31] Marc Kolanz, "Beryllium History and Public Policy," *Public Health Reports*, July-August 2008, p. 426.

[32] Elizabeth M. Whelan, "Quackery Promoters Are Wrong. With Some Exceptions, Cancer Death Rates Are Declining," Quackwatch Web site, www.quackwatch.org.

[33] "Everything Doesn't Cause Cancer," American Institute for Cancer Research, November 2007, www.aicr.com.

[34] Faguet, *op. cit.*, p. 96.

[35] Quoted in Richard A. Rettig, *Cancer Crusade: The Story of The National Cancer Act of 1971* (2005), p. 79.

[36] "Estimates of Funding for Various Disease, Conditions, Research Areas," National Institutes of Health, Feb. 5, 2008, www.nih.gov/news/fundingresearchareas.htm. For background, see Rettig, *op. cit.*, and Faguet, *op. cit.* For additional background, see Adriel Bettelheim, "Cancer Treatments," *CQ Researcher*, Sept. 11, 1998, pp. 785-808, and Sarah Glazer, "Breast Cancer," *CQ Researcher*, June 27, 1997, pp. 553-576.

[37] Rettig, *op. cit.*, p. 277.

[38] Faguet, *op. cit.*, p. 78.

[39] *Ibid.*, p. 79.

[40] For background, see Bristol, *op. cit.*

[41] For background, see Robert N. Proctor, *Cancer Wars: How Politics Shape What We Know and Don't Know About Cancer* (1995).

[42] *Ibid.*, p. 42.

[43] American Chemistry Council, letter to National Toxicology Program Associate Director, Jan. 30, 2004, www.americanchemistry.com.

[44] Devra Davis, *The Secret History of the War on Cancer* (2007), p. 378.

[45] Quoted in Tara Parker-Pope, "Prominent Cancer Doctor Warns About Cellphones," "Well blog," *The New York Times* Web site, July 24, 2008, http://well.blogs.nytimes.com.

[46] Quoted in "Reaching for Control of Carcinogenic Chemicals," Environmental News Service, May 5, 2004, www.ens-newswire.com/ens/may2004/2004-05-05-02.asp.

[47] Joseph G. Acker, "Joe's Blog," Synthetic Organic Chemical Manufacturers Association Web site, Oct. 9, 2008, http://joesblog.socma.org.

FOR MORE INFORMATION

American Association for Cancer Research, 615 Chestnut St., 17th Floor, Philadelphia, PA 19106-4404; (215) 440-9300; www.aacr.org. Promotes and disseminates research on cancer.

American Cancer Society, 901 E St., N.W., #500, Washington, DC 20004; (202) 661-5700; www.cancer.org. Promotes elimination of cancer.

American Chemistry Council, 1300 Wilson Blvd., Arlington, VA 22209; (703) 741-5000; www.americanchemistry.com. Represents leading chemical companies, including significant business groups such as the Plastics Division and Chlorine Chemistry Division.

American Council on Science and Health, 1995 Broadway, 2nd Floor, New York, NY 10023-5860; (212) 362-7044; www.acsh.org. Disseminates information on environmental-health questions, supporting a cautious approach to regulation.

American Institute for Cancer Research, 1759 R St., N.W., Washington, DC 20009; (202) 328-7744; www.aicr.org. Supports and disseminates research into the roles of diet, physical activity and weight management in cancer prevention.

American Society of Clinical Oncology, 1900 Duke St., #200, Alexandria, VA 22314; (703) 299-0150; www.asco.org. Advocates research and improved cancer care.

Cancer Prevention Coalition, c/o University of Illinois at Chicago School of Public Health, MC 922, 2121 West Taylor St., Chicago, IL 60612; (312) 996-2297; www.preventcancer.org. Seeks more attention to cancer prevention and tighter regulation of potential environmental carcinogens.

Collaborative on Health and the Environment, c/o Commonweal, P.O. Box 316, Bolinas, CA 94924; www.healthandenvironment.org. A coalition concerned with potential health effects of toxins and chemicals in the environment.

National Cancer Institute, 31 Center Dr., Bldg. 31, #11A48, MSC-2590, Bethesda, MD 20892-2590; (301) 496-5615; www.cancer.gov. Federal agency that conducts and funds research on cancer.

Science Daily, www.sciencedaily.com/news/health_medicine/cancer. An advertising-supported online publication that carries dozens of reports on cancer research.

Science and Environmental Health Network, 217 Welch Ave., Suite 101, Ames, IA 50014; (515) 268-0600; www.sehn.org. Advocates use of the "precautionary principle" as a new basis for environmental and public health policy.

Skin Deep, www.cosmeticsdatabase.com. Web site maintained by the activist nonprofit Environmental Working Group, which rates the safety of cosmetics and personal-care products.

[48] *Ibid.*

[49] Sen. Edward M. Kennedy, statement before Senate Health, Education, Labor, and Pensions Committee, May 8, 2008, http://kennedy.senate/gov.

[50] "Senators Dodd, Reed Seek to Improve Sunscreen Safety Standards," press release from office of Sen. Christopher Dodd, Aug. 1, 2008, http://dodd.senate.gov/index.php?q=node/4527.

[51] The Obama-Biden Plan to Combat Cancer, www.barackobama.com.

[52] Faguet, *op. cit.*, p. 182.

[53] Frank A. Sloan and Hellen Gelband, eds., *Cancer Control Opportunities in Low- and Middle-Income Countries*, Committee on Cancer Control in Low- and Middle-Income Countries (2007), National Academy of Sciences, p. 9.

Bibliography

Selected Sources

Books

Davis, Devra, *The Secret History of the War on Cancer*, Basic Books, 2007.

An epidemiology professor at the University of Pittsburgh's Graduate School of Public Health says prevention and the role of environmental risks — especially industrial products like chemicals and radiation — have been deliberately ignored for economic reasons throughout the war on cancer.

Faguet, Guy B., *The War on Cancer: An Anatomy of Failure, A Blueprint for the Future*, Springer, 2008.

A hematologist, oncologist and professor emeritus at the Medical College of Georgia delves into the history of cancer research and treatment — particularly how financial incentives affect treatment strategies — and argues that the war on cancer demands a significant overhaul.

Rettig, Richard A., *et al.*, *False Hope: Bone Marrow Transplantation for Breast Cancer*, Oxford University Press, 2007.

A group of health-care analysts chronicle how over-enthusiastic oncologists, the media and lawsuits against insurers helped to fuel the popularity of an unapproved, risky therapy for breast cancer, which was eventually proved useless and unsafe.

Welch, H. Gilbert, *Should I Be Tested for Cancer? Maybe Not and Here's Why*, University of California Press, 2006.

A professor of medicine at Dartmouth Medical School examines how screening apparently healthy people for cancer can result in some cancers being missed and some patients being exposed to invasive, unnecessary procedures for conditions that would never progress to cancer.

Articles

Abelson, Reed, "Quickly Vetted, Treatment Is Offered to Patients," *The New York Times*, Oct. 26, 2008, p. A1.

The Food and Drug Administration's process for approving some cancer treatments, such as radiation, is much less rigorous than the agency's scrutiny of experimental drugs.

Begley, Sharon, "Where Are the Cures?" *Newsweek*, Nov. 10, 2008, p. 56.

Few biomedical discoveries about cancer ever turn into effective treatments or prevention strategies, partly because scientific insights rarely suggest practical application and because turning bench-science findings into drugs or devices that can be tested on humans gets little support.

Parker-Pope, Tara, "Early Test for Cancer Isn't Always Best Course," *The New York Times*, Aug. 12, 2008, p. F5.

The United States Preventive Services Task Force recommends that prostate-cancer screening be stopped at age 75 and that doctors advise men of all ages of both the risks and benefits of screening, which can lead to false positives and treatments that can cause incontinence and impotence.

Saporito, Bill, "He Won His Battle With Cancer. So Why Are Millions of Americans Still Losing Theirs?" *Time*, Sept. 15, 2008, p. 36.

Private groups are trying to ensure that cancer funding is strategically used to produce cures.

Reports and Studies

"Cancer and the Environment: What You Need to Know, What You Can Do," National Cancer Institute/National Institute of Environmental Health Sciences, August 2003, www.niehs.nih.gov/health/docs/cancer-enviro.pdf.

As many as two-thirds of all cancers are linked to environmental factors ranging from cigarette smoking and lack of exercise to air pollutants and pesticides, and many if not most such cancers are probably preventable.

"Food, Nutrition, Physical Activity and the Prevention of Cancer: A Global Perspective," American Institute for Cancer Research/World Cancer Research Fund, 2007, www.dietandcancerreport.org.

An expert panel dissects the evidence on the carcinogenic or cancer-fighting effects of various diets and exercise patterns around the world and recommends prevention strategies.

"Promoting Healthy Lifestyles: Policy, Program, and Personal Recommendations for Reducing Cancer Risk," President's Cancer Panel, National Cancer Institute, 2006-2007 Annual Report, Aug. 2007, http://deainfo.nci.nih.gov/advisory/pcp/pcp07rpt/pcp07rpt.pdf.

A presidentially appointed panel of cancer experts and advocates find that federal state, and local government policies promote unhealthy eating and lack of exercise and that government officials haven't done enough to end tobacco use.

Gray, Janet, ed., "State of the Evidence: The Connection Between Breast Cancer and the Environment," Breast Cancer Fund, 2008, www.breastcancerfund.org.

A nonprofit concerned with environmental health argues that high levels of radiation and synthetic-chemical use connected with industrial society have increased the incidence of breast cancer over the past half century.

The Next Step:

Additional Articles from Current Periodicals

Cancer Drugs

Grace, Kerry E., "Expanded Gardasil Use on Hold," ***The Wall Street Journal*****, Jan. 9, 2009, www.wsj.com.**
The Food and Drug Administration is waiting for more data from Merck before approving a drug that prevents cervical cancer in women ages 27 to 45.

Hitti, Miranda, "Patrick Swayze Opens Up About Pancreatic Cancer," ***WebMD.com*****, Jan. 7, 2009.**
Actor Patrick Swayze is trying an experimental drug as part of his pancreatic cancer treatment.

Carcinogens

Bakalar, Nicholas, "Smokeless Tobacco on Par With Cigarettes," ***The New York Times*****, Aug. 21, 2007, p. F6.**
A new study finds that smokeless tobacco may be as potent as cigarettes in delivering nicotine and carcinogens.

Chandler, Kim, "State Proposes Stricter Rule for Carcinogens in Waterways," ***Birmingham News*** **(Alabama), Dec. 15, 2007, p. 1D.**
The Alabama Environmental Management Commission has voted to reduce the amount of cancer-causing carcinogens in state waterways.

Cone, Marla, "Common Chemicals Linked to Breast Cancer," ***Los Angeles Times*****, May 14, 2007, p. A1.**
Some chemicals identified as breast carcinogens are regulated to protect public health, but many of those in consumer products are not.

Eilperin, Juliet, "EPA Rejects Carcinogenic Wood Preservative for Home Use," ***The Washington Post*****, Jan. 9, 2007, p. A3.**
Federal officials have rejected an industry bid to use a known carcinogen as a preservative in lumber amid fears of increased cancer risk for plant workers.

Prevention

Ackerman, Todd, "$35 Million Gift Boosts Cancer Fight," ***Houston Chronicle*****, May 15, 2008, p. B1.**
A Houston energy magnate has given the University of Texas $35 million to boost efforts to prevent cancer.

Breen, Kim, "Perry Ready for Texas to Be Major Player in Cancer Fight," ***Dallas Morning News*****, June 14, 2007, p. 1B.**
Texas Gov. Rick Perry has signed legislation for a $3 billion plan to establish the Cancer Prevention and Research Institute of Texas.

Moreno, Sylvia, "Thinking Prevention," ***The Washington Post*****, May 13, 2008, p. HE1.**
The Cancer Preventorium at the Washington Hospital Center is aimed at drawing in low-income Latino women for prevention.

Wangsness, Lisa, "Patrick Seeks $72M Hike in Health Aid," ***The Boston Globe*****, Feb. 26, 2007, p. A1.**
Massachusetts Gov. Deval Patrick has announced an increase in the budget for public health spending, largely to expand cancer prevention services.

Screening

Alonso-Zaldivar, Ricardo, "FDA Scientists Complain to Obama of 'Corruption,' " The Associated Press, Jan. 8, 2009.
A group of federal scientists says corrupt practices at the Food and Drug Administration are leading to inefficient cancer-detection devices being approved.

Johnson, David A., "Colonoscopies Save Lives," ***Chicago Sun Times*****, May 7, 2007, p. A40.**
About 90 percent of the colon cancer deaths could have been prevented by proper screening.

Parker-Pope, Tara, "Panel Urges End to Screening for Prostate Cancer at Age 75," ***The New York Times*****, Aug. 5, 2008, p. A1.**
The U.S. Preventive Services Task Force says screening men 75 and older for prostate cancer causes more harm than good.

Rubin, Rita, "Screening Tests May Miss Prostate Cancer in Obese Patients," ***USA Today*****, Nov. 21, 2007, p. 11D.**
High blood volumes may cause some popular screening tests to miss certain cancers in overweight men.

CITING *CQ RESEARCHER*

Sample formats for citing these reports in a bibliography include the ones listed below. Preferred styles and formats vary, so please check with your instructor or professor.

MLA STYLE

Jost, Kenneth. "Rethinking the Death Penalty." CQ Researcher 16 Nov. 2001: 945-68.

APA STYLE

Jost, K. (2001, November 16). Rethinking the death penalty. *CQ Researcher, 11,* 945-968.

CHICAGO STYLE

Jost, Kenneth. "Rethinking the Death Penalty." *CQ Researcher,* November 16, 2001, 945-968.

CHAPTER

10

Battling HIV/AIDS

By Nellie Bristol

Excerpted from the CQ Researcher. Nellie Bristol. (October 26, 2007). "Battling HIV/AIDS." *CQ Researcher*, 889-912.

Battling HIV/AIDS

BY NELLIE BRISTOL

THE ISSUES

In the last 11 years, AIDS has killed Collins Omondi's parents, seven of his uncles, six aunts and five cousins. [1] The 28-year-old Kenyan is a member of the Luo ethnic group, whose men have one of the highest AIDS death rates in Kenya. Twenty-four percent of Luo men are infected with HIV, compared to 7 percent of Kenyan men nationwide. [2] Omondi blames the toll on the tribe's tradition of not routinely circumcising boys. [3]

Although circumcision lowers HIV infection rates by about 60 percent, the Council of Luo Tribal Elders opposes changing customs to include the procedure.

"But along the beaches of Lake Victoria, where fishermen push their colorful sailboats into the waves before dawn each day, many express a willingness to leave this tradition behind if it means surviving an epidemic that seems to have no end," writes *Washington Post* correspondent Craig Timberg. [4]

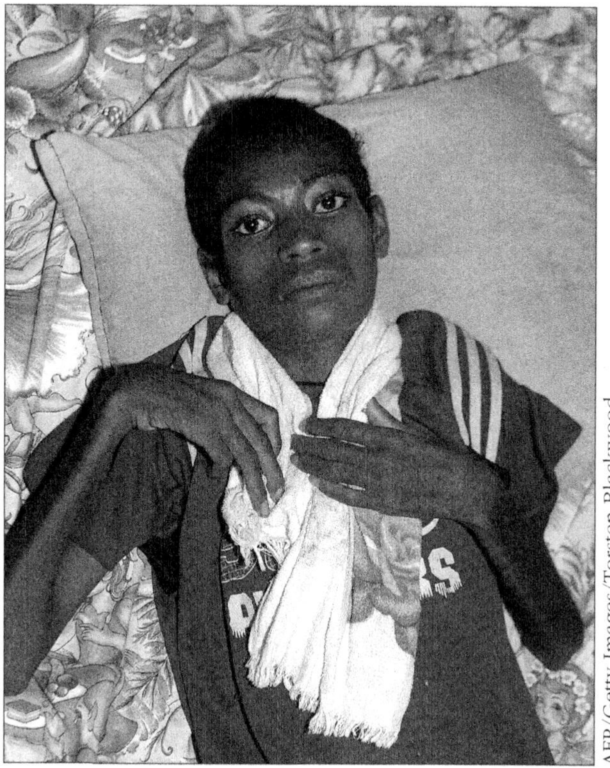

AFP/Getty Images/Torsten Blackwood

Aisi Lucas, a 13-year-old AIDS sufferer in Papua New Guinea, awaits treatment in Port Moresby General Hospital last August. Life-prolonging antiretroviral (ARV) drugs can help HIV/AIDS sufferers, but only 28 percent of those who need drugs receive them. With shortages of drugs and health-care workers and no vaccine in sight, experts are renewing calls for greater disease-prevention efforts, many focused on changing cultural norms, such as unprotected sex and lack of circumcision.

Two-thirds of the world's 40 million HIV/AIDS cases are in economically deprived sub-Saharan Africa — many in the southern African countries of Swaziland, Botswana, Lesotho and South Africa — and 72 percent of the 3 million people who died from AIDS in 2006 were Africans. [5]

Billions of dollars have been expended in the last seven years to provide life-prolonging antiretroviral (ARV) drugs to HIV/AIDS sufferers worldwide. Yet only 28 percent of those who need the drugs receive them, and the rate of new infections continues to outpace treatment at an alarming rate. [6]

"Spectacular advances" have been made in new HIV/AIDS therapies and access to treatment, says Anthony Fauci, director of the National Institute of Allergy and Infectious Diseases (NIAID). Nonetheless, he notes, "We are losing the numbers games."

The new mantra among AIDS experts has become: "We can't treat our way out of this disease."

Indeed, expanded treatment — in Africa and other developing regions — faces towering obstacles, including weak health systems in places where drugs are most needed. The most acute problem is a lack of medical personnel.

"The fact that the world is now short well over 4 million health-care workers . . . is all too often ignored," writes Council on Foreign Relations Senior Fellow for Global Health Laurie Garrett. [7] Africa, for example, bears 24 percent of the world's burden of disease but has only 3 percent of the global health workforce and 1 percent of its physicians. [8]

As this harsh reality settles over the AIDS community — and with no HIV vaccine in sight — experts are renewing calls for greater disease-prevention efforts, many focused on changing cultural norms such as those of the Luo tribe. But while providing medical care and traditional vaccines is daunting enough in impoverished parts of the world, changing behavior patterns that are driving the spread of AIDS may be even more difficult, says Christopher Elias, president of PATH, an international health organization. "Behavioral interventions require more effort to sustain," he says.

Having multiple sexual partners is among the behaviors known to feed the epidemic, along with the early onset of sexual activity, transfusions using tainted blood and the use of unsterilized medical and drug-injecting equipment.

But a major underlying driver of the epidemic "is the real disenfranchisement of women and women's rights" in male-dominated countries, says Fauci. "Women not only cannot protect themselves against the infection, but when they try to they get thrown out of the house, they get beaten, etc."

Changing the status quo, Fauci says, will require strong, concerted leadership in affected communities. "There has to be a reevaluation of centuries-old customs, of the relationship be-

Most AIDS Deaths Are in Poorer Nations

Two million people in low-income countries died from HIV/AIDS in 2005, or about 7 percent of all deaths in that group, according to projections (top). In high-income countries, HIV/AIDS didn't even register as one of the top 10 causes of death (bottom).

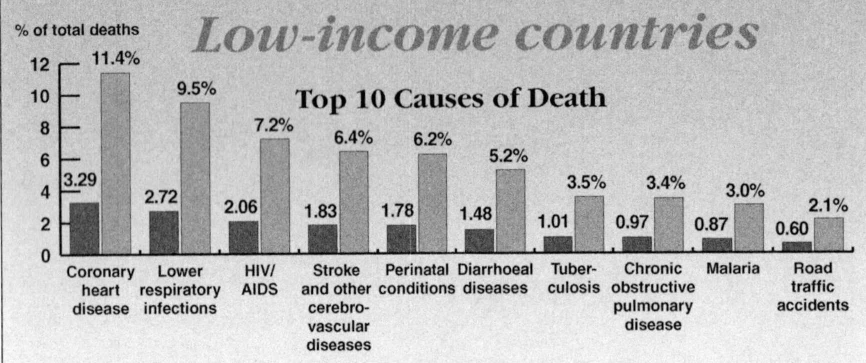

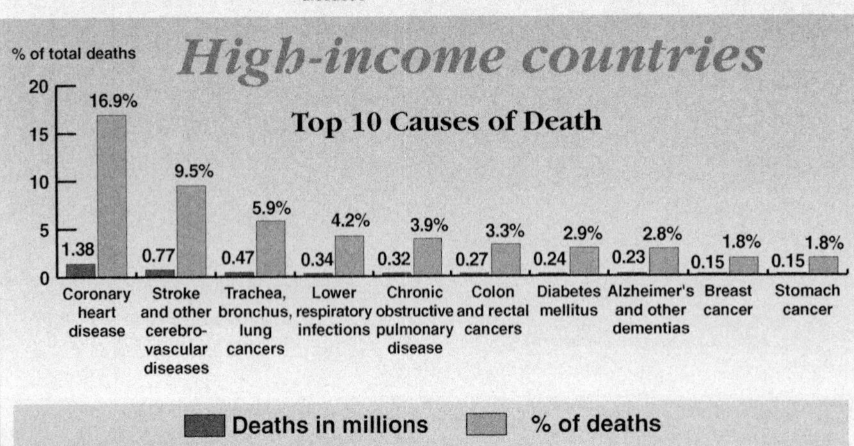

Source: World Health Organization, www.who.int

tween men and women," he says. "That is not going to be easy to change with money, and even with leadership it's difficult to change."

The stakes could not be higher. The carnage the disease is causing in many countries has been likened to an African holocaust and a weapon of mass destruction. [9] The virus has killed more than 25 million worldwide since 1981. Life expectancy has been cut nearly in half in some affected areas. Sixteen African countries had male life expectancies of 45 or less in 2005. [10]

The disease is particularly devastating because it strikes working-age people at the peak of their economic strength. Forty percent of new infections in 2006 affected victims ages 15-24, [11] contributing to shortages of desperately needed teachers and health-care workers. [12] Food shortages have developed in some African villages because there are not enough healthy adults to plant or harvest crops. AIDS has also left at least 12 million orphans in its wake — children who have lost parents to the disease and often suffer from it themselves. (*See sidebar, p. 902.*)

While some African countries are showing declines in national prevalence rates, "such trends are currently neither strong nor widespread enough to diminish the epidemic's overall impact in this region," according to UNAIDS. [13]

There also is concern about rising infection rates in Eastern Europe, Central Asia and the Far East. Russia and Ukraine have the largest HIV epidemics in Europe, accounting for about 90 percent of all cases in the region. [14] Almost two-thirds of reported cases in Eastern Europe were caused by non-sterile drug-injecting equipment. [15] Like a deadly game of Whac-A-Mole, the epidemic is popping up in countries that seemed to have it under control. Thailand, for example, served as a model for confronting the disease among sex workers but is now seeing rising infection rates among teenagers. [16]

In the United States, the number of new infections per year is holding steady at about 40,000 after peaking at 150,000 in the 1980s. [17] There were about 17,000 U.S. deaths from AIDS-related causes in 2005 — and more than 550,000 since 1981. About one-quarter of those infected with HIV in the United States don't know they have it. African-Americans are particularly affected by HIV/AIDS. More than 2 percent of all African-Americans are HIV positive — the highest rate of any racial or ethnic group. [18] Black women accounted for 66 percent of new AIDS cases among American women in 2005. [19] Most women are infected through "high-risk heterosexual contact," such as having unprotected sex, according to the Centers for Disease Control and Prevention (CDC). [20]

"Black and Hispanic women accounted for 81 percent of the women living with HIV/AIDS in 2005 who acquired HIV through high-risk heterosexual contact," the CDC says. "Lack of HIV knowledge, lower perception of risk, drug or alcohol use and different interpretations of safer sex may contribute to this disproportion. Relationship dynamics also play a role. For example, some women may not insist on condom use because they fear that their partner will physically abuse them or leave them," the agency adds. [21]

HIV/AIDS is one of the most high-profile examples of social and health inequities worldwide. While AIDS first came to public attention in the United States, it was stopped from becoming a generalized epidemic, though it remains a pressing problem in some communities. As with most diseases, however, the virus thrives among the disenfranchised and resourceless, becoming entrenched among those without the means to protect themselves.

But HIV also afflicts the affluent. UNAIDS Executive Director Peter Piot notes that one of the most efficient transmitters of the disease in China — where the disease is on the rise — is the 3Ms: Mobile Men with Money. "And I would add, mobile men without money, too," he says. "AIDS is not just a disease of poverty; AIDS is a disease of inequality." [22]

As the developed world seeks to help countries ravaged by HIV/AIDS, here are some of the issues being considered:

Number of Infected Women on the Rise

The percentage of women with HIV has increased in the developing world in the past several years, dramatically in some regions. Eastern Europe and Central Asia experienced a nearly 300 percent increase; in Asia it was 70 percent. Although increases were less significant in sub-Saharan Africa and the Caribbean, more than half of the adults living with HIV in both regions were women in 2006.

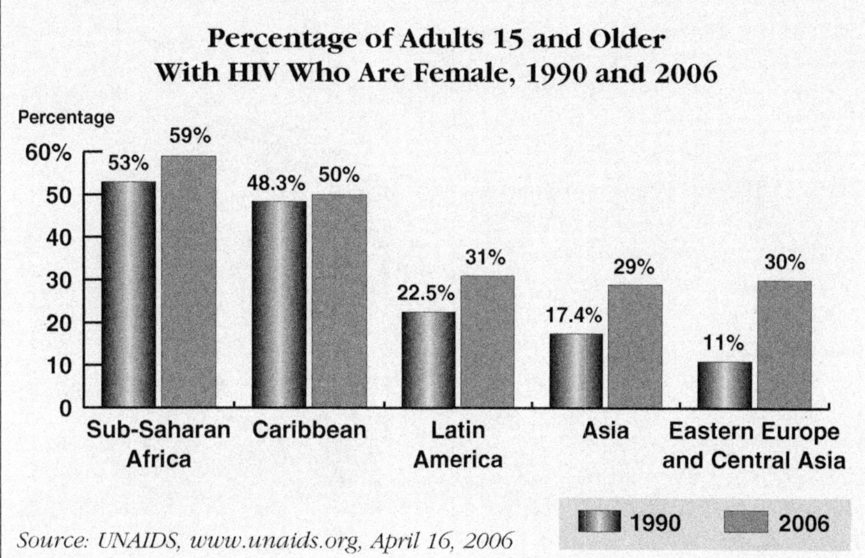

Source: UNAIDS, www.unaids.org, April 16, 2006

Is too much money being spent on AIDS to the detriment of other health issues?

Seven years ago, Piot of UNAIDS attended an international AIDS conference in Durban, South Africa, and "called for a [funding] shift from the M word to the B word — from millions to billions." At the time, major-donor country funding for global HIV/AIDS was about $749 million. [23]

In response, Piot recalls, some of the donors said "that somebody in my position should not make these kinds of irresponsible statements, and that in any case that money is not there." [24]

But over the years, more money was found. In 2007, an estimated $10 billion will be spent on AIDS-related prevention, treatment and care in low- and middle-income countries. Despite the additional resources, however, the effort to stem the global AIDS epidemic is butting up against broader, and seemingly intractable, social and economic problems, including poverty, poor access to clean water and proper nutrition and gender-based inequalities. More directly, the effort is being hampered by weak health systems and a shortage of health-care workers, managers and facilities.

As the initial euphoria of the ARV ramp-up dies down and the disease continues to spread, public health and AIDS experts consider the AIDS-reduction effort to be at a critical fork in the road: Should billions of dollars continue to be earmarked for AIDS-only efforts or should funds be allotted more broadly to strengthening health-systems, improving living conditions for women and general development?

Council on Foreign Relations Senior Fellow Garrett argues for altering disease-specific goals of current global health-care efforts. Too often, she writes, "aid is tied to short-term numerical targets such as increasing the number of people receiving specific drugs. . . . Few donors seem to understand that it will take at least a full generation (if not two or three) to substantially improve public health — and that efforts should focus less on particular diseases than on broad measures that affect populations' well-being." The world community, she argues, "should focus on achieving two basic goals: increased maternal survival and increased overall life expectancy. Why? Because if these two markers rise, it means a population's other problems are also improving."

"Where the water is safe to drink, mosquito populations are under control, immunization is routinely available and delivered with sterile syringes and food is nutritional and affordable, children thrive," she continues. "If any one of those factors is absent, large percentages of children perish before their fifth birthdays." Mosquito-borne malaria is a major killer of children in Africa and other developing countries. [25]

Garrett's arguments are countered by anthropologist and physician Paul Farmer, a founding director of the medical/social-justice group Partners in Health (PIH), which maintains world-famous clinics in Haiti. He argues that the new resources and "enthusiasm about global health" largely fueled by attention to HIV/AIDS can help even out health-care disparities between rich and poor. [26]

Farmer also cautions against following the model of classic development aid. "It is well known in development circles that huge amounts of aid have often brought few improvements to the lives of the world's poorest," he writes. Indeed, he suggests, a first principle for the emerging global health movement might well be, "Do not emulate the mainstream aid industry."

HIV/AIDS programs are improving health facilities and attracting and retaining health personnel in places desperately in need of both. In Haiti, Farmer notes, "As hospitals are refurbished and become something more than charnel houses, and as medicines are made available, some doctors and nurses are returning to the rural public-sector institutions in which we work."

Farmer disputes a suggested correlation between increased HIV/AIDS funding and a drop in virtually all other health indicators in Haiti. He attributes the decrease to government instability and related health-system disruptions.

The U.S. government's main global AIDS initiative — the President's Emergency Plan for AIDS Relief (PEPFAR) — has been criticized for establishing parallel heath-care systems wherein HIV/AIDS patients receive care in clean, well-equipped facilities with sufficient medical staff while patients suffering other diseases are less well attended, if they receive care at all. *

Global Funding Hits $8.9 Billion in 2006

More than two-thirds of the estimated $8.9 billion spent globally on HIV/AIDS in 2006 was donated to other countries. About 31 percent was in-country aid.

Global HIV/AIDS Funding, 2006

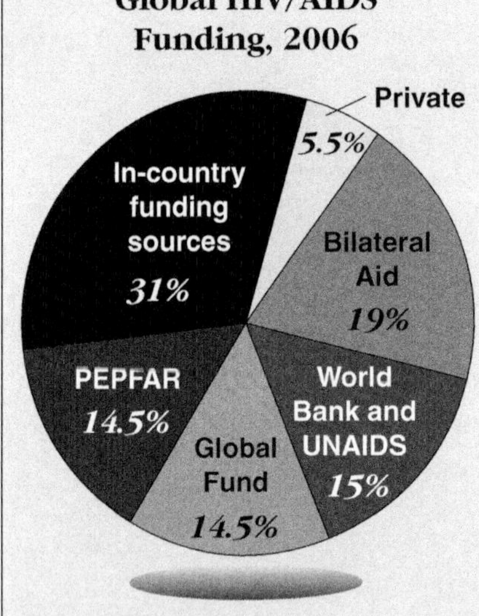

** Totals do not add to 100 due to rounding.*

Source: Global Health Council, www.globalhealth.org

But U.S. Global AIDS Coordinator Mark Dybul argues that while the data remain spotty, efforts to reduce HIV/AIDS have improved other services as well. For example, he says, 50 percent of hospital admissions in some areas are for HIV/AIDS-related care. Reducing those admissions through PEPFAR-funded prevention and treatment frees up resources for other diseases.

A study in three African countries found PEPFAR and other major funders had caused mixed effects on health systems. While some evidence indicated that both indigenous health-care workers and non-governmental organizations (NGOs) are pulling away from other needs to focus on HIV/AIDS, the study also found that upgrades in work environments had boosted workers' motivation. [27]

Similar findings were reported by a recent Institute of Medicine (IOM) review of the program. While PEPFAR may contribute to "internal brain drain" in some countries — pulling workers away from other public health programs — overall, the program is "making health systems stronger, not weakening them," said Jaime Sepulveda, who chaired the IOM committee. [28]

InterAction, an umbrella group for non-governmental organizations, along with other groups is urging PEPFAR to adopt "a more comprehensive, holistic approach" to HIV/AIDS that would allow the money to support non-medical needs of infected individuals, including food and housing. [29]

Should more money be devoted to prevention?

The rewards of heightened prevention efforts could be great. "A comprehensive, scaled-up HIV-prevention response would avert more than half of all new infections projected to occur between 2005 and 2015," UNAIDS predicts. However, it notes that while many countries are on target to reach anti-retroviral-access goals, "progress towards prevention targets appears to be less marked, underscoring the urgent need for intensification of prevention efforts." Achieving universal access to prevention programs by 2010 would cost $15 billion in 2010 alone, UNAIDS estimates. [30] The agency notes that $10 billion will be spent in 2007 for AIDS prevention, treatment and care combined. (*See graph, p. 904.*)

Recent research says prevention ultimately could be a cost-saver. Averting new infections at the rate cited by UNAIDS would cost $122 billion over the 10-year period but would reduce fu-

* PEPFAR was authorized in 2003 for $15 billion over five years. The money was to be used for HIV-AIDS prevention and treatment in countries hardest hit by the disease. President Bush wants to double the funding levels — to $30 billion — when it comes up for reauthorization in 2008.

ture need for care and treatment, a key study shows. "Our analysis suggests that it will cost about $3,900 to prevent each new infection but that this will produce a savings of $4,700 in foregone treatment and care costs," researchers predict.[31]

PEPFAR devotes 55 percent of funding to treatment, 15 percent to care, and 10 percent for orphans and vulnerable children. The remaining 20 percent is slotted for prevention, "of which . . . at least 33 percent should be expended for abstinence-until marriage programs."[32]

As policy makers consider the program's future, prevention spending will be a key issue. "The first PEPFAR program changed the world forever by initiating treatment," says Rep. Nita M. Lowey, D-N.Y., chairwoman of the House Appropriations Subcommittee on State, Foreign Operations and Related Programs. "Our next program must reflect a true commitment to prevention."

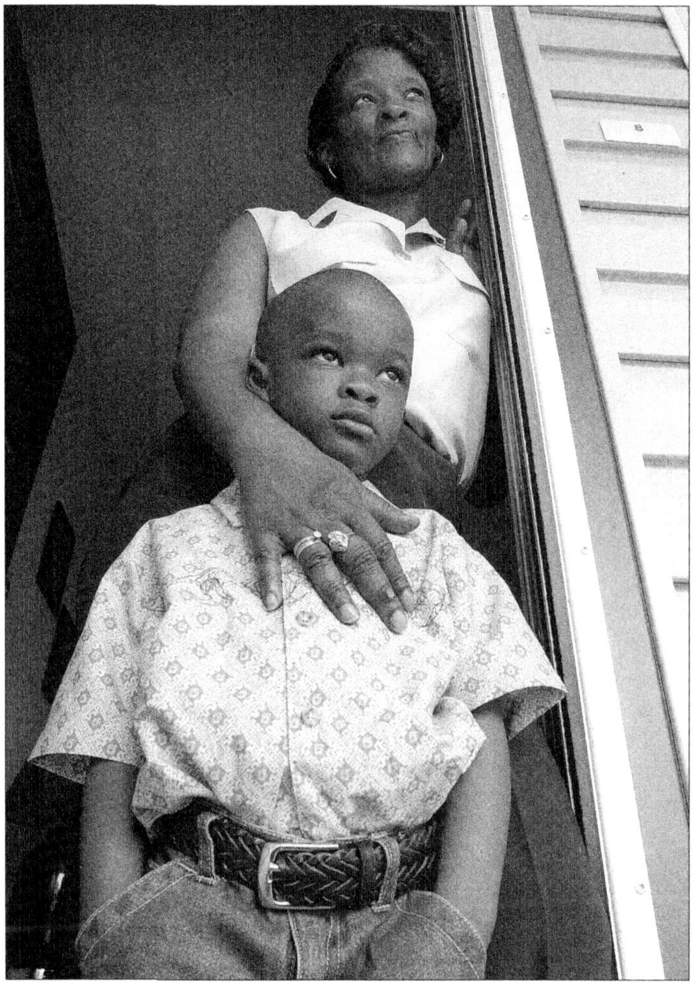

AP Photo/Dave Martin

African-Americans like AIDS sufferer Lawanda Bridges, of Ensley, Ala., are particularly affected by HIV/AIDS. More than 2 percent of all African-Americans are HIV positive — the highest rate of any racial or ethnic group. In the U.S. the number of new infections per year is holding at about 40,000 after peaking at 150,000 in the 1980s. There were about 17,000 U.S. deaths from AIDS-related causes in 2005.

UNAIDS Executive Director Piot agrees. "Greater investment in prevention is absolutely essential," he says.

But Elias of PATH says funding for prevention should not come at the expense of continued treatment access. "The challenge is not to see prevention and treatment as either-or choices but rather as highly synergistic components of the same national AIDS-control program," he says. Greater access to treatment will encourage people to get tested since there will be something they can do to improve their lives if they test positive, he adds.

NIAID's Fauci says public health experts know which prevention methods work. They include behavior modification, such as reducing numbers of sexual partners and delaying the onset of sexual activity. Also key is screening the blood supply, providing clean needles to injecting drug users, condom use and reducing mother-to-child transmission through available drugs.

"Despite these proven modalities, if you look throughout the world as little as 5 percent and at the most 10-15 percent of the people who could benefit from prevention modalities have access to them," Fauci says. Over the next 10 years, millions of new infections could be prevented "if we just used the [methods] that we know work," he adds.

The Global HIV Prevention Working Group says the key is to ramp up and sustain current programs. "To realize the promise of available HIV-prevention tools, they must be brought to scale," the group says.[33] "This means that the appropriate mix of evidence-based HIV-prevention strategies must achieve sufficient coverage, intensity and duration to have optimal public health impact." The group says scale-up efforts are hampered by inadequate financing, misallocation of resources, limits on health-system capacity, service fragmentation, stigma and discrimination.

But another huge factor is human nature. "The very, very difficult things that need to be done are more in the realm of customs, societal leadership and traditional practices," Fauci says.

The difficulties were illuminated recently by UNAIDS Executive Director Piot. Research shows that the social custom of having multiple, concurrent partnerships is vastly intensifying the HIV/AIDS epidemic, especially in Africa. Polygamy is still allowed in many African countries, and one study of behavior in Botswana, for instance, showed that nearly one in three sexually active men had multiple concurrent sex partners, as did 14 percent of women. The rate was 44 percent for men under 25.[34] Piot says UNAIDS is working to address the issue,

Global Funding Hits $10 Billion

Annual HIV/AIDS funding has increased by nearly 10 times over the past decade, reaching an estimated $10 billion in 2007. Donations from foundations and initiatives such as the Gates Foundation, UNAIDS and the President's Emergency Plan for AIDS Relief (PEPFAR) fueled the growth.

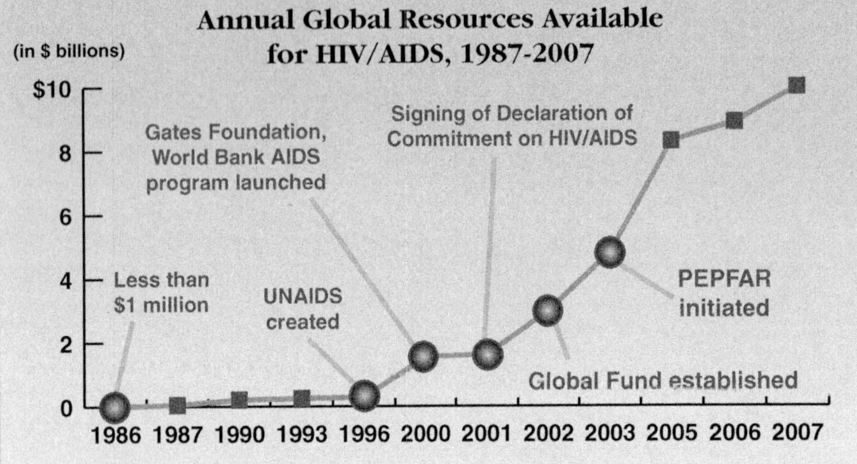

Source: "Financial Resources Required to Achieve Universal Access to HIV Prevention, Treatment, Care and Support," UNAIDS, September 2007

but he says, "We're struggling with the how, to be honest."

"It's about changing societal norms," Piot says. "That's not in the domain of public health anymore." Changing the behavior could have unforeseen consequences, including reducing the economic circumstances of the families involved. He calls for the engagement of cultural anthropologists and political scientists to further study the situation and make recommendations. He notes that far less HIV/AIDS money has been spent on behavior research than on treatment evaluation. [35]

Even with solid research, Piot adds, the adoption of known protective strategies is difficult. With circumcision, for example, "The step from . . . clinical trials to the real world is enormous," he says.

U.S. AIDS Coordinator Dybul also acknowledges the difficulty of studying and encouraging behavior change. "It's much more complicated science than measuring [immune cell] counts or viral load." But, he says, behavior change is possible anywhere and is correlated with drops and plateaus in infection rates. "It's something that bothers me frequently when I hear other people talk," he says. "It's almost as if [they are saying], 'Oh, those poor uneducated Africans can't possibly change their behavior' — it's a little appalling actually." He adds, "Small reductions in [the number of sexual] partners can actually radically change an epidemic."

But prevention strategies also tend to inflame ideological battles. "It's much easier politically to develop some degree of consensus about treatment because it doesn't have the same type of emotionally and ideologically charged controversy around it," says Maurice Middleberg, vice president for public policy at the Global Health Council, a U.S.-based alliance of NGOs, foundations, corporations, government agencies and academic institutions that studies world health problems.

PEPFAR provides a prime example. While supporting the program's ABC model (Abstinence, Be Faithful and Condom use), conservatives argue that the message needs to be weighted toward sexual abstinence and have restricted the program's funding for certain activities to ensure the focus on abstinence. If condoms are emphasized equally, they say, the result is a mixed message to young people about engaging in sexual activity.

But the approach has created a prolonged backlash among some AIDS groups, who say the abstinence message is ineffective and funding restrictions create unworkable constraints. PEPFAR also does not provide funding for needle exchanges, which other organizations endorse, and it has policies that hamper work with prostitutes, some groups say.

Middleberg says the debates are outdated and the AIDS epidemic needs every proven prevention method available. "The debate is, frankly, silly," he says. "The A, the B, the A, the B, the C . . . that's not the point." Ideology, he says, must take a back seat to implementing the most effective strategies tailored to the pattern of the epidemic in a particular area.

"I don't get red in the face about abstinence," he says, "because if data in a particular country are telling us that early sexual [activity] is contributing to the spread of the disease, then we ought to do something about it. Does that mean it's the only thing we should do? Does that mean that condoms are bad? No."

Donors, he says, should stop pushing their "pet interventions" and allow those closest to the epidemic to make program decisions. "Stop making up ideas in Washington or London or Paris or anywhere else about 'this is the magic bullet,'" he says. "Always the question should be, 'What does the particular country or context require?' and programs should be designed responsive to that. That's the whole key to this."

Should more resources be devoted to women?

"Current AIDS responses do not, on the whole, tackle the social, cultural and economic factors that put women at risk of HIV and that unduly burden them with the epidemic's consequences," according to UNAIDS' Global Coalition on Women and AIDS. [36]

"The world's governments have repeatedly declared their commitment to improve the status of women and acknowledged the linkage with HIV," the group continued, but by and large their efforts have been "small-scale, half-hearted and haphazard. It's time the world's leaders lived up to their promises." The group is seeking "a massive scaling up of AIDS responses for women and girls," including resources to adapt AIDS strategies to women, expand access to education, sexual and reproductive health, prenatal care and prevention of mother-to-child transmission. [37]

On the prevention technology front, AIDS experts and researchers in recent years have increased their focus on interventions that could be controlled by women — including virus-killing microbicides women could use vaginally — and female condoms. But microbicide trials so far have yielded little success. Two advanced trials were discontinued in January when results showed the products might increase vulnerability to infection. [38] The female condom appears to be effective in preventing pregnancy and sexually transmitted diseases, but it is more expensive than the male version and not commonly used. [39]

Experts call for more funding for female-controlled prevention methods. "Calculations done by analysts show that microbicide research is getting about half the funding that it should be," said Anna Forbes of the Global Campaign for Microbicides. "Calculations estimate that the field should be getting about $280 million, but is only getting about $168 million in funding per year." [40]

Funding Gap to Widen

Global spending on HIV/AIDS totaled $8.9 billion in 2006, or 40 percent short of global needs. While spending is expected to reach $10 billion this year, the estimated shortfall in 2008 is expected to increase to 55 percent. Prevention-related activities account for more than half of resource needs.

Resource Needs and Estimated Global Spending for HIV/AIDS, 2006-2008

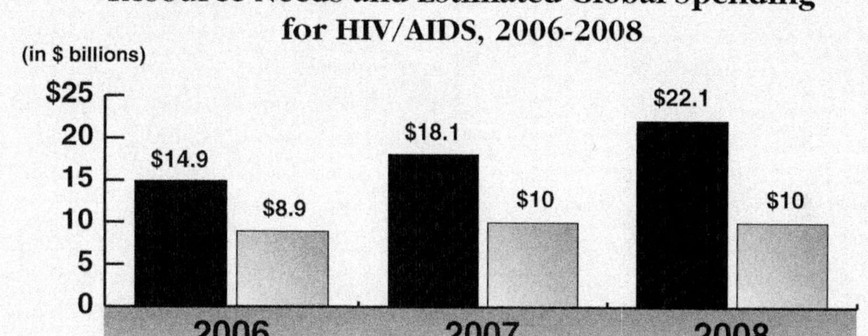

** Includes prevention-related activities, treatment and care components, support for orphans and vulnerable children, and program and administrative costs*

Source: Global Health Council, www.globalhealth.org

"Women are more biologically, socially and economically vulnerable to HIV infection than men," said Anjali Nayyar of the International AIDS Vaccine Initiative. "Women often do not seek counseling and testing and will usually seek treatment much later than a man. The HIV/AIDS epidemic, therefore, clearly highlights the gender inequality that continues to exist globally." [41]

The number of women infected with HIV has grown steadily over the last 25 years. (*See graph, p. 893.*) Worldwide, 48 percent of adults living with HIV are women — a total of 17.7 million. The figure is 13.3 million in sub-Saharan Africa, or 59 percent of all adults with HIV/AIDS. [42] Among young people in sub-Saharan African, three girls are infected for every boy.

Women are more susceptible than men to HIV infection in sexual transmission. In the developing world, infection also can be spread by unsterilized equipment used during genital mutilation or childbirth, or through tainted blood transfusions. [43] Women also are considered to have less control over HIV-prevention methods including use of condoms and partner fidelity. HIV risk was also found to be higher for women with violent or controlling partners. [44]

"I don't think there's any question in anyone's mind that gender inequality fuels this," says PEPFAR's Dybul, but he's not sure more money is the answer. PEPFAR already devotes 61 percent of care and treatment funds to women and 69 percent of counseling and testing funds. "I don't know if we need more resources. I think we need a lot more emphasis on the issue from a cultural perspective, which is something we can't do alone," he says. The focus also needs to be on older men who pressure younger women to have sex and on "predatory younger men," he says.

"Unless there are more resources in general and unless there's more emphasis on these cultural issues in countries and in communities, it's going to be really hard to reverse some of these things," he adds.

While PEPFAR supports programs aimed specifically at women, including counseling, testing and collecting data to determine barriers to program use, it also targets men as a way of protecting women. "Practices such as multiple and concurrent sex partners, cross-generation sex and transactional sex increase vulnerability to HIV infections, particularly among women and girls," program documents say. "The Emergency Plan supports the activities of community- and faith-based organizations to change social norms that perpetuate male violence against women, train couples in negotiation and conflict resolution and strengthen policy and legal frameworks that outlaw gender-based violence." Other programs counsel boys and men on "positive norms," alcohol and substance abuse and teach men in the armed forces about "responsible male behavior." [45] ■

BACKGROUND

Mystery in L.A.

AIDS was first identified in the United States in 1981, when five young men in Los Angeles developed a rare form of pneumonia. Other cases were found in New York. Initially thought to only affect gay men, the mysterious and deadly disease was dubbed Gay-Related Immune Deficiency, or GRID. When it was discovered in heterosexual women, initially mostly drug users, hemophiliacs and Haitian refugees, the CDC renamed it Acquired Immune Deficiency Syndrome (AIDS).

Two years later, the human immunodeficiency virus (HIV) was identified as the cause of AIDS. It is transmitted when a mucous membrane or the bloodstream comes in direct contact with a body fluid containing the virus, including blood, semen, vaginal fluid and breast milk. Transmission generally is through sex, blood transfusion, contaminated hypodermic needles or mother-to-child exchange during pregnancy, childbirth or breast feeding.

By the mid-1980s, public awareness of the disease in the United States and other Western countries had begun to grow, spurred by the death in 1985 of movie star Rock Hudson, the first major public figure to succumb to AIDS. [46] Mechanisms were developed to clean the blood supply, and the public health and gay communities marshaled the resources to address the epidemic among homosexual men. Despite the effort, 300,669 AIDS-infected men who have sex with men have died since the beginning of the epidemic, accounting for 57 percent of all AIDS-related deaths in the U.S. [47]

Despite the obvious vulnerability for all populations, stigma associated with the disease based on its sexual transmission and connection with gay men, created reluctance on the part of many policy makers to acknowledge and confront the disease. "While the gay label would fall, the misconception and stigma in which it was conceived would linger — a distorted prism through which wide swaths of Americans would perceive the disease through its flight," wrote author Greg Behrman. [48] U.S. funding for AIDS-related activities was $100 million in 1984. [49]

In Africa, meanwhile, the disease attacked nearly equal proportions of men and women from the beginning. Even in the early 1980s, the specter of large-scale heterosexual transmission created alarm among researchers, who saw the potential for a public-health crisis of enormous proportions.

So many African women were infected with AIDS, said UNAIDS' Piot, that "it said to me, it's heterosexual. That means that everyone is at risk. . . . Until then, I never thought a whole country, a whole population could be involved." [50]

U.S. health policy, however, focused largely on domestic HIV through the 1990s. Antiretroviral therapy became available in 1995, effectively turning a diagnosis from a death sentence to a chronic disease in Western countries. Meanwhile, education campaigns helped to limit the spread of the virus. The infection peaked in the 1980s at about 150,000 new infections; today the number of new infections in the United States is holding steady at about 40,000 per year. [51]

But in Africa the epidemic exploded. While some countries took aggressive leadership, notably Uganda and Senegal, many didn't. The prohibitive expense of drugs, coupled with poor health-services delivery, made access to antiretrovirals dismally low in the developing world.

PEPFAR

The President's Emergency Plan for AIDS Relief is among three organizations that provide the bulk of international HIV/AIDS funding. The other two are the Global Fund to Fight AIDS, Tuberculosis and Malaria and the World Bank's Multi-Country AIDS Program (MAP).

After an initially slow response from the U.S., President George W. Bush launched PEPFAR — considered to be the largest single disease-prevention and treatment initiative ever undertaken by a single country. Proposed in his 2003 State of the Union address, PEPFAR promised $15 billion over five years for AIDS care and prevention in the hardest-hit countries. Established by the 2003 U.S. Leadership Against HIV/AIDS, Tuberculosis and Malaria Act, PEPFAR aims to provide 2 million people with antiretroviral treatment,

Continued on p. 900

Chronology

1980s AIDS first appears and develops into global crisis. U.S. annual incidence peaks at 150,000.

June 1981
Centers for Disease Control and Prevention (CDC) documents first cases of immune-system disorder in homosexual men in Los Angeles, calls it GRID — gay related immune disorder.

July 1982
After determining the disease also occurs in heterosexuals, CDC renames it AIDS — acquired immune deficiency syndrome.

1983
CDC and National Institutes of Health scientists identify AIDS patients in Zaire. . . . Evidence suggests heterosexual contact spreads the virus.

1984
Scientists isolate AIDS virus, later named human immunodeficiency virus (HIV).

1985
Food and Drug Administration (FDA) approves first blood tests to detect HIV antibodies. . . . Movie star Rock Hudson dies of AIDS.

1988
FDA approves first anti-AIDS drug, AZT. Senegal begins successful AIDS-prevention campaign. . . . Five million people in sub-Saharan Africa have HIV or AIDS.

1990s AIDS begins spreading through developing world; progress is made on treatments.

1990
Central Intelligence Agency predicts 45 million people will be infected by 2000. . . . Congress enacts Ryan White Comprehensive AIDS Resources Emergency (CARE) Act.

1991
Basketball star Earvin "Magic" Johnson says he is HIV-positive. . . . Ten million people have HIV/AIDS in sub-Saharan Africa.

1992
AIDS prevention campaign begins in Uganda, reduces HIV infection rate by the late 1990s.

1995
First protease inhibitors, or antiretroviral drugs, are released.

1996
UNAIDS established to advocate for global action. . . . More than 20 million Africans have HIV or AIDS. . . . Ryan White CARE Act reauthorized.

1997
Antiretrovirals reduce AIDS-related deaths in U.S. by more than 40 percent vs. prior year.

1999
First human vaccine trial in developing country begins in Thailand. . . . Number of people with HIV/AIDS in sub-Saharan Africa approaches 25 million.

2000s Donors in developed world give billions for HIV/AIDS prevention, care and treatment programs. Experts call for increased prevention efforts.

2000
U.N. Security Council declares HIV/AIDS a security threat. . . . 13th International AIDS Conference heightens awareness of pandemic. . . . South African President Thabo Mbeki denies HIV causes AIDS. . . . President Bill Clinton signs law authorizing $300 million for AIDS prevention in developing world. . . . World Bank creates $500 million AIDS fund for sub-Saharan Africa.

June 2001
U.N. General Assembly convenes first special session on AIDS.

2002
HIV is leading cause of death worldwide among people ages 15-59. . . . Women comprise about half of all adults with HIV/AIDS. . . . Global Fund to Fight AIDS, Tuberculosis and Malaria approves first grants.

January 2003
President George W. Bush announces President's Emergency Plan for AIDS Relief (PEPFAR), promises $15 billion in hardest-hit countries. . . . William J. Clinton Presidential Foundation negotiates lower prices for HIV/AIDS drugs for developing countries. . . . World Health Organization (WHO) launches "3 by 5" AIDS initiative to treat 3 million people by 2005.

2004
UNAIDS launches Global Coalition on Women and AIDS.

January 2005
FDA approves HIV drug regimen under new, expedited review process.

December 2006
Congress reauthorizes Ryan White CARE Act for third time.

March 2007
WHO, UNAIDS endorse male circumcision for AIDS prevention. . . . Bush urges Congress to double PEPFAR funding to $30 billion.

HIV and TB Form Lethal Pair

"HIV is driving the TB epidemic."

The number of tuberculosis (TB) cases worldwide increased from 6.5 million new cases in 1990 to 8.8 million in 2005. [1] Experts attribute the rise to the increasing number of HIV-infected individuals, whose compromised immune systems make them up to 50 percent more likely to develop TB than individuals without HIV. [2]

"HIV is driving the TB epidemic in general," says Mario Raviglione, director of the World Health Organization's Stop TB Department. The susceptibility of HIV-positive individuals to TB depends on the degree to which the virus has compromised their immune systems, Raviglione explains. Experts describe HIV as "telescoping" the TB epidemic because TB develops more often and quicker in HIV-infected individuals than non-infected people.

Once known as consumption because it caused its victims to waste away, TB is among the oldest and most lethal of human afflictions. Dubbed the "captain of all these men of death" by 17th-century English writer John Bunyan, TB at its peak killed one in every four people in the United States. [3]

TB killed more than 1.5 million people in 2005, the vast majority in developing countries. Overall, one-third of the world's population is infected with TB, but mainly in a latent form. [4] Among people who are not HIV positive, only 5-10 percent of those infected with TB will develop the disease. [5]

While generally considered a lung disease, TB also can affect other body parts, including the central nervous system. TB is curable, but confirming diagnoses is difficult, and the drug regimen is intensive, often taking more than six months. Without treatment, half of those who develop the disease die from it. [6]

An estimated one-third of the 40 million people living with HIV/AIDS are co-infected with TB. [7] "HIV and TB form a lethal combination, each speeding the other's progress," according to the World Health Organization. In addition, TB is harder to diagnose in HIV-positive people, the disease progresses faster and TB occurs earlier in the course of HIV infection than many other opportunistic infections. [8] Without proper treatment 90 percent of people living with HIV/AIDS die within months of contracting TB. [9]

Also complicating TB treatment is the rise since the 1980s of drug-resistant forms, known as multidrug resistant TB (MDR-TB) and extensively drug resistant TB (XDR-TB). The new strains, Raviglione says, take treatment "almost virtually to the pre-antibiotic era."

While HIV is not fuelling drug-resistant forms per se, Raviglione says the new TB strains are particularly deadly for HIV-positive individuals and HIV helps the virulent strains spread faster in some areas. XDR-TB, considered by some to be untreatable, killed 52 of 53 infected patients in rural South African hospitals in late 2005 and early 2006. [10] While XDR-TB is also increasing in Russia and China, health experts are particularly alarmed about the high HIV rates in Africa. [11]

TB has been on the wane in developed countries for some time making it difficult for advocates to generate funding to fight the disease. The Washington-based Global Health Council estimates TB required global expenditures of $3.5 billion to $4.5 billion in 2007, but only half that amount was available.

The reality of drug-resistant TB was brought home to Americans when infected Atlanta lawyer Andrew Speaker boarded several overseas flights last summer, raising an international ruckus. Speaker was first thought to have XDR-TB, but his diagnosis was later changed to the more treatable MDR-TB. Speaker's controversial flights nonetheless focused U.S. attention on the disease that has been worrying global health experts for years. Both the House and Senate are now considering bills that boost funding for global TB efforts. [12]

Noting the connection between the first U.S. drug-resistant TB scare and the increased funding, Raviglione quips, "We need 10 Mr. Speakers every month."

---

[1] World Health Organization, "Global Tuberculosis Control: Surveillance Planning, Financing," 2006, www.who.int/tb/publications/global_report/en/index.html.

[2] World Health Organization, WHO Stop TB Partnership, "Can You Imagine a World Without TB? We Can," www.who.int/tb/en/index.html.

[3] Daniel Epstein, "Tuberculosis: 'The Captain of All These Men of Death,' " *Perspectives in Health*, 1996 Pan American Health Organization, www.paho.org/English/DD/PIN/Number1_article5.htm.

[4] World Health Organization, "Tuberculosis Fact Sheet," revised March 2007, www.who.int/mediacentre/factsheets/fs104/en/index.html.

[5] *Ibid.*

[6] Global Health Council, "Infectious Diseases," www.globalhealth.org/view_top.php3?id=228.

[7] Kaiser Family Foundation, "Tuberculosis," www.globalhealthreporting.org/tb.asp.

[8] World Health Organization, "Frequently asked questions about TB and HIV," www.who.int/tb/challenges/hiv/faq/en/index.html.

[9] www.theglobalfund.org/en/files/about/replenishment/disease_report_en.pdf.

[10] Michael Wines, "Virulent TB in South Africa May Imperil Millions," *The New York Times*, Jan. 28, 2007.

[11] *Ibid.*

[12] Adam Graham-Silverman, "Tuberculosis Measure, USIAD Nomination on Senate Foreign Relations Agenda," *CQ Today*, Sept. 10, 2007.

Continued from p. 898

prevent 7 million new infections and provide support care for 10 million people. The program is overseen by the U.S. Office of Global AIDS Coordinator (OGAC).

Author Behrman ascribes the change in U.S. policy to several factors. He says the Christian right, although sometimes brutal towards the gay sufferers of AIDS in America, began to push for treatment in developing countries particularly to stem mother-to-child transmission. In addition, the administration was looking for ways to soften the nation's image during the Iraq War. Behrman also credits U2 lead singer Bono, who lobbied both on Capitol Hill and at the White

House. At the same time, AIDS activists were pushing drug companies to lower their antiretroviral drug prices or allow generic versions of them to be manufactured. [52]

Public health experts consider PEPFAR a success. "The most significant infusion of leadership, of money and commitment, has come from the United States, through PEPFAR, and I would say that U.S. leadership has truly transformed the global response to AIDS and the course of the epidemic. . . . It really enabled us to make a qualitative and a quantum leap forward," says UNAIDS' Piot. [53] The United States was the largest AIDS-assistance donor in the world in 2006, providing 41 percent of disbursements, mainly through PEPFAR and the Global Fund. [54]

According to program data, PEPFAR has supported ARVs for more than 1.1 million infected individuals and prevention of mother-to-child HIV transmission for more than 6 million pregnancies. Further, PEPFAR says it supported more than 18.6 million counseling and testing sessions, provided care for more than 2 million orphans and vulnerable children, helped build and refurbish labs and health centers and provided funding for health personnel. All told, the program says it supported prevention activities that reached 61.6 million people.

Despite its achievements, PEPFAR has been harshly criticized, particularly for its focus on abstinence in HIV/AIDS prevention. PEPFAR touts the "ABC" approach to prevention — Abstinence until marriage, Be faithful and use Condoms, which it says is modeled after a successful Ugandan effort. The act creating the program specifies that 20 percent of PEPFAR spending be appropriated for prevention activities — and a third of that must be devoted to abstinence-until-marriage programs.

Critics argue the abstinence requirement smacks of heavy-handed social engineering and hampers effective programs in the field. The Government Accountability Office (GAO) agreed on the second point. In April 2006, the watchdog agency said despite OGAC efforts to clarify the requirement, and exemptions for smaller programs, the funding restrictions have "presented challenges for country teams." Further, it said, "to meet the abstinence-until-marriage spending requirement, teams have in some cases reduced or cut funding for certain prevention programs, such as comprehensive programs for certain populations." Continuing to apply the restriction, it added, could "further challenge country teams' ability to address local prevention needs." [55] An Institute of Medicine's assessment was similar. [56]

PEPFAR also was chastised for its slow approval of generic drugs, which critics said benefited U.S. drug companies while limiting the availability of treatment. In January 2005, GAO supported the claims. It found PEPFAR included a smaller number of ARVs than other major HIV/AIDS initiatives "and does not include some [fixed dose combinations] that are preferred by most of the focus countries because they can simplify treatment." [57] IOM also concurred on this finding. PEPFAR has since expedited approval of generic drugs, according to US AIDS Coordinator Dybul. [58]

The program also will not fund needle-exchange programs, said to reduce transmission among drug users, and will not fund programs that do not explicitly oppose prostitution and sex trafficking. Groups in the field argue that the provisions hamper their ability to work with populations at highest-risk of developing the virus.

The Global Fund to Fight AIDS

The Global Fund to Fight AIDS, Tuberculosis and Malaria, was created in 2002 as a unique public-private funding agency to help low- and middle-income countries. Established as a private foundation in Geneva, the fund was championed by U.N. Secretary General Kofi Annan in 2000. The U.S. pledged $200 million to the future fund in May 2001. [59] It is now the largest funding organization for the three diseases, providing 20 percent of the donor funding for AIDS-related prevention and treatment, 64 percent for malaria and 70 percent for tuberculosis. [60]

The United States is the fund's major donor, having paid more than $2.5 billion toward its $8.6 billion in paid pledges. Other top governmental contributors are France, the European Union, Italy, Japan and the UK. The largest private donor is the Bill & Melinda Gates Foundation, which has paid $350 million to the fund. (*See box, p. 904.*) [61]

The fund makes grants to applicants but stays out of program implementation. The approach was designed to be "country driven," primarily by groups in funded countries. Recipient programs are closely monitored, and some countries have had funding discontinued based on poor performance reviews. While generally well received, the fund has been criticized for not providing enough technical support for programs.

The Multi-Country AIDS Program (MAP), established in 2000, is one of many World Bank HIV/AIDS programs. [62] It aims to provide long-term support for disease-related activities and to "encourage recipient governments to focus attention on developing and implementing a national response," according to the Center for Global Development. MAP has committed $1.2 billion to 29 countries and $107 million to four sub-regional projects. [63] The effort has funded 49,000 faith-based and community-based sub-projects by non-governmental organizations.

Vaccine Development

Twenty-three years ago, Health and Human Services Secretary Margaret Heckler predicted early success on an AIDS vaccine. "We hope to have such a vaccine ready for testing in approx-

Continued on p. 903

'On the Floor of the Hut Were 32 Orphaned Children'

AIDS ravages families in sub-Saharan Africa.

In 2003, the U.N. secretary general's special envoy for HIV/AIDS in Africa, Stephen Lewis, witnessed a numbing scene in Zamibia:

"[We] were taken to a village where the orphan population was described as out of control. As a vivid example of that, we entered a home and encountered the following: To the immediate left of the door sat the 84-year-old patriarch, entirely blind. Inside the hut sat his two wives, visibly frail, one 76, the other 78. Between them they had given birth to nine children; eight were now dead. The ninth, alas, was clearly dying. On the floor of the hut, jammed together with barely room to move or breathe, were 32 orphaned children ranging in age from 2 to 16. . . . It is now commonplace that grandmothers are the caregivers for orphans." [1]

As many as 15 million children worldwide have lost at least one parent to AIDS. [2] Of those, 12 million live in sub-Saharan Africa. [3] The number of AIDS orphans is expected to almost double in the next 10 years. [4]

Orphans typically suffer from emotional distress, removal from their homes and communities and loss of resources, including their family's land. [5] They have had to care for one and sometimes two chronically ill parents. They are more likely than other orphans to lose both of their parents since the parents likely infected each other with HIV. They face a future of increased vulnerability and decreased opportunity.

"One important concern is that orphans will acquire less education because they may have caregivers who cannot afford the costs of schooling, they may be needed for economic activities or their caregivers may have less interest in their welfare," a UNICEF report notes. [6]

Moreover, orphans are often stigmatized, which "can expose them to even greater risks, limited access to health care and schooling and possible rejection by family, friends and community members." [7] In Central and Eastern Europe, and other regions, HIV-positive children are at increased risk of abandonment. In Russia 20-25 percent of children born to HIV-positive mothers are abandoned at birth. [8]

In most places, extended families care for orphaned children. But the burden is crushing some already-struggling communities and households. "The AIDS epidemic contributes to deepening poverty in many communities, since the burden of caring for the vast majority of orphans falls on already-overstretched extended families; women or grandparents with the most meager resources," UNICEF reports. [9] "Such households are expected to earn 31 percent less than other households."

When children cannot be cared for by the family, UNICEF recommends protecting and expanding adoption possibilities and also making known the possibility of institutionalization, and its use as a last resort. [10]

"In the view of most child- and human-development experts, institutional settings are typically inadequate and even unjustifiable," the group reports. Limitations include lack of personal care and interaction. Institutionalized children frequently have trouble integrating into society and lack cultural and practical knowledge and skills. In addition, residential forms of care are five-to-20-times more expensive, not including buildings and infrastructure. In Tanzania it costs $1,000 per month to support a child in an institution — six times the cost of foster care.

Other support options being developed include group fostering, where a paid caregiver lives with a group of children that often includes siblings. Structures also are being developed to help the increasing number of child-headed households. In Rwanda, for example, the Association of Child Headed Households supports children with food, housing and economic opportunities. [11]

With the number of AIDS orphans expected to explode in the next decade — along with the epidemic — experts are concerned not only about the children's welfare but also the fabric of society itself.

"What is often overlooked is the ripple effect the epidemic will have on future governance, social structures and growth of the worst-hit countries in sub-Saharan Africa," the United Nations says. "Dramatically higher mortality rates will result in the depletion of much of the labour force, both in urban and rural areas, with the losses having profound impact on the very foundations of economies and state administration." [12]

---

[1] Stephen Lewis, "Opening Address of the XIIIth International Conference on AIDS and STIs in Africa," Sept. 21, 2003, www.stephenlewisfoundation.org/news_item.cfm?news=402&year=2003.

[2] UNAIDS, UNICEF, USAID, "Children on the Brink 2004," http://data.unaids.org/pub/GlobalReport/2006/2006_GR_CH04_en.pdf.

[3] *Ibid.*

[4] President's Emergency Plan for AIDS Relief, "Orphans and Vulnerable Children," updated August 2007, www.pepfar.gov/pepfar/press/82280.htm.

[5] UNICEF, "Africa's Orphaned and Vulnerable Generation: Children Affected by AIDS," 2006, www.unicef.org/publications/index_35645.html.

[6] *Ibid.*

[7] UNICEF Innocenti Research Center, "Caring for Children Affected by HIV and AIDS," *Innocenti Insight,* November 2006, www.unicef-irc.org/cgi-bin/unicef/Lunga.sql?ProductID=472.

[8] *Ibid.*

[9] UNICEF, "AIDS Orphans in Sub-Saharan Africa: a Looming Threat to Future Generations," 2006, www.un.org/events/tenstories/story.asp?storyID=400.

[10] UNICEF Innocenti Research Center, *op. cit.*

[11] *Ibid.*

[12] UNICEF, *op. cit.*

Continued from p. 901

imately two years," she told reporters in 1984. [64]

"The implication was that it was going to be quick and easy," says Wayne Koff, vice president for research and development at the International AIDS Vaccine Initiative (IAVI). But none of the many vaccines that have been tested has proven effective, and experts predict a comprehensive formulation is still years away. Some suggest one may not be possible at all. [65]

NIAID's Fauci says the failure is largely scientific. "We develop vaccines by mimicking natural infection," he explains. Researchers examine survivors of a disease and design vaccines to elicit responses that clear the infection from the body. Most diseases kill only a small percentage of their victims. For example, 85 percent of those who contract smallpox recover spontaneously, Fauci says, as do 98 percent of those who contract the polio virus. "Even with the deadliest disease, the body has told us through centuries of experience it has the capability of preventing and blocking infection," Fauci says. But with HIV — "unbelievably" — Fauci says, "there hasn't been a single documented case of spontaneous eradication and recovery." That leaves researchers with little to work with in figuring out how to stimulate an immune response.

Vaccine researchers started out with confidence when the human immunodeficiency virus was first isolated in 1984. "In the early days, people felt it would be easy to make an AIDS vaccine because there was a revolution going on in the biotech field — particularly in vaccines," Koff says. Researchers were coming off recent success with the hepatitis B vaccine using the concept of neutralizing antibodies. The vaccine stimulates the body to create antibodies that attack infectious agents and inhibit their infectivity and virulence.

Like AIDS, hepatitis B is blood-borne and sexually transmitted, and researchers thought the same concept could be used to create an HIV vaccine. Researchers rapidly identified the outer protein of the virus, and initial trials began in 1987. The approach seemed to work. "A lot of it had a lot of parallels to the preclinical work that had been done on the hepatitis B vaccine," Koff says.

But in the early 1990s "the roof caved in," he says. Researchers discovered that while the vaccine formulations worked in laboratory strains of the virus, they had no effect on the virus found in infected humans. "It was as if the virus was just laughing at the antibody, and it was just growing merrily along," Koff recalls.

That was a major turning point for AIDS vaccine development. "If you're watching the movie of HIV, that's when all the music changes from happy-go-lucky to the ominous sounds of 'Psycho,' or something," he says.

The setback pointed the bulk of AIDS vaccine research onto a different approach. Instead of an AIDS vaccine that prevents infection through the use of neutralizing antibodies, researchers began focusing on the other arm of the immune system: so-called cell-mediated immunity. But instead of preventing infection, these vaccines — if administered before infection occurs — should reduce the seriousness of the infection and the chance of transmission. All of the more than 30 AIDS vaccine trials now being conducted worldwide use the cell mediated approach. [66]

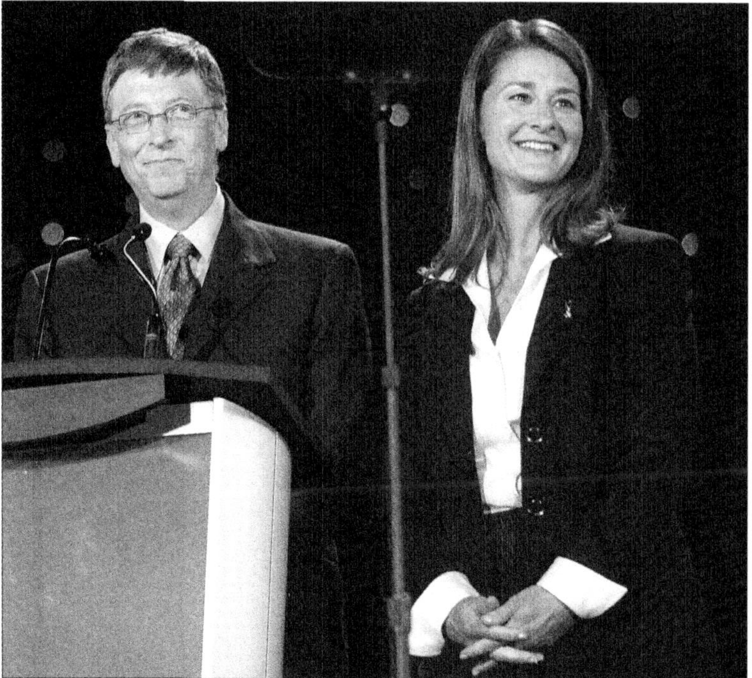

AP Photo/Adrian Wyld

Bill and Melinda Gates address the International AIDS Conference in Toronto in August 2006. As the world's leading private donor to the HIV/AIDS fight, their foundation has provided $1.8 billion since its founding in 2000.

"Current vaccine research suggests that the first licensable vaccines may be effective only in a modest proportion of those vaccinated and may induce a different kind of immune response," wrote researchers at the Futures Institute. [67] The response "would not eliminate HIV infection entirely but would keep the amount of viruses at a low level so that the vaccinated person would be less likely to transmit HIV to a partner and would also have a slower progression to AIDS via control of the viral load at a reduced 'set point.' "

The partially effective vaccine would require a different public health approach than previous vaccines because it would have to be delivered with continued focus on prevention efforts. "If licensed, such a vaccine will have to be delivered

Private Donors Commit Billions to Fight

Gates Foundation tops list with $1.8 billion.

Gates Foundation — The world's top private donor, by far, to the HIV/AIDS fight is the Bill & Melinda Gates Foundation. In 2006 alone, it committed $736 million to programs and grantees — 75 percent of all funds committed by U.S. philanthropies. Other top donors in 2006 were the Bristol-Myers Squib Foundation ($28 million), The Ford Foundation ($21 million), Abbott Laboratories Fund ($19 million) and MAC AIDS Fund and MAC Cosmetics ($16 million). International efforts received 90 percent of U.S. philanthropic funding. [1]

Since its inception in 2000, the Gates Foundation has spent $1.8 billion on HIV- and tuberculosis-related activities. [2] Its HIV/AIDS efforts focus on research on HIV vaccines, microbidicides and other preventive therapies and supporting large-scale prevention initiatives. [3] It also has committed $258 million to address HIV/AIDS in India under its Avahan program. [4] In July, 2006, the foundation began a series of grants to create an international network of research consortia focused on accelerating HIV vaccine development. [5]

Clinton Foundation — The William J. Clinton Foundation's HIV/AIDS Initiative (CHAI) worked with UNITAID, a global health financing organization, to reach agreements with pharmaceutical manufacturers to reduce the price of HIV/AIDS drugs. Finalized May 8, 2007, agreements with Cipla and Matrix resulted in reductions for 16 medicines including second-line drugs and a "gold-standard one pill, once daily first-line drug. The agreement was one of several negotiated by CHAI over the years. Launched in 2002, the Clinton program also works with countries to address health systems issues and increase HIV/AIDS services in rural areas and to children. [6]

---

[1] Funders Concerned About AIDS, "US Philanthropic Commitments for HIV/AIDS: 2005 & 2006," www.fcaaids.org/publications/Publications_Mapping.htm.

[2] Bill & Melinda Gates Foundation, "Global Health," www.gatesfoundation.org/GlobalHealth/Pri_Diseases/HIVAIDS/Grants/default.htm?showYear=2007.

[3] Bill & Melinda Gates Foundation, "Grantmaking Priorities for HIV/AIDS," www.gatesfoundation.org/GlobalHealth/Pri_Diseases/HIVAIDS/HIV_Grantmaking.htm.

[4] Bill & Melinda Gates Foundation, "Avahan: India AIDS Initiative," www.gatesfoundation.org/GlobalHealth/Pri_Diseases/HIVAIDS/HIVProgramsPartnerships/Avahan.

[5] Bill & Melinda Gates Foundation, "Foundation Fund Major New Collaboration to Accelerate HIV Vaccine Development," July 19, 2006, www.gatesfoundation.org/GlobalHealth/Pri_Diseases/HIVAIDS/Announcements/Announce-060719.htm.

[6] William J. Clinton Foundation, "Clinton Foundation HIV/AIDS Initiative," www.clintonfoundation.org/cf-pgm-hs-ai-home.htm.

as part of a comprehensive, multifaceted prevention program," writes Margaret Johnston, director of the Vaccine Research Program at the NIAID. [68]

The partially effective formulation may prove to be a tougher sell to the countries that would have to supply the financial and human resources needed to disseminate the vaccine. Although even a partially effective vaccine is still years off, the IAVI has begun preparing developing countries to roll it out as soon as it's available.

"We want to make sure it's not dismissed because it's not 100 percent effective," says Robert Hecht, the group's senior vice president of public policy. Discussions with country leaders have mostly been positive, he adds. "The more they know about the idea of a potentially partially effective vaccine, the more interested they are actually in exploring what it might mean for their country," he says.

A vaccine with 50 percent efficacy provided to 30 percent of the population would help avoid 17 million new infections, according to research. [69]

Also impeding vaccine progress is drug company reluctance to invest in a risky proposition. "When it comes to HIV, many [major pharmaceutical companies] have been slow to participate, in part because there is so much uncertainty about which approach is most promising and in part because the return on the massive investment required is likely to be small, especially as compared with the profits created by blockbuster drugs such as statins or antidepressants," wrote Howard Markel, director of the Center for the History of Medicine at the University of Michigan. [70]

Nonetheless, funding for vaccine research and development is increasing. In 2005 total global investment in an HIV vaccine was $759 million, up 11.3 percent from 2004. [71] Governments fund 88 percent of the R&D total, the commercial sector 10 percent and philanthropies the remaining 2 percent. [72] ■

CURRENT SITUATION

Reauthorizing PEPFAR

PEPFAR expires in September 2008, and President Bush is proposing reauthorizing and funding the program at $30 billion for the 2009-2013 period. Reauthorization has bipartisan support. "The legislation [PEPFAR] produced by our committee has yielded dramatic results," said House Foreign Affairs Committee Chairman Tom Lantos, D-Calif. "But the task for the next five years is not only to solidify these gains, but to reorient the program so that our efforts to combat HIV/AIDS will be sustainable for generations to come." [73]

Continued on p. 906

At Issue:

Does U.S. patent policy delay developing countries' access to affordable, new HIV/AIDS drugs?

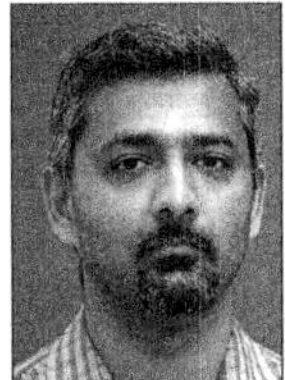

DR. BUDDHIMA LOKUGE
U.S. MANAGER, CAMPAIGN FOR ACCESS TO ESSENTIAL MEDICINES, DOCTORS WITHOUT BORDERS/MÉDECINS SANS FRONTIÈRES

WRITTEN FOR *CQ RESEARCHER*, OCTOBER 2007

yes

As doctors, we've seen the costs of pharmaceutical patent barriers for years. More than 25 million people have died of HIV/AIDS — the majority in the developing world — even though effective therapies existed for more than a decade.

While there are many obstacles to the wide use of antiretrovirals (ARVs) in the developing world, price has been a major barrier. As the pandemic spread in the late 1990s, our teams sent people with HIV/AIDS home to die because patents made ARVs unaffordable.

International advocacy and competition from generic manufacturers dramatically transformed the landscape. In 2000-2001, the huge price drop of generic ARVs (from more than $10,000 for patented versions to less than $100 per patient per year for standard first-line ARV therapy) has led to the treatment of nearly 2 million people in the developing world.

While efforts to put more patients on first-line treatment continue, the next crisis is already here. Toxicities and naturally forming resistance require patients to be switched to alternative ARVs, which are more widely patented and cost between five and 22 times as much as first-line treatments.

The "Doha Declaration" of 2001 placed health over trade. Yet developing countries trying to obtain affordable generic drugs are still met with threats and sanctions. In November 2006, Thailand's Ministry of Health issued compulsory licenses to obtain versions of three patented medicines, including two next-generation HIV therapies. The licenses improved access. They also prompted several members of Congress to complain to the U.S. Trade Representative, landing Thailand on a "watch list;" U.S.-based Abbott Laboratories even withdrew new drug registrations there. Such actions have a chilling effect on the use of legal flexibilities by developing nations.

Overriding the AIDS crisis is this important question: Have international trade rules requiring all countries to give 20-year patent terms sparked medical innovation needed by the developing world? As our doctors struggle to confront diseases like TB with diagnostics from the 1880s and 50-year-old medicines, we see little evidence of this.

Falsely linking innovation with increased IP protection does not justify threats against countries trying to improve access to life-saving medicines. As doctors struggling to provide essential care to patients in the developing world, we expect U.S. patent and trade policy to encourage access and innovation, not stymie it.

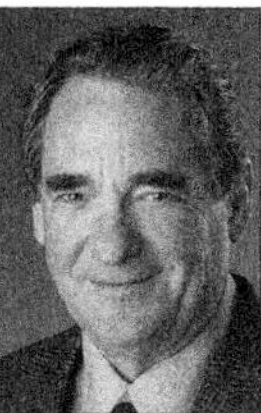

BILLY TAUZIN
PRESIDENT, PHARMACEUTICAL RESEARCH AND MANUFACTURERS OF AMERICA (PHRMA)

WRITTEN FOR *CQ RESEARCHER*, OCTOBER 2007

no

America's biopharmaceutical research companies are proud of the HIV/AIDS therapies they have developed, and they continue to invest in developing new and better treatments. Continued investment is important because this deadly virus is constantly mutating and developing resistance to existing medicines. If the pipeline dries up, patients will die.

Already, 22 HIV/AIDS medicines are available, and another 35 new antiretrovirals and 19 vaccines are in development. All this is supported by patent protections that provide researchers with needed incentives to inspire medical innovation.

Critics claim that U.S. patent protections somehow inhibit development of new HIV/AIDS medicines or prevent patients from obtaining the medicines. This is not supported by the facts.

There are very few patents on HIV/AIDS medicines in the poorest countries hardest hit by the disease. Where patents do exist in these countries, historically most biopharmaceutical research companies have chosen not to enforce their patent rights or have provided these medicines at not-for-profit prices. Additionally, companies have developed a large number of donation programs to facilitate access to their medicines.

Indeed, it is striking to note that India — with world-class domestic antiretrovirals production — had fewer than 7 percent of patients in treatment out of almost 3 million infected with the virus as of 2005. Patent protection clearly is not been the reason India's patients did not have access to medicines.

The primary mission of biopharmaceutical research companies is to develop innovative new medicines. Without the promise of reliable patents and intellectual-property protection, there is a significant question whether any of the existing HIV/AIDS medications would be available.

Attacks on patent protection do little to address the core challenge often confronting HIV/AIDS patients around the world — poor health-care infrastructure and delivery systems. Once cutting-edge therapies are developed, a stable and accessible health system is critical to get those therapies to patients.

Certainly, we can and must do more to ensure that HIV/AIDS patients get the medicines they need. Biopharmaceutical research companies are working to do just that. But the best way is for the world community to work together to improve health-care delivery and distribution systems, hospitals, and the education of health-care professionals. The research pharmaceutical industry supports these efforts.

Continued from p. 904

The call for making the program sustainable is coming from many quarters, but the difficulty will be how. "At the strategic level, authorizers will need to consider how the objectives and scope of the initiative might change and how the program fits within the evolving context of global health and development assistance," write researchers at the Center for Strategic and International Studies. "PEPFAR was conceived as an emergency response, with priority emphasis on getting resources to the field quickly and providing antiretroviral treatment to those in need. Today, HIV/AIDS remains an urgent global problem, but there is growing recognition that the United States will need to broaden its approach to one that responds with the urgency required, but one that also lays more fully the foundation of a long-term, sustainable health and development commitment." [74]

AIDS activists and global health experts are encouraging Congress to reauthorize PEPFAR based on the Institute of Medicine's suggestions, which called for a sustainable, broader commitment. "U.S. efforts should move from focusing on emergency relief to long-term strategic planning and capacity building," said the IOM's PEPFAR committee Chairman Sepulveda. The report also recommends that prevention programs be evidence-based and linked to national information on the epidemic. IOM also says PEPFAR should help better coordinate services by working more closely with other countries, donors and program implementers.

In its recommendations for reauthorization, UNAIDS calls for expanding the number of countries receiving high levels of PEPFAR support. While it currently provides some support to more than 100 nations, the current program focuses on 15 countries. The U.N. group also calls for localized response to the epidemic and more emphasis on prevention, increased support for women and girls and resources to strengthen health systems. In a veiled criticism of the abstinence-only provisions, it suggests, "acknowledging that any strategy that includes the word 'only' is a bad strategy." [75]

Sexual Abstinence

UNAIDS isn't alone in pushing for eliminating restrictions on prevention funding, which means a showdown is likely during the PEPFAR reauthorization process. Provisions striking the sexual-abstinence provision already are included in fiscal year 2008 appropriations legislation.

The problem with the abstinence approach, says PATH's Elias, is that it's "an ideological position. It's basically saying that one of these approaches is better than the others when in fact what we need is a balanced approach of all the different strategies that an individual or a community can use to avoid HIV infection. Abstinence doesn't really work for the married woman who's monogamous herself but whose husband is off visiting sex workers. It's not a practical prevention strategy for her."

Congressional conservatives are likely to fight for the abstinence provisions. "They are absolutely essential, and they remain essential," says Rep. Chris Smith, R-N.J. Other donors may be pushing more for condom use, says Smith, one of the original supporters of the PEPFAR legislation, but he says the United States has greatly bolstered the abstinence message. "Behavioral change is the answer to ending their epidemic," he says.

PEPFAR's funding approach is also praised by some African health leaders. "ABC . . . is evidence-based and is not driven by PEPFAR but by African countries, which is critical for sustainability," said Richard Kamwi, Namibia's minister of Health and Social Services. "Condom programmes receive support from numerous partners, making PEPFAR support for a balanced ABC portfolio all the more necessary." [76]

OGAC's Dybul agrees. Early in the epidemic there was too much focus on concentrated epidemics involving sex workers and other temporary sexual relationships, he says. In those cases, encouraging fidelity and condom use made the most sense. But in some places, especially Africa, the epidemic was generalized to the larger population from the beginning. "We still need A, B and C as part of a response to a generalized epidemic," he says.

Even so, he says, the original PEPFAR legislation may be too restrictive. He says reauthorizing legislation introduced by Sen. Richard G. Lugar, R-Ind., "strikes the right balance."

Under Lugar's bill, at least 50 percent of PEPFAR funds used for the prevention of sexual transmission of AIDS "shall be dedicated to abstinence and fidelity as components of a comprehensive approach including abstinence, fidelity and the correct and consistent use of condoms, consistent with other provisions of the law and the epidemiology of HIV infection in a given country." New prevention modalities would not be included in determining compliance, it stipulates.

Nicole Bates, the director of government relations at the Global Health Council, says that while the Lugar language is "generally better" than current law, it still includes restrictions that could impede local flexibility.

Paul Zeitz, executive director of the Global AIDS Alliance, says the reauthorization should include more than the president's proposed $30 billion. He notes that Congress is likely to appropriate $6.4 billion in fiscal 2008. To continue that funding through the next five-year cycle would total $32 billion. Additional funds are needed to expand gender-equality, sexual and reproductive health programs and efforts to improve health systems and workforces. PEPFAR funding also should be flexible enough to support food and clean-water programs, he said. His group and many others in the global health community are pushing for a $50 billion authorization.

Zeitz also urges more balanced U.S. funding for the Global Fund and PEPFAR. As originally envisioned by some, he says, U.S. support for HIV/AIDS programs would be more evenly split between the bilateral PEPFAR program and mechanisms like the Global Fund that are more multilateral in approach. Instead, he says, the U.S. is "hyper-unilateral," with the bulk of HIV/AIDS global funding allotted to PEPFAR. The Kaiser Family Foundation calculates 16 percent of U.S. global AIDS funding went to the Global Fund and the remainder to PEPFAR in fiscal 2007. While allotting the funding to PEPFAR ensures U.S. control and credit, the Global Fund is considered to work in a more coordinated fashion with recipient countries.

In the United States, meanwhile, the Ryan White Program — named for an HIV-infected Indiana teenager who died in 1990 — provides funding to cities and states, health-care providers and other organizations to fund care for uninsured patients. [77]

The program was reauthorized for a third five-year period in December 2006, but some recipients and advocates say the new version expands the regions eligible for money while allowing less assistance for support programs like meals and legal aid.

"We have a growing population of needy patients and a growing cost of care and the funding is not keeping pace," said Jennifer Kates, vice president and director of HIV policy at the Kaiser Family Foundation. "If we have someone in South Carolina not getting medicine and someone in San Francisco not getting housing, how do we choose?" [78] Congressional supporters of the change and administration officials say they need to ensure funding is available for medical care first and ancillary support second.

There are also concerns that HIV/AIDS patients may be getting short shrift under some programs in the Medicare drug benefit. *The New York Times* reported on Oct. 7 that some of the private insurance companies contracting with Medicare have improperly terminated coverage for HIV/AIDS patients. [79] Medicare officials said the abuses are being corrected. ■

OUTLOOK

Prevention Is Key

The AIDS epidemic will require huge investments in treatment, prevention, care and vaccine and microbicide development for the foreseeable future. Millions more infected individuals will receive ARVs, a regime that will continue for the rest of their lives. UNAIDS estimates that despite the vast increases in AIDS-related resources, there is still an $8.1 billion funding gap between what is available and what is needed for 2007, a disparity expected to grow. In addition, improved drugs will be necessary to ward against resistance. [80]

"We still need to have a robust pipeline of new drugs because whenever you have to give drugs essentially for the life of the patient, there will always be important issues of the evolution of resistance" and drug intolerance, NIAID's Fauci notes.

Leaders in affected countries need to take stronger roles in promoting prevention, he says, because they bear ultimate responsibility for solving the AIDS dilemma. He cites good leadership in Uganda and other places but also says there has been an "appalling lack of leadership" as well as "contradictory" and "counterproductive activity on the part of South Africa."

South Africa, which has one of the highest HIV/AIDS infection rates in the world, has been criticized for its anemic response to the disease. Its health minister has consistently questioned the safety of ARVs. [81] She told an international group last year that beetroot and garlic will treat the virus. [82] A Roman Catholic archbishop in Mozambique recently declared his belief that Western-donated condoms are infected with HIV. [83]

But Fauci attributes many leadership lapses to "other confounding problems" facing low- and middle-income countries: "You don't blame them for not focusing only on preventing HIV infection when a million of their children and their babies die each year of malaria, and they have 1.6 million deaths from tuberculosis and hundreds of thousands of deaths from diarrheal disease and respiratory disease."

As the AIDS epidemic continues unabated and costs mount, U.S. AIDS Coordinator Dybul worries about dwindling interest in the disease. "AIDS fatigue worries me a lot," he says.

He also calls for increased focus on subtle variations in the disease in geographic regions. The key, he says, is to assess "in a country, where your last 1,000 infections come from and target [interventions] to that — not where were your last 1,000 new infections five years ago. Where are they today, and how do we in a very nimble way react? If we're not careful around that, it's going to be years before we can catch up on our mistakes."

Prevention, he adds, will dictate how the disease progresses. "Prevention is ultimately the key to where we'll be in 10 years, and [deciding] what combination of prevention modalities we need going forward to get us to a point where we can bring infections down as much as possible."

The expertise is available, he says, but he wonders about the will. "I know we can do all that — the question is will we?" he asks.

Vaccine supporters remain determined despite the cancellation recently of one of the most promising clinical trials. [84] The formulation, developed by Merck, was shown to be ineffective. Nonetheless, IAVI's Koff predicts "incremental progress" on the cell-mediated formula. Progress on a true 100 percent effective prevention vaccine is trickier. "The unknown is when will you crack the neutralizing antibody problem," he says.

It is an area where "we need an invention" to produce an effective product. He adds that recent investments in several consortia devoted to developing a neutralizing antibody vaccine will "really optimize the potential for innovation and invention."

Despite the challenges and frustrations, he says, a vaccine is essential. "Simply saying that we're going to end this epidemic, or make a major impact on it, with the antiretrovirals or education alone is you know a little bit of Kumbaya and Pollyanna," he says. Other prevention strategies are all part of the package, but "to really make a significant impact on blunting the epidemic, you're going to need the vaccine." ■

Notes

[1] Craig Timberg, "HIV Loosens Tribe's Resistance to Circumcision: Many Kenyans See Survival at Stake," *The Washington Post*, Sept. 7, 2007.

[2] Craig Timberg, "Anti-AIDS Program to Fund Circumcision: U.S. Initiative Targets African Men," *The Washington Post*, Aug. 20, 2007.

[3] Timberg, Sept. 7, 2007, *op. cit.*

[4] *Ibid.*

[5] "2006 AIDS Epidemic Update," Joint United Nations Programme on HIV/AIDS (UNAIDS), September 2007, www.unaids.org/en/HIV_data/2006GlobalReport/default.asp.

[6] "Toward Universal Access," WHO, UNAIDS, UNICEF, April 2007.

[7] Laurie Garrett, "The Challenge of Global Health," *Foreign Affairs*, January/February 2007.

[8] Pape Gaye, President, IntraHealth International, "Where Have all the Health Workers Gone," Global Health Council, September 2007.

[9] "Tragedy and Hope: Africa's Struggle Against HIV/AIDS," United Nations Africa Renewal Online, June 2004, www.un.org/ecosocdev/geninfo/afrec/subjindx/aids_africa.pdf.

[10] "Life Expectancy — Male 2005," Kaiser Family Foundation, www.globalhealthfacts.org/topic.jsp?i=79.

[11] UNAIDS, *op. cit.*

[12] Kaiser Family Foundation "The Global HIV/AIDS Epidemic," June 2007, www.kff.org/hivaids/3030.cfm.

[13] UNAIDS, *op. cit.*

[14] *Ibid.*

[15] *Ibid.*

[16] Nick Cumming-Bruce, "Thailand Faces New AIDS Threat," *International Herald Tribune*, Nov. 27, 2005.

[17] Kaiser Family Foundation, "The HIV/AIDS Epidemic in the United States," July 2007, www.kff.org/hivaids/3029.cfm.

[18] *Ibid.*

[19] *Ibid.*

[20] "HIV/AIDS Among Women," Revised June 2007, Centers for Disease Control and Prevention, www.cdc.gov/hiv/topics/women/resources/factsheets/women.htm.

[21] *Ibid.*

[22] Peter Piot, presentation at Woodrow Wilson Center, Sept. 24, 2007.

[23] "Spending on the HIV/AIDS Epidemic: Global Spending on HIV/AIDS in Resource-Poor Settings," Kaiser Family Foundation, July 2002, www.kff.org/hivaids/20020706a-index.cfm.

[24] Piot, *op. cit.*

[25] Garrett, *op. cit.*

[26] Paul Farmer, "From 'Marvelous Momentum' to Health Care for All: Success is Possible with the Right Programs," *Foreign Affairs*, March/April 2007.

[27] John Novak, "System-Wide Effects of Global Health Initiatives: Evidence from Ethiopia, Malawi and Benin," www.iom.edu/Object.File/Master/42/755/PEPFAR%20WSP%20Novak%205-1-07.pdf.

[28] Michael McCarthy, "Report Calls for Changes in US Global AIDS Effort," *The Lancet*, April 17, 2007.

[29] "A Development Approach to AIDS," *InterAction*, May 2006.

[30] "Financial Resources Required to Achieve Universal Access to HIV Prevention, Treat, Care and Support," UNAIDS, Sept. 28, 2007, http://data.unaids.org/pub/Report/2007/20070925_advocacy_grne2_en.pdf.

[31] John Stover, *et al.*, "The Global Impact of Scaling up HIV/AIDS Prevention Programs in Low and Middle-Income Countries" *Sciencexpress*, Feb. 2, 2006.

[32] The United States Leadership Against HIV/AIDS, Tuberculosis and Malaria Act of 2003, Public Law 108-05, 108th Congress.

[33] "Bringing HIV Prevention to Scale: An Urgent Global Priority," Global HIV Prevention Working Group, June 2007, w.globalhivprevention.org. Also see David Masci, "Aiding Africa," *CQ Researcher*, Aug. 29, 2003, pp. 697-720.

[34] Craig Timberg, "Speeding HIV's Deadly Spread: Multiple Concurrent Partners Drive Disease in Southern Africa," *The Washington Post*, March 2, 2007, p. A1, www.washingtonpost.com/wp-dyn/content/article/2007/03/01/AR2007030101607.html.

[35] Piot, *op. cit.*

[36] "Keeping the promise: an agenda for action on women and AIDS," UNAIDS Global Coalition on Women and AIDS, 2006, http://womenandaids.unaids.

[37] *Ibid.*

[38] "Phase III Trials of Cellulose Sulphate Microbicide for HIV Prevention Closed," *Eurekalert*, Jan. 31, 2007.

[39] B. Shane, "The Female Condom: Significant Potential For STI and Pregnancy Prevention," Outlook, PATH, May 2006, www.path.org/publications/pub.php?id=1266.

[40] Roxanne Nelson, "Female-Initiated Prevention Strategies Key to Tackling HIV," The Lancet Infectious Diseases, October, 2007.

[41] Quoted in Nelson, *op. cit.*

[42] "Global Summary of the AIDS Epidemic," UNAIDS, December 2006.

[43] Mary Katherine Keown, "Female Genital Mutilation Linked to AIDS," thestar.com, Sept. 1, 2007, www.thestar.com/living/Health/article/250720.

[44] Kristin Dunkle, *et al.*, "Gender-based Violence, Relationship Power, and Risk of HIV Infection in Women Attending Antenatal Clinics in South Africa," *The Lancet*, May 2004.

[45] "Gender," PEPFAR, updated July 2007, www.pepfar.gov/pepfar/press/76365.htm.

[46] For background, see David Masci, "Global AIDS Crisis," *CQ Researcher*, Oct. 13, 2000, pp. 809-832, and Adriel Bettelheim, "AIDS Update," *CQ Researcher*, Dec. 4, 1998, pp. 1049-1072.

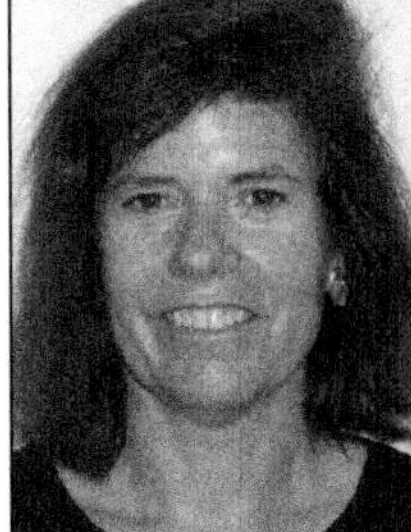

About the Author

Nellie Bristol is a veteran Capitol Hill reporter who has covered health policy in Washington for more than 20 years. She now writes for *The Lancet*, *The British Medical Journal* and the *Journal of Disaster Medicine and Public Health Preparedness*. She graduated in American studies from The George Washington University, where she is now working toward a master's degree in public health.

[47] "HIV/AIDS Among Men Who Have Sex With Men," revised June, 2007, Centers for Disease Control and Prevention, www.cdc.gov/hiv/topics/msm/resources/factsheets/msm.htm.
[48] Greg Berhman, *The Invisible People* (2004), p. 6.
[49] "New Hope, Old Challenges in AIDS Fight," CNN.com, Nov. 24, 2004, www.cnn.com/2004/HEALTH/11/23/overview.
[50] Barton Gellman, "The World Shunned Signs of the Coming Plague," *The Washington Post*, July 5, 2000.
[51] "HIV/AIDS Basic Information," Centers for Disease Control and Prevention, www.cdc.gov/hiv/topics/basic.
[52] Garrett, *op. cit.*
[53] Piot, *op. cit.*
[54] "Financing the Response to AIDS in Low- and Middle-Income Countries 2006," Kaiser Family Foundation, June 5, 2007, www.kff.org/hivaids/7347.cfm.
[55] "Spending Requirement Presents Challenge for Allocating Prevention Funding Under the President's Emergency Plan for AIDS Relief," Government Accountability Office, April 2006, www.gao.gov/new.items/d06395.pdf.
[56] "PEPFAR Implementation: Progress and Promise," Institute of Medicine, March 30, 2007, www.iom.edu/CMS/3783/24770/41804.aspx.
[57] "Global AIDS Epidemic: Selection of antiretroviral medications provided under the U.S. Emergency Plan is limited," Government Accountability Office, January 2005.
[58] Bob Roehr, "IOM Gives PEPFAR Passing Grade," *Medscape Medical News*, April 2, 2007.
[59] "History of the Fund in Detail," *The Global Fund*, www.theglobalfund.org.
[60] Michael McCarthy, "The Global Fund: 5 years on," *The Lancet*, July 2007.
[61] "Pledges," updated Sept. 24, 2007, Global Fund to Fight AIDS, Tuberculosis and Malaria, www.theglobalfund.org/en/funds_raised/commitments.
[62] Oomman Nandini, "Overview of the World Bank's Response to the HIV/AIDS Epidemic in Africa, with a Focus on the Multi-Country HIV/AIDS Program (MAP), Center for Global Development, www.cgdev.org/section/initiatives/_active/hivmonitor/funding/map.
[63] The World Bank, "Multi Country HIV/AIDS Program (MAP)," http://web.worldbank.org/wbsite/external/topics/exthealthnutritionandpopulation/exthivaids/0,,menupk:376477~pagepk:149018~pipk:149093~thesitepk:376471,00.html.
[64] "Targeting AIDS," "NewsHour with Jim Lehrer," June 27, 2001.
[65] Richard Horton, "AIDS: The Elusive Vaccine," *The New York Review of Books*, Sept. 23, 2004, www.nybookds.com/articles/17400.
[66] For background, see "AIDS Vaccine Blueprint 2006," International AIDS Vaccine Initiative, www.iavi.org/viewfile.cfm?fid=41059.
[67] John Stover, *et al.*, "The impact of an AIDS vaccine in developing countries: A new model and initial results," *Health Affairs*, July/August 2007.
[68] Margaret Johnston, "Current concepts: an HIV vaccine — evolving concepts," *The New England Journal of Medicine*, May 17, 2007.
[69] Stover, *et al.*, *op. cit.*
[70] Howard Markel, "The search for effective HIV vaccines," *The New England Journal of Medicine*, Aug. 25, 2005.
[71] "Adding it all Up: Funding for HIV Vaccine and Microbicide Research and Development Between 2000 and 2005," International AIDS Vaccine Initiative, www.hivresourcetracking.org.
[72] *Ibid.*
[73] Rep. Tom Lantos, opening statement, House Foreign Affairs Committee hearing, Oct. 1, 2007.
[74] Stephen J. Morrison, *et al.*, "Advancing U.S. Leadership on Global HIV/AIDS: Opportunities in the PEPFAR Reauthorization Process," Center for Strategic and International Studies, May 4, 2007, www.csis.org/component/option,com_csis_pubs/task,view/id,3873.
[75] "PEPFAR: Roadmap to Reauthorization," UNAIDS, Sept. 18, 2007.
[76] Richard Kamwi, *et al.*, "PEPFAR and HIV in Africa," *The Lancet*, June 17, 2006.
[77] Kaiser Family Foundation "The Ryan White Program" March 2007, www.kff.org/hivaids/7582.cfm.
[78] Erik Eckhold, "HIV Patients Anxious as Support Programs Cut," *The New York Times*, Aug. 1, 2007.
[79] Robert Pear, "Medicare Audits Show Problems in Private Plans," *The New York Times*, Oct. 7, 2007.
[80] UNAIDS, Sept. 28, 2007, *op. cit.*
[81] Michael Wines, "South Africa Official Is Accused, but Not Investigated," *The New York Times*, Aug. 21, 2007.
[82] Adam Graham-Silverman, "Stigmas Dog AIDS Relief Effort," *CQ Weekly*, Oct. 8, 2007.
[83] *Ibid.*
[84] Lawrence Altman and Andrew Pollack, "Failure of Vaccine Test Is Setback in AIDS Fight," *The New York Times*, Sept. 22, 2007.

FOR MORE INFORMATION

Global AIDS Alliance, 1413 K St., N.W., 4th Floor, Washington, DC 20005; (202) 789-0432; www.globalaidsalliance.org. Works with civil-society groups, relief agencies and faith-based organizations to fight AIDS in developing nations.

Global Health Council, 1111 19th St., N.W., Suite 1120, Washington, DC 20036; (202) 833-5900; www.globalhealth.org. An alliance of NGOs, foundations, corporations, government agencies and academic institutions that reports on world health problems.

Global HIV Prevention Working Group, www.globalhivprevention.org. International panel of experts and advocates seeking HIV prevention.

Joint United Nations Programme on HIV/AIDS, 20, Avenue Appia, CH-1211 Geneva 27, Switzerland; +41-22-791-3666; www.unaids.org. Coordinates the global response to AIDS by U.N. organizations.

Kaiser Family Foundation, 2400 Sand Hill Road, Menlo Park, CA 94025; (650) 854-9400; www.kff.org. Studies major U.S. and global health-care issues.

National Institute of Allergy and Infectious Diseases, 6610 Rockledge Dr., MSC 6612, Bethesda, MD 20892-6612; (301) 496-5717; www.niaid.nih.gov. Conducts and supports research on immunologic, infectious and allergic diseases.

Office of the U.S. Global AIDS Coordinator, 2100 Pennsylvania Ave., N.W., Suite 200, Washington, DC 20522; (202) 663-2440; www.pepfar.gov. Coordinates and oversees the U.S. response to global HIV/AIDS.

PATH, 1455 N.W. Leary Way, Seattle, WA 98107; (206) 285-3500; www.path.org. Works to create sustainable and culturally relevant ways communities worldwide can break cycles of poor health.

Bibliography

Selected Sources

Books

Garrett, Laurie, *The Coming Plague: Newly Emerging Diseases in a World Out of Balance*, Farrar, Straus and Giroux, 1994.
A former science writer for *Newsday* and now a senior fellow for global health at the Council on Foreign Relations recounts global researchers' efforts to understand HIV/AIDS.

Behrman, Greg, *The Invisible People: How the US Has Slept Through the Global AIDS Pandemic, the Greatest Humanitarian Catastrophe of Our Time*, Free Press, 2004.
A fellow at the Carr Center for Human Rights Policy at Harvard's Kennedy School of Government details the U.S. political reaction to the AIDS crisis from 1983 to 2003.

Articles

Brubaker, Bill, "The Limits of $100 Million," *The Washington Post*, Dec. 29, 2000, p A1.
Brubaker's report about drug company reactions to the AIDS epidemic is the last article in a series.

Gellman, Barton, "A Turning Point that Left Millions Behind," *The Washington Post*, Dec. 28, 2007, p A1.
Gellman looks at drug discounts for developing world access to antiretrovirals.

Gellman, Barton, "An Unequal Calculus of Life and Death," *The Washington Post*, Dec. 27, 2000, p A1.
Gellman details efforts to provide access to antiretrovirals.

Gellman, Barton, "The Belated Global Response to AIDS in Africa," *The Washington Post*, July 5, 2000, p A1.
Gellman discusses the developing world's slow reaction to the growing global HIV/AIDS crisis.

Jeter, Jon, "South Africa's Advances Jeopardized by AIDS," *The Washington Post*, July 2, 2000, p A1.
Jeter discusses South Africa's response to the pandemic as part of a series on HIV/AIDS.

Vick, Karl, "Disease Spread Faster Than the Word," *The Washington Post*, July 7, 2000, p A1.
Vick describes the Kenyan community's response to the disease.

Reports and Studies

"AIDS Vaccine Blueprint 2006: Actions to strengthen Global Research and Development," International AIDS Vaccine Initiative, 2006.
A leading AIDS vaccine group outlines the needs and promises for vaccine development.

"Bringing HIV Prevention to Scale: An Urgent Global Priority," Global HIV Prevention Working Group, June 2007.
Leading public health experts, clinicians, biomedical and behavioral researchers, advocates and people affected by HIV/AIDS discuss successful prevention efforts and how to expand them.

"Financial Resources Required to Achieve Universal Access to HIV Prevention, Treatment, Care and Support," UNAIDS, Sept. 26, 2007.
The U.N. AIDS group discusses resource needs to scale up access to AIDS services.

"Global Summary of the AIDS epidemic," UNAIDS, December 2006.
Details the latest trends in the AIDS epidemic.

"HIV and AIDS-United States, 1981-2000," Centers for Disease Control and Prevention, June 2001.
The CDC provides a brief history and epidemiological updates.

"The Impact of AIDS," U.N. Department of Economic and Social Affairs, Population Division, Sept. 16, 2004.
The report summarizes the effects of HIV/AIDS on families, communities and economies.

"The Multisectoral Impact of the HIV/AIDS Epidemic — A Primer," Kaiser Family Foundation, July 23, 2007.
A compilation of data reveals the impact of HIV/AIDS on population structure, demographics, households, business and public sectors and macroeconomics.

"Outlook: The Female Condom: Significant Potential for STI and Pregnancy Prevention," USAID, UNFPA, PATH, May 2006.
A report by three international groups discusses the efficacy and adoption issues surrounding female condoms.

"PEPFAR Implementation: Progress and Promise," Institute of Medicine, March 2007.
A well-regarded independent panel reviews the U.S. global AIDS program and makes recommendations for improvement.

"PEPFAR Reauthorization Recommendations from Global AIDS Experts," Global Health Council, Sept. 26, 2007.
A leading health group outlines 11 recommendations for the next five years of the U.S. global AIDS program.

"Towards Universal Access: Scaling Up Priority; HIV/AIDS Interventions in the Health Sector," WHO, UNAIDS, UNICEF, April 2007.
A progress report summarizes the current status of HIV/AIDS programs and makes recommendations to improve them.

The Next Step:

Additional Articles from Current Periodicals

Prevention Initiatives

Carroll, James, "Outlawed AIDS Prevention," *Boston Globe*, May 1, 2006, p. A13.

The Roman Catholic Church has been hesitant to promote contraceptive methods in AIDS prevention amid concerns over compromising its moral principles.

Preciphs, Joi, and Marni Leff Kottle, "Report: Speed AIDS Prevention in Poor Nations," *The Philadelphia Inquirer*, Aug. 16, 2006, p. A4.

The Global HIV Prevention Group recommends the immediate training of health workers in poor nations in order to avoid delays between the completion of AIDS research and the distribution of new prevention tools.

Russell, Sabin, "Prevention Evolves Into Wider Array of Options," *The San Francisco Chronicle*, June 4, 2006, p. E3.

Biomedical options must accompany behavioral change if new HIV infections are to be reduced.

Zeller, Shawn, "Prevention Bows to Politics in AIDS War," *CQ Weekly*, Dec. 11, 2006, p. 3258.

The nonpartisan Center for Public Integrity reports that spending on prevention programs has declined in key target countries over the past two years.

Spending Debates

Gerstenzang, James, "Bush Seeks Boost in AIDS Spending," *Los Angeles Times*, May 31, 2007, p. A12.

President Bush is expected to ask Congress to increase U.S. support in the global fight against HIV/AIDS to $30 billion over the next five years, doubling the current commitment.

Stewart, Nikita, "HIV-AIDS Agency at Risk of Losing Funds for the Poor," *The Washington Post*, April 21, 2006, p. B3.

Although federal funds are available for spending on poor patients with HIV/AIDS, small nonprofits do not have enough time or staff to administer their programs.

Timberg, Craig, "U.N. Urges Quadrupling of Global AIDS Spending to Meet 2010 Treatment Goal," *The Washington Post*, Sept. 26, 2007, p. A20.

UNAIDS has called for the international community to spend $40 billion annually on AIDS by 2010 in order to reach the U.N. goal of providing universal treatment.

Werner, Erica, "Conflict Develops Between Urban, Rural States As Congress Rewrites HIV/AIDS Spending," The Associated Press, April 22, 2006.

AIDS patients in the Northeast and California get more funds per capita than those in the South, where activists are lobbying for a greater share.

Tuberculosis

"Stopping Tuberculosis Proves Hard to Do," *The Lancet*, March 24, 2007, p. 965.

There is a mounting danger that HIV infection will accelerate the spread of tuberculosis (TB) into a global epidemic.

Altman, Lawrence K., M.D., "Rise of a Deadly TB Reveals a Global System in Crisis," *The New York Times*, March 20, 2007, p. F1.

A drug-resistant form of tuberculosis has been described by the World Health Organization as a grave public health threat because of its potential to kill HIV-infected individuals.

Manning, Anita, "U.S. Stays Vigilant Against TB," *USA Today*, March 22, 2007, p. 4D.

U.S. health organizations are seeking new and better drugs and programs to treat HIV and TB simultaneously.

Women

"The Not-So-Fair Sex," *The Economist*, June 20, 2007, p. 91.

Recent research in Africa suggests that women may be more responsible for spreading AIDS than previously believed.

Gates, Melinda French, "What Women Really Need," *Newsweek*, May 15, 2006, p. 66.

The world has been slow to invest in HIV-prevention tools that could easily be initiated by women in the developing world.

Parenthoen, Isabel, "AIDS: Women and Children in Brunt of Pandemic," Agence France-Presse, Aug. 18, 2006.

The number of women worldwide infected with AIDS has now reached just about the same number as men.

CITING *CQ RESEARCHER*

Sample formats for citing these reports in a bibliography include the ones listed below. Preferred styles and formats vary, so please check with your instructor or professor.

MLA STYLE

Jost, Kenneth. "Rethinking the Death Penalty." CQ Researcher 16 Nov. 2001: 945-68.

APA STYLE

Jost, K. (2001, November 16). Rethinking the death penalty. *CQ Researcher, 11*, 945-968.

CHICAGO STYLE

Jost, Kenneth. "Rethinking the Death Penalty." *CQ Researcher*, November 16, 2001, 945-968.

CHAPTER

11

Fighting Superbugs

By Marcia Clemmitt

Excerpted from the CQ Researcher. Marcia Clemmitt. (August 24, 2007). "Fighting Superbugs." *CQ Researcher*, 673-696.

Fighting Superbugs

BY MARCIA CLEMMITT

THE ISSUES

In late January, 12-year-old Carlos Don — a sixth-grader in Ramona, Calif., who loved playing football and racing motorcycles — returned from several days at a school-sponsored trip with flulike symptoms. The local urgent-care center diagnosed pneumonia and assured his parents he'd be fine once antibiotics kicked in.

But within days Carlos was hospitalized and breathing with the aid of a ventilator. On Feb. 4, with his heart, lungs and other organs too damaged to function, he was taken off the ventilator. The cause of death was an often-fatal bacteria widely known as MRSA (methicillin-resistant staphylococcus aureus). [1]

Staph infections were once easily treatable with antibiotics. Over the past few decades, however, more staph bacteria and other pathogens — microbes that make us sick — have evolved into bacteria that are resistant to antibiotics like methicillin and cephalosporin — dubbed superbugs.

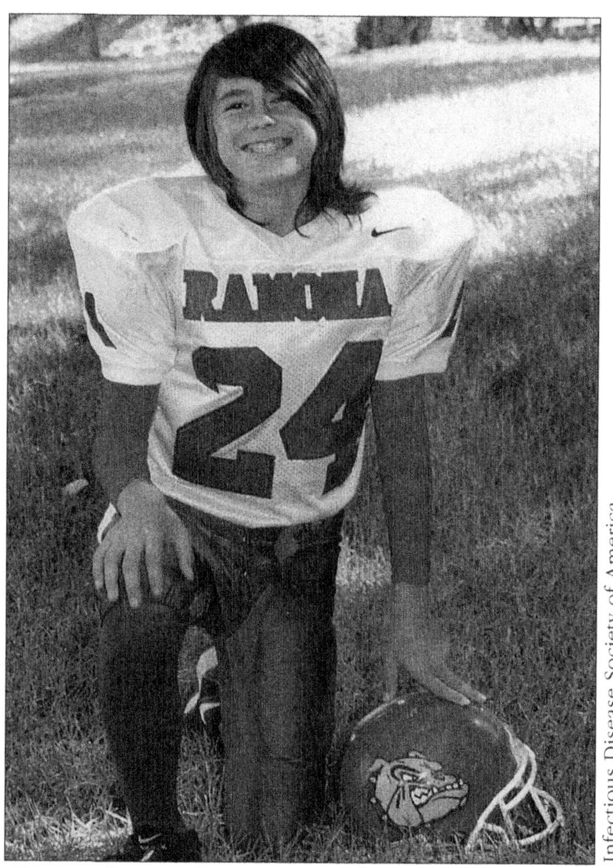

Infectious Disease Society of America

Doctors diagnosed pneumonia when 12-year-old Carlos Don, of Ramona, Calif., became ill in late January, but his flulike symptoms actually were caused by the antibiotic-resistant staph infection known as MRSA, and he died on Feb. 4. Once easily treated, staph infections have become drug resistant. A resistant pathogen that often afflicts wounded soldiers in Iraq has forced many infected limbs to be amputated.

Until recently, MRSA mainly infected hospital patients. Today, however, many resistant bacteria are acquired outside hospitals, like the staph infection Carlos contracted. Known as CA-MRSA (community-acquired MRSA), it seems to be even more dangerous than its hospital-acquired cousin, HA-MRSA.

An antibiotic is designed to kill specific bacteria, but they can mutate and become resistant to the drug. Over time, such antibiotic-resistant bacteria can survive and multiply, producing an entire population of bugs that are difficult or impossible to kill with existing antibiotics, especially frequently used antibiotics. * (To reduce the chance that bacteria will become resistant, doctors urge patients to take all the antibiotics they are prescribed, even after an infection has been cleared up, because not using all the prescribed pills tends to kill off just the weaker bugs, leaving behind the stronger, more resistant bacteria.)

Shortly after antibiotics came into use in the 1940s, scientists and doctors observed that some bugs developed resistance, but only now are they beginning to understand the true scope of the danger from superbugs. Each antibiotic is "like a tank of gasoline," good for only so many uses, says John H. Powers, former lead medical officer for Antimicrobial Drug Development and Resistance Initiatives at the Food and Drug Administration (FDA).

"When it runs out, it runs out," says Powers, now senior medical scientist at Maryland-based SAIC Frederick, Inc., a research contractor for the National Institute of Allergy and Infectious Diseases.

Community-acquired MRSA may be the most frightening of the newly resistant pathogens, as Dee Dee Wallace, a 47-year-old mother of two in Mahotah, Wis., discovered late last year when she developed several skin infections. Her doctors thought they were minor, but after a "little red bump" on Wallace's knee "turned into white blisters," then "deep bone pain," doctors cultured her infection and discovered drug-resistant "flesh-eating" staph, she says.

Even the surgery that removed a chunk of her abscessed flesh — "down to where my husband could see the muscle lying on the bone" — didn't end Wallace's troubles. The bug lingered, eventually becoming resistant to vancomycin, the main antibiotic used to treat MRSA today, and it was months before she fully recovered.

A pediatrician's similar lack of awareness of CA-MRSA last year nearly claimed the life of a toddler from Santee, Calif., a San Diego suburb. The one-and-a-half-year-old, who'd never even had a cold, grew bloated and lethargic, his nostrils flaring as he struggled for breath, recalls his father, Scott Smith.

* Antibiotics kill bacteria but not viruses, such as the common cold, flu and HIV/AIDS.

Few States Require Hospital Infection Reports

Only 17 states require hospitals to report infection rates or infection information. Twenty-seven states and Washington, D.C., have similar legislation pending. With the rise of "superbugs," patient-safety advocates say it's more important than ever for patients to pressure hospitals to control the spread of infections.

State Requirements for Reporting Hospital Infection Rates

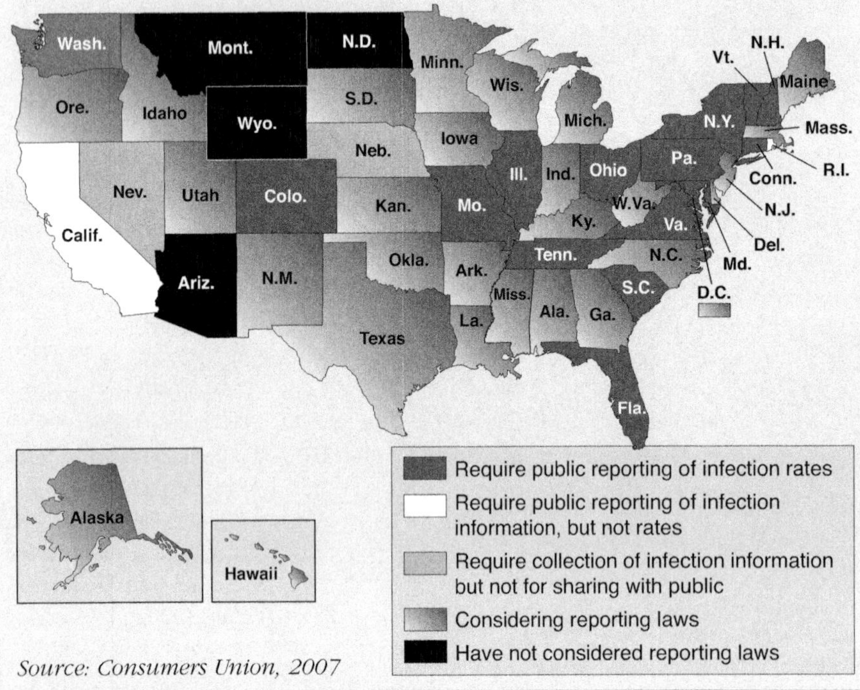

Source: Consumers Union, 2007

"We felt something was terribly wrong," but Bryce's pediatrician "said we were typical new parents" and repeatedly advised that they take the baby home and stop worrying, Smith says. Early on New Year's Day, with Bryce's condition worsening, his parents took him to the emergency room, where staff immediately suspected MRSA.

After a 55-day hospital stay — and surgery to remove part of his lung, through which the infection had eaten a hole — Bryce went home. He had to be given methadone to wean him from the narcotics he'd been sedated with during his long hospital stay, which included 49 days in intensive care.

The Smiths have switched doctors, and "our new pediatrician says she sees a case [of CA-MRSA] almost weekly," Smith says.

Hospital-acquired MRSA is also on the rise. According to a 2007 study by the Association for Professionals in Infection Control and Epidemiology, 34 out of every 1,000 hospital patients (3.4 percent) have active HA-MRSA infections; another 12 patients are "colonized" with the bug, which means they could contract or spread the disease. That amounts to up to 1.2 million patients infected annually and between 48,000 and 119,000 deaths — far more than epidemiologists previously thought. A study released in 2005 by the U.S. Centers for Disease Control and Prevention (CDC) found that only 3.9 of every 1,000 patients (0.39 percent) had active MRSA infections. [2] At a minimum, treating HA-MRSA costs the United States between $3 billion and $4 billion annually. [3]

In fact, all bacteria — not just MRSA — and other microbes like viruses and fungi are becoming resistant to antimicrobial drugs. But antibiotic-resistant bacteria are causing the most concern, because most have been successfully treated with antibiotics for decades, while treating other kinds of microbes has been less successful.

Among other dangerous bacteria showing resistance, *klebsiella pneumoniae* can cause several kinds of urinary-tract and wound infections in hospitalized people, says Michael Feldgarden, research director of the Boston-based Alliance for the Prudent Use of Antibiotics. And if *klebsiella* develops resistance, Feldgarden explains, "a whole bunch of other organisms" will begin developing resistance as well.

Another hospital-based resistant pathogen, *acinetobacter*, has afflicted many soldiers wounded in the Iraq War, often forcing infected limbs to be amputated. [4] "It's totally resistant to all antibiotics but doesn't have the virulence of MRSA," says Harold Standiford, medical director of infection control and antimicrobial effectiveness at the University of Maryland Medical Center in Baltimore.

And tuberculosis (TB) — which kills 2 million worldwide a year, more than any other infectious disease — is becoming increasingly resistant. In the five years from 2000 to 2005, multidrug-resistant TB (MDR-TB) increased from 275,000 cases to at least 460,000, mostly in Russia, China and India. [5]

Inadequately treated MDR-TB may evolve further into "extensively drug-resistant" TB (XDR-TB), which is impervious to almost all drugs. It was the initial diagnosis given to Atlanta lawyer Andrew Speaker, who made headlines around the world in May for sneaking back into the United States after learning of his diagnosis — potentially exposing his fellow airline passengers to TB. Speaker claimed he feared he would die if he stayed in Europe, where he had honeymooned against doctors' advice.

Only 30 to 50 percent of patients with XDR-TB recover from the deadly illness. [6] Speaker was later found to have MDR-TB, not the lethal XDR variety. [7]

Not long ago, it was widely assumed that when a drug lost its potency, another would soon be available to replace it. But today "there are so few new drugs in the pipeline that if we don't act to prolong the effectiveness of the drugs we've got, then we're in trouble," says Robert Guidos, director of policy and government relations at the Infectious Disease Society of America.

Although doctors know that overuse of antibiotics promotes resistance, controlling excessive antibiotic use has proven difficult. In many developing countries, for example, access to antibiotics is unregulated, says John McGowan, a professor of epidemiology at Emory University's Rollins School of Public Health in Atlanta. "You can walk into a pharmacy and get whatever you want" without a prescription.

Moreover, he says, countries like the United States promote resistance by creating "an artificial division" between individual care and the care given by public-health agencies. Private physicians often feel compelled to dose patients with the strongest, newest antibiotics, he explains, while public-health agencies want doctors to reserve such drugs for the toughest cases in order to prevent resistance from increasing.

Curbing the spread of infections through careful hygiene and isolation of the sick is crucial to slowing the spread of resistant microbes. But there is little consensus about what, if any, infection-control measures public-health agencies should impose.

"It's tough to make rules when everybody is not in agreement," says Standiford. For example, while he says it is important to screen at least some incoming hospital patients for MRSA — even if they show no signs of infection — he's unsure exactly who should be screened — surgical intensive-care patients, all intensive-care patients or some other group?

Antibiotics are also widely used on farms, not only to treat diseases that can spread to humans but also to increase animal growth rates, keep infection from breaking out in crowded barns and prevent crops from developing infections. [8]

Fighting Drug Resistance in Hospitals

Fewer than 60 percent of U.S. hospitals follow recommended guidelines for antimicrobial use, according to a recent survey of infection-control personnel. And only 27 percent hand out guidelines for treatment of infectious diseases.

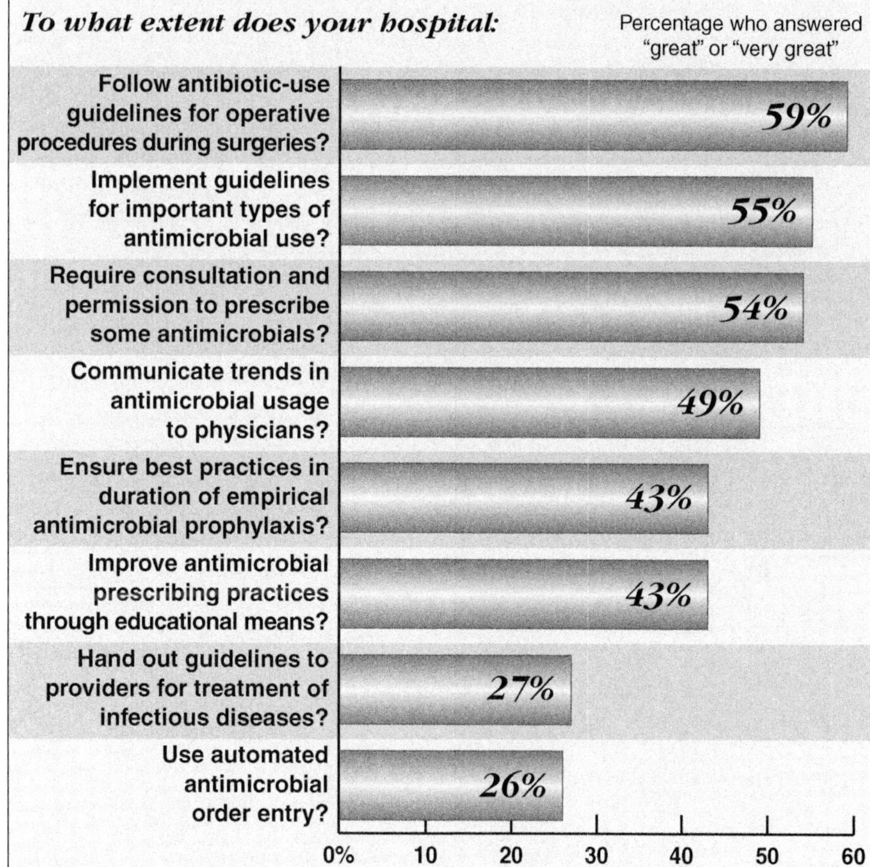

Source: Alan J. Zillich, et al., "Antimicrobial Use Control Measures to Prevent and Control Antimicrobial Resistance in US Hospitals," Infection Control and Hospital Epidemiology, *October 2006; 448 infection-control practitioners responded.*

How to Avoid Drug-Resistant Bugs

Hand washing is crucial

As antibiotics grow less effective, hygiene once again assumes a key role in protecting health.

Raised in an age before antibiotics, "Our grandparents told us, 'Wash your hands. Period. Wash before you eat. Wash after you go to the bathroom,'" says Stuart Levy, a professor of microbiology at Tufts University School of Medicine in Boston. Now, as the ability of antibiotics to treat infections wanes, those days are back, he says. "In developing countries, that means giving people clean water. For us, it means 'Wash.' "

Here are some other tips for staying healthy:

- Be especially careful about hygiene in moist, sweaty environments, like gyms. Athletic locker rooms, including in major-league professional sports, have become breeding grounds for dangerous bugs like methicillin-resistant staphylococcus aureus (MRSA). "You shouldn't be sharing clothes or towels or personal items like razors," says Jane D. Siegel, a pediatric infectious-disease specialist at the University of Texas' Southwestern Medical Center in Dallas.
- Avoid sharing personal objects like cell phones, too. Alla Lulu, a sophomore biology major at the University of Arizona (UA), picked up a nasty face rash after borrowing a friend's phone, said Charles Gerba, a professor of environmental microbiology at UA and Lulu's uncle. The phone carried staph bacteria. [1]
- Avoid products like special soaps and detergents that contain antibacterials like the chemical triclosan. "There's no benefit to it over plain, old soap, and it drives resistance, so we need to be careful," says Allison Aiello, assistant professor of epidemiology at the University of Michigan School of Public Health. These antibacterials, which are hard to avoid, leave residues that continue killing at a low rate, thus driving bacteria to become resistant. In a recent survey 76 percent of liquid soaps contained triclosan, and 30 percent of bar soaps contained triclocarban, according to the Alliance for the Prudent Use of Antibiotics. [2] For tough cleanups, traditional antiseptics like alcohol, peroxide and bleach are the better choice. They kill quickly and leave no residue, so they're unlikely to increase resistance. Antibacterials like triclosan do have legitimate uses in health-care situations.
- Don't demand that your doctor give you an antibiotic, but if one is prescribed, take it for as long as directed. Otherwise, partly resistant bacteria still in your body can multiply and grow more resistant. [3]
- Don't take anyone else's antibiotic. It may not be appropriate for your illness and will kill off beneficial bacteria in your body. [4] "You've got hundreds of millions of bacteria in your intestines, and they ain't bothering you," says John H. Powers, former lead medical officer for the Food and Drug Administration's Antimicrobial Drug Development and Resistance Initiatives. In fact, many carry out important jobs, such as synthesizing vitamins like Vitamin K, used in blood clotting, he says. "Bugs get a bad rap. They're only bad if they get in the wrong place."
- If you're hospitalized, have someone there with you, especially on weekends and at night, says Lisa McGiffert, director of the Stop Hospital Infections project at Consumers Union. Hospital staff members might wash their hands and then touch the bed or a tray before touching you, but that shouldn't happen, says McGiffert. "You want them to go straight from the hand gel to you," she says. Health-care workers "know that and they mean to do it right, so they won't mind being reminded."
- When you have surgery scheduled, don't be afraid to ask the surgeon about the hospital's infection rate, says William Schaffner, chair of preventive medicine at the Vanderbilt University School of Medicine. Hospitals should also be able to tell you their hand-hygiene compliance rate, and you should ask, he says. "It is important to have a conversation with your surgeon," says McGiffert. "Just ask, 'Can you tell me what you do to prevent infections?' You should get a number of answers," including these: give antibiotics within 60 minutes of surgery; use the right antibiotic for the surgery; clip rather than shave the body pre-operation; keep the body warm during surgery and stop antibiotics within 24 hours of the surgery.

"You have to be your own advocate," says Dee Dee Wallace, a 47-year-old Wisconsin mom who had a life-threatening brush with a resistant skin infection this year that doctors responded to slowly. "You have to say, 'I don't think this is right.' You know your own body. Stick up for yourself. Don't let them say, 'Go home, you'll be fine.' "

---

[1] Quoted in Yusra Tekbali, *Arizona Daily Wildcat*, University of Arizona, "University Wire," Aug. 1, 2007.

[2] "Antibacterial Agents," APUA, www.tufts.edu/med/apua/Q&A_antibacterials.html.

[3] "When and How to Take Antibiotics," Alliance for the Prudent Use of Antibiotics, www.tufts.edu/med/apua/Patients/How2Take.html.

[4] *Ibid.*

But the amount of antibiotics used in agriculture is heavily disputed, primarily because no government agency collects the data. While most experts agree farms use many more antibiotics than humans do, debate rages over how seriously farm antibiotics affect human health. And while foodborne bacteria can grow resistant, few foodborne diseases are as virulent as MRSA. Moreover, benign resistant bacteria can transfer their resistance to pathogens, but there is no clear evidence that agricultural antibiotics have accelerated drug resistance among human pathogens like MRSA.

Several bills pending in Congress address resistance, as does at least one major bill in the works but not yet introduced. The proposals include incentives for drug companies to discover new antibiotics, stricter limits on farm use of antibiotics, a strengthened federal role in studying resistant infections and programs to combat them. Democratic leaders of the House and Senate health committees hope at least some of the provisions will be enacted this year, but action on the measures stalled during the summer while Congress debated other issues, including expansion of children's health insurance.

As lawmakers and infectious-disease specialists confront the rising tide of drug resistance, here are some of the questions being asked:

Should government agencies do more to combat superbugs?

With antibiotic-resistant bacteria on the rise — hospital-acquired MRSA, for example, soared from about 3 percent of hospital staph infections in 1980 to nearly 60 percent in 2004 — most experts agree the government should spend more on disease-surveillance and anti-resistance efforts. Moreover, they say hospitals, doctors and the drug industry aren't doing enough to stem the tide of resistance. But debate rages over whether they should be required to do more.

Ideally, Congress should establish an antibiotic-resistance coordinator who reports directly to the secretary of Health and Human Services (HHS), says Guidos of the infectious disease society. A direct line to the Cabinet is vital, he says, because other departments — including Defense, Veterans Affairs and Agriculture — also have roles to play.

Most other industrialized countries keep stricter tabs on how antibiotics are used — both for humans and agriculture — says Feldgarden of the Alliance for the Prudent Use of Antibiotics. Without knowing exactly what's being used and how, it's difficult to trace the cause and effect for microbes developing resistance or to issue accurate guidelines and alerts to hospitals and doctors, he says.

Incidence of MRSA Rose Steadily

The percentage of staph infections resistant to methicillin and other antibiotics has increased from less than 4 percent to nearly 60 percent in 2004.

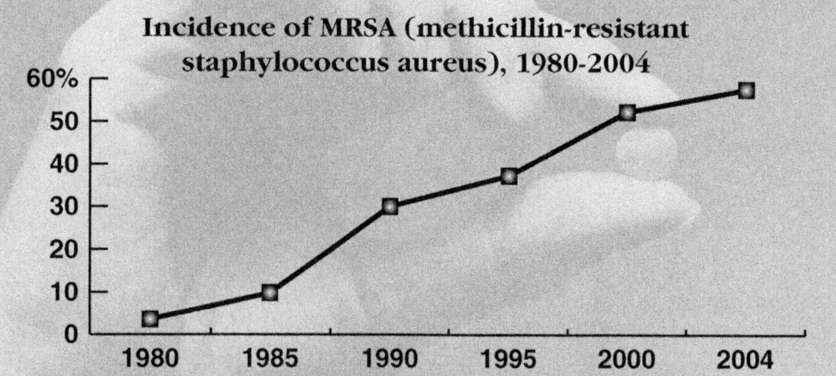

Source: "Bad Bugs, No Drugs As Antibiotic Discovery Stagnates . . . A Public Health Crisis Brews," Infectious Disease Society of America, 2007

The U.S. data-gathering effort — the National Antibiotic Resistance Monitoring System (NARMS) — is "run on a shoestring" by three agencies, Feldgarden says, and data in some of their reports "are three years behind," so scientists can't get a real handle on how resistance is developing today. In addition, the agencies don't have authority to collect some of the data that would be most useful, he says.

"There are a lot of stakeholders with conflicting interests," he says, such as antibiotics manufacturers, who are unwilling to see their sales data made public.

But Neil Fishman, an associate professor of medicine at the University of Pennsylvania School of Medicine, says the government could gather much more information without compromising business secrets. "I don't care what Dr. Smith prescribes," he says. "I just need his state's use."

States also should be required to report incidents of MRSA, says Brian Currie, senior medical director of the Montefiore Medical Center at the Albert Einstein College of Medicine in Bronx, N.Y. "There's mandatory reporting for other communicable diseases in every state," he says, and MRSA should be on the list.

The private sector has not shown that it's able or willing to control infections or head off antibiotic resistance on its own, says Feldgarden. "We've got slightly more staph, and MRSA is going through the roof," he says, yet there has been no "forceful government intervention," such as shutting down hospitals. "The idea has been, 'Let doctors practice medicine.' But at some point, you have to say, 'You guys don't get to call the shots any more.' "

Yet, he warns, regulations would need to avoid unfairly scapegoating some hospitals. "If you're a hospital with an elderly population, you'll have a lot of MRSA even if you're doing a good job," he says. "So you can't just set a percentage level and tell people, 'Above that, and you're in trouble.' "

The High Cost of Hospital Infections

The cost to treat a patient with a hospital-acquired infection in Pennsylvania in 2004 was $60,678— more than seven times the cost of treating an uninfected patient.

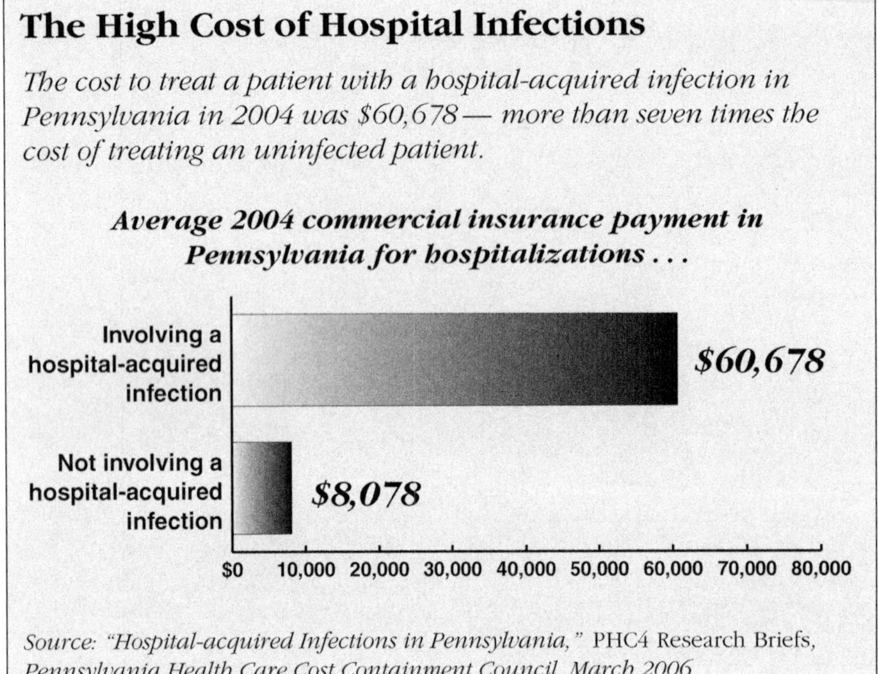

Source: "Hospital-acquired Infections in Pennsylvania," PHC4 Research Briefs, *Pennsylvania Health Care Cost Containment Council, March 2006*

The Netherlands, for instance, has instituted "search and destroy" tactics in MRSA cases, says Feldgarden. Patients infected with MRSA are isolated, MRSA-colonized health-care employees are furloughed with pay and their families and pets are also checked and treated. The country's MRSA rate has dropped to 1 percent of its hospital-based staph infections, "while ours is 50 percent," he says.

However, the CDC doesn't have the authority to do what the Netherlands did, Feldgarden says.

Traditionally, states are the primary regulators of health care in the United States, but that approach can fail, says Feldgarden. "In the many tri-state areas, infections jump state lines," he says.

Whether or not they envision a stronger government role in fighting resistance, many analysts concede that private institutions aren't making much headway. For example, medical education has not focused much on resistance prevention, says Elaine Larson, associate dean of research at the Columbia University School of Nursing in New York City and director of the Center for Interdisciplinary Research on Antimicrobial Resistance.

Still, she and others remain skeptical of government efforts to force change.

Given Americans' predominantly private health system and their love affair with high-tech solutions, it's been difficult to develop a national policy that dissuades doctors from prescribing the most expensive, newest antibiotic first, says Larson. "I don't think a change is going to happen voluntarily," she says. Nevertheless, she's "not a big proponent" of legislating solutions because "it can take forever to change laws while microbes mutate very fast."

Even Fishman says the data do not yet support mandatory universal screening for MRSA. Universal screening "is the right strategy in some settings," he says, such as in academic medical centers that see the sickest patients. "But it might not be the correct strategy for a community hospital with low MRSA rates."

In addition, neither the Society for Healthcare Epidemiology of America nor the Association for Professionals in Infection Control and Epidemiology supports mandatory screening of patients showing no symptoms of active infection with MRSA or other antimicrobial-resistant pathogens. They fear any legislation would be written too narrowly and would not be flexible enough to apply to a newly developing resistance.

"Legislation in general is not sufficiently flexible to permit rapid response to local epidemiological trends," the groups maintain. [9]

Should the government make it easier for drug companies to bring new antibiotics to market?

With few if any new antibiotics being developed, some infectious-disease experts say the government should ease drug companies' path to creating new products. But other drug analysts argue that safety and public-health priorities must not be compromised.

"There are no drugs coming through the pipeline," says Guidos at the infectious disease society. With diseases like MRSA spreading, the government should consider major monetary incentives for companies to develop new antimicrobials, he says. For example, companies could be given a "wild card" patent extension — additional time to exclusively market some other lucrative drug they've developed — in exchange for developing the less profitable antibiotic. Drug patents run for 20 years from the date a patent application is filed.

From drug companies' standpoint, curbing antibiotic overuse makes drug development economically risky in the anti-infective field, says William Schaffner, chairman of preventive medicine at the Vanderbilt University School of Medicine in Nashville, Tenn. "As soon as one is developed, we immediately tell doctors, 'Don't use it, you dopes,' " he says. "We don't do that with Fords. I know of no other new product for which people say out in chorus, 'Don't use it.' "

Antibiotic development is further complicated by its heavy dependence on small producers, says Michael Bonney, CEO of Cubist Pharmaceuticals in Lexington, Mass. And unlike big pharmaceutical companies, smaller firms depend on the capital markets for borrowing funds for research and development, says Bonney, whose small company specializes in antibiotics for hospital-based infections.

"Lenders aren't devoted to antibacterials" and will put their dollars elsewhere if they don't see the promise of good returns, he says. "They pay a lot of attention to what's happening in Washington." Few small companies will be able to obtain cash to develop antibiotics if the law doesn't assure lenders they'll eventually make money, he says.

The federal government could buy and stockpile a new drug until resistance appears, Bonney says. But stockpiling "would have to work in concert with extending [the developer's] market exclusivity" for more years, so the company — not a generic competitor — would make money once the drug was in demand.

To offset the low profitability of so-called orphan drugs — which target serious diseases affecting fewer than 200,000 people — Congress in 1983 created development incentives for drugmakers. The law could be tweaked to help spur antibiotic development, says Michael Kurilla, director of the office of biodefense research affairs and associate director of biodefense product development at the National Institute of Allergy and Infectious Diseases.

Today, drugs for illnesses that affect populations just above the orphan-drug cutoff get no breaks, says Kurilla. "If you're at 250,000 patients or 10 million, it's all the same." A "sliding scale" of incentives might support antibiotic development, he says.

Some pharmaceutical scientists argue the FDA is more concerned about safety today than in the 1950s and '60s — the golden age of antibiotic development — making the discovery of new drugs more challenging. The FDA should give more weight during the approval process to the potential benefits of new antibiotics instead of nixing those that show modest safety risks, says Jeffrey D. Alder, vice president of drug discovery and evaluation at Cubist.

"Some infectious diseases have a very high kill rate" — as high as 70 to 90 percent for staph aureus in the blood, for example — says Alder. "In those cases, almost everyone would say they'd want to be treated, even if it meant nausea" or some other side effect.

But some infectious-disease experts are wary of suggesting that companies don't have enough financial incentives, or that the FDA should make it easier to get antibiotics approved.

SAIC Fredericks' Powers, the former FDA infectious-disease officer, argues against offering financial carrots unless they're carefully targeted at companies developing antibiotics for virulent resistant infections like MRSA, not for self-resolving conditions like sinusitis. "The places where we need new antibiotics are very specific situations," he says.

He's skeptical of incentives because the FDA earlier had tried hard to make it easier for companies to develop antibiotics, but rather than stimulating development of drugs to treat more serious diseases, most companies focused on relatively minor problems like sinusitis, ear infections and bronchitis — most of which clear up on their own.

Some drug analysts also question the wisdom of further easing any FDA standards to help companies bring antibiotics to market.

For instance, in 2004 the agency approved the antibiotic Ketek — manufactured by the French firm Sanofi-Aventis — as a drug that might head off resistance in treating pneumonia, bronchitis and sinusitis. The company had tested the drug using FDA clinical-trial guidelines designed to speed approvals of new antibiotics.

The agency abandoned the guidelines as inadequate before Ketek received its final approval, but the drug was approved anyway because the agency felt it needed "to stand by prior agreements with industry," said David B. Ross, a clinical assistant professor at George Washington University School of Medicine and Health Sciences in Washington and a former FDA physician who helped in reviewing Ketek. [10]

In 2006, the drug was linked to severe liver damage and failure in a small number of patients, but the agency was reluctant to react too strongly for fear of discouraging antibiotic development. For example, after a Ketek user died of liver failure, the FDA's only formal response was a few paragraphs in "an internal safety review written months later," said Ross. The FDA didn't re-label the drug to warn about liver damage until 16 months after the first report and didn't withdraw approval until Feb. 12, 2007 — a day before congressional hearings on Ketek's safety were to be held, he said.

The Ketek case suggests the agency, at least in some cases, has paid too little attention to antibiotics' downsides, said Ross. [11]

Powers says that rather than paying too much attention to the adverse effects of antibiotics — such as allergic reactions — the FDA and the medical community focus too much on the "inferred benefits" of antibiotics, which Powers says are often unproven. One pediatrician told Powers that he "will treat a million kids for ear infections to prevent one case of meningitis," Powers says. "I said, 'And you'll kill 10 with allergic reactions.' "

Powers also rejects drug company claims that testing is too costly. An antibiotic trial, he points out, only requires about 200 subjects, while a trial for a cardiac drug requires 10,000. "People say the FDA should lower the [testing] standards. But they already have."

Should Congress limit the use of antibiotics in farming?

Debate is fierce over antibiotic use in farming.

Because food animals like cows and chickens largely are raised today crammed into tight quarters rather than in open fields or pastures, antibiotics are used both to treat and to prevent communicable diseases.[12] Animals also get low doses of antibiotics to promote faster growth, and many crops are sprayed with antibiotics to kill bacteria. Consequently, most food — from milk to potatoes to beef — is likely to contain at least traces of the drugs. Food produced organically is prohibited from containing antibiotics.[13]

Advocates of stricter limits on farm use of antibiotics argue that, to slow development of antibiotic resistance among human pathogens, antibiotic use should be cut back. Farm animals can become reservoirs of resistant bacteria, they point out, and non-pathogenic bacteria can pass their resistance to bacteria that do make people sick.

But veterinary-drug manufacturers and farmers say there are few proven links between antibiotics used in farming and life-threatening drug-resistant infections in humans and that clamping down would lead to more foodborne illness. Epidemiological studies don't show that antibiotic-resistant bacteria in farm animals increase resistance in dangerous human diseases, says Michael Doyle, director of the Center for Food Safety at the University of Georgia.

Even if the illnesses humans sometimes pick up from food were to become antibiotic resistant, they are far less serious than other resistant pathogens like MRSA, he adds. "How many people have had untreatable foodborne illnesses? You can count them on two hands," he says. "You may have seen more hospitalizations, but you don't have deaths. I'm just not seeing the data to tell me that this is a public-health hazard like MRSA."

However, scientists at the National Institutes of Health's Fogarty International Center, which studies global health issues, say farm use of antibiotics can contribute significantly to drug-resistant disease in humans, even if the illness isn't life-threatening.

In a 2005 paper, infectious-disease ecologist David L. Smith and his colleagues compared the incidence of VRE — vancomycin-resistant *enterococci* — in humans in Europe and in the United States. They found that in the late 1990s in Europe — where vancomycin was used in hospitals and the related antibiotic avoparcin was used on farms — VRE rates outside the hospitals ranged from 2 to 12 percent of all enteroccus infections. Meanwhile, in the United States — where vancomycin was heavily used in hospitals but no avoparcin was used on farms — community VRE rates were below 1 percent. And community rates of VRE declined after the European Union banned avoparcin, demonstrating that agricultural antibiotics did contribute to VRE showing up in humans, said Smith.[14]

Europe has restricted use of agricultural antibiotics for the past decade. "We are never willing to accept that you first have to create a lot of dead people before you intervene," said Henrik C. Wegner, director of both the World Health Organization's Collaborating Centre for Antimicrobial Research and Foodborne Pathogens and the Danish Institute for Food and Veterinary Research. "From our perspective, this is first and foremost a preventive action. It is not acceptable to sit and wait for the next MRSA."[15]

Moreover, he added, Denmark has had "fewer healthy people in the community who carry VRE in their guts since we stopped using growth promoters" on farms.

Many infectious-disease experts want the United States to follow Europe's lead in banning much antibiotic use on farms. "It's embarrassing that we're way behind Europe," says Columbia University's Larson.

Others complain the impact of agricultural antibiotics on resistance gets an undeserved pass in the United States. "Agribusiness is off the public radar screen," says Currie of Montefiore Medical Center. "We've had antibiotics developed where the resistance was high before the drug was [even] released," he says, because related drugs were already being used in agriculture.

At the very least, agricultural antibiotic users should release data on what drugs farms are using and how, says Guidos of the infectious disease society. "The animal-drug industry says [various] reported volume-of-use numbers are inflated," he says, "but we say, 'Prove it.' We want to see what is really going on."

Agriculture analysts say, however, that limiting antibiotics in farming would drive up the rate of foodborne illnesses, outweighing any so-far-undiscovered benefits for limiting their use. "When the European Union cut off some of the antibiotics used as growth promoters, more animals got sick," and the infected animals could pass the illnesses to consumers, says the University of Georgia's Doyle.

Indeed, some farm advocates and scientists say not enough attention is paid to the value of antibiotics on farms. "Antibiotics help farmers keep animals healthy with less strain on the environment," according to the Animal Health Institute, an association of animal-drug manufacturers. "More meat can be raised [on less land] with fewer animals because of the growth-promoting qualities of antibiotics."[16]

Ian Phillips, a professor of biological and chemical sciences at the University of London, says research suggests the added risk to human health caused by antibiotics being used as growth promoters "is small." But "the benefit to human health from their use, hitherto largely ignored, might

Continued on p. 684

Chronology

1940s-1950s

Penicillin becomes the first widely available antibiotic, used to treat soldiers in World War II whose infected wounds would otherwise be deadly. By the mid-1940s, the first penicillin-resistant staph bacteria are found.

1940
Oxford University pathologist Howard Florey isolates pure penicillin and demonstrates that it kills a wide range of pathogens, including strep and gonorrhea.

1943
Drug companies begin to mass-produce penicillin.

1958
American molecular geneticist Joshua Lederberg wins Nobel Prize in medicine for demonstrating bacteria's ability to exchange genetic material, which helps spread resistance.

1960s

Fast-developing resistance to antibiotics like tetracycline is spotted, but a large number of new antibiotics enter the market.

1960
Methicillin is introduced in Great Britain.

1961
The first methicillin-resistant staph aureus infection (MRSA) turns up in a British hospital.

1963
MRSA appears in Denmark.

1967
Penicillin-resistant strep pneumonia is found in New Guinea.

1970s-1980s

Antibiotics are routinely prescribed for cold-like illnesses, even when they aren't bacterial. U.S. soldiers return from the Vietnam War with penicillin-resistant gonorrhea. People increasingly have weakened immune systems and need stronger antibiotics as more cancer patients are successfully treated, organ transplants increase and HIV/AIDS appears.

1977
South African doctor Michael Jacobs finds a strep *pneumoniae* bacterium that resists every available drug.

1983
The first hospital-acquired intestinal infection becomes penicillin resistant. . . . Eighteen people in the Midwest are hospitalized with multi-drug-resistant salmonella food poisoning after eating beef from cows given antibiotics.

1986
Sweden bans use of antibiotics to make farm animals grow faster.

1990s

Big drug firms pull resources away from infectious-disease research. MRSA turns up outside hospitals.

1992
Antibiotic-resistant bacterial infections kill record 13,000 hospital patients.

1998
Denmark taxes antibiotics used as animal-growth promoters. . . . European Union bans use of antibiotic used in humans for animal growth.

1999
Federal Interagency Task Force on Antimicrobial Resistance is launched.

2000s

More microbes become resistant, but public-health efforts to combat resistance lag.

2000
Congress reauthorizes Public Health Services Act, enabling federal government to take stronger steps to combat resistance, but the measure is never funded.

2001
Terrorism-related anthrax scare leads some Americans to take the high-powered antibiotic Cipro "just in case" and stockpile it in their homes.

2003
Drug-resistant *acinetobacter* infects Iraq War wounded in military hospitals, leading to many amputations.

2005
France bans 12 sore-throat medications containing topical antibiotics.

2006
European Union bans using any antibiotic to promote animal growth. . . . Ketek, an antibiotic to treat bronchitis, pneumonia and sinusitis, is linked to severe liver damage.

2007
Cases of multiple-drug-resistant tuberculosis (TB) quadruple in South Africa's Western Cape Province. . . . World Health Organization launches plan to fight drug-resistant TB. . . . Scientists find avian-flu virus is naturally evolving resistance to anti-flu drugs. . . . Study finds 10 times as many MRSA cases in U.S. hospitals as previously thought. . . . Food and Drug Administration mulls approval of a new antibiotic for respiratory disease in cows, although infectious-disease experts argue the drug could create more resistant pathogens since similar antibiotics are used in human medicine.

Doctors Turning to Ancient Remedies for Infections

Honey and copper doorknobs are said to work wonders

With superbugs developing resistance to many antibiotic drugs, doctors are trying out some old anti-infective remedies in hopes of finding additional tools to fight infection. Meanwhile, the search for new antibiotics goes on, with some scientists hoping to exploit the millions of microbial species — many in remote environments like hot springs or the sea bottom — for new kinds of antibiotic action.

Most future anti-infective drugs are likely to bypass killing bacteria, antibiotic-style, in favor of blocking their sickness-inducing properties. Microbes would be less likely to develop resistance to such drugs.

Honey was known to have anti-infective properties as far back as the ancient Mesopotamian kingdom of Sumer, 5,000 years ago. Today some doctors are using it again.

Jennifer Eddy, an assistant professor of family medicine at the University of Wisconsin School of Medicine, dressed an elderly diabetic man's ulcerated foot in honey-soaked gauze after the sore was attacked by drug-resistant bacteria, and amputation seemed the only option. In two weeks, the blackened foot began to heal, and a year later, the man was walking again. "I've used honey in a dozen cases since then," said Eddy. "I've yet to have one that didn't improve." [1] Some research suggests that bacteria are unlikely to become resistant to honey.

Another ancient antibacterial remedy — copper — is getting a trial in a British hospital. Healers in ancient Egypt, Greece and Rome all recognized copper's infection-killing properties and used it to treat wounds. Despite its history of discouraging the growth of germs, however, little copper is found in modern hospitals, which gleam with stainless steel, even though germs can remain active on steel for days.

Now the Selly Oak Hospital in Birmingham, England, is testing whether replacing stainless steel fittings like door handles, bathtub faucets, toilet flush handles and grab bars with copper can help cut the spread of infections. The hospital was chosen for the trial in part because soldiers wounded in Iraq had become infected with MRSA while being treated in the facility. [2]

In the early 20th century, biologists discovered a way to treat infections using bacteriophages — viruses that invade certain species of bacterial cells and cause them to burst and die. The therapy was pioneered at Paris' Pasteur Institute and the Institute of Microbiology in Tbilisi, capital of the Soviet Republic of Georgia, home of George Eliava, one of the scientists who discovered bacteriophages. Eliava discovered the tiny killers when he returned after three days to look at a microscope slide of river water that had contained cholera bacteria and found the slide bacteria-free. [3]

In World War II, Soviet military medics used the viruses to treat infected wounds on the battlefield, and German Gen. Erwin Rommel's troops used phage therapy against infections in hot North Africa, where infection-causing bacteria thrive.

But as antibiotics came into wide use after the war, bacteriophage therapy was largely forgotten. Georgian scientists and doctors continued studying and even treating patients with phages, but lack of money gradually crippled their research. Today, however, phage research is making a comeback, as superbugs strip traditional antibiotics of their power.

For example, researchers at the Massachusetts Institute of Technology and Boston University are using DNA technology

Continued from p. 682

more than counterbalance this." For instance, Phillips said, banning farm antibiotics except to treat sick animals has put more unhealthy animals into the human food chain in Europe. [17]

In another assessment, Phillips and other epidemiologists found the risk of increased antibiotic resistance related to antibiotic use in chickens "is small" compared to the increase in human foodborne illnesses that would result if the chickens' antibiotics were cut.

"Immediately following the removal of the antibiotic, animal illness levels might be expected to increase," they said, potentially making more people who ate the chicken sick. [18] ■

BACKGROUND

Bacterial World

Almost as soon as antibiotics came into use, microbes began developing resistance to them. [19]

In the 1940s and '50s, when penicillin was first used, it could kill most bacteria. But as early as 1945, the drug's discoverer, British bacteriologist Alexander Fleming, warned in a *New York Times* interview that misusing penicillin could quickly lead to the evolution of mutant bacterial strains not susceptible to the medicine, an outcome he'd already verified.

In the 1960s, when the antibiotic tetracycline was routinely prescribed for teenagers' acne, resistant bacteria turned up in patients "within a few weeks," says Columbia University's Larson.

That resistance develops quickly among microbes isn't surprising. The world is chock full of bacteria — and other microscopic organisms like fungi — "all fighting for their environmental niche," says SAIC Fredericks' Powers, the former lead infectious-disease officer at FDA. In fact, virtually all antibiotics today were derived from organisms that evolved to have bacteria-killing or bacteria-growth-to alter bacteriophages to produce enzymes that can kill specific infectious bacteria like *e. coli.* [4] The Food and Drug Administration also recently approved a bacteriophage product for food-processing companies to use to eliminate the dangerous foodborne microbe *listeria.* [5]

Meanwhile, new antibiotics still lurk in nature, waiting to be discovered, says Jeffrey D. Alder, vice president of drug discovery and evaluation at Cubist Pharmaceuticals in Lexington, Mass.

Only one in 100,000,000,000,000,000,000,000,000 (1 in 10 to the 25th power) of the world's microbes has been screened for antibiotic action, says Alder. Most of the vast number remaining grow in airless environments, in a narrow temperature range, or in difficult-to-access places. Earth's more remote and unusual environments could be the source for new antibiotic discoveries, some scientists believe.

The University of Hawaii, for example, hopes to set up a drug-discovery center "to take advantage of their unique isolated environment" that's home to hordes of unstudied microbes in hot springs, ocean thermal vents and the like, says Alder. DNA techniques make it possible to discover antibiotic and other microbial properties more easily than in the past, he says.

But most future anti-infective drugs will be developed according to a new paradigm, says Michael Kurilla, director of the office of biodefense research affairs at the National Institute of Allergy and Infectious Diseases. Lost in medicine's long love affair with antibiotics is the fact that "you're really interested in curing a disease, not killing an organism," Kurilla says. Shifting the focus from killing bugs to blocking their sickness-causing toxins — as a tetanus shot or anthrax vaccine do — may be the best approach for future drug discovery.

"If we take care of the toxin," and your immune system is strong, "your body can clear" the bacteria on its own, says Kurilla.

Paratek Pharmaceuticals, a small Boston-based company started by Stuart B. Levy, a microbiology professor at Tufts University School of Medicine, takes such an approach. Paratek focuses on a protein that can inactivate the process by which bacteria cause illness. "The bacteria doesn't need it to live and grow, so because you aren't inhibiting the bacteria's survival, you're not selecting against it," and resistance is much less likely to develop, Levy says.

But so far, financial backers are hard to come by for novel approaches, Levy says. "Everybody loves the story. But when it comes to plunking the money down, they go to the guy next door who has an antibiotic."

[1] Quoted in Brandon Keim, "Honey Remedy Could Save Limbs," *Wired*, Nov. 11, 2006.

[2] Philippe Naughton, "Hospital Gets Copper Fittings in MRSA Trial," *The Times online*, March 13, 2007, www.timesonline.co.uk/tol/news/uk/article1509513.ece.

[3] For background, see Richard Martin, "How Ravenous Soviet Viruses Will Save the World," *Wired*, October 2003, www.wired.com/wired/archive/11.10/phages_pr.html.

[4] Brandon Klein, "Scientists Build Bacteria-Killing Organisms From Scratch," *Wired Science*, Wired Blog Network, July 10, 2007.

[5] "FDA Extends GRAS Approval LISTEX to All Food Products," *Food Ingredients First*, May 7, 2007, www.foodingredientsfirst.com.

inhibiting properties. "The bugs actually invented the antibiotics" in their evolutionary struggle for survival, Powers says.

Microbes abound in the environment, and they multiply quickly. "When we are born, 100 percent of our cells are mammalian," says Barry I. Eisenstein, senior vice president for medical affairs at Cubist Pharmaceuticals. "By the time we are 1 month old, only 10 percent [of our cells] are." That's because most of the cells in and on the body are bacterial — hundreds of trillions of them.

And, under optimal conditions, a single bacterium can produce a billion offspring in a single day. Furthermore, "out of a million bacteria, every one will have a mutation," any one of which might allow that cell and its offspring to survive exposure to an antibiotic, says N. Kent Peters, program officer for antibacterial resistance at the National Institute of Allergy and Infectious Diseases (NIAID).

Doctors' Orders

The good news is that, "everywhere you measure, there's been improvement in antibiotic use," says Schaffner, Vanderbilt's preventive medicine chairman. But while the message is getting through, and many doctors are becoming warier prescribers, "it's not enough," he says. "We are not going to get a stream of antibiotics that will rescue us." [20]

New antibiotics aren't forthcoming, in part, because the easy-to-find ones were discovered long ago. Today's huge pharmaceutical companies increasingly are focused on high-profit drugs that patients take for chronic conditions, while small firms have trouble funding drug development at all and thus tend to seek more specialized niches.

"Why should we be investing in anti-infectives when people take them for seven to 10 days, while they'll take chronic-disease drugs" — such as antidepressants or cholesterol drugs — "for the rest of their lives?" an executive at the large pharmaceutical company Eli Lilly once asked Cubist's Eisenstein, who directed infectious-disease research at Lilly in the early 1990s.

Ironically, systematic technical improvements in the drug-development process also act as a barrier to finding new antibiotics.

Chemists find new drugs by testing compounds from pharmaceutical companies' vast libraries of chemicals, explains Kurilla, the director of biodefense research affairs at NIAID. But as companies have refined their collections, "they've evolved a series of ideas about what makes a compound 'druggable' " — meaning that it is absorbable and capable of penetrating human cells or entering the brain, he says.

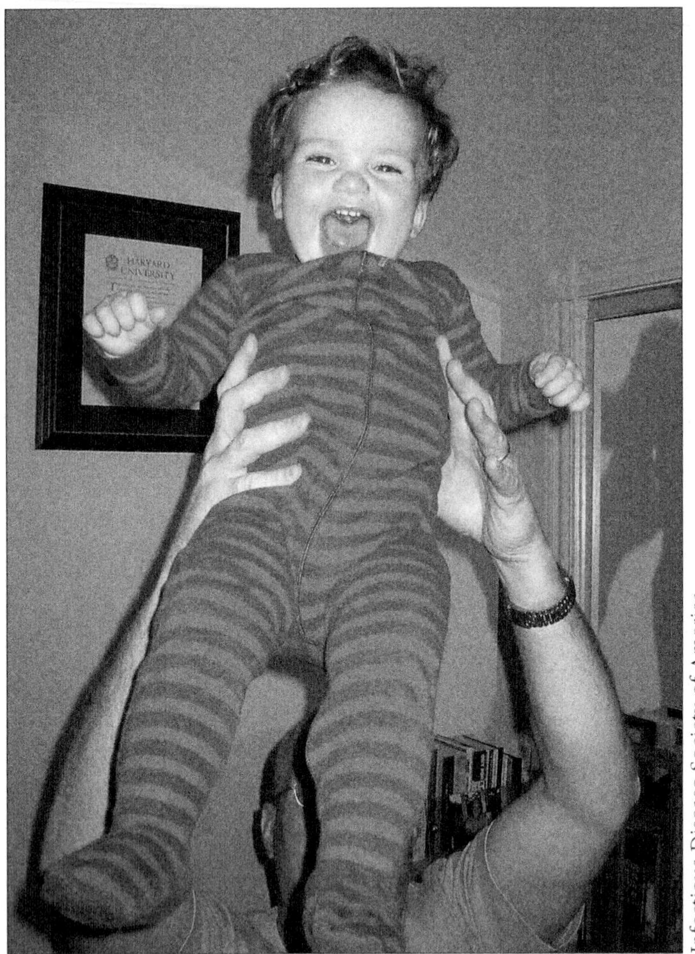

Infectious Disease Society of America

Simon Macario appeared to have a minor throat infection, but one morning he awoke screaming with pain. "By 10 that night he was dead" from MRSA, which was attacking his organs, says his mother. Until recently, MRSA mainly infected hospital patients. Today, however, many resistant bacteria are acquired outside hospitals and seem more dangerous than hospital-acquired infections.

"If you asked a chemist today if [the antibiotic chemicals] tetracycline or cephalosporin could be drugs, he'd say no," says Kurilla, because today's pharmaceutical chemists focus almost entirely on compounds that show potential for creating drugs that interact with human cells, such as the cholesterol-reducing drug Lipitor or the antihistamine Claritin. Chemicals with the potential to interact with bacteria — as antibiotics must — have been weeded out of the drug-discovery labs to make screening chemicals for drug potential more efficient, he says.

The U.S. medical system also has built-in barriers to reducing the use of antibiotics. For instance, patients know antibiotics are wonder drugs and ask for them — even when their infections are viral, and antibiotics won't work. "It takes longer for a physician to explain why an antibiotic isn't a good idea" than to simply prescribe one, even if it's not indicated, says Larson, the associate dean of research at Columbia.

As a result, about 28 percent of doctors say they would order an antibiotic if a patient had a chest cold — a viral illness — says Feldgarden of the Alliance for the Prudent Use of Antibiotics, and the percentage doubles in the case of bronchitis. Furthermore, prescribing habits inexplicably worsen as doctors-in-training advance through their medical education, he says.

Indeed, a study in the late 1990s showed that one of five U.S. prescriptions is for an antimicrobial drug, and 95 percent of them are unnecessary, Feldgarden says. Another study showed that doctors prescribe antibiotics for children's colds and earaches 65 percent of the time if they believe that parents expect them to, but only 12 percent if they don't. [21]

"Prescribing practices are difficult to change, so we need an array of interventions," says Vanderbilt's Schaffner.

Funds have been lacking for "social-marketing" campaigns to help change public attitudes. For instance, the Centers for Disease Control and Prevention (CDC) has developed a consumer-awareness program dubbed "Get Smart" but doesn't have enough money to launch it, says Ralph Gonzales, a professor of medicine, epidemiology and biostatistics at the University of California, San Francisco.

Gonzales tested a similar advertising campaign in Denver that raised public awareness by about 10 percent and cost about $150,000 to implement. The dent in attitudes is significant enough to lower antibiotic use, which would save money for insurance companies and Medicare and improve public health, says Gonzales. But only a few private insurers and cities have expressed interest.

Development of Antibacterials on the Decline

The number of antibiotic drugs approved in the United States has steadily declined in the past quarter-century, reflecting lack of interest by drug firms and the fact that many key drugs already have been developed.

Number of Approved Antibacterials in the U.S., 1983-2007

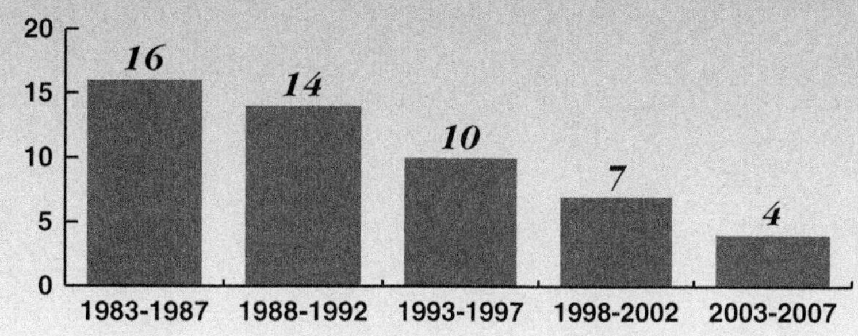

Source: "Bad Bugs, No Drugs As Antibiotic Discovery Stagnates . . . A Public Health Crisis Brews," Infectious Diseases Society of America, 2007

The University of Pennsylvania's Fishman says the lack of quick, cheap diagnostic tests to identify what's making a patient sick is also a problem. "It's 2007, and we can only determine the cause of pneumonia 50 percent of the time, if we're lucky," he says. Thus, doctors often have to guess at the cause of an infection and use broad-spectrum antibiotics that kill multiple kinds of bacteria rather than an antibiotic narrowly targeting one bacteria. But broad-spectrum antibiotics should be reserved for resistant cases, Fishman says.

Technical hurdles have bedeviled development of quick, accurate diagnostics, such as the difficulty — or sometimes the impossibility — of growing some bacteria and viruses in the lab. The National Institute of Allergy and Infectious Diseases (NIAID) is pushing for development of diagnostics as fast as it can, "but cost is still an issue" in implementing them, says NIAID program officer Peters.

"Even when diagnostic tests work, though, many physicians are reluctant to narrow the therapy" once they get a diagnosis if they've already started treatment with another antibiotic, Fishman says. "In America, we tend not to stop the treatment."

"Education alone doesn't work" in changing prescribing behavior, says Donald Goldmann, a professor of infectious diseases at the Harvard School of Public Health and senior vice president of the Institute for Healthcare Improvement, which supports quality-improvement initiatives for health-care institutions. In fact, he says, physicians "will fudge" even when systems exist to warn doctors away from some drugs. One study found an "epidemic" of pneumonia at a hospital where doctors discovered they could prescribe a certain drug only if they "checked a box for pneumonia" on a prescription order form, he says.

The best intervention is "strong decision support" — good, specific information provided at the time and place of prescribing — and "tough feedback" showing doctors how they're doing compared to other physicians, Goldmann says.

U.S. doctors who treat patients outside of hospitals, however, are tied into few if any systems offering feedback, Schaffner says, making it even more difficult to mold non-hospital physician behavior. Some health-maintenance organizations and a few fledgling state Medicaid efforts, however, have made headway, he says. "Physicians really need to know what the standard of practice is and how they measure up to it," says Schaffner. "When they do, a light goes on."

Drug companies' "gross overpromotion" of the latest antibiotics exacerbates the problem, says Sidney Wolfe, director of the Health Research Group at the consumer organization Public Citizen. For example, after CDC guidelines declared that azithromycin (trade name Zithromax) should not be either a first- or a second-choice treatment for ear infections, the drug's manufacturer, Pfizer, "brought in academics to subvert the guideline," says Wolfe, who obtained and publicized an internal Pfizer memo about the policy.

The company's heavy promotion, including sponsoring the children's television program "Sesame Street" — "brought to you by the letter Z as in Zithromax" — made the drug the fifth most commonly prescribed in the United States by 2003. Nineteen states sued Pfizer to stop the promotion, but the $6 million in fines Pfizer paid was dwarfed by the $1.5 billion it earned in 2003 from Zithromax sales alone.[22]

At the federal level, the FDA has no authority to levy fines for overpromotion and can't regulate prescription-writing, but Wolfe says health-care payers, especially Medicare and Medicaid, should crack down on doctors' unjustified use of overhyped new antibiotics.

"I've been urging FDA to do more education" on prescribing, but not much has happened, says Wolfe. "CDC and the Centers for Medicare and Medicaid Services do some, but it is inadequate to counterbalance the vast amounts of advertising."

How Superbugs Develop Resistance Quickly

Speed and flexibility help them mutate

Bacteria can become resistant to antibiotics even if they have never come in contact with a human-made antibiotic. (Antibiotic drugs are derived from naturally occurring microbes that excrete substances that can kill bacteria or interfere with some of their vital natural processes.)

For example, wild animals in Australia have little or no exposure to antibiotics, but a study of *e. coli* bacteria from kangaroos and wombats found that 3 percent were resistant to the antibiotic amoxicillin. And hospital patients in India, Turkey and Poland were infected with methicillin-resistant *staphylococcus aureus* — MRSA — even before the antibiotic methicillin had been used in those countries. [1]

Large numbers of resistant bacteria usually don't evolve, however, until after the bacteria come in contact with the antibiotic. And over the years, scientists have discovered some traits that allow bacteria to evolve into a resistant population quickly, such as:

- **Speed.** Bacteria can evolve quickly partly because they reproduce so quickly. A human population can double about every 20 years. "For bacteria, it's every 20 minutes," says Barry I. Eisenstein senior vice president for medical affairs at Cubist Pharmaceuticals, in Lexington, Mass.
- **Exchangeability.** Many resistant bacteria can pass on their resistance genes to other bacteria, even if they're of different species. Humans' guts are filled with harmless bacteria that can block antibiotics. That's no problem unless a disease-causing bug enters the gut. Then the harmless but resistant bugs may pass their resistance to the dangerous bacteria, making them resistant, too. Often what's transferred is a "plasmid" — a hunk of DNA that isn't part of the bug's regular DNA — and some plasmids can carry resistance genes for several kinds of antibiotics. A bacterium that picks them up becomes a "superbug," resistant to more than one drug. A potential route to new antibiotic treatments would be drugs that block plasmid transfer, says N. Kent Peters, program officer for antibacterial resistance at the National Institute for Allergy and Infectious Diseases (NIAID).
- **Tendency to mutate.** In nature's ongoing war among microbes, mutant offspring with better ways to survive allow a species to evolve to overcome enemies. In recent years, scientists have found that something even more complicated occurs. When some bacteria are under pressure, such as from a dose of antibiotics, their offspring actually have more genetic mutations than usual, thus increasing the species' chance of evolving a means to survive, says Michael Kurilla, director of the office of biodefense research affairs at NIAID. A few researchers are exploring ways to block mutations, Kurilla says. When bacteria are under attack from an antibiotic that doesn't kill them, they "don't sit on their duffs," says Eisenstein. "They become more promiscuous," exchanging more genes with other nearby bacteria, which ups the chance they'll produce resistant offspring that can survive.

[1] Peter J. Collignon, "Antibiotic Resistance," *Medical Journal of Australia*, Sept. 16, 2002, p. 325, www.mja.com.au/public/issues/177_06_160902/co110836_fm.html.

Ounce of Prevention

Since fewer antibiotics will be prescribed if fewer people get sick, curtailing the spread of infectious disease is key in fighting antibiotic resistance. [23]

In the past, resistant pathogens spread mainly in hospitals. But today an especially virulent strain of MRSA has emerged outside of hospitals, making infection control even tougher.

"Every hospital in the country has a policy for handling MRSA," but "we have failed dismally" in getting a handle on it, says Montefiore Medical Center's Currie. "A lot of the guidance on infection control is not data-based."

The University of Maryland's medical center now screens everyone checking into its nine intensive-care units for MRSA, whether the patient shows signs of infection or not. "There's debate in the United States over whether [such] 'active surveillance' works," says medical director Standiford. "I believe it does and that it saves money in the long run" by identifying the "reservoirs of infection" — non-symptomatic patients who can spread the bug. "Every time you get MRSA in the bloodstream, it costs the hospital $20,000 at least" because the patient's stay is so much longer.

In hospitals, the confining of infected patients once halted the spread of contagion, but with the number of infections growing, many hospitals don't have enough separate areas to confine patients, says Allison Aiello, an assistant professor of epidemiology at the University of Michigan School of Public Health.

And with the new, highly virulent strain of MRSA popping up in the community, infection control becomes even harder. More patients already have a resistant infection when they enter a hospital, and no one knows how the CA-MRSA strain spreads, says Robert Daum, a professor of pediatrics at the University of Chicago.

During the past decade, the federal government has taken stabs at attacking the antimicrobial-resistance problem but hasn't sustained its support. In 1999 the CDC established a Federal Interagency Task Force to Combat Microbial Resistance, which issued an action plan in 2001. [24] The inadequately funded panel, however, has the tools to do little "but issue an annual laundry list of uncoordinated activities," says Guidos of the Infectious Disease Society of America.

In 2000, Sen. Edward M. Kennedy, D-Mass., and former Sen. Majority Leader Bill Frist, R-Tenn., a cardiac surgeon, authorized $40 million in annual funding for resistance research and federal initiatives like the task force. But Congress never appropriated any funds, says Guidos. In 2001, for example, then-Rep. Sherrod Brown, D-Ohio — now a senator — and Sen. Orrin Hatch, R-Utah, sponsored legislation to fund the programs, "but no funding ever came," Guidos says.

Moreover, jurisdictional struggles between the CDC and the states makes surveillance of resistance difficult, says Feldgarden at the Alliance for the Prudent Use of Antibiotics. Too often, "there's a one-way highway for information. It goes up to the CDC and then doesn't get back to the states," he says. And states don't always hold up their end of the reporting bargain, he adds. "Unless they get money, states don't want to play nice with the CDC."

The CDC and state public-health agencies already issue many disease-surveillance reports, and "diseases don't go away. So if you want to add something" — such as resistance — "you need to add money," Feldgarden explains. But in recent years states haven't been adding money for public health.

"It's ridiculous that CVS [pharmacy] knows more about the [birthday] cards I send to my mother" than health agencies know about developing infectious outbreaks, says Feldgarden. "Real-time reporting is essential, because once you're beyond the anecdote stage, look out."

In any case, the states, the federal government and private organizations are unlikely to do much to institute anti-resistance measures until they get clear proof that they can save both lives and money, says Stuart B. Levy, a professor of microbiology at Tufts University School of Medicine in Boston. The Massachusetts Department of Public Health, for instance, is "very receptive" and is launching its own surveillance system, but doing it "on a shoestring," he says,

The Alliance for the Prudent Use of Antibiotics, which Levy founded, is mining hospital records for what it says will be the first solid statistics on the dollar cost of resistant infections. The CDC's current cost data "are all wrong" because the agency did not have access to the hospital cost information that tells the real story, says Christopher Spivey, the alliance's manager for business development and communications. The real costs are "quite breathtaking, much bigger than we thought," he says. He could not predict exactly when the data will be available. ■

CURRENT SITUATION

Under the Radar

Unlike in previous decades, MRSA is now invading facilities such as sports locker rooms, jails and day-care centers and threatens even healthy people, says University of Chicago pediatrics professor Daum, and it's more potent than hospital-acquired MRSA. After first turning up in a handful of cases, community-acquired (CA) MRSA has seen "an explosive increase over the past 10 years in city after city," he says, beginning in the Midwest and Texas, then spreading to the West Coast and finally in the East. "And when it comes, it doesn't leave."

Today "perfectly healthy people are coming in with MRSA infections," he says, whereas in the past they developed only in hospitalized patients.

And many times the victims have never heard of the disease. "When we got the cause of [our son's] death, I had never heard of MRSA," recalls Everly Macario, a public-health researcher and writer in Chicago whose year-and-a-half-old son Simon died of CA-MRSA in 2004. The child, who had appeared to have a minor throat infection, awoke screaming with pain one morning. Doctors later discovered that toxins from the bacteria were attacking his organs. "By 10 that night he was dead," Macario says.

While hospitals still have a tough time containing traditional, hospital-acquired MRSA in their facilities, containing the community-acquired version — which causes more severe illness and appears to be more contagious — presents a more daunting challenge, says Daum. And CA-MRSA is beginning to spread to hospitals.

State public-health agencies didn't immediately realize that the new MRSA was a public-health problem, because they thought it was hospital-related, says Daum. But the "CDC is now really on board with the idea that this is something new," he says.

And as Macario found, no one is safe. "My parents are scientists, so I'm anal about washing hands," she says. "In my own home I want everything to be immaculate. I had breast fed Simon for a year, and he was up to date on all his inoculations."

Scientists don't know how CA-MRSA is spread, says Daum. For example, "I don't know what the role of inanimate objects is," such as whether the bacteria can survive and spread to other people if a person with an abscess, for example, sits on a doctor's table, he says.

"Staph is an amazing foe," Daum says. Some bacteria are easy to fight because they have limited ways to carry out certain functions, such as adhering to human cells. If the immune system counters that method, it can neutralize the bug. But staph has multiple means of accomplishing some basic functions, making it much more formidable, he points out. And while vaccines usually stimulate the immune system to produce a key antibody that can stop a microbe, he says, "staph is not going to yield to an approach like that."

Legislation Uncertain

Efforts to shore up the federal response to drug resistance are moving forward in Congress, but it's not clear how much legislation — if any — will be enacted this year.

Both the House and the Senate have passed FDA-overhaul measures that also provide incentives for developing antibiotics. The bills would make orphan drugs eligible for special federal grants and contracts and offer longer periods for companies to retain exclusive rights to market their new antibiotics before they can be sold by generic-drug makers.

House and Senate lawmakers must still reconcile differences between the two versions, but a joint conference panel has yet to be appointed, partly because a bitter fight over children's health insurance has stalled progress of health legislation. [25]

Bills also are pending that would ban many uses of agricultural antibiotics, an especially contentious issue.

Finally, Rep. John Matheson, D-Utah, plans to introduce a measure establishing initiatives to jump-start federal efforts to combat resistance. Among other provisions, the bill would give the CDC task force greater authority; establish a surveillance network covering several geographic regions; provide incentives for development of new antimicrobials and require drug companies marketing new antibiotics to explain whether the drugs would increase resistance and if so, what steps would be taken to retard the spread of resistance.

Many infectious-disease experts — and especially the Infectious Disease Society of America (IDSA) — have pressed Congress to strengthen the federal government's anti-resistance efforts and offered suggestions to Matheson and others about what legislation should contain. "I have a lot of hope for the Matheson bill," says the University of Pennsylvania's Fishman, who chairs IDSA's Antibiotic Resistance Working Group. "There's a need to coordinate and oversee research, and a need for increased funding in all areas related to resistance, and it's critical to do it now."

To ease the bill's passage, Matheson probably will not make many specific demands on the private sector. Even so, the bill's introduction has been stalled for months.

The Democratic leaders of the two health committees hope to discuss both the farm-antibiotics measure and Matheson's bill, possibly in connection with the yet-to-be-held conference on the FDA bills. But the FDA bills' slow movement leaves the fate of the antibiotic legislation unclear.

Meanwhile, many states are moving to require hospitals to publicly report how many of their patients contract infections in hospitals.

Consumers Union has pushed for such laws over the past three-and-a-half years, and the effort is working, says Lisa McGiffert, director of the group's Stop Hospital Infections project. Hospital-related infections, including resistant ones, have been going on for decades "because there hasn't been a public outcry," she says.

To date, bills have been filed in 45 states, 17 of which require hospitals to report information about what infections their patients contract in their facilities, McGiffert says. Other states have voluntary reporting systems, but she prefers mandatory systems because they can be standardized so consumers can understand what the data mean. Four states — Pennsylvania, Missouri, Florida and Vermont — publish their reports online.

But most of the reporting requirements don't yet include antibiotic-resistant infections. "Data on resistant strains will come next," she says, as states perfect their systems. ■

OUTLOOK

Beyond Antibiotics

Without decisive action, drug resistance can only get worse, warn infectious-disease experts.

The drug-resistance issue "is at a tipping point right now, and I see it escalating dramatically and exponentially," says Associate Professor of Medicine Fishman at the University of Pennsylvania.

Despite her young son's death, public-health researcher Macario is optimistic but still wary about the future. "There are campaigns to urge prudent prescribing," she says, so "sometimes I think: 'There's hope. We can all rally together.' " But humans have a defense mechanism in which they say to themselves, " 'It won't happen to me.' "

"Without aggressive collaboration, we may be faced with a public-health crisis and return to the pre-antibiotic era," warns the Alliance for Prudent Use of Antibiotics in a paper laying out guidelines for medical practitioners. [26]

Continued on p. 692

At Issue:

Should tighter restrictions be placed on antibiotics in animals?

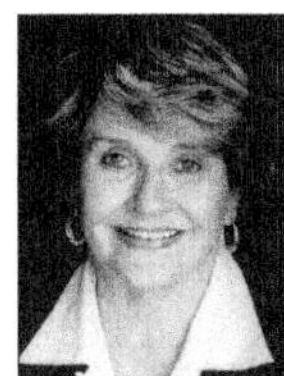

REP. LOUISE M. SLAUGHTER, D-N.Y.
CHAIR, HOUSE RULES COMMITTEE

WRITTEN FOR *CQ RESEARCHER*, AUGUST 2007

yes

The overprescription and overuse of antibiotics has produced an increasingly widespread number of resistant microbes. Current global trends, including urbanization and global travel and trade, have increased the demand for antibiotics worldwide. That, in turn, has increased the opportunities for antibiotic misuse. Additionally, although more and more bacteria have become resistant to the limited availability of treatments, research and development of new antibiotics has been scarce.

Antibiotic resistance already has been labeled a top concern by the Centers for Disease Control and Prevention and a "crisis" by the World Health Organization. Bacterial infections resistant to existing treatments increase health-care costs by $4 billion to $5 billion each year. Two million Americans acquire a bacterial infection annually during stays at hospitals. Seventy percent of the infections they contract are resistant to the drugs prescribed for treatment, and 38 patients die every day as a result.

As a microbiologist, I have always been concerned that our nation's health policies have done little to deter microbial drug resistance. The question of how we can preserve the effectiveness of existing antibiotics is complex but demands an immediate response.

One area in which it is both feasible and logical to limit antibiotic overuse is in production of food animals. In North America and Europe, an estimated 50 percent of all antibiotics are used in food-producing animals and poultry. Much of this is not for treating sick animals but for preventing disease and promoting growth. As a result, huge numbers of animals are regularly exposed to subtherapeutic concentrations of antibiotics, with disastrous results.

To address this problem, I am the proud sponsor of the Preservation of Antibiotics for Medical Treatment Act, which would phase out antibiotics use in livestock for growth or preventative purposes unless manufacturers could prove such uses don't endanger public health. It would also provide federal funds to help farmers adopt other approaches to preventing illness among their herds, such as cleaner housing and natural supplements. This bill would not restrict the use of antibiotics to treat sick pets or other animals not used for food.

Options exist to combat the growing public-health threat from drug-resistant bacteria. We must reevaluate how we use antibiotics, beginning with situations we can control. Our ultimate goal should be the elimination of practices that threaten the health and well-being of our citizens. The lessons of the past are plain for all to see. If we ignore them, we will risk making antibiotic treatments a thing of the past.

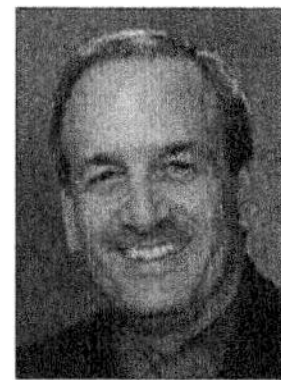

RICHARD CARNEVALE
VICE PRESIDENT, REGULATORY, SCIENTIFIC AND INTERNATIONAL AFFAIRS, ANIMAL HEALTH INSTITUTE

WRITTEN FOR *CQ RESEARCHER*, AUGUST 2007

no

Bans on antibiotics used to keep animals healthy have proven to be counterproductive. The United States should not risk animal health and human health by repeating these mistakes.

Following Denmark's ban on using antibiotics for growth promotion, the increase in animal illness and death in that country required veterinarians to nearly double their use of antibiotics to treat diseases.

The current U.S. regulatory system provides many layers of protection to ensure the safest possible use of antibiotics to keep animals healthy:

- The pre-market review process used by the Food and Drug Administration (FDA) to review antibiotics is arguably more stringent than the review of antibiotics for humans. Sponsors must demonstrate safety for both animals and the humans who consume the meat from treated animals. Also, measures imposed in 2003 require sponsors, prior to product approval, to assess the risk of resistant bacteria being transferred from animals to humans.
- Post-approval risk assessments that have been conducted and published by FDA, sponsors and researchers.
- Food-safety monitoring programs that have been established by government agencies and sponsors to track the development of antibiotic-resistant bacteria.
- Responsible-use programs that are specific to the different livestock species give veterinarians and producers specific guidelines to safely and properly use antibiotics in their health management systems.
- Pathogen-reduction programs that have successfully led to documented reductions in pathogens on meat, contributing to decreased foodborne illness.

Recent literature demonstrates the benefits of using antibiotics to keep animals healthy and the risks of letting politicians ban uses. These papers show that when antibiotics are removed without a careful assessment of the consequences, there is an increased risk of meat containing the kinds of pathogens that make people sick. Allowing producers to carefully use antibiotics to keep their animals healthy is important to our food safety system.

The FDA has in place a rigorous, science-based process for the approval of new animal drugs. This review process, combined with post-approval monitoring, risk assessments and adherence to proper-use principles, allows producers to use antibiotics to keep animals healthy, contribute to a safe food supply and minimize the risk of resistant bacteria transferring from animals to humans.

Continued from p. 690

Nevertheless, a Chicken-Little-sky-is-falling attitude isn't warranted, since 20th- and 21st-century medicine has already developed many more tools besides antibiotics to combat infectious disease, says former FDA infectious-disease officer Powers. Despite headlines declaring the contrary, "we won't go back to the pre-antibiotic era," he says. Evidence for this comes from the fact that better public health and health care had already made many infectious diseases more tractable, even before the discovery of antibiotics, he says. For example, between 1935 and 1945 — before the public introduction of penicillin — mortality from pneumonia in industrialized countries had already dropped from 70 percent to 40 percent, and medical progress in non-antibiotic areas will continue, he says.

Meanwhile, researchers continue to seek new antibiotics, exploring for undiscovered, natural antimicrobial excretions from microbes in remote environments like the Amazon jungle, deserts and the ocean floor. They also are using genetic technology to screen for more "targets" within bacteria to attack with drugs. And some researchers are using DNA techniques to explore the antibiotic effects of microbes that can't be grown in the lab, by transferring genetic material from microbes that don't grow in the lab into other microbes that can be grown and studied there, says Kurilla, of the National Institute of Allergy and Infectious Diseases.

Future infectious-disease drugs may act on the human host rather than on the microbes, says Kurilla. Today's scientists hope someday to be able to identify host targets in human cells that will block the ability of a bacterium to complete its life cycle and produce an infection, he says.

Some small companies already are researching this area, while " 'big pharma' is watching from the sidelines," he says. If the research pans out, large pharmaceutical companies' chemical libraries — which primarily contain chemicals suitable for interacting with human cells — would become a richer resource for anti-infective drugs, he says.

Focusing on the host would "sidestep resistance," because bacteria would have a harder time producing the complex group of mutations needed to bypass a change in their human host, Kurilla says.

Up to now, infectious-disease medicine has focused too much on throwing antibiotics at infections, then depending on pharmaceutical companies to develop a new antibiotic when resistance and new infectious ills pop up, says Montefiore Medical Center's Currie. But with new antibiotics harder and harder to find, in the future that paradigm must change, he says.

"We should have a five- or 10-year goal of learning to pry ourselves" from the antibiotic-resistance treadmill, "kind of the equivalent of the Manhattan Project to build an atom bomb in five years," Currie says. ■

About the Author

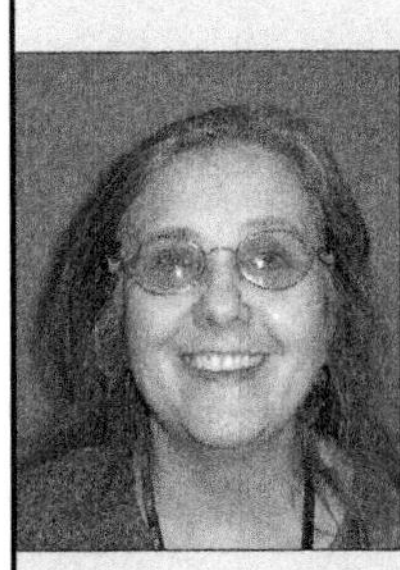

Staff writer **Marcia Clemmitt** is a veteran social-policy reporter who previously served as editor in chief of *Medicine & Health* and staff writer for *The Scientist*. She has also been a high-school math and physics teacher. She holds a liberal arts and sciences degree from St. John's College, Annapolis, and a master's degree in English from Georgetown University. Her recent reports include "Climate Change," "Health Care Costs," "Cyber Socializing" and "Prison Health Care."

Notes

1 For background, see "Severe Methicillin-Resistant Staphylococcus aureus Community-Acquired Pneumonia Associated with Influenza — Louisiana and Georgia, December 2006-January 2007," *Morbidity and Mortality Weekly Report*, Centers for Disease Control and Prevention, www.cdc.gov/mmwr/preview/mmwrhtml/mm5614a1.htm, April 13, 2007.

2 Judith Graham, "Hospital Infections on the Rise," *Chicago Tribune*, June 25, 2007, p. C1.

3 "Guide to the Elimination of Methicillin-Resistant Staphylococcus Aureus (MRSA) Transmission in Hospital Settings," Association for Professionals in Infection Control and Epidemiology, www.apic.org/Content/NavigationMenu/GovernmentAdvocacy/Methicillin ResistantStaphylococcusAureusMRSA/Resources/MRSAguide.pdf, March 2007.

4 For background, see Steve Silberman, "The Invisible Enemy," *Wired*, February 2007, www.wired.com/wired/archive/15.02/enemy.html?pg=2&topic=enemy&topic_set=.

5 Christopher J. Lettieri, "The Emergence and Impact of Extensively Drug-Resistant Tuberculosis," Medscape Pulmonary Medicine Web site, www.medscape.com/pulmonarymedicine, May 31, 2007.

6 Kathleen S. Swendiman and Nancy Lee Jones, "Extensively Drug-Resistant Tuberculosis (XDR-TB): Quarantine and Isolation, Congressional Research Service, June 5, 2007.

7 For background, see Lawrence K. Altman, "Traveler's TB Not as Severe as Officials Thought," *The New York Times*, July 4, 2007, p. A11.

8 For background, see Richard E. Isaacson and Mary E. Torrence, "The Role of Antibiotics in Agriculture," American Academy of Microbiology, www.asmusa.org, 2002; "Antimicrobial Resistance: Implications for the Food System," *Comprehensive Reviews in Food Science and Food Safety*, July 2006, pp. 71-137.

9 "SHEA/APIC: Talking Points on Legislative Mandates for Active Surveillance for MRSA and VRE in the United States," Society for

Healthcare Epidemiology of America, www.shea-online.org/Assets/files/Active_SurveillanceTalking_Points.pdf.

[10] *Ibid.*

[11] David B. Ross, "The FDA and the Case of Ketek," *The New England Journal of Medicine*, April 19, 2007, p. 1601.

[12] For background, see Jennifer Weeks, "Factory Farms," *CQ Researcher*, Jan. 12, 2007, pp. 25-48.

[13] For background, see Kathy Koch, "Food Safety Battle: Organic vs. Biotech," *CQ Researcher*, Sept. 4, 1998, pp. 761-784.

[14] David L. Smith, Jonathan Dushoff and J. Glenn Morris, Jr., "Agricultural Antibiotics and Human Health," in Public Library of Science, Medicine, www.pubmedcentral.nih.gov/articlerender.fcgi?artid=1167557, August 2005.

[15] Quoted in Madeline Drexler, "APUA One-on-One: The Danish Experiment," *APUA Newsletter*, Alliance for the Prudent Use of Antibiotics, Issue No. 2, 2004, p. 1, www.tufts.edu/med/apua/Newsletter/APUA_v22n2.pdf.

[16] "The Antibiotics Debate: Antibiotics and the Environment," Animal Health Institute, www.ahi.org.

[17] Ian Phillips, "Withdrawal of Growth-Promoting Antibiotics in Europe and its Effects in Relation to Human Health," *International Journal of Antimicrobial Agents*, 2007 (in press).

[18] Randall S. Singer, *et al.*, "Modeling the Relationship Between Food Animal Health and Human Foodborne Illness," *Preventive Veterinary Medicine*, 2007, p. 186.

[19] For background, see Adriel Bettelheim, "Drug-resistant Bacteria," *CQ Researcher*, June 4, 1999, pp. 473-496; Stuart B. Levy, *The Antibiotic Paradox*, second edition (2002); Abigail A. Salyers and Dixie D. Whitt, *Revenge of the Microbes: How Bacterial Resistance Is Undermining the Antibiotic Miracle* (2005).

[20] For background, see Donald E. Low, "Changing Trends in Antimicrobial-Resistant Pneumococci: It's Not All Bad News," *Clinical Infectious Diseases*, Supplement 4, 2005, pp. S228-233.

[21] "Frequently Asked Questions: Get Smart: Know When Antibiotics Work," Centers for Disease Control and Prevention, www.cdc.gov/drugresistance/community/faqs.htm.

[22] Barbara Mintzes, "Pharmaceutical Promotion and Prevention of Antibiotic Resistance," October 2005, www.pasteur.fr/applications/euroconf/antiinfectionstherapies/7_Mintzes_abstract_.pdf.

[23] For background, see Betsy McCaughey, "Unnecessary Deaths: The Human and Financial Costs of Hospital Infections," Committee to Reduce Infection Deaths, www.hospitalinfection.org, 2006.

[24] For background, see "The 2001 Federal Interagency Action Plan to Combat Antimicrobial Resistance," Union of Concerned Scientists, www.ucusa.org.

[25] For background, see Alex Wayne, "Tough Negotiations Ahead on Children's Health Expansion, Medicare," *CQ Today*, Aug. 2, 2007.

[26] "Antibiotic Resistance: Careful Antibiotic Use Can Help Control the Growing Problem," APUA, www.tufts.edu/med/apua/Practitioners/ABRcontrol.html.

FOR MORE INFORMATION

Acinetobacter Baumannii; www.acinetobacter.org. Web site run by individuals concerned about drug-resistant infections affecting U.S. soldiers.

Animal Health Institute, 1325 G St., N.W., #700, Washington, DC 20005-3104; (202) 637-2440; www.ahi.org. Organization of companies that manufacture veterinary drugs; advocates for farm use of antibiotics.

Alliance for the Prudent Use of Antibiotics, 75 Kneeland St., Boston, MA 02111-1901; (617) 636-0966; www.tufts.edu/med/apua/index.html. International group that supports research and projects to combat antimicrobial resistance.

Association for Professionals in Infection Control and Epidemiology, 1275 K St., N.W., Suite 1000, Washington, DC 20005-4006; (202) 789-1890; www.apic.org. Professional society that conducts research and education on resistance.

Centers for Disease Control and Prevention, Antimicrobial Resistance Program, 1600 Clifton Rd, Atlanta, GA 30333; (404) 639-3534; www.cdc.gov/drugresistance. Federal agency that coordinates the U.S. response to antimicrobial resistance.

DANMAP; www.danmap.org. A Danish agency that monitors antibiotic use in Denmark, the first country to enact strong government controls over all antibiotics.

Extending the Cure, Resources for the Future, 1616 P St., N.W., Washington, DC 20003; (202)-328-5000; www.extendingthecure.org. Analyzes economic and other policy options for extending antibiotics' effectiveness.

Infectious Disease Society of America, 1300 Wilson Blvd., Suite 300, Arlington, VA 22209; (703) 299-0200; www.idsociety.org. Physicians' group that makes policy recommendations for combating resistance.

Institute of Food Technologists, 1025 Connecticut Ave., N.W., Suite 503, Washington, DC 20036-5422; (202) 466-5980; www.ift.org/cms/. Food scientists' group that studies antibiotic use from the point of view of food production.

Keep Antibiotics Working, P.O. Box 14590, Chicago, IL 60614; (773) 525-4952; www.keepantibioticsworking.com. Nonprofit group that combats drug resistance.

MRSA Notes; www.mrsanotes.com. Posts news updates and links about drug-resistant staph infections.

Society for Healthcare Epidemiology of America, 1300 Wilson Blvd., Suite 300, Arlington, VA 22209; (703) 684-1006; www.shea-online.org. Provides information and advocacy on antimicrobial resistance.

Stop Hospital Infections, Consumers Union; www.consumersunion.org/campaigns/stophospitalinfections/learn.html. Consumer group that advocates for state laws requiring hospitals to publicly report rates of infection.

Bibliography

Selected Sources

Books

Levy, Stuart B., *The Antibiotic Paradox*, second edition, Perseus Publishing, 2002.

A microbiology professor at the Tufts University School of Medicine explains the basic biology of bacteria and details the history of antibiotic use and misuse that is increasing the prevalence of drug resistance.

Salyers, Abigail A., and Dixie D. Whitt, *Revenge of the Microbes: How Bacterial Resistance Is Undermining the Antibiotic Miracle*, American Society for Microbiology Press, 2005.

Microbiology professors at the University of Illinois, Urbana-Champaign, chronicle the rise of resistance microorganisms and the hazards they pose to the health-care system.

Articles

Bryant, Howard, "Blitzing Microbial Infections," *The Washington Post*, Aug. 3, 2006, p. E1.

Five cases of drug-resistant staph infections turned up among members of the Washington Redskins in a two-year period, and drug-resistant infections are growing common in sports franchises. Steps the team has taken to combat infections include a new Jacuzzi with germ-killing ultraviolet light and locker-room benches with individual stools for each player.

Hester, Tom Jr., The Associated Press, "As Woman Marvels at Recovery, New Jersey Targets 'Superbug' Infections," *Newsday.com*, Aug. 2, 2007.

Gov. Jon Corzine, D-N.J., signs legislation requiring hospitals to screen patients for methicillin-resistant staph aureus (MRSA), implement new controls to prevent the spread of infections and report MRSA cases to the state.

Langreth, Robert, and Matthew Herper, "Biotech Engages in Germ Warfare," *Wired*, June 9, 2006, www.wired.com/print/medtech/health/news/2006/06/71110.

As antibiotic-resistance increases, small biotechnology companies are looking for new ways to combat bacterial infections.

Silberman, Steve, "The Invisible Enemy," *Wired*, February 2007, www.wired.com/wired/archive/15.02/enemy.html.

Soldiers wounded in Iraq encounter a severe drug-resistant infection — *acinetobacter baumannii* — during treatment in military medical facilities.

Von Bubnoff, Andreas, "Seeking New Antibiotics in Nature's Backyard," *Cell*, Dec. 1, 2006, p. 867.

Scientists are using DNA techniques and other new approaches to test the potential antibiotic effects of previously unstudied microbes from unusual environments.

Weiss, Rick, "FDA Rules Override Warnings About Drug," *The Washington Post*, March 4, 2007, p. A1.

A Food and Drug Administration advisory panel recommended rejecting a request to approve the antibiotic cefquinome for use in cattle because of the danger that more bacteria will become drug resistant, but the FDA argues that its drug-approval rules override those considerations.

Reports and Studies

***Antibiotic Resistance: Federal Agencies Need to Better Focus Efforts to Address Risk to Humans From Antibiotic Use in Animals*, Government Accountability Office, April 2004.**

Congress' nonpartisan auditing office finds federal agencies aren't doing enough to pin down the precise health risks posed by antibiotic use on farms.

***Bad Bugs, No Drugs*, Infectious Diseases Society of America, July 2004.**

Infectious-disease researchers argue that antimicrobial resistance is approaching a crisis and recommend that Congress provide incentives for companies to develop new antibiotics.

***Impacts of Antibiotic-Resistant Bacteria*, Office of Technology Assessment, www.theblackvault.com/documents/ota/Ota_1/DATA/1995/9503.PDF, September 1995.**

A nonpartisan federal agency reports on the history of antibiotic resistance and discusses federal policy options to combat it.

***The Resistance Phenomenon in Microbes and Infectious Disease Vectors: Implications for Human Health and Strategies for Containment*, Forum on Emerging Infections, National Academy of Sciences, www.nap.ed/catalog/10651.html, 2003.**

A national expert panel discusses the science of developing resistance and strategies to control it, including economic approaches, health-care system changes and emerging technologies like bacteriophages.

Isaacson, Richard E., and Mary E. Torrence, *The Role of Antibiotics in Agriculture*, American Academy of Microbiology, 2002.

Microbiologists describe the long-running, contentious debate over how strictly governments should control antibiotic use on farms, concluding that science-based policy in the field is difficult to develop.

Laxminarayan, Ramanan, and Anup Malani, *Extending the Cure, Resources for the Future*, www.extendingthecure.org/research_and_downloads.html, 2007.

Economists who specialize in maximizing environmental resources analyze the human and scientific factors leading to increased antimicrobial resistance and discuss policy options.

The Next Step:

Additional Articles from Current Periodicals

Antibiotic Approvals and Bans

Harris, Gardiner, "Approval of Antibiotic Worried Safety Officials," *The New York Times*, July 19, 2006, p. A15.
A Food and Drug Administration (FDA) official has concluded that a controversial antibiotic made by the French drug company Sanofi-Aventis should be withdrawn, citing the drug's apparent ineffectiveness.

Kaufman, Marc, "Bayer Seeks Reprieve for Animal Antibiotic," *The Washington Post*, Sept. 2, 2005, p. A4.
Bayer Corp. has asked the FDA to allow it to keep selling Baytril, its controversial animal antibiotic, while it fights the ban in federal court.

Yee, Daniel, "As Gonorrhea Joins List of 'Superbugs,' CDC Recommends New Drug for Treating It," The Associated Press, April 12, 2007.
The Centers for Disease Control and Prevention has recommended that cephalosporin be used to treat gonorrhea because the disease has become resistant to older antibiotics.

Antibiotics in Farming

Herskovits, Zara, "The Tide Turns In Battle to Rid Farms of Antibiotics," *The Boston Globe*, Aug. 22, 2005, p. C1.
The federal government and the farming industry are attempting to protect the effectiveness of antibiotics in humans by restricting their use in farm animals.

Lamb, Gregory M., "Avian-Flu Concerns Push Bans On Drugs for Animals," *The Christian Science Monitor*, April 19, 2006, p. 14.
The FDA has proposed a prohibition on antiviral drug use in farm animals, suggesting the practice could hinder the drugs' effectiveness against avian flu.

Schmeltzer, John, "Organics' Edge Questioned," *Chicago Tribune*, June 26, 2006, p. B1.
Antibiotic-free foods are not necessarily better for human consumption, according to a study by the Institute of Food Technologists.

Weise, Elizabeth, " 'Natural' Chickens Take Flight," *USA Today*, Jan. 24, 2006, p. 5D.
Four of the top 10 poultry producers in the United States say they have stopped using antibiotics to make their chickens grow faster and bigger.

Government Intervention

"Government Alleges Iowa Dairy Sold Cows with Antibiotics In Meat," The Associated Press, Aug. 10, 2007.
The federal government has filed a complaint alleging that an Iowa dairy has violated FDA guidelines by selling culled cows with more than the allowable amount of antibiotics in their systems.

Graham, Judith, " 'Super Bug' Bill Targets Hospitals," *Chicago Tribune*, April 30, 2007, p. A1.
Illinois may become the first state to require hospitals to implement programs that combat the drug-resistant bacterium MRSA (methicillin-resistant staphylococcus aureus).

Patton, Zach, "Bad Bugs," *Governing*, May 2007, p. 50.
The Infectious Disease Society of America's "Bad Bugs, No Drugs" campaign is lobbying Congress to create incentives for developing new bacteria-fighting drugs.

Other Treatments

"Sticky Solution," *The Economist*, April 28, 2007, p. 92.
A doctor in Germany has discovered that honey may be effective in the battle against superbugs.

Feinmann, Jane, "Now Wash Your Hands . . .," *Financial Times*, April 7, 2007, p. 11.
A silver-bullet solution to antibiotic-resistant bugs is a long way away; maintaining the basics of personal hygiene is arguably the best current solution.

MacGregor, Hilary E., "A Closer Look: Anti-Listeria Spray," *Los Angeles Times*, Aug. 28, 2006, p. F1.
The FDA has approved certain bacteriophages to be sprayed on meats in order to prevent listeriosis, the deadliest of all foodborne illnesses in the United States.

CITING *CQ RESEARCHER*

Sample formats for citing these reports in a bibliography include the ones listed below. Preferred styles and formats vary, so please check with your instructor or professor.

MLA STYLE

Jost, Kenneth. "Rethinking the Death Penalty." CQ Researcher 16 Nov. 2001: 945-68.

APA STYLE

Jost, K. (2001, November 16). Rethinking the death penalty. *CQ Researcher, 11*, 945-968.

CHICAGO STYLE

Jost, Kenneth. "Rethinking the Death Penalty." *CQ Researcher*, November 16, 2001, 945-968.

CHAPTER

12

Regulating Toxic Chemicals

By Jennifer Weeks

Excerpted from the CQ Researcher. Jennifer Weeks. (January 23, 2009). "Regulating Toxic Chemicals."
CQ Researcher, 49-72.

Regulating Toxic Chemicals

BY JENNIFER WEEKS

THE ISSUES

In October 2007, the Eastman Chemical Co. of Kingsport, Tenn., introduced Tritan, a new plastic boasting "faster molding cycles compared to many other types of transparent polymers," plus enhanced durability and high gloss. [1]

But Tritan had another feature that made the plastics market take special notice: The new resin did not contain bisphenol A (BPA), a chemical widely found in rigid plastic products like food containers and baby bottles.

BPA has been used in consumer products for decades, although researchers have known since the 1930s that in mammals the chemical mimics estrogen, the natural hormone that regulates female sexual development and reproductive cycles. Endocrine disruption, as the effect is known, has been linked to developmental, reproductive and other problems in wildlife and laboratory animals, and some researchers believe it has a similar impact in humans. [2]

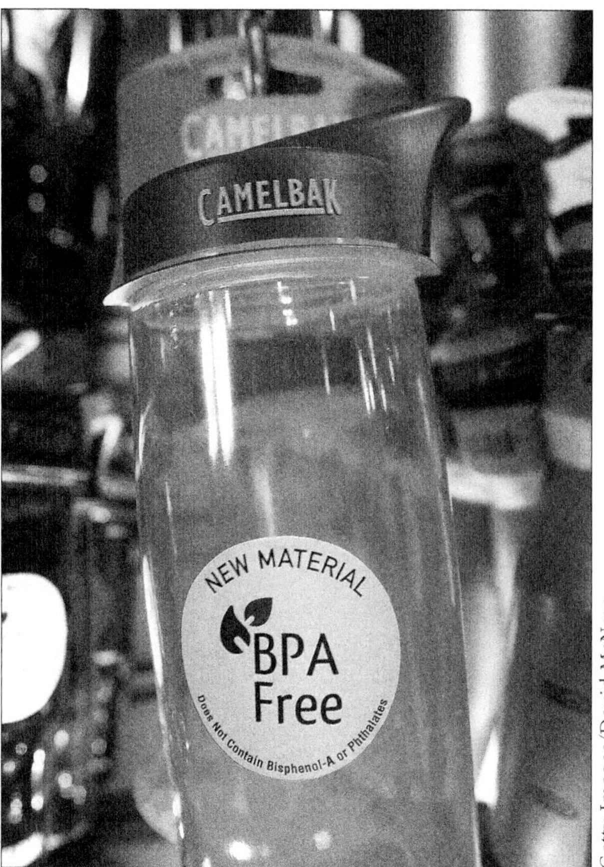

Getty Images/David McNew

Concern about exposure to the chemical bisphenol A (BPA), widely used in hundreds of products, is prompting consumers and retailers to switch to BPA-free products. The National Toxicology Program warned recently that BPA poses some concern for "effects on the brain, behavior and prostate gland in fetuses, infants and children." Wal-Mart, Target, and other large companies have stopped selling products containing BPA.

Until the late 1990s scientists thought BPA was only harmful at high doses, but then some studies showed that quantities as low as a few parts per billion could have toxic effects. They also demonstrated that BPA could leach from bottles and can linings into infant formula and food. [3] Then in 2008 the federally funded National Toxicology Program warned that current exposure levels to BPA posed some concern for "effects on the brain, behavior and prostate gland in fetuses, infants and children." [4] In contrast, the Food and Drug Administration (FDA), which regulates exposure to BPA from food packaging, maintained it was safe.

Consumers and retailers opted to be safe rather than sorry, especially after Canada banned BPA from baby bottles in April. Wal-Mart, Target, REI, Costco and other large companies pulled products containing BPA from their shelves or found substitutes. Many of these stores now sell hard plastic water bottles made with Tritan copolyester, prominently marked as BPA-free.

"They're selling fantastically," says Carolyn Beem, public affairs manager for L.L. Bean, the Maine outdoor retailer. "We're not experts in science, but we are experts in listening and responding to our customers. With all of the reports out there, it seemed like a good time to start again." In March 2008 Eastman expanded Tritan production to keep up with demand. [5]

In addition to BPA, environmentalists and consumer advocates warn that many other materials in commercial products may be harmful to human health, including:

- polyvinyl chloride (PVC) plastic, used in items such as shower curtains and water pipes;
- phthalates, a group of chemicals used to make plastics soft and pliable; and
- polybrominated diphenylethers (PBDEs), chemicals added to foams and fabrics as flame retardants.

In addition, some consumer goods contain materials widely known to be toxic, such as lead in popular brands of lipstick. [6]

"Consumers assume when they buy a product that someone has vetted it to make sure it's safe, but that doesn't always happen," says Sarah Janssen, a physician and environmental health expert at the Natural Resources Defense Council (NRDC), an advocacy group. "They're at a disadvantage because most of the important information isn't even on the label."

Humans are exposed to many potentially harmful substances in their daily lives, from air and water pollutants to household contaminants like mold and dust. Over time some of these exposures may cause cancer or other serious problems, such as birth defects or organ damage. Some of these illnesses result from lifestyle choices: for example, smoking, inactivity and obesity are major causes of cancer in the United States. [7] But workers and consumers also can be exposed unknowingly to risky materials that are legally used in commercial products.

Human exposure to toxic chemicals is controlled by several different agencies, depending on how the chemical is used and where people come in contact with it. The Environmental Protection Agency (EPA) regulates industrial chemicals and pesticides, while the FDA controls food additives, drugs and cosmetics and the Consumer Product Safety Commission (CPSC) oversees thousands of other consumer goods, from personal care products to toys. Workplace exposure to chemicals is regulated by the Occupational Safety and Health Administration (OSHA). Some materials must be tested for toxicity before marketing, but in other cases manufacturers merely have to notify regulators that they are going to start producing them.

WARNING
UNSAFE WATERS
YOU SHOULD NOT SWIM
IN THESE WATERS
YOU SHOULD NOT EAT FISH
FROM THESE WATERS

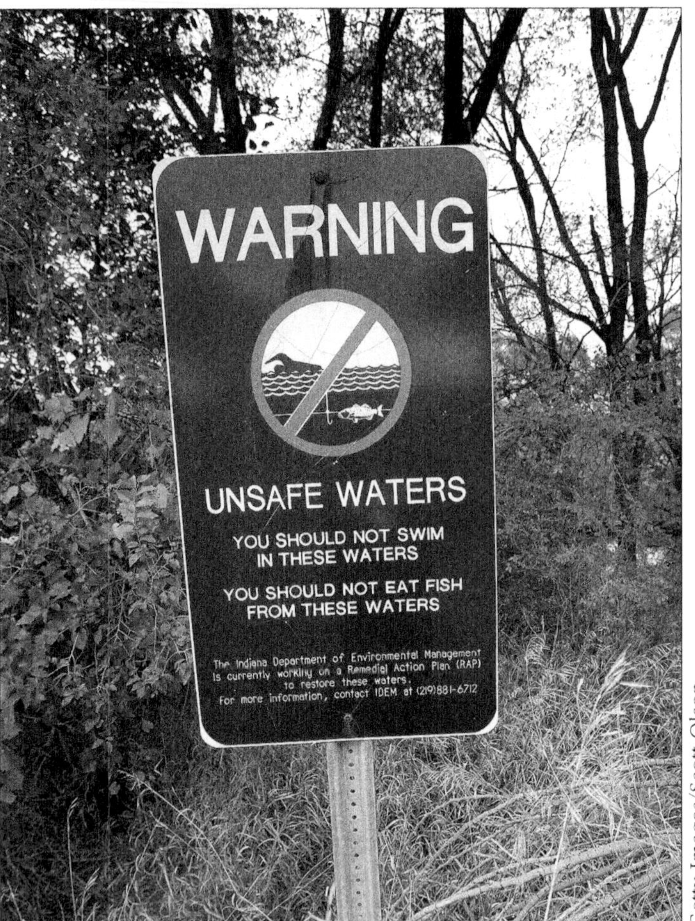

Getty Images/Scott Olson

A sign warns that dangerous industrial chemicals were dumped in a lake near Gary, Ind. In 1979 the Environmental Protection Agency banned production of polychlorinated biphenyls (PCBs), which cause cancer and birth defects in laboratory animals, and set timetables for phasing out their use in various industries.

Many experts think federal policy should be more consistent. "The agencies have very different approaches because they are covered by laws that find wildly varying levels of risk acceptable," says David Michaels, a professor of environmental and occupational health at George Washington University and a former assistant secretary of Energy. "We should be thinking about ways to harmonize standards across these agencies, because their actions affect each other. They allow different levels of exposure for many of the same chemicals."

Chemical manufacturers say the Toxic Substances Control Act (TSCA) — the core law that regulates industrial chemicals — is working. "TSCA has protected human health and the environment," says Michael Walls, managing director for regulatory and technical affairs at the American Chemistry Council (ACC), a chemical industry trade group. "There are areas where we can reform it, and we're encouraged that proposals have been offered to amend the law, not to replace it." The chemical industry is working with EPA to make more data available on hazards from widely used chemicals and assess how chemical exposures affect children's health.

Many critics worry that it is too easy for new materials to enter commerce before their effects have been well studied. They are especially concerned about the growing field of nanotechnology, which uses microscopic particles to enhance products ranging from sunscreen to medications. Reducing materials to the nano scale makes it easier to apply them precisely: for example, chemotherapy drugs can be targeted directly at tumors. But materials acquire new properties at this scale, and scientists are still analyzing the toxicity of many nanomaterials.

"Nanotechnology is taking our understanding of what makes something harmful and how we deal with that, and turning it upside down," said Andrew Maynard, chief science advisor to the Project on Emerging Nanotechnologies, in April 2008 congressional testimony. "New, engineered nanomaterials are prized for their unconventional properties. But these same properties may also lead to new ways of causing harm to people and the environment." [8]

In 2007 the European Union (EU) launched a new system for regulating chemicals that differs markedly from the U.S. approach. Under the REACH (Registration, Evaluation, Authorization and Restriction of Chemicals) policy, companies that produce or import chemicals in large volumes have to register their products with the EU and provide data on their properties and uses. Chemicals must be shown to be safe before they can enter commerce. U.S. companies doing business in Europe have to comply with the directive. [9] (*See sidebar, p. 62.*)

REACH is based on the so-called precautionary principle, which can be traced back through history but was articulated as a basis for environmental regulation at an international conference in 1998: "When an activity raises threats of harm to the environment or human health, precautionary measures should be taken even if some cause-and-effect relationships are not fully established scientifically." [10]

In contrast, many U.S. laws require regulators to produce scientific evidence that a substance is harmful before it can be removed from the market. Environmental and health advocates want the United States to adopt a more precautionary approach to regulation. But critics say the precautionary principle is too vague to be a viable basis for regulation and fails to balance risks and benefits. (*See "At Issue," p. 65.*)

For example, EPA banned use of the insecticide DDT in the U.S. in 1972 because it harmed the environment, but in 2006 the World Health Organization endorsed DDT for controlling mosquito-borne malaria in developing countries. [11] Some environmental groups want DDT banned worldwide, along with other persistent organic pollutants, but other advocates — including health experts — say it should remain in use until safer alternatives are developed. [12]

As Congress, regulators, businesses and advocates debate how to protect consumers from harmful exposures, here are some issues they are considering:

Concerns Linger Over Exposure to Bisphenol A

Scientists say they have "negligible concern" to "some concern" about the health effects of exposure to bisphenol A, a chemical commonly used in the production of plastics.

The National Toxicology Program uses the following five-level scale of concern for adverse effects from exposure to BPA:

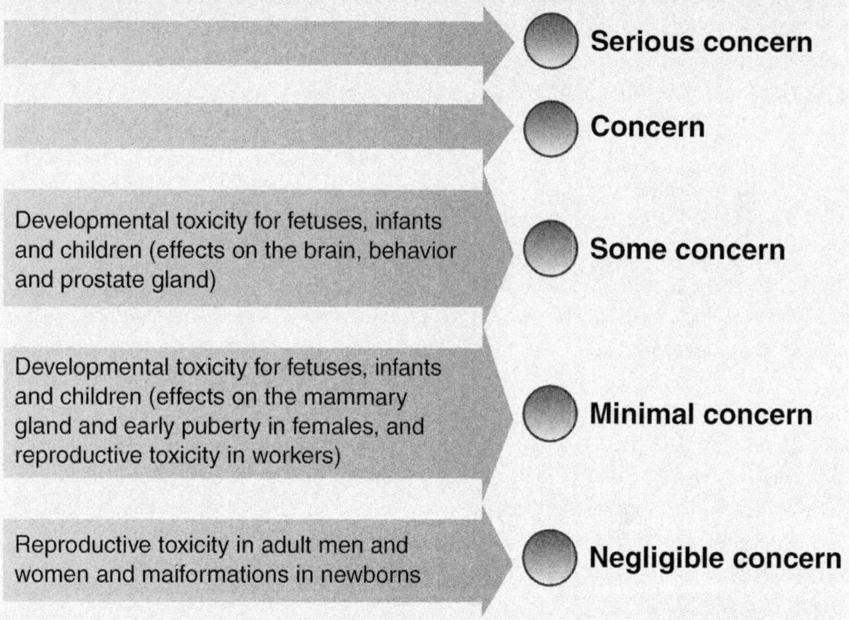

Effects	Level of concern
	Serious concern
	Concern
Developmental toxicity for fetuses, infants and children (effects on the brain, behavior and prostate gland)	**Some concern**
Developmental toxicity for fetuses, infants and children (effects on the mammary gland and early puberty in females, and reproductive toxicity in workers)	**Minimal concern**
Reproductive toxicity in adult men and women and maiformations in newborns	**Negligible concern**

How to Reduce Your Exposure to Bisphenol A:

- Don't microwave polycarbonate plastic food containers. Bisphenol A may break down from repeated use at high temperatures.
- Avoid plastic containers with the number 7 on the bottom. (www.recyclenow.org/r_plastics.html)
- Don't wash polycarbonate plastic containers in the dishwasher with harsh detergents.
- Reduce your use of canned foods.
- When possible, opt for glass, porcelain or stainless steel containers, especially for hot foods or liquids.
- Use infant formula bottles and toys that are bisphenol A-free.

Source: National Toxicology Program

Do we know enough about chemical risks?

Chemicals are central to the economy and to many products that Americans associate with modern living. They underpin a $637 billion industry in the United States and generated over $135 billion in export revenues as of 2006. [13] Innovations in chemistry have contributed to technical advances such as composite materials for vehicles, stronger adhesives, faster microprocessors for computers and recyclable plastics.

Core responsibility for regulating the massive chemical industry falls to the EPA, which is authorized under the Toxic Substances Control Act of 1976 (TSCA) to collect information about industrial chemicals from manufacturers and to limit or ban those that pose unreasonable risks. [14] Today EPA has some 82,000 chemicals in its TSCA inventory, of which about 62,000 were already in use when the law was passed. On average, more than 700 new chemicals are introduced each year. [15]

Although TSCA gives EPA the power to review chemicals already in commerce, the testing burden falls mainly on the agency rather than on manufacturers. As a result, EPA has required testing for fewer than 200 of the 62,000 chemicals that were in commerce in the 1970s. TSCA also requires the agency to show substantial evidence that a substance already in use poses an unreasonable risk in order to limit its use. EPA has banned only five chemicals or classes of chemicals under TSCA, and one of these efforts was overruled by a federal court in 1991. [16]

For new chemicals, manufacturers have to notify EPA before they start production and provide information on production volumes, expected uses and any test data that they have. However, most companies do not voluntarily test their products. Instead of testing new chemicals directly, EPA uses scientific models to compare their properties to similar existing chemicals and identify potential hazards. According to the Government Accountability Office (GAO), these reviews have led to actions that reduced risks from over 3,600 new chemicals. [17]

Critics say that the U.S. needs a broader and more proactive policy for regulating chemicals. "Our approach is barbaric and out of date. We used to be the leader decades ago, but now we're behind," says Lois Gibbs, founder and director of the Center for Health, Environment & Justice. In the late 1970s Gibbs organized homeowners in Niagara Falls, N.Y., after learning that their neighborhood had been built on top of a leaking toxic waste dump called Love Canal; after two years, the federal government relocated the families.

"The U.S. is much more science-bound than other countries. There's a presumption that we understand all of the harmful interactions from exposure to toxics, but we don't," Gibbs argues. "Industry doesn't want anything changed until there's proof beyond the shadow of a doubt that it will cause harm, but we're just not that smart."

Manufacturers say that the U.S. regulatory system is fundamentally sound. "TSCA gives EPA broad authority to collect information, order testing, prohibit new uses of a substance and label or ban substances," says Walls at the American Chemistry Council. "We can enhance it to promote more systematic review and give the public more information about what chemicals are being produced." Under a program called the High Production Volume (HPV) Challenge, launched in 1998, chemical companies are voluntarily testing about 2,800 chemicals that are produced or imported in quantities of at least 1 million pounds per year and providing the information to EPA. About 1,400 data sets have been completed to date.

But GAO, while calling the HPV Challenge "laudable," has concluded that TSCA makes it too expensive and time-consuming for EPA to review chemical hazards. [18] In order to force companies to do testing EPA has to issue a regulation, a process that can take several years. "Given the difficulties involved in requiring testing, EPA officials do not believe that TSCA provides an effective means for testing a large number of existing chemicals," GAO reported in 2006. As a solution, it recommended empowering EPA to require companies to do chemical testing and provide the data to regulators.

Both EPA and FDA also need better testing methods in order to regulate toxic substances effectively. Scientists agree that current approaches, which rely heavily on animal testing, are too slow and expensive to cover hundreds of new chemicals each year and are not well-suited to predict harm from very low doses. "We need to bring our methodologies into the 21st century by making them less animal-intensive and getting higher throughputs," or testing many substances quickly, says John Bucher, associate director of the federally funded National Toxicology Program (NTP), which studies the impact of chemicals on human health.

Current test methods typically give rats or mice large doses of chemicals, look for end points like cancer or organ damage and then extrapolate those responses from animals to humans — a complex and often controversial process. A 2007 report by the National Research Council called for a new approach focused on "toxicity pathways" — changes that occur in networks of cells due to chemical exposure and which eventually may lead to adverse health effects. For example, exposure might initially cause hormone levels to change or tissues to become inflamed. The study recommended developing rapid systems for testing chemicals in cell cultures to identify toxicity pathways — a shift that it predicted would greatly reduce the need for animal testing and focus more attention on human biology and exposures. [19]

The NTP shares this vision, says Bucher. "These would be short-term assays [tests] with very simple readouts that could be run 24/7 just by punching buttons and would give a signature of biological interactions that a particular chemical would have," he says. "We hope that certain structures will be related to particular chemical classes and that that will let us make judgments about which chemicals should go through more sophisticated studies or should not be authorized for significant human exposures."

Are we commercializing nanotechnologies too quickly?

Many nanoscale materials (particles as small as 1/100,000th of the width of a human hair) have unique chemical, physical or biological characteristics that are different from larger particles of the same materials. Because they have distinctive properties such as high electrical conductivity, nanomaterials have special uses and are showing up in hundreds of consumer products, from kitchenware with antibacterial silver coatings to paints impregnated with silica particles that repel graffiti.

Consumer advocates worry that some of these applications could pose health risks, and that government agencies do not know enough about nanomaterials to regulate them effectively. An EPA fact sheet states the challenge bluntly: "At this early stage of the development of nanotechnology, there are few detailed studies on the effects of nanoscale materials in the body or the environment . . . it is not yet possible to make broad conclusions about which nanoscale substances may pose risks." [20]

Twenty-six federal agencies, including EPA, FDA and the CPSC, participate in the National Nanotechnology Initiative, a federal program that supports research on promising applications of nanotechnology and on environmental health and safety (EHS) issues. From fiscal 2005 through 2008, these agencies spent an estimated $180 million on research to address EHS questions. [21]

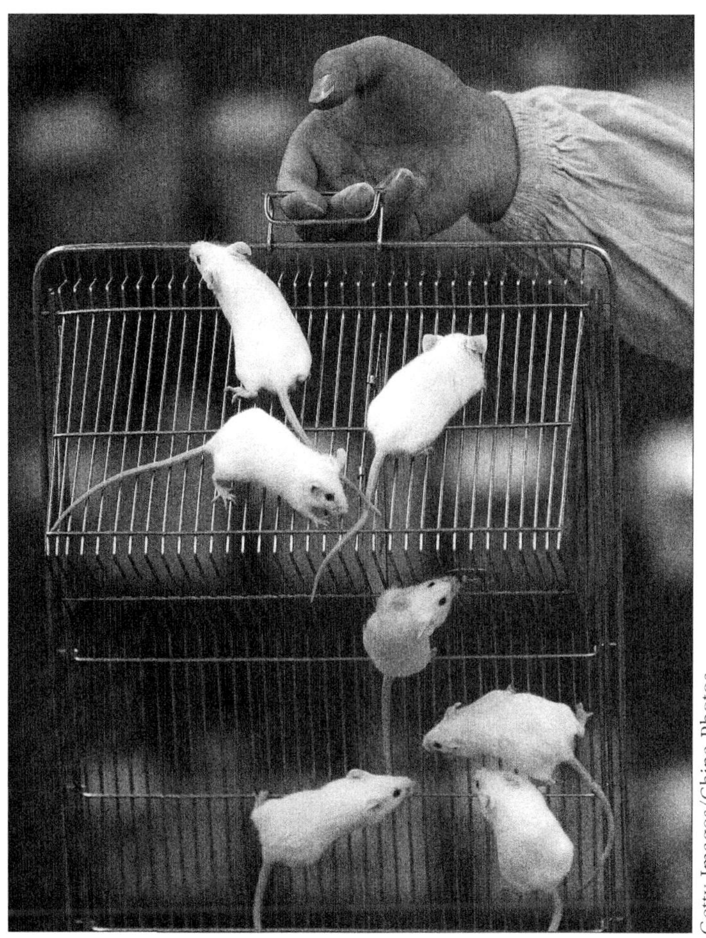

Getty Images/China Photos

Scientists agree that animal testing is generally too slow and expensive to cover hundreds of new chemicals each year and is not well-suited to predict harm from very low doses. The National Research Council has called for testing chemicals in cell cultures, a shift it predicted would greatly reduce the need for animal testing.

But keeping up with this fast-growing field is challenging for regulators. "I do not pretend to understand nanotechnology, and our agency does not pretend to have a grasp on this complicated subject either," CPSC Commissioner Thomas H. Moore told a Senate subcommittee in March 2007. "For fiscal year 2007, we were only able to devote $20,000 in funds to do a literature review on nanotechnology. Other agencies are asking for, and getting, millions of dollars for research in this area." [22]

Four months later an FDA task force report on regulating nanomaterials pointed out that because of their unique properties, the agency might need new testing equipment and methods to predict how they will react in body tissues. [23] Other agencies studying nanotechnologies confirm they often behave in surprising ways. "It is a daily occurrence in our labs that one of our standard assays doesn't work because of the unusual properties of these nanomaterials," said Scott E. McNeil, director of the National Cancer Institute's Nanotechnology Characterization Laboratory, at a conference last March. [24]

Some watchdog groups want to stop the marketing of nanoproducts until they are proven safe. Last May a coalition of health, environmental, and consumer groups petitioned EPA to control products containing nano-silver, which is highly effective at killing bacteria, fungi and other microorganisms. Because of this property, nanosilver has been added to garments (to kill odor), food storage containers, soaps, air purifiers and dozens of other products.

The petitioners argued that nanosilver in the environment could kill plants, benign microbes, fish and other aquatic species and might also threaten human health. They called on EPA to regulate the material as a pesticide and require comprehensive safety testing before any products containing it could be marketed. [25]

At a minimum, critics say, manufacturers should be required to label products containing nanoparticles so that consumers can choose whether or not to buy them. A study by Consumers Union found that four out of five sunscreens that claimed to be nano-free actually contained nanoparticles

Use of Nanotechnology Is Increasing

More than 800 consumer products containing nanomaterials were in the marketplace as of August 2008 — nearly quadruple the amount from just two years earlier. Some 60 percent of the products were related to health and fitness.

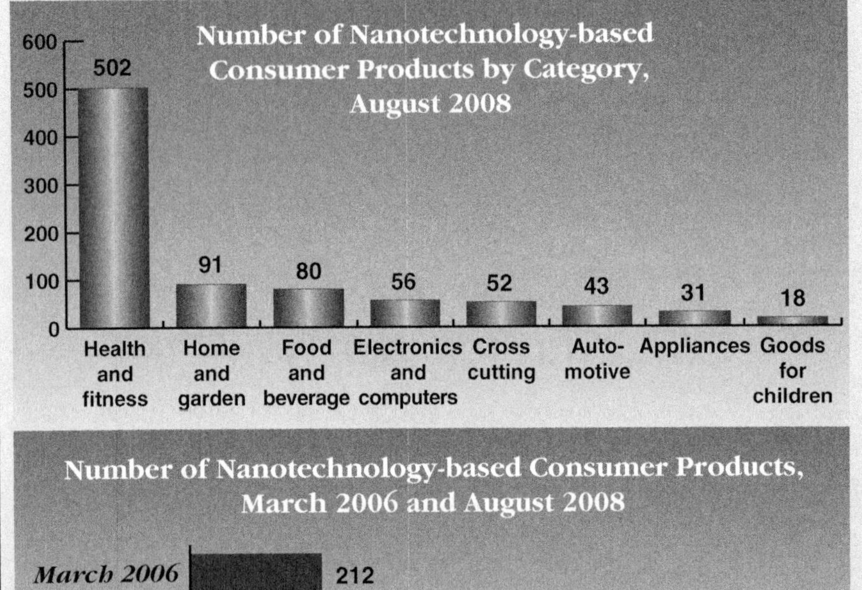

Source: The Project on Emerging Nanotechnologies, Woodrow Wilson International Center for Scholars

of titanium dioxide and/or zinc oxide, two compounds that help protect against ultraviolet radiation. [26]

"Size matters. Materials at the nanoscale should be considered new particles and have to go through new safety assessments," says Michael Hansen, senior staff scientist at Consumers Union. "Right now, it's assumed that if a material has been tested for bulk applications, it's safe. But when you reduce things to such small sizes, their behavior and surface area can change drastically. You can't assume that something safe at the macro scale is safe at the nano scale."

Some experts say that health concerns may be exaggerated. "When we started looking at them, we found that the properties of nanomaterials in products, such as particle size, often were different from what manufacturers said they were. People didn't always know what they were studying," says the NTP's Bucher. "We completely characterized the materials we were working with and then administered them to animals in ways that might mimic human exposures. Our studies suggest that some risks are lower than reports in the literature have suggested."

For example, according to Bucher, many reports predicted that titanium dioxide in sunscreen would penetrate skin readily, but the NTP concluded that won't happen unless the skin is cut or scraped. However, he cautions, this does not prove that all nanomaterials are harmless. "Every product is going to be different," he says.

Even if many nanomaterials are harmless, weak and underfunded regulatory agencies may have trouble distinguishing benign products from risky ones. Marla Felcher, an expert on marketing and consumer issues at Harvard University's Kennedy School of Government, says the Consumer Product Safety Commission is unprepared for the challenge. "CPSC is playing catch-up," she says. "More than half of the nanotechnology goods on the market come under its jurisdiction, and the funding it has to work with is a drop in the bucket."

But Felcher says the CPSC needs more than additional staffing and funding to ensure that nanomaterials in consumer products are safe. It also needs new authority to make manufacturers identify products that contain these substances and to impose mandatory safety standards for products based on new technologies, she says. (Today the agency relies on industry to develop and comply with voluntary safety standards). [27]

Hansen is hopeful the EPA will regulate nano-silver as a pesticide, but he says the FDA has so far refused to agree that nanomaterials are categorically different from their conventional counterparts. "The biggest exposures come from items that you put on or in your body and that contain free [non-bound] nanoparticles, like food ingredients and personal care products," says Hansen. "Scientific studies are saying that these materials need to be regulated."

Would stricter regulations hurt manufacturers and consumers?

Regulating chemicals in consumer products more stringently would affect chemical companies and manufacturers that use those chemicals to make retail goods. Chemical toxicity testing is expensive, and many business leaders say that substitutes for widely used materials like BPA will be more expensive and could produce inferior products. Health, environmental and consumer groups respond that safer products don't always cost much more, and in any case are worth a cost premium.

Even if a chemical poses risks, only some uses may require substitutes. "Health and safety concerns about a chemical like BPA are dictated as much by how it's used as by its chemistry. I'm more concerned about using it in baby bottles than in auto parts or compact discs," says Terry Collins, a professor of chemistry and director of the Institute for Green Science at Carnegie Mellon University.

Industry representatives say the risks of BPA have been widely studied and that removing it from food containers, as many critics urge, will be difficult. "BPA has been part of epoxy resin can linings for more than 50 years, and that's why we have canned goods with long shelf lives," says Steven Hentges, executive director of the American Chemistry Council's Polycarbonate/BPA Global Group. These linings prevent metallic flavors from migrating into food and keep acidic foods like tomatoes from corroding the cans.

"Substitutes have to be safer than what's being replaced, and no alternatives have been as thoroughly tested as BPA" says Hentges. The European Food Safety Authority concluded last July that BPA was safe in food packages. Canada banned BPA in baby bottles as a precautionary measure and declared it a toxic substance, but has not removed the material from food packaging for adults. Canadian regulators are funding studies to see whether further steps are needed to limit how much BPA is released into the environment. [28]

But other options exist. Many Americans buy juices, soups, sauces and chopped tomatoes in brick-shaped cartons, which were originally introduced in Europe. These containers, which are about 75 percent paper, 20 percent polyethylene plastic and 5 percent aluminum, typically cost more than canned goods, but foods packaged this way retain more color and flavor than canned foods because the food and the container are sterilized separately. The boxes can be recycled with milk and juice cartons. [29]

"There also are ways to can food so that it doesn't contain such high levels of BPA," says Janssen at the Natural Resources Defense Council. "Japan set voluntary standards for reducing BPA use in canned food, and now a lot of Japanese canned goods have a polyethylene layer inside that seals the epoxy resin lining so that BPA doesn't migrate into food. Industry should be thinking about more sustainable techniques instead of fighting to maintain the status quo."

Chemical companies and consumer advocates are also debating risks associated with phthalates, especially in children's toys. In 1998 a coalition of environmental and consumer groups petitioned the CPSC to ban toys that contained phthalates and were designed for children under age 6, citing studies suggesting that these materials could be toxic and the fact that young children commonly chewed on soft plastic toys. An expert panel convened by the commission found some risk from the phthalate DINP and asked toy makers to remove phthalates from toys voluntarily. According to the American Chemistry Council most companies removed phthalates from teethers, rattlers and pacifiers. [30]

The European Union also studied phthalates and imposed a temporary ban on six forms of the chemicals in toys and teething items in 1999. In 2005 it made the ban permanent, requiring manufacturers to eliminate three phthalates (DEHP, DBP and BBP) from all toys and to remove three others (DINP, DIDP and DNOP) from toys and child-care items that could be mouthed by children. [31]

EU regulators acted in response to studies that suggested, but did not prove, that exposure to phthalates could have toxic effects or cause abnormal reproductive development, especially in boys. A 2005 study in the United States reached a similar conclusion, but a U.S. government review panel found that animal studies that showed a connection were not necessarily applicable to people. [32] However, California, Washington and Vermont passed state-level bans. In 2008 Congress permanently banned DEHP, DBP and BBP from toys and set an interim ban on the other three types pending a safety review by the CPSC. [33]

Many businesses opposed the measure. "[M]anufacturers would be forced to use more expensive alternatives that may subject them to additional safety and legal liability concerns, and consumers would be exposed to products containing alternatives that have not been approved for use in children's products by any federal agency," the U.S. Chamber of Commerce wrote to Senate members early in 2008. [34]

Chemical industry representatives maintain that scientific evidence shows phthalates to be safe. "The pro-regulatory side considers phthalates guilty until proven innocent. They want to act even though the data is not conclusive," says Allen Blakey, vice president of the Vinyl Institute, a trade group for companies that manufacture vinyl and vinyl products (many of which contain phthalates to make them soft and flexible).

But toy manufacturers seem to be adapting to phthalate restrictions. Observers predicted the U.S. ban could drive some of China's small and uncompetitive toy manufacturers out of business, but other Chinese companies already make toys with phthalates for U.S. markets and without them for sale in the EU. [35] BASF, a major German chemical company, still produces DEHP in the United States but developed a new plasticized version called Hexamoll DINCH, which it markets to toy makers as a product "whose health safety is beyond all question" and "an ideal solution to adapting their products to the requirements of the new EU regulation." [36] ■

BACKGROUND

Reactive Regulation

Through the 19th century, as the United States grew from a nation of small-scale farmers into an industrial powerhouse, few standards protected people from hazardous materials. And even when government began to regulate dangerous products and substances in the early 20th century, controls were almost always put in place belatedly after scandals or disasters.

Muckraking journalist Upton Sinclair spurred passage of early consumer-protection laws with his 1906 novel *The Jungle*, which described filthy conditions in Chicago's meatpacking industry. Simultaneously, a series of articles in *Collier's* magazine spotlighted false claims and unsafe ingredients in so-called patent (non-prescription) medicines. Many of these concoctions were sold as cure-alls for numerous diseases but contained addictive substances like cocaine, heroin or alcohol. "[F]raud, exploited by the skillfulest [sic] of advertising bunco men, is the basis of the trade," author Samuel Hopkins Adams charged. [37]

In response Congress passed the Meatpacking Act and the first Food and Drug Act, which authorized government regulators to inspect meat processing plants and to seize products that were mislabeled or contained harmful or spoiled ingredients. However, manufacturers were not required to list all of the ingredients in foods or medicines or submit any information to the government before marketing them.

In 1933 the Food and Drug Administration proposed a complete revision of the Food and Drug Act, but Congress failed to act until 107 people in 15 states died in 1937 after taking elixir of sulfanilamide for strep infections. A chemist had created a liquid form of sulfanilamide, a new and effective prescription medicine, by dissolving the powdered medication in diethylene glycol, a chemical normally used as antifreeze, which he failed to realize was poisonous. [38] This tragedy spurred passage of the Federal Food, Drug, and Cosmetic Act, which required new drugs to be tested for safety before marketing.

As Congress debated safety standards, the fast-growing chemical industry was inventing myriad new materials. Important chemical products developed in the 1920s and '30s included polychlorinated biphenyls (PCBs), used as coolants and lubricants; synthetic estrogens (female hormones); and organic pesticides like the mosquito-killer DDT. Nineteenth-century inventors had already discovered many basic types of plastic, and by World War II these materials were widely used in applications including cellophane, vinyl, nylon and Teflon coatings.

During this period the labor movement gained strength as workers formed unions and won the right to collective bargaining. One of their priorities was making workplaces safer. Government agencies started to regulate safety, initially focusing on industries like mining and manufacturing, where workers were frequently injured by machinery, fires and explosions. Toxic exposure was also emerging as a serious hazard. For example, by the 1930s manufacturers knew that workers who inhaled silica dust or asbestos had high rates of lung disease, and medical researchers were starting to connect asbestos inhalation with cancer.

Under President Franklin D. Roosevelt (1933-1945), the Labor Department worked with industry and unions to improve workplace safety, mainly through voluntary safety codes and better training programs. During the economic boom of the 1950s occupational safety became a more established professional field, but it focused on traumatic injuries such as falls or machine accidents rather than exposure to dangerous materials. In one industrial hygienist's words, it was hard to draw attention to safety issues "unless people saw the blood drip." [39]

New Guardians

As corporations shifted from wartime manufacturing to civilian products, new materials streamed into commercial use, including vaccines, food additives, pesticides and herbicides and an avalanche of consumer goods. Most Americans welcomed these products, but research soon showed that some were unsafe.

By the late 1950s government regulators had banned more than a dozen food additives because they caused cancer, organ damage or other toxic effects in animals. [40] In 1958 Congress adopted the Delaney Clause, which barred all food additives that had been shown to cause cancer in laboratory animals. Six years later Surgeon General Luther Terry released a report stating that smoking caused cancer, and Congress passed a law requiring cigarette packs to carry health warning labels. [41] However, the tobacco industry — which had created its own scientific arm, the Tobacco Industry Research Committee, to refute incriminating studies — argued that smoking was a personal choice, and successfully lobbied against any limits on cigarette advertising or marketing.

By this time other toxic exposures were in the news. Rachel Carson's 1962 bestseller *Silent Spring* warned that persistent organic pesticides like DDT were accumulating in the environment, harming fish and birds and contaminating food supplies. In the same year it was disclosed that thousands of babies in Asia, Africa and Europe had been born with deformed or missing limbs after their mothers took thalidomide, a new sedative that the FDA was then close to approving for sale in the United States.

Continued on p. 61

Chronology

1900-1960

Government begins regulating consumer goods to protect buyers; fast-growing chemical industry produces thousands of materials that are quickly put to use.

1906
Congress authorizes federal inspections of meatpacking plants and outlaws adulterated or mislabeled foods and drugs.

1929
Chemical companies start making polychlorinated biphenyls (PCBs).

1930
Food and Drug Administration (FDA) is established. . . . Studies show asbestos can cause cancer.

1938
After tainted medicine kills 105 people, Congress passes Food, Drug and Cosmetic Act, requirng food additives and drugs to be proven safe. . . . British scientists produce diethylstilbestrol (DES), a synthetic estrogen, which is approved to treat gynecological ailments.

1939
Swiss chemist Paul Müller discovers that the synthetic chemical DDT is an effective insect killer. Müller later wins Nobel Prize after DDT-B is widely used to protect troops from typhus and malaria during World War II.

1954
Cigarette manufacturers create Tobacco Industry Research Council in response to scientific findings of health threats from smoking.

1958
Delaney Clause to Food, Drug and Cosmetic Act bans food additives that cause cancer in animals.

1960-1980

New agencies protect consumers and workers from hazardous substances. Studies find popular chemicals can harm health.

1962
Rachel Carson's bestseller *Silent Spring* warns of environmental and health threats from DDT.

1964
Surgeon general declares smoking hazardous to health; warning labels are required on cigarettes.

1970
Environmental Protection Agency (EPA) is created.

1971
Occupational Safety and Health Administration (OSHA) is established. . . . DES is linked to vaginal cancer.

1972
Consumer Product Safety Commission (CPSC) is established. . . . EPA bans DDT.

1976
Toxic Substances Control Act (TSCA) authorizes EPA to regulate chemicals but exempts 62,000 substances.

1977
CPSC bans nearly all uses of lead paint, including on toys.

1980-2000

Anti-regulatory forces challenge new, protective standards.

1980
Supreme Court's "benzene decision" says OSHA must show significant risks before limiting a chemical's use.

1983
OSHA requires employers to show workers how to use toxic chemicals.

1986
California mandates warning labels for products with chemicals that cause cancer or birth defects.

1990
Congress requires leaded gasoline to be phased out by 1996.

1996
Food Quality Protection Act tightens standard for pesticide residues in food and requires special protection for infants and children.

1997
Study finds bisphenol A (BPA) alters reproductive development in mice.

2000-Present

Support grows for natural and organic products.

2000
National Nanotechnology Initiative is launched.

2003
Congress approves $3.7 billion over four years for nanotech research, but only a small amount is earmarked for studying health impacts.

2007
European Union's REACH chemical regulation enters into force.

2008
Congress strengthens CPSC and bans lead and six phthalates from children's toys. . . . Canada bans BPA from baby bottles. . . . FDA committee concludes BPA is not harmful in food packaging, but the agency's review panel faults the study's methods.

Americans' Bodies Contain Over 100 Chemicals

Some cause cancer and other health problems.

Studies indicate that all human beings alive today carry traces of many industrial chemicals in their bodies. Some of these substances enter during fetal development or infanthood, carried by maternal blood and breast milk. In addition, we inhale airborne pollutants, ingest pesticide residues and chemical additives with our food and drinking water and absorb others through our skin. Exposure can happen in the workplace, outdoors or inside homes and schools.

Some so-called "chemical body burdens" in humans are harmless, but others can cause cancer, birth defects, developmental problems and other serious health impacts. Many are still being studied. The presence of a chemical in the body does not necessarily mean it will cause harm, but scientists say chemical exposure is pervasive in modern society, and they underscore the importance of testing widely used chemicals for toxic effects.

"I find it remarkable that in this day and age one of the primary ways by which the toxic effects of chemicals are discovered is still the 'body in the morgue' method," writes epidemiologist and former assistant secretary of Energy David Michaels. "An industrial worker dies from some very unusual condition, and we ask why. Well, some of us ask."

For example, Michaels notes, chemical companies that make diacetyl (the main ingredient in artificial butter flavor) did not know that breathing the compound could cause lung damage until workers in popcorn factories became ill. Manufacturers had been required to test diacetyl as a food ingredient, but not as an airborne contaminant in the workplace. [1]

According to a 2005 report from the Centers for Disease Control and Prevention (CDC), well over 100 chemicals are present in Americans at detectable levels, including heavy metals like cadmium and mercury, phthalates and many pesticides. Levels of some chemicals have fallen in recent years, notably lead (which has been banned from gasoline and house paint) and substances found in secondhand cigarette smoke. [2]

Others are more worrisome. For example, the CDC found that almost 6 percent of women of childbearing age had blood levels of mercury that were borderline dangerous. Mercury is a potent neurotoxin that can cause birth defects, nervous system damage and other harmful effects. It is emitted into the air from sources including coal-burning power plants and incinerators, then falls back to the surface and concentrates in the food chain. Humans are exposed mainly by eating fish that contain high amounts of mercury.

Another 2005 study commissioned by two advocacy organizations, Commonweal and the Environmental Working Group, tested umbilical cord blood from 10 babies born in U.S. hospitals during the previous year. Researchers found an average of 200 industrial chemicals and pollutants in the samples, including mercury, environmental pollutants known as dioxins and pesticides. This study showed that pollutants cross the placenta from mother to fetus as infants grow in utero, exposing the gestating infants to a complex mixture of chemicals during critical months of development. [3]

AFP/Getty Images/Andre Forget

An Inuit woman in Iqaluit, Nunavut, Canada, dries a caribou skin. Toxic chemicals remain a major threat to traditional ways of life in the Arctic.

Living far from industrial sources does not necessarily make people safer from exposures. Indigenous peoples in the Arctic have some of the highest body concentrations of mercury, PCBs and other pollutants of any region on the planet, thanks to global wind patterns and ocean currents that carry pollutants to the poles. Inuit, Aleut, and other native people in Greenland, Alaska and Canada eat large quantities of locally caught meat and fish, which contain high concentrations of chemicals. [4]

Recent studies show that concentrations of some toxins in Arctic food animals are stabilizing, thanks to international agreements limiting use of some of the most hazardous chemicals. [5] However, toxic chemicals remain a major threat to Arctic indigenous peoples' traditional way of life — an ironic fate for people who neither produce nor use most of these products.

[1] David Michaels, *Doubt Is Their Product: How Industry's Assault on Science Threatens Your Health* (Oxford University Press, 2008), p. 247.

[2] "Third National Report on Human Exposure to Environmental Chemicals," 2005, www.cdc.gov/exposurereport/report.htm, and "Spotlight on Mercury," both Centers for Disease Control and Prevention, www.cdc.gov/Exposure Report/pdf/factsheet_mercury.pdf.

[3] "Body Burden — The Pollution in Newborns," *Environmental Working Group*, July 14, 2005, http://archive.ewg.org/reports/bodyburden2/contentindex.php.

[4] Marla Cone, *Silent Snow: The Slow Poisoning of the Arctic* (2006).

[5] "Toxic Chemical Levels Finally Dropping in Arctic Food Animals, New Study Shows," The Canadian Press news agency, July 14, 2008.

Continued from p. 58

In 1965 consumer activist Ralph Nader amplified pressure on the government to regulate dangerous products with his book *Unsafe at Any Speed*, which attacked U.S. automakers for refusing to include safety devices like seat belts and filling cars with confusing and distracting features. [42] The book and subsequent congressional hearings generated new safety requirements and oversight agencies for passenger cars.

The Nixon administration created other agencies to regulate industry more tightly and protect consumers, including the Environmental Protection Agency (EPA) in 1970, the Occupational Safety and Health Administration (OSHA) in 1971 and the Consumer Product Safety Commission (CPSC) in 1972. Along with the FDA, each of the new agencies had some responsibility for protecting workers and the public from toxic threats, although the scope of their powers varied.

During the 1970s federal regulators passed some important protective measures. EPA banned DDT use in 1972 because of its harmful environmental impacts. In 1979 the agency banned production of PCBs, which had been shown to cause cancer and birth defects in laboratory animals, and set timetables for phasing out their use in various industries. In 1977 the CPSC banned lead paint and its use on toys and furniture. OSHA set occupational exposure standards for many hazardous substances and developed requirements (finalized in the early 1980s) for businesses to identify and label hazardous chemicals in the workplace and tell employees how to use them safely.

The Polluted Arctic

Atmospheric and ocean currents carry persistent organic pollutants around the world far from their sources and concentrate them in some regions, notably the Arctic, where they are a threat to indigenous peoples and wildlife. Even relatively "clean" air from non-industrial areas contains low levels of pesticides and other chemicals.

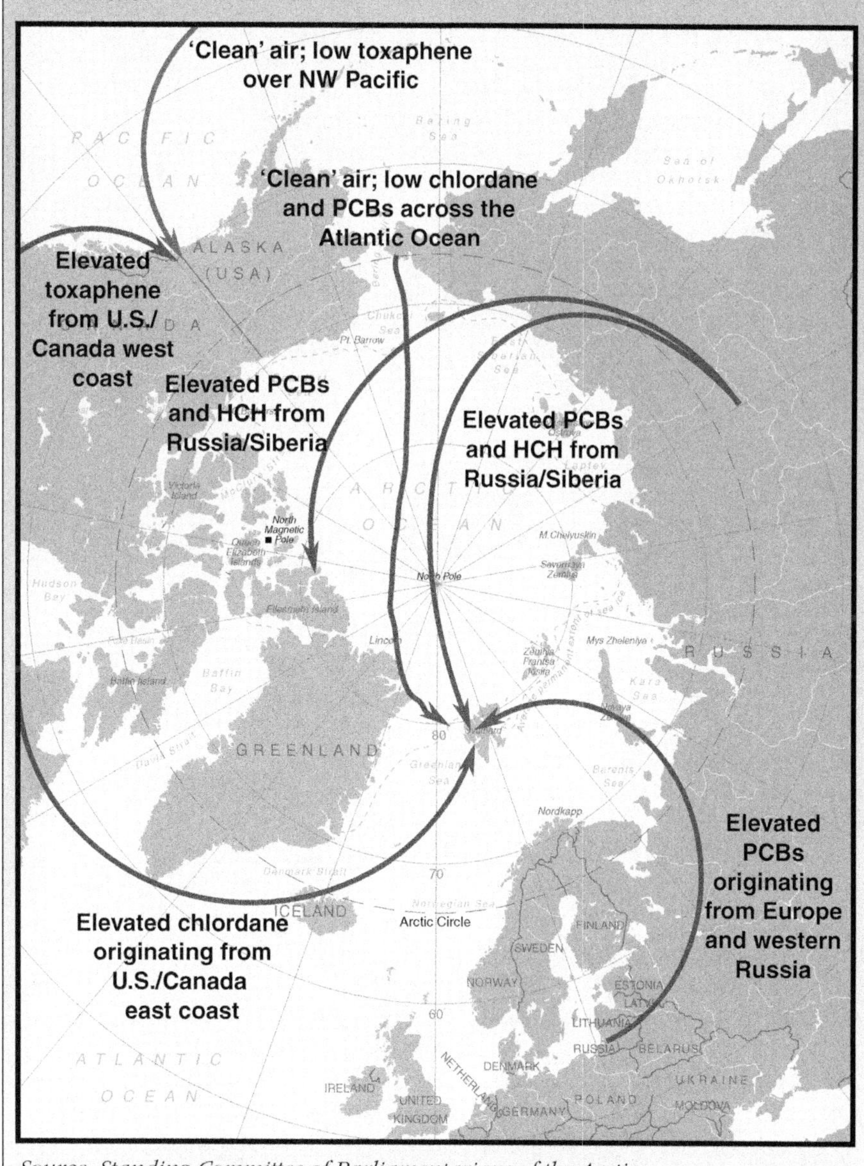

Source: Standing Committee of Parliamentarians of the Arctic

Business Pushes Back

Many controls adopted in the 1970s made the environment cleaner and improved public health. But industry and conservative politicians argued that government regulators were becoming high-handed and that excessive regulations slowed economic growth. President Ronald Reagan (1981-1989) made reducing government's power a centerpiece of his administration, cutting budgets at EPA, OSHA and CPSC and appointing officials who were hostile to regulation.

European Regulators Take 'Precautionary' Approach

Chemical companies must show products are safe.

Chemicals are big business in Europe as well as in the United States, but the European Union (EU) has taken a sharply different approach to regulating chemical risks. In 2007 the EU's new REACH policy (Registration, Evaluation, Authorization, and Restriction of Chemicals) went into effect. In the United States, regulators must show that chemicals pose risks to human health or the environment before they can limit their production or use. But REACH takes essentially the opposite approach: Companies must show that chemicals will not harm human health or the environment before they can be marketed.

During an 11-year phase-in period, businesses that produce or import any chemical into the EU in quantities greater than one metric ton per year will have to register it with the new European Chemicals Agency and submit information about its physical and chemical properties, how it will be made, how to use it safely and how it affects human health and the environment. More detailed information is required for chemicals that are produced in larger volumes. EU officials estimate that about 30,000 chemicals now in use will be subject to REACH. [1]

Manufacturers of chemicals deemed to pose especially high risks — such as those that cause cancer, birth defects or endocrine disruption or that persist and are toxic in the environment — will have to apply to the European Commission for authorization. They will have to show that it is not technically or economically feasible to use safer substitutes, and that the risks from using the chemical can be controlled. REACH allows regulators to ban or restrict the use of chemicals that pose unacceptable risks to human health or the environment and limits the amount of health-related data that manufacturers can shield as proprietary information.

Many U.S. health and environmental advocates say REACH is a better model for regulating hazardous substances than the Toxic Substances Control Act (TSCA), and that the U.S. should emulate Europe by moving in a more precautionary direction. "TSCA is really ineffective and needs to be updated," says Sarah Janssen, a scientist at the Natural Resources Defense Council. "It limits EPA's ability to request toxicity information from manufacturers; there are thousands of chemicals on the market now without toxicity information; and there's no requirement for companies to notify EPA if they increase production or start using chemicals in new ways. REACH isn't perfect, but it's definitely a lot better than what we have, which is basically a free-for-all."

U.S. chemical companies and the Bush administration lobbied hard against REACH, arguing that it was too complex and expensive, posed a barrier to foreign exporters outside of Europe and could cause American workers to lose their jobs. C. Boyden

Reagan also required the White House Office of Management and Budget to review proposed new rules — a policy that his successors continued — and signed an executive order directing agencies not to issue new ones unless their potential benefits to society were greater than their costs. [43] Many policy experts agreed that cost-benefit analysis was a useful tool for setting priorities, but others worried that health and environmental benefits were hard to quantify and would be undervalued.

Critics charged the Reagan administration with leading a "retreat from safety." "The agencies no longer respond to the needs of unorganized victims of technological hazards. Instead, they service the business executives and stockholders who are responsible for the hazards," wrote Joan Claybrook, president of the Nader-founded activist group Public Citizen and former head of the National Highway Traffic Safety Administration, in 1984. [44]

In this climate some of the most significant new steps were so-called right-to-know policies, which did not limit the use of risky materials but gave people more information about potential exposures. After methyl isocyanate, a deadly industrial gas, leaked from a chemical plant in Bhopal, India, in 1984 (killing some 4,000 people) and a plant in West Virginia the next year (with no deaths), Congress passed the Emergency Planning and Community Right to Know Act in 1986. The law required companies to tell EPA and state officials what hazardous chemicals were used in significant quantities at their plants and to notify emergency responders about any chemical releases.

Another major step in 1986 was the passage in California of Proposition 65, a ballot initiative that directed the state to publish an annual list of chemicals used in California that were known to cause cancer, birth defects or other reproductive harms. Businesses had to warn people before exposing them to significant risks from listed chemicals — for example, by putting warning labels on processed food or signs in workplaces where listed substances were used. [45]

The Clinton administration (1993-2001) was more receptive to new health and safety regulations than its predecessors. FDA Commissioner David Kessler declared cigarettes to be "drug delivery devices," an acknowledgment that nicotine was addictive, and called for limiting marketing and sales to young people. In 1996 Clinton signed the Food Quality Protection Act, which tightened standards for pesticide residues in foods and required EPA to consider children's higher sensitivity to these chemicals when it set tolerance levels.

In 1998 the administration called for chemical companies to perform

Gray, the U.S. ambassador to the EU, said REACH would "be hell for American multinationals. . . . Our position is if we don't stop it, it will multiply like kudzu." [2] Now, however, U.S. manufacturers are reformulating their products for sale in Europe and preparing to register them.

Michael Walls, managing director at the American Chemistry Council, the main U.S. chemical industry trade group, acknowledges that REACH breaks some valuable ground. "It's raised the issue of how we assure safe use, and it's promoted dialogue about how certain chemicals are used in sectors like electronics, automobiles and aerospace," he says. But, Walls argues, REACH does not pay enough attention to how chemicals are used, which is one determinant of how risky they are. "There are some opportunities to consider specific uses, but chemicals are identified for regulation specifically based on hazardous characteristics, and we don't think that's the way to prioritize," he says.

No regulatory decisions have been made under REACH yet. A preregistration phase for existing chemicals ended last November, and regulators now are considering which substances should require authorization before they can be used. By December 2010 companies must submit data on high-volume chemicals (those produced in quantities over 1,000 metric tons per year) and highly toxic chemicals produced in smaller quantities. "REACH is still untested and unproven, and we have concerns about whether some of its provisions are workable," says Walls.

But some activists already would like to make REACH even more stringent. For example, Janssen argues the system does not pay enough attention to endocrine-disrupting chemicals. "Some chemicals aren't produced in very big volumes, but they have serious impacts at very low volumes," she says. "Hormones work in the parts-per-billion to parts-per-trillion range in your body — very small doses have really big impacts." And REACH does not explicitly cover nanomaterials, although manufacturers who want to use an existing chemical substance at the nano level will have to supply additional information on the nanoform's specific properties and describe measures to minimize risks from them. [3]

[1] "Chemical Regulation: Comparison of U.S. and Recently Enacted European Union Approaches to Protect Against the Risks of Toxic Chemicals," U.S. Government Accountability Office, August 2007.

[2] Mark Schapiro, *Exposed: The Toxic Chemistry of Everyday Products and What's at Stake for American Power* (2007), p. 253.

[3] "REACH and Nanomaterials," European Commission, http://ec.europa.eu/enterprise/reach/reach/more_info/nanomaterials/index_en.htm.

voluntary toxicity testing on chemicals in use that had not been tested — and threatened to require it if industry did not comply. Subsequently the EPA, the chemical industry and the advocacy group Environmental Defense announced the High Production Volume (HPV) Challenge, which aimed to complete toxicity testing by 2004 on about 2,800 industrial chemicals made or imported into the U.S. in large quantities.

Along with cancer and birth defects, Americans started to hear in the 1990s about so-called endocrine disruptors — chemicals that interfered with hormones responsible for regulating biological processes throughout the body, such as brain growth and sexual development. Scientists were finding evidence that endocrine disruptors were causing reproductive abnormalities, population declines and other negative impacts in wildlife. Some studies linked pesticides that mimicked estrogen, the female sex hormone, with increased risk of breast cancer.

Other researchers were alarmed by falling human sperm counts. "Every man sitting in this room today is half the man his grandfather was," University of Florida zoologist Louis Guillette told a Senate committee in 1993. "Are our children going to be half the men we are?" Three years later, the best-selling book *Our Stolen Future* argued that endocrine disruptors posed pervasive health risks but that federal controls on toxic chemicals were overly focused on detecting and controlling cancer risks. "The assumptions about toxicity and disease that have framed our thinking for the past three decades are inappropriate and act as obstacles to understanding a different kind of damage," the authors contended. [46]

New Worries

Under President George W. Bush (2001-2009), momentum once again swung from strong regulation to voluntary compliance strategies in which companies agreed to police themselves. With pro-business officials in charge at many regulatory agencies and limited budgets, the pace of federal regulation dropped sharply. Rulemaking fell by more than 50 percent at FDA and 57 percent at EPA between 2001 and 2008 compared with those agencies' records during the Clinton administration. OSHA withdrew more than a dozen regulations that had been proposed under Clinton and delayed taking action on silica dust after identifying it as a workplace health threat. [47]

Conservative advocates generally supported the shift to deregulation, arguing that excessive health and safety regulations were burdens on the economy and often were not the most effective way to protect public health or the environment. "Regulations unquestionably force the issue, but usually at a very high cost to the economy and to property rights," wrote American Enterprise Institute analyst Steven Hayward in 2008. "This kind of bureaucratic environmentalism has about played itself out, and is decreasingly relevant to the local environmental problems that remain to be tackled." [48]

At the same time, however, consumers and even some large industries were asking federal agencies for more regulation. From 2007 through mid-2008 a string of product scares made headlines, including U.S.-grown spinach carrying hazardous bacteria, imported pet food and seafood adulterated with chemicals, and recalls of toys found to contain lead paint. [49] Many of these products, including the tainted pet food and toys, came from China, while contaminated fish was shipped from China and other countries in Asia and from Latin America. In May 2008 FDA Commissioner Andrew von Eschenbach asked Congress for $275 million in immediate funding to improve oversight of drugs, medical products and imported food. [50]

Two months later Congress passed the Consumer Product Safety Act of 2008, which overhauled the CPSC and increased its staffing, required toys and other children's products to be tested for safety before they entered the market and banned lead and several types of phthalates from children's products. "This reform is much needed, long overdue and necessary to ensure that CPSC can successfully ensure the safety of consumer products," said Rachel Weintraub, director of product safety and senior counsel at the Consumer Federation of America. ■

CURRENT SITUATION

FDA and BPA

As debate continues over potential health risks from BPA, the FDA is at the center of controversy. Last August the agency released a draft assessment concluding that BPA in food packaging did not pose a health risk. But an advisory panel that reviewed the draft report found a number of flaws, such as omitting studies suggesting BPA could have harmful effects, using too few infant formula samples and not considering cumulative exposures. The reviewers concluded that "the Margins of Safety defined by the FDA as 'adequate' are, in fact, inadequate." [51] (A margin of safety is the gap between the lowest dose of BPA expected to cause harm and the actual exposure that scientists expect to occur.)

The FDA is reviewing these arguments and has pledged to provide a response by this February. "FDA agrees that, due to the uncertainties raised in some studies relating to the Potential effects of low-dose exposure to bisphenol A, additional research would be valuable," says agency spokesperson Michael Herndon. "[The agency] is already moving forward with planned research to address the potential low-dose effects of bisphenol A, and we will carefully evaluate the findings of these studies."

Critics argue the FDA has deliberately downplayed low-dose exposures to avoid having to issue new regulations. "We're replaying what happened with lead regulation," says Carnegie Mellon chemistry Professor Terry Collins. "Trade associations fought against banning lead from house paint and gasoline for 70 years by beating up doctors who said lead was bad for children and funding studies that only looked at high doses. EPA chose for years not to look at risks from ultra-low doses, and FDA is doing the same thing now. It's very confusing to the public, and these impacts are showing up across the population."

The National Toxicology Program's Bucher agrees that the FDA needs new methods to evaluate BPA. "The academic studies that found effects at low doses assessed exposures to very fine degrees," he says. "FDA's guidelines for industry studies don't require such detail, and they're just not adequate to pick up subtle changes that can occur from low-dose exposures, such as behavior differences between male and female mouse pups."

The NTP is still trying to answer important questions about BPA, says Bucher: "We know what doses animals receive in studies, but we don't know much about where it goes and how much of it reaches different tissues, or how quickly it's eliminated from the body. It's not eliminated as quickly in young animals as in older ones, and we think that's true in humans as well." He expects that the NTP will soon initiate a study to see whether prenatal exposure to BPA can lead to cancer. "Earlier studies started dosing in young adults, but clearly the most sensitive periods are earlier than that," Bucher adds.

Activist Congress

Although research is ongoing, some members of Congress have already called for new limits on chemicals in consumer products, starting with a ban on BPA in food and beverage containers. Several legislators cited a November 2008 study by the *Milwaukee Journal Sentinel* that found plastic products labeled as "microwave safe" leached potentially harmful doses of BPA when they were heated. "Parents always err on the side of caution when it comes to their kids' health. We think the law should do the same," said Sen. Charles E. Schumer, D-NY. [52] He introduced legislation in

Continued on p. 66

At Issue:

Does the precautionary principle make us safer?

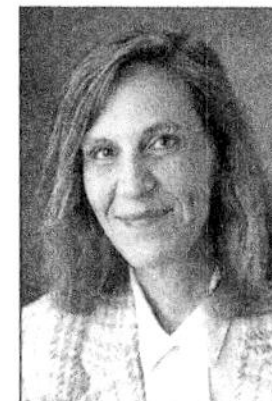

WENDY E. WAGNER
PROFESSOR OF LAW
UNIVERSITY OF TEXAS

WRITTEN FOR *CQ RESEARCHER*, JANUARY 2009

yes

The regulation of chemicals in the United States epitomizes what can go wrong when a legal system adopts a non-precautionary approach. Under the Toxic Substances Control Act (TSCA), manufacturers are not required to do any pre- or post-market testing on their chemicals unless mandated by the Environmental Protection Agency. At the same time, there are few to no rewards under the act for producing safer or better-tested chemicals, at least with regard to latent hazards.

In fact, chemical manufacturers that do voluntarily test their chemicals may put themselves at a competitive disadvantage: They not only produce evidence that can be used against them by regulators and plaintiffs' attorneys but also dedicate resources to testing that are unlikely to be recouped in sales — either because the testing reveals unwelcome risks or because the positive results cannot be validated readily by consumers or investors.

The TSCA's non-precautionary approach is partly to blame for the resulting ignorance about the long-term safety of most chemicals and for the lack of incentives to develop safer, "greener" chemicals. Over the 30-year-plus history of the legislation, EPA has required testing for fewer than 200 chemicals. Most of the remaining 75,000 chemicals produced during that period are essentially unrestricted and unreviewed with regard to their health and environmental impacts. While such a counter-productive regulatory scheme would seem at first blush a perfect candidate for public-spirited reform, the highest-stakes participants in toxics policy are the chemical manufacturers, who not surprisingly have become well-organized and steadfast in their opposition to reform.

Fortunately, the European Union's REACH directive will produce valuable toxicity information on chemicals, whether U.S. manufacturers want it or not. Through its mandatory testing requirements, REACH (registration, evaluation, authorization and restriction of chemicals) may also generate incentives for safer chemical substitutes.

In the United States, the precautionary features of REACH could be supplemented by creating additional rewards for producing safer chemicals. For example, EPA could preside over petitions filed by manufacturers seeking regulatory certification of a chemical's superiority relative to its competitors. Pitting manufacturers against one another through such adjudication will help draw out information on the toxicity of chemicals and reward greener chemical companies, while at the same time undermining the unified resistance of chemical manufacturers to modifications in TSCA's non-precautionary approach.

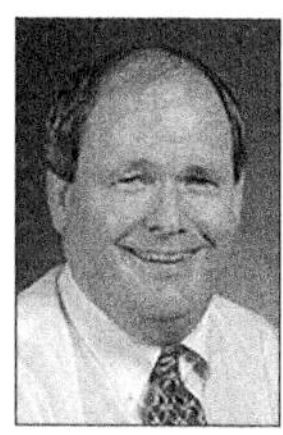

GARY MARCHANT
PROFESSOR OF LAW
ARIZONA STATE UNIVERSITY

WRITTEN FOR *CQ RESEARCHER*, JANUARY 2009

no

The precautionary principle (PP) attempts to address a serious problem: How should we deal with uncertain risks? Bisphenol A, Teflon, thimerosal in vaccines, melamine in baby formula and phthalates in fire retardants are just some of the uncertain risks on the front pages of newspapers today. Which ones should we restrict now, and which should we just study more before taking action?

Unfortunately, the PP fails to provide a coherent or useful answer to this critical question. The problem, as H. L. Mencken once noted: "[t]here is always an easy solution to every human problem — neat, plausible, and wrong."

Since originating in Europe approximately 40 years ago, the PP is now binding law in Europe, Canada, Australia and several Asian nations, has been incorporated in over 60 international treaties and has been adopted by several U.S. cities. Yet, the PP is problematic, especially when enacted as a binding legal rule. First, there is no standard or official definition of "the" precautionary principle, and dozens of unofficial versions exist. Which version applies will make a huge difference in many decisions.

Second, available interpretations of the PP offer no clear guidance on key questions, such as what manufacturers must do to satisfy the PP and how costs are factored in. Without answering these fundamental questions, the PP opens the door to arbitrary decisions motivated by political bias, protectionism and other inappropriate motives, rather than objective scientific evidence of risk.

Thus, relying on the PP, Norway banned Kellogg's Corn Flakes because the added vitamins could theoretically harm some ultra-susceptible person. France banned Red Bull energy drinks because the caffeine might harm pregnant women (but did not ban coffee or wine) and Denmark banned cranberry fruit drinks because vitamin C might harm some people.

More tragically, Zambia cited the PP to deny U.S. food aid to its starving population because of the possible presence of genetically modified corn (which Americans routinely eat with no apparent consequences). The European Union even used the PP to justify governmental subsidization of the coal industry, even though coal is not generally perceived as the most environmentally friendly energy source. With the PP, however, no further explanation is needed.

Finally, the PP fails to consider that many new technologies, such as biotechnology and nanotechnology, offer the promise of enormous benefits, including health and environmental gains. By failing to consider these effects, the PP fails its own test for seeking to prohibit dangerous innovations.

Continued from p. 64

2008 that would have banned BPA from products designed for children ages 7 and under, while Rep. Edward J. Markey, D-Mass., introduced a House bill that would have eliminated BPA from all food and beverage packaging. [53]

At least 13 states are also considering BPA bans. However, one such proposal failed in California in August 2008. Food processors, chemical manufacturers and packaging companies opposed the bill, which would have banned use of BPA in products for children ages 3 and under. "California's legislators made the right decision for consumers," said the American Chemistry Council's Hentges.

Another 2008 congressional bill that is likely to be reintroduced, the Kid-Safe Chemicals Act, would require more sweeping reforms to the Toxic Substances Control Act and the chemical-testing process. [54] The measure seeks to "eliminate the exposure of all children, workers, consumers and sensitive subgroups to harmful chemicals distributed in commerce by calendar year 2020." The measure would:

- require industry to demonstrate that chemicals in use are safe;
- authorize EPA to require additional testing for health effects at low doses and for nanomaterials;
- expand analysis by the Centers for Disease Control and Prevention (CDC) of chemical residues in humans; and
- provide new funds to promote safer alternatives.

"It is critical that we modernize our nation's chemical safety laws," said Rep. Henry A. Waxman, D-Calif., a sponsor of the House bill and the new chair of the Energy and Commerce Committee. "The Kid-Safe Chemicals Act will deliver what its name implies — a non-toxic environment for our children."

Another chemical issue on Congress's agenda is reauthorization of the National Nanotechnology Initiative (NNI), which coordinates nanotechnology research by federal agencies. The House passed a reauthorization bill with little controversy in 2008, but nanotechnology may face a bumpier ride in the Senate. In December 2008 the National Research Council released a review of NNI's research plan for studying potential health and environmental risks of nanotechnologies. While the study did not address whether current uses of nanomaterials posed risks to the public, it found that NNI did not have an adequate strategy for answering that question.

NNI's plan "does not describe a clear strategy for nano-risk research. It lacks input from a diverse stakeholder group, and it lacks essential elements, such as a vision and a clear set of objectives, a comprehensive assessment of the state of the science, a plan or road map that describes how research progress will be measured, and the estimated resources required to conduct such research," the NRC review stated. [55]

Making Exceptions

Banning products does not always end debate over them. Bans on phthalates in children's products under the 2008 Consumer Product Safety Improvement Act were scheduled to start on Feb. 10, 2009, but lawyers representing toy wholesalers and retailers wrote to the CPSC in late 2008 that the ban would impose "significant financial hardship" on their clients — especially if they were left with useless products after the deadline passed.

In response CPSC General Counsel Cheryl Falvey held that the law did not contain a "clear statement of unambiguous intent" to apply the ban to existing toys, so manufacturers could keep selling items in their inventories that contained the proscribed materials. [56] Two advocacy groups, the Natural Resources Defense Council and Public Citizen, filed suit against the agency, arguing that all items containing the phthalates in question should be removed from shelves by the February 2009 deadline. "The CPSC decision will generate and prolong exposure to known hormone-disrupting chemicals. . . . There is no way for [consumers] to know whether products on store shelves after the ban date contain phthalates or not," the groups argued. [57]

Many toy vendors and manufacturers also say the law's Feb. 10 deadline for applying tough, new lead levels could cost them heavily. By that date toys may contain no more than 600 parts per million by weight of lead, a trace amount that will ratchet further down over time. Falvey ruled in November that unlike the phthalate ban, the new lead ban (which was worded differently in the law) did apply to existing toys. But some toy company owners said that testing their entire inventories for lead would be extremely expensive, and that retailers might send entire shipments back if there were worries about whether some items met the standard. [58] According to the CDC, only certified laboratories can test toys accurately for lead. [59]

Another proposed ban, on polyvinyl chloride (PVC) plastics, passed through the California Assembly and two Senate committees last year but then stalled in the Senate Appropriations Committee. PVC is used for many applications, including water pipes, medical tubing and numerous types of packaging. But critics like the Center for Health, Environment, and Justice (CHEJ) call PVC "poison plastic" because it can release chemicals such as phthalates and dioxins (a family of persistent, toxic, chlorinated hydrocarbon chemicals) during its life cycle, and its production exposes workers to other hazardous materials.

Debate over the California bill showed the difficulty of making up-or-down decisions about substances that have many uses but also pose risks. As the bill moved through various committees, legislators exempted a number of products from the ban, including medical devices, packaging for medications and containers for petroleum products. "It's easy for attackers to dismiss PVC, but not so easy for the marketplace," says the Vinyl Institute's Blakey.

Many large manufacturers and retailers have adopted policies to phase out PVC in products or packaging, including Mattel, Nike, Sony, Target, Wal-Mart, K-Mart and Sears. But Blakey calls these steps responses to political pressure and argues that PVC products are safe. Retailers, he says, "are misinformed and pressured. They don't have a lot of staff to verify critiques, and they want the issue to go away."

Activists don't deny that they're pushing companies to drop PVC, but they say safer alternatives are available. "There are some substances that don't have substitutes, so we have to use them carefully. But there are all kinds of substitutes for PVC," says CHEJ President Lois Gibbs. The center published a guide in 2008 that lists dozens of sources for toys, clothing, mattresses and other goods made without PVC. (However, as the guide notes, the center does not endorse any of the listed substitute products, manufacturers, or retailers.) [60]

The Obama Administration

Many environmentalists are optimistic about what the newly inaugurated President Barack Obama will do about toxic chemicals. Obama has embraced green issues during his campaign and since his election. Although the economic meltdown undoubtedly will force Obama to pare down his campaign wish list, his transition team has been examining new environmental policies that could be adopted quickly, including some Clinton-era initiatives that could be resurrected.

During his inaugural speech on Jan. 20, Obama said he would "restore science to its rightful place" and has vowed to listen more closely to scientific advisers and environmental experts, whose advice the Bush administration often ignored or overruled. "I think we are in store for something new," said William Reilly, who led the Environmental Protection Agency under President George H. W. Bush. "His pledge to follow the science will be reassuring to a lot of people, including those who fear the regulators are going to run amok." [61]

Within hours after Obama's inauguration, his Chief of Staff Rahm Emmanuel ordered a halt on all work on unfinished Bush administration regulations until they can be reviewed by the new team. Bush issued 100 new rules after Obama was elected in November, including one that President Obama strenuously opposes, which would make it much harder for the government to regulate toxic substances and hazardous chemicals in the workplace. [62]

Earlier, Obama and four other senators had proposed a measure to block the new rule and wrote a letter urging the department to scrap it, saying it would "create serious obstacles to protecting workers from health hazards on the job." [63]

The administration probably will also reconsider a Jan. 15 EPA health advisory urging Americans not to drink water with more than 0.4 parts per billion (ppb) of perfluorooctanoic acid (PFOA) — a toxic chemical linked to cancer, liver damage and birth defects that is used to make Teflon and other non-stick coatings. [64]

Some scientists have urged limits as low as 0.02 parts per billion of PFOA, and, in fact, his pick to lead the EPA, New Jersey Environmental Protection Commissioner Lisa Jackson, recommended a level of 0.04 parts per billion in her state — 10 times stricter than the new federal limit.

Richard Wiles, executive director of the Environmental Working Group — a nonprofit organization that has pushed for stricter regulation of PFOA — said the EPA's new advisory was "essentially legalizing unsafe exposure levels. Nobody should have to drink a cancer-causing Teflon chemical in their water." [65] ■

OUTLOOK

Green Chemistry

The task of regulating the chemical industry's constant stream of new products for health and safety risks can seem hopelessly daunting. But some experts see a way: green chemistry, which seeks to design chemicals and chemical processes with reduced environmental impacts. [66]

Since the mid-1990s, green chemistry has developed into an active research field. The EPA provides grants, awards and fellowships for green chemistry achievements, and the American Chemical Society's Green Chemistry Institute works to advance green principles across all fields of chemical research. About a dozen U.S. universities offer green chemistry programs, and major corporations like GE and BASF are investing billions of dollars in green applications, such as alternative energy systems.

Winners of the EPA's green chemistry awards for 2008 included Battelle, which developed bio-based resins and toners for office copiers and printers. Made from soy and corn feedstocks instead of petroleum products, the inks are easier to remove from paper than conventional toner, which reduces the amount of energy needed to recycle waste paper. Another winner, Nalco, designed technology to monitor the water that circulates through many building cooling systems. The Nalco system adds chemicals to keep cooling water clean only when needed, saving water and energy and reducing the quantity of chemicals in discharged cooling water. [67]

Although the field is growing rapidly, Carnegie Mellon Professor Collins says government leadership is needed. "Federal investment in green chemistry is almost nonexistent, and we desperately need it," he says. "We need to prioritize hazards and figure out how to design against them." Collins recently invented an environmentally friendly catalyst that can break down harmful pollutants into less-toxic substances. [68]

The Green Chemistry Research and Development Act, which was passed by the House in 2007 and introduced in the Senate, would provide $188 million over three years for agencies to support research, development, education and training in green chemistry.

"Modern science keeps giving us new warnings about many of the chemicals we use every day, from home cleaning products to the food we put on our family's table," said Sen. John Kerry, D-Mass., a cosponsor of the Senate bill. "It's time for Washington to respond by helping to build a whole, new chemistry industry that's on a mission to make America greener."

Reducing serious risks is key, says Collins. "Green chemistry could exist without focusing on hazardous products, and it would probably do all kinds of nice little things. But to be authentic, it has to deal with hazards." ■

Notes

[1] "All About Eastman Tritan Copolyester," www.eastman.com/company/news_center/News_archive/2007.

[2] "Endocrine Disruptors," National Institute of Environmental Health Sciences, February 2007.

[3] "Timeline: BPA from Invention to Phase-Out," Environmental Working Group, April 22, 2008, www.ewg.org/node/26291/print.

[4] "Bisphenol A (BPA)," National Toxicology Program, September 2008, www.niehs.nih.gov/health/docs/bpa-factsheet.pdf.

[5] "Eastman Expanding Tritan Copolyester Capacity," Reuters, March 13, 2008. For background, see Jennifer Weeks, "Buying Green," *CQ Researcher*, Feb. 29, 2008, pp. 193-216.

[6] "A Poison Kiss: The Problem of Lead in Lipstick," Campaign for Safe Cosmetics, October 2007, www.safecosmetics.org/docUploads/A%20Poison%20Kiss.pdf.

[7] For background, see Marcia Clemmitt, "Preventing Cancer," *CQ Researcher*, Jan. 9, 2009, pp. 25-48.

[8] Testimony of Andrew D. Maynard before Committee on Science and Technology, U.S. House of Representatives, April 16, 2008, p. 5.

[9] For background, see Brian Beary, "The New Europe," *CQ Global Researcher*, August 2007, pp. 181-210, and Kenneth Jost, "Future of the European Union," *CQ Researcher*, Oct. 28, 2005, pp. 909-932.

[10] "Wingspread Statement on the Precautionary Principle," www.sehn.org/ppfaqs.html.

[11] "WHO gives indoor use of DDT a clean bill of health for controlling malaria," World Health Organization, Sept. 15, 2006.

[12] "Alternatives to DDT on International Radar," United Nations Environment Programme, November 2008.

[13] "The Business of Chemistry," American Chemistry Council, August 2007.

[14] Exceptions include pesticides, which EPA regulates under a separate law, and food additives, drugs, and cosmetics, which are controlled by the Food and Drug Administration.

[15] "Chemical Regulation: Actions Are Needed to Improve the Effectiveness of EPA's Chemical Review Program," U.S. Government Accountability Office, Aug. 2, 2006, p. 1.

[16] The five chemicals are PCBs, chlorofluorocarbons, dioxin, asbestos, and hexavalent chromium for use as a water treatment chemical. EPA's decision banning asbestos was reversed in *Corrosion Proof Fittings v. EPA*, 947 F. 2d 1201 (1991).

[17] GAO, *op. cit.*, p. 3.

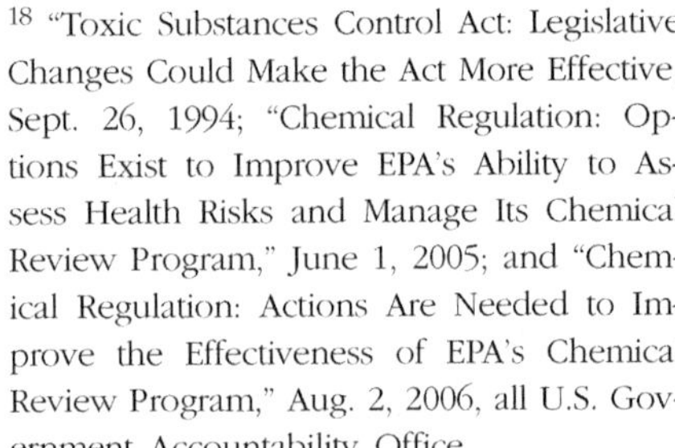

[18] "Toxic Substances Control Act: Legislative Changes Could Make the Act More Effective, Sept. 26, 1994; "Chemical Regulation: Options Exist to Improve EPA's Ability to Assess Health Risks and Manage Its Chemical Review Program," June 1, 2005; and "Chemical Regulation: Actions Are Needed to Improve the Effectiveness of EPA's Chemical Review Program," Aug. 2, 2006, all U.S. Government Accountability Office.

[19] "Toxicity Testing in the 21st Century: A Vision and a Strategy," National Research Council (2007), pp. 48-52.

[20] "Fact Sheet for Nanotechnology Under the Toxic Substances Control Act," U.S. Environmental Protection Agency, www.epa.gov/oppt/nano/nano-facts.htm.

[21] E. Clayton Teague, Director, National Nanotechnology Coordination Office, testimony before House Subcommittee on Research and Science Education, Oct. 31, 2007, pp. 1-4.

[22] Thomas H. Moore, Commissioner, Consumer Product Safety Commission, testimony before Senate Commerce Subcommittee on Consumer Affairs, Insurance, and Automotive Safety, March 21, 2007, p. 7.

[23] "Nanotechnology: A Report of the U.S. Food and Drug Administration Nanotechnology Task Force," July 25, 2007, pp. 12-15.

[24] David J. Hanson, "FDA Confronts Nanotechnology," *Chemical & Engineering News*, March 17, 2008.

[25] Online at www.nanoaction.org/nanoaction/doc/CTA_nano-silver%20petition__final_5_1_08.pdf.

[26] "No-Nano Sunscreens?" *Consumer Reports*, December 2008.

[27] E. Marla Felcher, "The Consumer Product Safety Commission and Nanotechnology," *PEN 14*, Project on Emerging Nanotechnologies, August 2008.

[28] "Baby Bottle Chemical Levels Safe, EU Agency Says," Reuters, July 23, 2008; "Health Canada Responds to Concerns Raised About Bisphenol A in Canned Food," Health Canada, May 29, 2008; "Canada Declares BPA a Health Hazard," *USA Today*, Oct. 18, 2008.

[29] Kate Murphy, "Business: Thinking Outside the Can," *The New York Times*, March 14, 2004; "Frequently Asked Questions," Hain Celestial Canada, www.hain-celestial.ca/index.php/faq/.

[30] For a chronology see "Phthalates and Children's Toys," American Chemistry Council, Phthalate Information Center, www.phthalates.org/yourhealth/childrens_toys.asp.

[31] "New EU Phthalates Directive Finalised," *Intertek Labtest*, July 2005.

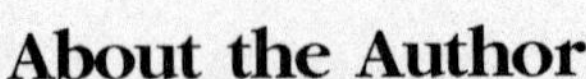

About the Author

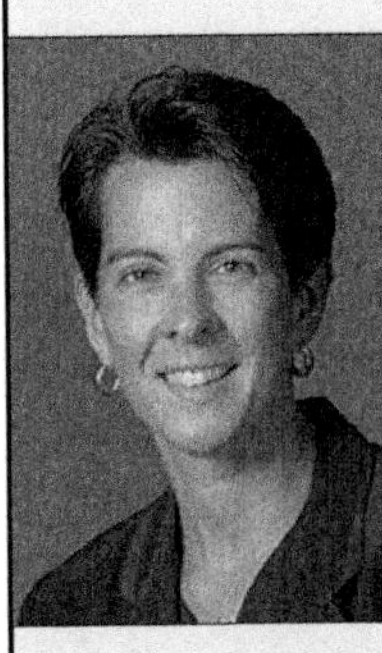

Jennifer Weeks is a *CQ Researcher* contributing writer in Watertown, Mass., who specializes in energy and environmental issues. She has written for *The Washington Post*, *The Boston Globe Magazine* and other publications, and has 15 years' experience as a public-policy analyst, lobbyist and congressional staffer. She has an A.B. degree from Williams College and master's degrees from the University of North Carolina and Harvard.

[32] Jocelyn Kaiser, "Panel Finds No Proof That Phthalates Harm Infant Reproductive Systems," *Science*, Oct. 21, 2005.

[33] "Congress Passes Consumer Product Safety Improvement Act," *Beveridge & Diamond*, July 31, 2008.

[34] Letter online at www.uschamber.com/issues/letters/2008/080304_phthalate_ban.htm.

[35] Bohan Loh and Judith Wang, "U.S. Ban To Shake up China Toy Sector," *ICIS News*, July 31, 2008; Mark Schapiro, *Exposed: The Toxic Chemistry of Everyday Products and What's at Stake for American Power* (2007), pp. 56-57.

[36] "A Plasticizer for Sensitive Applications," *Science Around Us*, BASF, June 2007.

[37] Samuel Hopkins Adams, "The Great American Fraud: Articles on the Nostrum Evil and Quacks," Reprinted from *Collier's Weekly* (Collier, 1905), p. 3.

[38] "Taste of Raspberries, Taste of Death: The 1937 Elixir Sulfanilamide Incident," *FDA Consumer Magazine*, U.S. Food and Drug Administration, June 1981.

[39] Gregg LaBar, "Seven Decades of Safety: Good Times Take Their Toll," *EHS Today*, Oct. 1, 2008.

[40] "Food Additives," Center for Science in the Public Interest, www.cspinet.org/reports/chemcuisine.htm#Food%20additive.

[41] "The Reports of the Surgeon General," National Library of Medicine, http://profiles.nlm.nih.gov/NN/Views/Exhibit/narrative/smoking.html.

[42] Ralph Nader, *Unsafe at Any Speed: The Designed-In Dangers of the American Automobile* (1965).

[43] Philip Shabecoff, "Reagan Order on Cost-Benefit Analysis Stirs Economic and Political Debate," *The New York Times*, Nov. 7, 1981.

[44] Joan Claybrook *et al.*, *Retreat From Safety: Reagan's Attack on America's Health* (1984), p. xi.

[45] "Proposition 65 in Plain Language," California Office of Environmental Health Hazard Assessment, www.oehha.org/prop65/background/p65plain.html.

[46] Theo Colborn, Dianne Dumanoski and John Peterson Myers, *Our Stolen Future: Are We Threatening Our Fertility, Intelligence, and Survival?* (1996).

[47] Stephen Labaton, "OSHA Leaves Worker Safety in Hands of Industry," *The New York Times*, April 25, 2007.

[48] Steven Hayward, "Happy Earth Day," *Human Events Online*, April 22, 2008.

[49] For background see Jennifer Weeks, "Fish Farming," *CQ Researcher*, July 27, 2007, pp. 625-648, and Peter Katel, "Consumer Safety," *CQ Researcher*, Oct. 12, 2007, pp. 841-864.

[50] Gardiner Harris, "F.D.A. Chief Writes Congress for Money," *New York*, May 14, 2008.

[51] "Scientific Peer-Review of the Draft Assessment of Bisphenol A for Use in Food Contact Applications," U.S. Food and Drug Administration Science Board Subcommittee on Bisphenol A, Oct. 31, 2008, p. 4.

[52] Meg Kissinger, "Lawmakers to Seek Ban on BPA," *Milwaukee Journal Sentinel*, Nov. 17, 2008.

[53] S. 2928, introduced April 29, 2008, and H.R. 6228, introduced June 10, 2008.

[54] S. 3040 and H.R. 6100, both introduced May 20, 2008.

[55] National Research Council, *Review of Federal Strategy for Nanotechnology-Related Environmental, Health, and Safety Research* (2008), prepublication version, p. 6.

[56] The letter and CPSC advisory opinion are online at www.cpsc.gov/LIBRARY/FOIA/advisory/320.pdf.

[57] The complaint is online at http://docs.nrdc.org/health/files/hea_08120401a.pdf.

[58] Melanie Trottman, "Vendors Urge Relaxed Lead-Safety Rule," *The Wall Street Journal*, Nov. 18, 2008.

[59] "Toys and Childhood Lead Exposure," Centers for Disease Control and Prevention, www.cdc.gov/nceh/lead/faq/toys.htm.

[60] "Pass Up the Poison Plastic," Center for Health, Environment and Justice, November 2008, www.besafenet.com/pvc/documents/PVC-Guide-1.pdf.

[61] Michael Hawthorne, "Change gets green light; His plans for environmental legislation may have big impact," *Chicago Tribune*, Nov. 19, 2008, p. C4.

[62] Robert Pear, "Bush Aides Rush to Enact a Rule Obama Opposes," *The New York Times*, Nov. 29, 2008, www.nytimes.com/2008/11/30/washington/30labor.html?ref=us.

[63] Quoted in *ibid*.

[64] See Michael Hawthorne, "U.S. warns of Teflon chemical in water," *Chicago Tribune*, Jan. 16, 2009, p. C18.

[65] *Ibid*.

[66] "Introduction to the Concept of Green Chemistry," U.S. Environmental Protection Agency, www.epa.gov/greenchemistry/pubs/about_gc.html.

[67] "Award Winners," U.S. Environmental Protection Agency, www.epa.gov/greenchemistry/pubs/pgcc/past.html.

[68] "Green Catalysts Provide Promise for Cleaning Toxins and Pollutants," *Science Daily*, Aug. 20, 2008.

FOR MORE INFORMATION

American Chemistry Council, 1300 Wilson Blvd., Arlington, VA 22209; (703) 741-5000; www.americanchemistry.com. The main trade organization for the U.S. chemical industry.

Center for Health, Environment and Justice, P.O. Box 6806, Falls Church, VA 22040; (703) 237-2249; www.chej.org. A grassroots advocacy group that works to protect communities from exposure to dangerous environmental chemicals.

Consumer Product Safety Commission, 4330 East West Highway, Bethesda, MD 20814; (301) 504-7921; www.cpsc.gov. The federal agency charged with protecting the public from unreasonable risks from products.

Consumers Union, 101 Truman Ave., Yonkers, NY 10703; (914) 378-2000; www.consumersunion.org. A nonprofit group that tests products.

National Nanotechnology Coordination Office, 4201 Wilson Blvd., Stafford II Room 405, Arlington, VA 22230; (703) 292-8626; www.nano.gov. Provides information about federal research and development of nanotechnologies.

National Toxicology Program, 111 T.W. Alexander Dr., Research Triangle Park, NC 27709; (919) 541-3665; http://ntp.niehs.nih.gov. A Department of Health and Human Services agency that studies the impact of chemicals on human health.

Project on Emerging Nanotechnologies, One Woodrow Wilson Plaza, 1300 Pennsylvania Ave., N.W., Washington, DC 20004; (202) 691-4282; www.nanotechproject.org. Provides independent, objective analysis of nanotechnology.

Project on Scientific Knowledge and Public Policy, 2100 M St., N.W., Suite 203, Washington, DC 20052; (202) 994-0774; www.defendingscience.org. Examines how science is used and misused in government decision-making.

Bibliography

Selected Sources

Books

Hilts, Philip J., *Protecting America's Health: The FDA, Business, and One Hundred Years of Regulation*, Knopf, 2003.
A health and science reporter traces the history of the Food and Drug Administration and business resistance to regulation.

Michaels, David, *Doubt Is Their Product: How Industry's Assault on Science Threatens Your Health*, Oxford University Press, 2008.
An epidemiologist and former assistant secretary of Energy criticizes what he calls the "product defense industry" for promoting doubt and uncertainty about whether unsafe products should be regulated.

Schapiro, Mark, *Exposed: The Toxic Chemistry of Everyday Products and What's at Stake for American Power*, Chelsea Green, 2007.
An investigative journalist argues that Europe is replacing the United States as a commercial leader by setting high standards that require manufacturers to develop safer products.

Shabecoff, Philip, and Alice Shabecoff, *Poisoned Profits: The Toxic Assault on Our Children*, Random House, 2008.
Two journalists link rising levels of childhood illness and death to toxic exposures in children's homes, schools and neighborhoods.

Articles

Cone, Marla, "A Greener Future," *Los Angeles Times*, Sept. 14 and 19, 2008.
Once an obscure subfield, green chemistry is slowly changing the chemical industry, but more funding and training are needed before it becomes the mainstream approach.

Henig, Robin Marantz, "Our Silver-Coated Future," *On Earth*, fall 2007.
Nano-silver, the most widely used nanomaterial, illustrates the need for safety testing and new regulations for nanotechnologies.

Hogue, Cheryl, "The Future of U.S. Chemical Regulation," *Chemical & Engineering News*, Jan. 8, 2007.
American Chemistry Council Managing Director Michael Walls and University of Massachusetts-Lowell Professor Joel Ticknor debate whether U.S. law regulating commercial chemicals is stringent enough.

Pereira, Joseph, "Protests Spur Stores to Seek Substitute for Vinyl in Toys," *The Wall Street Journal*, Feb. 12, 2008.
Under pressure from consumers and advocacy groups, toy makers are exploring substitute materials without vinyl or phthalates.

Rosenberg, Tina, "What the World Needs Now is DDT," *The New York Times Magazine*, April 11, 2004.
DDT is a cheap way to kill mosquitoes that carry malaria, but the pesticide's toxic reputation and the challenging logistics of effective spraying campaigns have made it hard for the countries that most need help to use it.

Spivak, Cary, Susanne Rust and Meg Kissinger, "Are Your Products Safe? You Can't Tell," *Milwaukee Journal Sentinel*, Nov. 25, 2007.
Shampoo, carpets, skin lotions, clothing and many other consumer products contain endocrine-disrupting chemicals that cause cancer and other health problems in laboratory animals. Critics call U.S. government efforts to regulate these substances "an abject failure."

Reports and Studies

"Chemical Regulation: Comparison of U.S. and Recently Enacted European Union Approaches to Protect Against the Risks of Toxic Chemicals," U.S. Government Accountability Office, Aug. 17, 2007.
The report compares U.S. chemical regulation under the Toxic Substances Control Act (TSCA) and the European Union's REACH directive.

"Third National Report on Human Exposure to Environmental Chemicals," Centers for Disease Control and Prevention, 2005, www.cdc.gov/exposurereport/report.htm.
This ongoing assessment of human exposure to environmental chemicals, based on human specimens such as blood and urine, finds that levels of some substances such as blood lead and secondhand cigarette smoke have fallen, but that many other chemicals are widely present throughout the U.S. population, including known hazardous substances.

"Toxicity Testing in the 21st Century: A Vision and a Strategy," National Research Council, 2008.
The council charts a course for making chemical toxicity testing faster, more affordable and more accurate while reducing reliance on animal studies.

Felcher, E. Marla, "The Consumer Product Safety Commission and Nanotechnology," Project on Emerging Nanotechnologies, August 2008, www.nanotechproject.org/process/assets/filed/7033/pen14.pdf.
An expert on business and consumer protection argues that the commission is ill-prepared to regulate nanomaterials in consumer products.

The Next Step:

Additional Articles from Current Periodicals

Body Chemicals

"Study: Oregonians Full of Toxic Chemicals," ***Confederated Umatilla Journal*** **(Oregon), December 2007, p. 9.**
A study concludes that Oregonians have at least nine and as many as 16 out of 29 toxic chemicals tested for in their bodies.

Rabb, Sara, "Air Pollution: Toxic Hot Spots," ***Pensacola News Journal*** **(Florida), March 9, 2008, p. 1A.**
A two-county area in Florida is trying to determine whether there's a connection between air pollution and elevated rates of health problems.

VanderHart, Dirk, "Monitoring Turns Up Toxins in Air Around School," ***Springfield News-Leader*** **(Missouri), Dec. 11, 2008, p. 1A.**
Long-term exposure to toxic air at a Missouri elementary school could produce increased instances of cancer.

Nanotechnologies

Fernholm, Ann, "Consumers Not Always Aware of Presence of Nanotechnology," ***The San Francisco Chronicle*****, May 12, 2008, p. D3.**
Three or four nanotechnology-based products enter the market annually, but it isn't easy to know if products contain nanoparticles.

Ruckelshaus, William, and J. Clarence Davies, "An EPA for the 21st Century," ***The Boston Globe*****, July 7, 2007, p. A9.**
Meeting the oversight challenges of nanotechnology — estimated to represent $2.6 trillion in manufactured goods by 2014 — requires the Environmental Protection Agency (EPA) to adapt more modern research methods.

Van, Jon, "Nanotechnology Could Be Basis of Future Cures," ***Chicago Tribune*****, April 23, 2007, p. C5.**
Nanotechnology has the potential to grow new tissue in order to treat conditions such as Alzheimer's or Parkinson's disease.

Products

Chambers, Jennifer, "Some Toys Have Toxic Chemicals," ***Detroit News*****, Nov. 26, 2008, p. 1B.**
Excessive amounts of toxic chemicals are present in many toys intended for children under age 3, according to the U.S. Public Research Group.

Dugan, John, "Students Find Toxic Chemicals," ***Marin Independent Journal*** **(California), May 10, 2008.**
Students at a California high school have discovered that toxic chemicals are present in many of the products used at their school.

Gathright, Alan, "Saying Yuck to Toxins in Toys, Protesters Chuck Rubber Ducks," ***Rocky Mountain News*** **(Colorado), May 21, 2008, p. 24.**
Phthalates are a class of toxic chemicals used to make plastic in baby teethers and are also present in industrial solvents, insecticides and paints.

Regulations

"State Panel Urges Cutting Chemicals in Products," The Associated Press, Dec. 16, 2008.
Gov. Arnold Schwarzenegger, R-Calif., wants California to force companies to disclose the chemicals they put in products and analyze their effects on the environment.

Coile, Zachary, "EPA Was Stymied By White House," ***The San Francisco Chronicle*****, April 30, 2008, p. A1.**
A congressional watchdog agency has concluded that the Bush administration has repeatedly intervened in the governmental scientific process for assessing the risks associated with toxic chemicals.

DePalma, Anthony, "E.P.A. Is Sued by 12 States Over Reports on Chemicals," ***The New York Times*****, Nov. 29, 2007, p. A25.**
Twelve states are suing the EPA for weakening regulations that for two decades have required businesses to report the toxic chemicals that they use, store and release.

Richardson, John, "Maine to Consider Tracking Toxins in Toys, Products," ***Portland Press Herald*****, Feb. 27, 2008, p. A1.**
Two bills in the Maine legislature would create lists of chemicals deemed to pose great threats to public health.

CITING *CQ* RESEARCHER

Sample formats for citing these reports in a bibliography include the ones listed below. Preferred styles and formats vary, so please check with your instructor or professor.

MLA STYLE

Jost, Kenneth. "Rethinking the Death Penalty." CQ Researcher 16 Nov. 2001: 945-68.

APA STYLE

Jost, K. (2001, November 16). Rethinking the death penalty. *CQ Researcher, 11,* 945-968.

CHICAGO STYLE

Jost, Kenneth. "Rethinking the Death Penalty." *CQ Researcher,* November 16, 2001, 945-968.

Printed in Great Britain
by Amazon

79492892R00174